Handbook of Leukemia

Handbook of Leukemia

Edited by Dylan Hill

hayle medical

New York

Hayle Medical,
750 Third Avenue, 9th Floor,
New York, NY 10017, USA

Visit us on the World Wide Web at:
www.haylemedical.com

ISBN: 978-1-63241-699-5

Printed in China.

Cataloging-in-Publication Data

Handbook of leukemia / edited by Dylan Hill.
p. cm.
Includes bibliographical references and index.
ISBN 978-1-63241-699-5
1. Leukemia. 2. Cancer. 3. Leucocytosis. I. Hill, Dylan.
RC643 .H36 2019
616.994 19--dc23

Table of Contents

Preface

Leukemia is a group of cancer, which occurs in the bone marrow and results in abnormal growth of white blood cells. Such cells are called blasts or leukemia cells. Bleeding and bruising, fever, tiredness and increased infections are some of the symptoms of leukemia. It can be classified as chronic lymphocytic leukemia, acute lymphoblastic leukemia, acute myeloid leukemia and chronic myeloid leukemia. The diagnosis of leukemia is usually determined by blood tests or though a bone marrow biopsy. A variety of factors may contribute to its incidence, among which are smoking, genetics, chemical exposure, etc. Leukemia is treated with a multi-drug chemotherapy regimen, pharmaceutical medication or with radiation therapy. A bone marrow transplant is also an important strategy to treat such a cancer. This book provides comprehensive insights into leukemia. It consists of contributions made by international experts. Coherent flow of topics, student-friendly language and extensive use of examples make this book an invaluable source of knowledge.

The information shared in this book is based on empirical researches made by veterans in this field of study. The elaborative information provided in this book will help the readers further their scope of knowledge leading to advancements in this field.

Finally, I would like to thank my fellow researchers who gave constructive feedback and my family members who supported me at every step of my research.

Editor

Acute Leukemia in Down Syndrome Children, A Morroccan Retrospective Review

Ayad A*, Kababri M, Kili A, Hsissen L, Khattab M

Pediatric Hematology and Oncology Center (CHOP), Rabat children's hospital, Morrocco

Abstract

Children with Down syndrome (DS) are at higher risk of developing acute leukemia and has been recognized to have unique clinical features and significant differences in treatment response and toxicity profiles compared to patients without Down syndrome. One of the challenges faced in treating children with Down syndrome and leukemia is balancing curative therapy against potential toxicities.

A retrospective review of the clinical features, treatment outcomes of DS children with acute leukemia was conducted in the Center for Pediatric Hematology and Oncology in rabat child hospital.(CHOP) from 2006 to 2016. This review included a total of 30 patients with DS. Ten were diagnosed with acute lymphoblastic leukemia and 20 had acute myeloid leukemia (AML). This study points out that investigators will have to carefully assess the balance between the antileukemic efficacy and treatment-related mortality of current chemotherapy regimens. Several studies are currently in progress that will answer some of the many questions raised in this field .

Keywords: Leukemia; Down syndrome; Chemotherapy; Toxicity

Introduction

Down syndrome (DS) is the commonest type of trisomy in live born infants, characterized by dysmorphic features and congenital abnormalities, such as heartdefects and cognitive impairment. It occurs in approximately 1 in 691 live births Patients with DS have a unique pattern of malignancy predisposition, with a higher incidence of developing leukemia than solid tumors Compared with the general population [1]. Children with DS are estimated to have 10 to 20 folds increased risk of developing leukemia, particularly acute myeloid leukemia (AML) Children with DS account for 8% to 14% of all pediatric AML cases, with up to 500- folds increased risk of developing acute megakaryoblastic leukemia compared with the general population [2]. Transient myeloproliferative disease (TMD), characterized by spontaneous regression of abnormal blasts, occurs in approximately 10% of neonates with DS. As for acute lymphoblastic leukemia (ALL), children with DS exhibit specific patterns ofimmunophenotype and cytogenetics, and they account for about 3% of all childhood ALL. Treatment of acute leukemia in children with DS is particularly challenging due to their high susceptibility to treatment-related toxicities Reducing treatment intensity seems to be beneficial for patients with DS. This study reviews the current knowledge and research questions regarding DS-associated acute leukemias.

Patients and Methods

We conducted a retrospective review on acute leukemia(ALL and AML) in children with DS in Rabat from 2006 to 2016. 30 Patients with DS were identified from the leukemia registry of the Center for Pediatric Hematology and Oncology in rabat child hospital (CHOP).

The center coordinates treatment protocols for all pediatric oncology patients below 18 years of age. Data on demographic, clinical features, important prognostic factors, treatment complications, and outcomes were collected retrospectively and additional information was supplemented from review of medical records using a uniform study sheet. The inclusion criteria were:

- DS phenotype and clinical feature of constitutional trisomy 21.
- Acute leukemia (lymphoblastic and myeloblastic), diagnosed on

Bone morrow aspiration with cytochemistry and immunophenotyping (the karyotype was mostly Is performed in patients with acute myeloblastic leukemia).

The mean follow-up duration of this cohort of patients was 2.3 years .Children with ALL were treated according to MARALL 2006 protocol (Figure1) And were given the standard risk treatment with lower dosage of most of the chemotherapy drugs espicially methotrexate during the consolidation phase by 25 to 30% Children with AML were treated according to the AML-MA 2011 protocol except for one patient who received the AML-MAROC 2006 protocol (Figures 2 and 3). They all had dose reduction of all chemotherapy agents by 25% to 50% ,

2 patients received only Ara-C during induction 1.

Results

Patient characteristics: All patients were born in morrocco and majority were from urban areas (27/30, 81%). For the remaining 3 Patients , they were all from the rural areas of the north of the country (ouazzane , tetouan and chefchaouen) three patients had parents cosanguinity ,and only 4 patients had health insurance the rest benefited from the Medical Insurance Plan for the Financially Underprivileged (RAMED) that allowed them to access to the same care facilities .

Treatment and treatment related complications: Treatment modification was documented in 18 patients who were treated according to the AML-Ma 2011 protocol. All of them suffered significant treatment-related toxicities after the initial induction courses, during

***Corresponding author:** Ayad A., Pediatric Hematology and Oncology Center (CHOP), Rabat children's hospital, Morrocco; E-mail: drayadanass@gmail.com

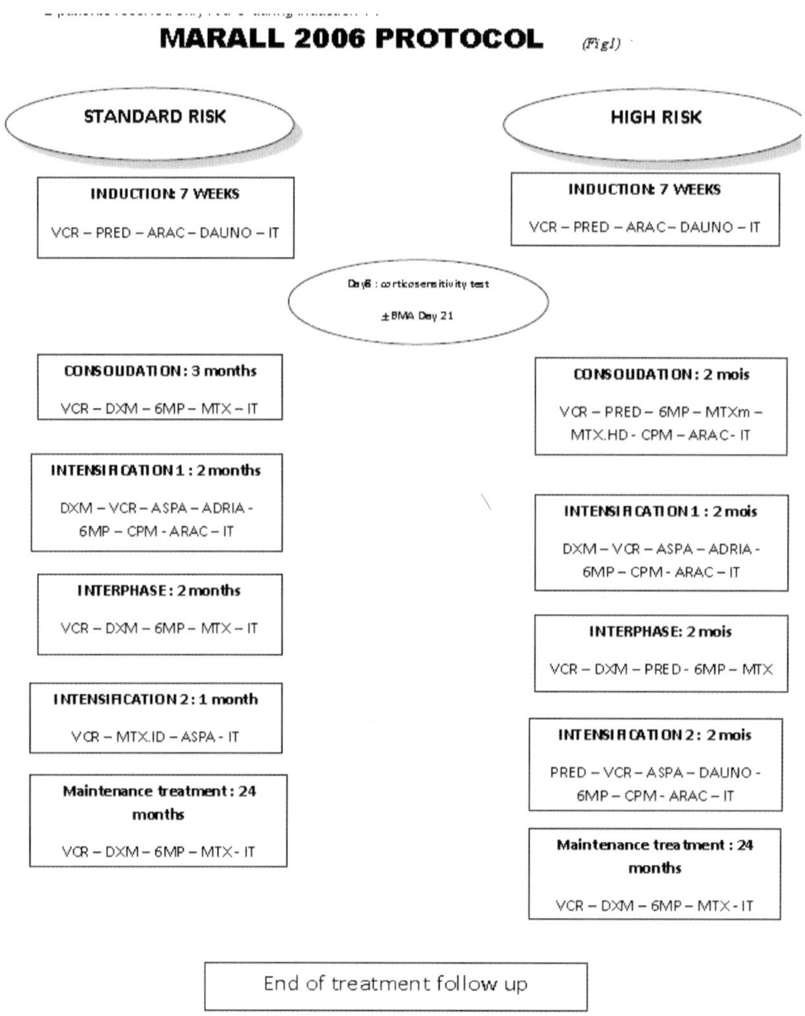

Figure 1: Children with ALL were treated according to MARALL 2006 protocol.

induction 1, 5 patients received only Ara-c and 3 others didn't receive daunomycin, all had 50% dose reduction and subsequently switched to less intensive consolidation treatment. For ALL, all patients had good response to the prednisolone prephase. 9 patients achieved morphologic remission after induction or consolidation and none received hematopoietic stem cell transplant. The most common treatment-related toxicity was severe mucositis (62.5% for ALL and 55% for AML), which responded positively with supportive management. One patient with ALL had severe chemotherapy-induced vomiting and was complicated by reflux oesophagitis and haematemesis which required extended omeprazole and ranitine treatment. Culture proven bacterial or fungal infections were common, being documented in 60% of ALL and 50% of AML patients.

One child with ALL developed hepatitis and jaundice during delayed intensification chemotherapy. The remaining delayed intensification chemotherapy was withheld and intrathecal chemotherapy was omitted subsequently in the maintenance phase. This patient did not have permanent liver damage on follow-up. Two patients with AML developed cellulitis of the hand and of the face for the second patient resulting in compartment syndrome requiring abscess drainage with extended parenteral antibiotic (flucloxacilline)One child with AML and underlying Tetralogy of Fallot experienced Acute lung oedema and pericardial effusion during induction chemotherapy. This patient eventually succumbed as a result of Cardiogenic shock and heart failure. Febrile neutropenia (FN) was common in all AML patients (100%) compared to ALL group (50%) and was defined as an axillary temperature measured as >38°C for once or as >37.5°C for at least one hour in patients who had an absolute neutrophil count (ANC) of <500/mm or who had an ANC between 500 and 1 000/mm3 and whose ANC was expected to decrease below 500/mm^3 in 24-48 hours. 12 of the FN episodes were fever of unknown origin, 30% were microbiologically documented infection. Of the microbiologically documented infections, 40% of them were caused by gram positive bacteria and 60% were by gram negative bacteria. Eight of 25 patients developed invasive fungal infection during treatmen t. FN was the cause of death in 1 patient. Types of antibiotics and Sites of infection are presented in (Tables 1 and 2). There were 10 patients with ALL and 20 with AML.The median age at diagnosis for the latter group was significantly younger (1.7 vs. 7.3 y, P=0.001). Transient myeloproliferative disease (TMD), was documented in one case of AML but none of the ALL patients. Congenital heart disease, the most common malformation associated with DS, was found more commonly in AML than ALL patients (78.9%

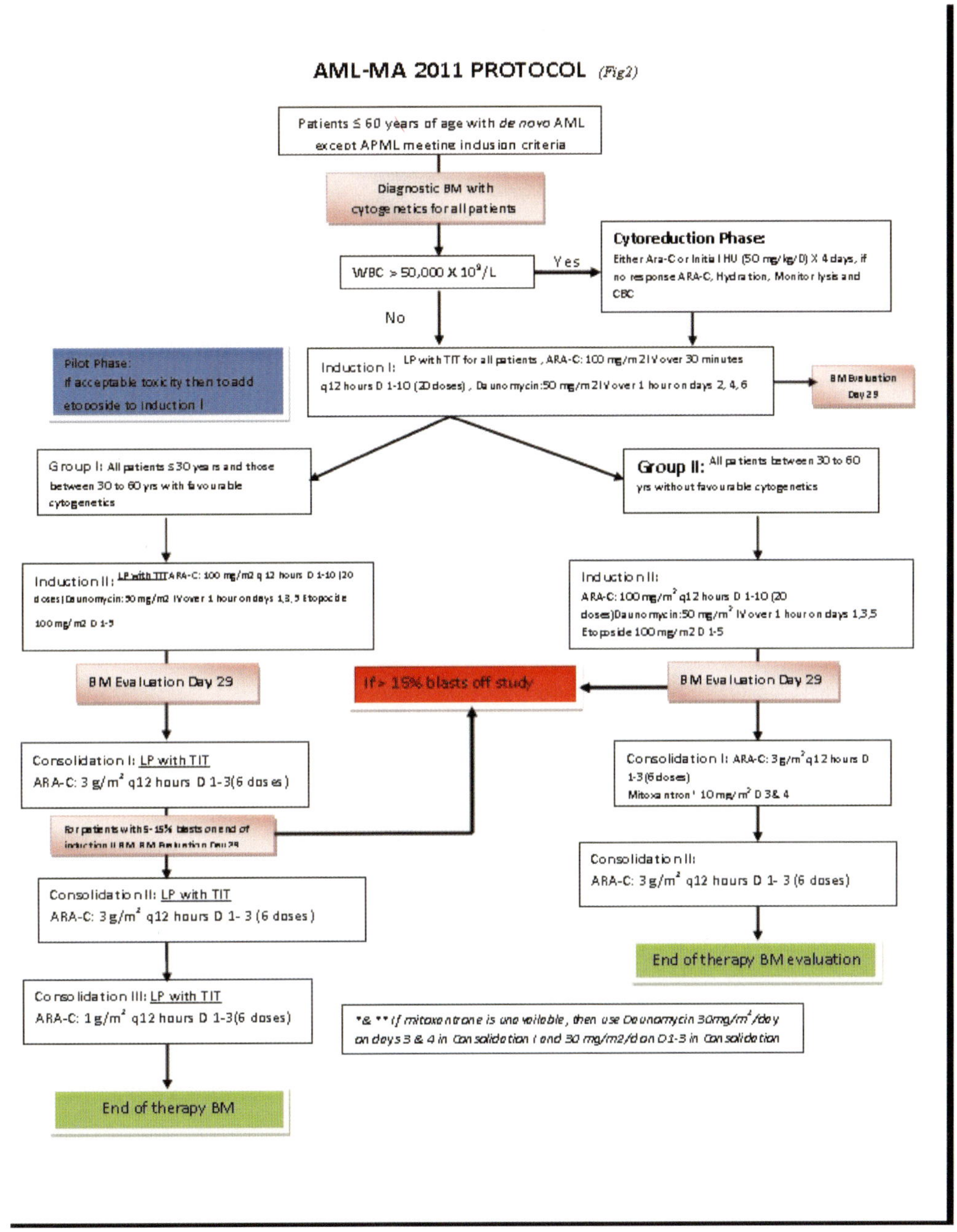

Figure 2: Children with AML were treated according to the AML-MA 2011 protocol.

Antibiotics	N	(%)
Ceftriaxone + Gentamycine	10	40
Ceftazidime + Amikacine	8	32
Metronidazole	3	12
Fluconazole	5	20
Vancomycine	6	24
Other	1	4

Table 1: Types of antibiotics used.

Site	N	(%)
Oral cavity infection	14	56
Respiratory tract infection	9	36
Blood stream infection	5	20
Urinary tract infection	2	8
Skin and soft tissue infection	1	4
Gastrointestinal tract infection	3	12

Table 2: Site of infection.

vs. 33.3%, P=0.026). The following cardiac defects were documented: atrial septal defect (n=12), patent ductus arteriosus (n=10), ventricular septal defect (n=3), atrioventricular canal defect (n=3), Tetralogy of Fallot (n=2), and complex cyanotic heart disease (n=1). Only 2 patients had congenital hypothyroidism . The common presenting features were anemia (51.7%), fever (48.3%), hepatosplenomegaly (41.4%), and bleeding symptoms (37.9%). One child with AML had pericardial effusion and high WBC of 100 000/mm^3 at diagnosis. None of the

Clinical and biological features n (%)			
	DS-ALL (N=10)	DS-AML (N= 20)	Total
Age (y)			
<1	0	1	1
1-3	1 (10)	17 (89.4)	18
4-9	6 (60)	1 (5.2)	7
>10	3 (30)	0	3
Median (range)	7.31 (3.12-15.98)	1.74 (0.61-4.08)	
Sex			
Male	5 (50)	12(60)	17
Female	5 (50)	8(40)	13
Presenting WBC			
<10	6 (60)	13 (65)	19
10-49	4 (40)	6(30)	10
50-99	0	1 (5)	1
>100	0	1 (5)	1
Congenital heart disease			
Yes	3 (33.3)	15 (75)	18
No	6 (66.6)	4 (20)	10
Unknown	1	0	1
Treatment protocol			
Treatment protocol			
MARALL 2006	10 (100)		10
AML-Ma 2011		9(95)	9
Other		1(5)	1
Toxicity			
Septicemia			
Yes	5 (62.5)	8 (40)	13
No	3 (37.5)	7 (35)	10
Unknown	2	5	7
Severe mucositis			
Yes	5 (62.5)	11 (55)	16
No	3 (37.5)	5(25)	8
Unknown	2	4	6
Febrile neutropenia			
Yes	5 (50)	20 (100)	25
No	4 (40)		4
Unknown	1		1
Transfusion			
Yes	5 (62.5)	15 (75)	20
No	3 (37.5)	3 (15)	6
Unknown	2	2	4
Treatment dose modification			
Yes	10 (100)	18 (90)	28
No			
Unknown		2	2

Figure 3: Microbiologically documented infections.

patients had central nervous system involvement at diagnosis. All patients with DS-ALL had B precursor ALL. Five of the 10 patients had additional cytogenetic abnormalities apart from constitutional trisomy 21. None had hyperdiploidy of >50 chromosomes. There was 2 patients with t(8 ;21), t(15 ;17),16q22 fusion and another one had 11q23 fusion. Among the 20 patients with AML, all had bone marrow aspiration classified as myeloid leukemia 10 were classified as FAB M7 subtype , 5 as FAB M6 , 2 patients had M0 (minimallydifferentiated) subtype.

For the 3 remaining the AML pathology could not be further classified.

Ten of the 19 patients had additional cytogenetic abnormalities, including monosomy 7, 5q deletions, and 7q deletions that are more commonly associated with myelodysplastic syndrome.

Outcome: Among the 30 cases we had there were 2 deaths in the ALL group (20%), The first patient had severe neutropenia and septicemia and died of multiorgan failure during intensification chemotherapy. The second patient died from disease relapse after he developed pulmonary tuberculosis during paliative chemotherapy (Table 3).

There were 4 deaths in the AML group (20%) The first was a one-year-old infant admitted with Generalized oedematous syndrome and digestive hemorrhage associated to a severe respiratory distress. He succumbed on the first day of hospitalization.

The second patient died from salmonella septicemia and septic shock during the third day of induction chemotherapy. The other patient was a 2 year-old child with Tetralogy of Fallot and succumbed from Cardiogenic shock and heart failure during induction 1.

The exact cause of death for the last patient was unknown due to incomplete data. There were no relapses among the AML patients. None of the 30 patients developed secondary malignancies.

Study group	Death	Complete remission	Relapse	Abondan of treatment	Lost of sight
AML	4	12	1	1	2
ALL	2	6	2	0	1
Total	6	18	3	1	3

Table 3: Outcomes of study groups.

For patients with DS-ALL the 5-year survival was 40% and respectively 60% for DS-AML Group

Discussion

This review paper covered a 10-year period and included a total of 30 patients with acute leukemia and DS and was mainly representative of the whole north area of Morocco. All of our patients were morrocan and from Arab ethnicity, and our findings would allow comparison with other cohorts to examine for the impact of ethnicity on disease outcome. The health care opportunities in morocco varies from regions to regions and Are mostly centralized in the main cities of the kingdom. Many women would not have had any antenatal care before their late presentation for obstetric care in Rabat or other hospital structure in the area with high-level maternity, this could explain the increased incidence of DS births and led to a proportionate increase in children with DS and acute leukemia.

Majority of our DS-ALL patients belonged to the standard risk group according to age and WBC count at diagnosis. Higher median age at diagnosis of 7.3 years compared with that of 5.6 years for the HKALL 97 cohort [3]. The presenting WBC were all below 50˙106/mm³. None of them had high-risk chromosomal translocations such as t(9;22) or t(4;11), and none had central nervous system involvement.

They were given a 4-drug induction therapy with prednisone , vincristine, Ara-c and Daunomycin and as well as intrathecal methotrexate. Following remission induction, therapy continues with a consolidation phase, an intensification phase, and maintenance. Chemotherapeutics during these phases may include cyclophosphamide, Ara-C, doxorubicin, mercaptopurine, vincristine, methotrexate and continued intrathecal chemotherapy .All patients achieved first remission after induction chemotherapy. Patients who eventually relapsed were all treated according to intermediate risk protocols. It has been documented that patients with DS-ALL has high risk of relapse and treatment-related mortality throughout the treatment period independent of the chemotherapy regime [4]. They are also at higher risk for infection-related mortality throughout all treatment phases [5]. Patients with DS–ALL tend to have poorer outcomes than those with No DS–ALL .One reason for previous treatment failures in children with DS–ALL is that these patients tend to develop toxic reactions to therapies In particular, a severe toxicity to methotrexate has been noted [6]. Methotrexate pharmacokinetics were analyzed retrospectively in children with ALL, comparing 44 with Down syndrome and 87 without the syndrome. Using non-linear mixed effect modeling, no differences in methotrexate pharmacokinetics were found between patients with and without Down syndrome which could explain the significantly higher proportion of children with Down syndrome who experienced methotrexate-induced toxicity.

The authors concluded that the higher toxicities suffered by Down syndrome patients are probably related to pharmacodynamic differences and that intermediate doses of methotrexate (such as 1-3 g/m²) can be used safely in Down syndrome children with ALL [7].

The increased in vitro sensitivity to chemotherapy observed in Down syndrome patients does not seem extend to those with ALL. Down syndrome lymphoblasts do not demonstrate greater sensitivity than non-Down syndrome cell lines to various chemotherapy agents. This biological characteristic can potentially account for the inferior outcome to therapy described in Down syndrome children with ALL in comparison to the outcome in non-Down syndrome children.

However, no significant differences in cytotoxicity to chemotherapy were found between fibroblasts from patients with or without Down syndrome. Other factors may account for the variation in chemotherapy response and toxicity and the molecular bases that contribute to these differences are not completely understood [8].

Indeed, our DS-ALL patients had poorer outcome than the DS-AML group. Another observation was that a substantial proportion of our patients had dose reduction from the standard ALL protocol, and disease relapse accounted for 1 of the 2 deaths in DS-ALL. However, we could not demonstrate any association between treatment reduction and relapse in our group .DS children with ML have a superior outcome when compared with children without DS who develop AML. Although all 12 DS children with AML enrolled on the original study POG 8498 achieved complete remission and were long survivors, subsequent publications, while noting the continuing evidence for the high curability (75% event-free survival [EFS] for DS-AML) [9].

In our review, the mean age of our patients with DS-AML were younger at presentation as compared with DS-ALL patients (1.74 vs.7.31 y). Distribution of morphological subtypes in AML-DS patients showed a predominance of AMKL-FAB M7 subtype (50%). The outcomes for childhood AML in our study is comparable with results from other study groups. The UK AML trials reported an overall 5-year OS as 65% in non-DS versus 76% in DS children [10]. The BFM group reported 7-year EFS and OS as 78% and 79%, respectively, for ML DS patients for the DS children on NOPHO-AML 93 protocol [11].

All of our patients had chemotherapy reduction using the AML-MA 2011 PROTOCOL , complications related to chemotherapy toxicity were frequent resulting in an increase in treatment-related mortality. We lower treatment intensity compared with the standard AML protocols. During induction 1 course the DS children didn't receive anthracyclines due to The increased risk of anthracycline-induced cardiac toxicity is potentially , although one patient died from congestive heart failure during day 2 of induction . At the time of analysis, all the patients who were treated on this protocol were able to adhere to the regimen without major complications.

On the short term efficacy appeared promising as 12 patients were able to achieve full remission, although long-term outcome is still uncertain. Treatment reduction for DS-AML appeared to have no adverse impact on disease outcome. This suggested that the reduction of treatment intensity was probably beneficial to DS-AML but not DS-ALL patients. The potential for reduced treatment intensity is based on the unique hypersensitivity of myeloid leukemia cells of DS patients to chemotherapy, when compared with AML cells from non-DS individuals, as demonstrated by various investigators [12]. This increased sensitivity to chemotherapy extends to agents with different mechanisms of action. Zwaan and colleagues have reported that myeloid blasts were significantly more sensitive to cytarabine, anthracyclines mitoxantrone, etoposide 6-thioguanine busulfan and vincristine than non-DS AML cells [13].

The major limitation for our study was the small sample size. There was also Poor adherence. To treatment protocols from some patients. Continued improvement of supportive care for these patients may also be a confounder on the incidence of treatment-related mortality. In contrast, long-term follow-up of these patients would allow better understanding of the late effects of disease and treatment in DS with leukemia. Due to its small sample size. Whether dose reduction of chemotherapy to reduce treatment-related mortality increases relapse remains unknown. The superior outcome in DS became obvious only after the inclusion of high-dose cytarabine in the treatment of childhood AML. Thus, the prevailing opinion is that two or more courses of high-dose cytarabine post–remission induction may be necessary for optimal therapy. However, the 100% EFS reportedby the POG investigators, based on the POG 8498 AML regimen, has not been duplicated in subsequent studies by POG or by other groups [14-15]. Plus the final four courses of conventional dose Ara-C, and sought to intensify the postinduction courses. At the same time, recognition of the unique responsiveness of AML in children with DS lead both to greater enrollment of DS cases on therapeutic studies and the recognition of risk for toxicity and the potential for mortality from infections. Gamis et al. [16] observed no increase in mortality rate in children with DS, but did observe high pulmonary toxicity during induction, including the need for ventilatory support and an increased incidence of mucositis and skin toxicity (perhaps from Ara-C). In our series the deaths occurred in an early phase and cannot be attributed to toxicity of chemotherapy but rather to a late arrival to the service for management.

Conclusion

The prognosis for DS-AML patients was superior to ALL-DS patients. Given the enhanced sensitivity of myeloid leukemic cells in these patients, dose-reductions in ML regimens for DS patients are easier accepted than for ALL regimens. The main side effects include mucositis, and an increased susceptibility to infections wich is mainly associated with high-dose methotrexate (MTX). An important aspect in treating children with DS is whether they have an increased risk of long-term cardiotoxicity following anthracycline exposure, given the fact that a significant proportion of DS children may have a compromised cardiac function because of congenital abnormalities to begin with.

In this study, there was no increased cardiotoxicity in DS children, but these children were treated with reduced dosages of anthracyclines. Finally, as there is still uncertainty in the optimal chemotherapeutic drug dosing for the entire pediatric DS population, new treatment methodologies will be especially crucial to help increase the remission rate for these children. Creating new risk group classifications based on patient cytogenetics may be one way to develop more specific chemotherapeutic drug dosing schedules for particular patient groups. Furthermore, focusing on integration of targeted non-cytotoxic agents, such as monoclonal antibodies may provide a better non-toxic treatment method for all Patients.

References

1. Rabin KR, Whitlock JA (2009) Malignancy in children with trisomy21. Oncologist. 14: 164-173.
2. Lange B (2000) The management of neoplastic disorders of haematopoiesis in children with Down's syndrome, Br. J. Haematol. 110: 512-524.
3. Li CK, Chik KW, Ha SY (2006) Improved outcome of acute lymphoblastic leukaemia treated by delayed intensification in Hong Kong children: HKALL 97 study. Hong Kong Med J. 12: 394- 400.
4. Buitenkamp TD, Izraeli S, Zimmermann M (2014) Acutelymphoblastic leukemia in children with Down syndrome: a retrospective analysis from the Ponte di Legno study group. Blood. 123: 70-77.
5. O'Connor D, Bate J, Wade R (2014) Infection-related mortality in children with acute lymphoblastic leukemia: an analysis of infectious deaths on UKALL2003. Blood. 124: 1056-1061.
6. Goto.H, Inukai T, Inoue H, Ogawa C, Fukushima T (2011) Acute lymphoblastic leukemia and Down syndrome: the collaborative study of the Tokyo Children's Cancer Study Group and the Kyushu Yamaguchi Children's Cancer Study Group, Int. J. Hematol. 93: 192-198.
7. Buitenkamp TD, Mathot RA, de Haas V, Pieters R, Zwaan CM, et al. (2010) Methotrexate-induced side effects are not due to differences in pharmacokinetics in children with Down syndrome and acute lymphoblastic leukemia. Haematologica. 95:1106-1113.
8. Valle M, Plon SE, Rabin KR (2009) Differential in vitro cytotoxicity does not explain increased host toxicities from chemotherapy in Down syndrome acute lymphoblastic leukemia. Leuk Res.33: 336-339.
9. Ravindranath Y, Yeager AM, Chang MN (1996) Autologous bone marrow transplantation versus intensive consolidation chemotherapy for acute myeloid leukemia in childhood: Pediatric Oncology Group. N Engl J Med. 334:1428-1434.
10. Rao A, Hills RK, Stiller C (2005) Treatment for myeloid leukemia of Down syndrome: population-based experience in the UK and results from the Medical Research Council AML 10 and AML 12 trials. Br J Haematol. 132: 576-583.
11. Blink M, Zimmermann M, Von Neuhoff C (2014) Normal karyotype is a poor prognostic factor in myeloid leukemia of Down syndrome: a retrospective, international study. Haematologica. 99: 299-307.
12. Frost BM, Gustafsson G, Larsson R (2000) Cellular cytotoxic drug sensitivity in children with acute leukemia and Down's syndrome: an explanation to differences in clinical outcome? [letter]. Leukemia.14: 943-944.
13. Zwaan CM, Kaspers GJL, Pieters R (2002) Different drug sensitivity profiles of acute myeloid and lymphoblastic leukemia and normal peripheral blood mononuclear cells, in children with and without Down syndrome. Blood. 99: 245-251.
14. Lie SO, Jonmundsson G, Mellander L (1996) A population-based study of 272 children with acute myeloid leukaemia treated on two consecutive protocols with different intensity: Best outcome in girls, infants, and children with Down's syndrome - Nordic Society of Paediatric Haematology and Oncology (NOPHO). Br J Haematol 94: 82-88.
15. Creutzig U, Ritter J, Vormoor J (1996) Myelodysplasia and acute myelogenous leukemia in Down's syndrome: A report of 40 children of the AML-BFM Study Group. Leukemia 10:1677-1686.
16. Gamis AS, Alonzo TA, Buxton A (2003) Increased age at diagnosis has a significantly negative effect on outcome in children with Down's syndrome and acute myeloid leukemia: A report from the Children's Cancer Group Study, CCG-2891. J Clin Oncol 21: 3415-3422.

Myeloid Neoplasms Associated with t(3;12)(q26.2;p13) Are Clinically Aggressive and Frequently Harbor *FLT3* Mutations: A Report of 8 Cases

Xiaohong I. Wang[1], Xinyan Lu[1], C. Cameron Yin[1], Lian Zhao[1], Carlos E. Bueso-Ramos[1], L. Jeffrey Medeiros[1], Shaoying Li[2], Heesun J. Rogers[3], Eric D. Hsi[3] and Pei Lin[1]*

[1]*Department of Hematopathology, The University of Texas MD Anderson Cancer Center, Houston, Texas, 77030, USA*
[2]*Department of Pathology, Vanderbilt University School of Medicine, Nashville, Tennessee, 37235, USA*
[3]*Department of Clinical Pathology, Cleveland Clinic Foundation, Cleveland, Ohio, 44195, USA*

Abstract

The t(3;12)(q26.2;p13) involving *EVI1* and *ETV* 6 is a rare recurrent translocation that has been identified in myeloid neoplasms. The clinicopathologic features of these are not well characterized.

We identified 5 cases of acute myeloid leukemia (AML) and 3 cases of myelodysplastic syndrome (MDS) associated with t(3;12)(q26.2;p13). There were 5 men and 3 women, with a median age of 60 years. The AML cases included 2 *de novo*, 2 arising from prior MDS and 1 relapsed AML. The median bone marrow blast count was 50% (range, 35-91%). Dysplasia was noted in all cases. Of the 3 MDS cases, two were classified as refractory anemia with excess blasts and one therapy related. Two that had follow up data rapidly evolved to AML within 6 months.

Conventional cytogenetic analysis showed t(3;12)(q26.2;p13) in all neoplasms and additional abnormalities in 5 patients, Including chromosome 7 abnormalities in 3 patients. Fluorescence *in situ* hybridization confirmed *ETV6* rearrangement in all 3 cases assessed and *EVI1* rearrangement in both cases assessed. *FLT3-ITD* was identified in 3 of 5 cases assessed. The median overall survival was 12 months (range, 7-58 months).

We conclude that t(3;12) can occur as either a primary or secondary event in myeloid neoplasms. The t(3;12) is associated with multilineage dysplasia, chromosome 7 aberrations and an aggressive clinical course.

Keywords: Myeloid neoplasms; t(3;12)(q26.2;p13); *EVI1; MECOM; ETV6; FLT3;* Chromosome 7

Introduction

Disruption of chromosome locus 3q26 is an uncommon recurrent cytogenetic abnormality that occurs in a small percentage of cases of acute myeloid leukemia (AML) or myelodysplastic syndrome (MDS). The ecotropic viral integration site 1 (*EVI1)* gene, located on chromosome 3q26.2, also known as *MECOM* gene, has been shown to be activated in at least a subset of these meyleoid neoplasms. *EVI1* is activated in various AML associated cytogenetic abnormalities, such as inv(3)(q21q26.2) or t(3;3)(q21;q26.2)/*EVI1-GATA1.*

The t(3;12)(q26.2;p13) is a rare recurrent event in cases of AML, MDS, and blast phase of CML [1-3]. The *ETV6* gene (ETS variant 6), also called Translocation Ets Leukemia (*TEL*), is located on 12p13 and encodes for a transcription factor that is a target of deletions and translocations in both myeloid and lymphoid malignancies. Various partner genes in reciprocal translocations involving 12p13 have been described. *ETV6* rearrangements are much less frequent in myeloid neoplasms [4].

The clinical and molecular features of myeloid neoplasms associated with t(3;12)(q26.2; p13) are not as well understood as those associated with inv(3)/t(3;3). In this study, we comprehensively described features of 8 patient with myeloid neoplasms associated with t(3;12)(q26.2; p13).

Materials and Methods

We searched the database of the Clinical Cytogenetics Laboratory for cases of myeloid neoplasms associated with t(3;12)(q26.2;p13) detected by conventional cytogenetic analysis. Two cases were also obtained from the Department of Pathology, Vanderbilt University School of Medicine and Cleveland Clinic, respectively. The diagnosis was based on the 2008 WHO criteria. Wright-Giemsa-stained bone marrow (BM) aspirate smears and touch imprints and H&E-stained core biopsy and clot sections were reviewed. This study was conducted according to an institutional review board-approved protocol.

Multicolor flow cytometry immunophenotypic analysis was performed on BM aspirate specimens using a FACScan instrument (Becton-Dickinson, San Jose, Calif) as described previously [5]. The blast population was gated using right-angle side scatter and CD45 expression. The panel of monoclonal antibodies included reagents specific for CD3, CD5, CD7, CD13, CD14, CD19, CD33, CD34, CD38, CD64, CD117, HLA-DR, TdT, and myeloperoxidase (Becton-Dickinson).

BM aspirate specimens were analyzed by conventional cytogenetic analysis as described previously [6]. Karyotypes were reported according to the 2013 International System for Human Cytogenetic Nomenclature [7].

***Corresponding author:** Pei Lin, Department of Hematopathology, The University of Texas MD Anderson Cancer Center, 1515 Holcombe Boulevard, Unit 72, Houston, Texas 77030-4009, USA; E-mail: peilin@mdanderson org

Fluorescence *in Situ* Hybridization (FISH) was performed using a LSI *ETV6* dual color, breakapart probe (Vysis-Abbott Molecular, Inc), which hybridizes to band 12p13. The *EVI1* dual-color, breakapart DNA probe (Leica/Kreatech Inc.) was used to detect *EVI1* gene rearrangement at 3q26. For each specimen, 200 interphases were analyzed. The FISH images were captured and analyzed by Applied Imaging software- Cyto Vision software (Leica, Inc).

Analyses for *FLT3* Internal Tandem Duplication (*ITD*) and codon 835/836 point mutation were performed by polymerase chain reaction (PCR)-based amplification of genomic DNA and capillary electrophoresis as described previously [8]. Codons 12, 13, and 61 of *KRAS* and *NRAS* were sequenced following PCR amplification using Sanger sequencing or a pyrosequencing-based method as previously described [9]. *NPM1* mutations spanning codons 956 to 971 of exon 12 were detected by PCR followed by capillary electrophoresis as described previously [10]. *KIT D816V* mutation was detected by direct Sanger sequencing on an ABI Prism 3100 Genetic Analyzer [10,11].

The overall survival (OS) was calculated from date of diagnosis of either MDS or AML associated with t(3;12)(q26.2;p13) until death from any cause or date of last follow-up.

Results

Clinical findings

The clinical and morphological features are summarized in Table 1. Of the 8 patients with t(3;12)(q26.2;p13), there were 5 men and 3 women, with a median age of 60 years (range, 33-79 years). Presenting symptoms include fever, chills, general malaise, weakness and night sweats (cases 1, 2), fatigue (cases 3, 5, 6, 8), gum bleeding (case 4) and upper airway infection (case 7). Physical exam found lymphadenopathy (cases 1, 4) and a palpable spleen (case 1). None had myeloid sarcoma involving soft tissue at the diagnosis. Five cases were classified as AML and 3 cases MDS. All patients had anemia with a median hemoglobin level of 8.9 g/dL (range, 6.8 to 12.3 g/dL [68-123 g/L]; reference range, 14-18 g/dL [140-180 g/L] for men and 12-14 g/dL [120-140 g/L] for women) and thrombocytopenia with a median platelet count of 52 × 10^9/L (range, 24-111 × 10^9/L; reference range, 140-440 × 10^9/L). The median white blood cell (WBC) count was 62.6 k/uL (rang, 1.9-129.5 k/uL) for the 5 cases of AML with a median peripheral blood blast count of 31% (range, 21-88%). The patients with MDS had a median WBC of 4.0 k/uL (range, 1.8-7.6 k/uL) with a median peripheral blood blast count of 1% (range, 0% to 3%).

Serum chemistry results were generally unremarkable except the lactate dehydrogenase level was elevated in 2 of 6 patients assessed: 489 IU/L and 4183 IU/L, respectively, (reference range, 313-618 IU/L). The β2-microglobulin level was elevated in 1 patient, 7.3 mg/L (reference range, 0.6-2.0 mg/L).

Morphologic findings

Peripheral blood smears showed circulating blasts in 7/8 cases (range, 1%-88%), anemia with mild to moderate anisopoikilocytosis (5/6 cases), nucleated red blood cells (2/5 cases), absolute monocytosis (3/5 cases).

BM smears showed multilineage dysplasia in all 8 cases. Five of 8 (63%) cases showed megakaryocytic hypoplasia. Small hypolobated

Case number	1	2	3	4	5	6	7	8
Age/gender	34/M	54/M	58/M	79/M	70/F	61/F	33/F	61/M
Diagnosis	AML, M1	AML, M5a	AML-MRC	AML-MRC	Recurrent AML	RAEB-1	RAEB-2	t- MDS
Peripheral Blood								
WBC (k/uL)	129.5	113	8.9	62.6	1.9	7.6	1.8	4
Hemoglobin (g/dL)	6.8	8.1	8.5	8.2	12.3	9.3	9.3	9.8
Platelet count (k/uL)	68	74	70	33	111	30	36	24
Peripheral blood blast count	88%	21%	32%	31%	10%	3%	1%	0%
Bone Marrow								
Bone marrow cellularity	95%	100%	60%	95%	70%	60%	40%	50%
Bone marrow blasts	91%	63%	45%	35%	50%	8%	18%	1%
Granulocytic series	Decreased, dysplastic	Dysplastic	Dysplastic	Dysplastic	Decreased, dysplastic	Dysplastic	Decreased, dysplastic	Dysplastic
Erythroid series	Decreased, dysplastic	Decreased, dysplastic	Decreased, dysplastic	Decreased, dysplastic	Decreased, dysplastic	Dysplastic	Decreased, dysplastic	Increased, dysplastic
Megakaryocytic series	Decreased, dysplastic	Decreased, dysplastic	Dysplastic	Dysplastic	Decreased, dysplastic	Dysplastic	Decreased, dysplastic	Decreased, dysplastic
Molecular Results								
FLT3 ITD mutation	Positive	Positive	Negative	Positive	NA	NA	Negative	NA
KRAS mutation	Negative	Negative	Negative	Positive (G12D)	NA	NA	NA	Positive (G12A)
NRAS mutation	NA	Negative	Negative	Positive (G13D)	NA	NA	NA	NA
KIT D816V	Negative	NA	Positive	Negative	NA	NA	NA	NA
NPM1 mutation	Negative	NA	NA	NA	NA	NA	NA	NA
Treatment and Survival								
Multiagent chemotherapy	Yes	Yes	Yes	Yes	Yes	Yes	NA	Yes
BM transplantation	Yes	Yes	No	No	No	No	NA	Yes
Overall (Months)	58	17	7	7	7	11	NA	12
Alive/deceased	Alive	Deceased	Deceased	Deceased	Alive	Deceased	NA	Deceased

NA: not available, MRC: myelodysplasia related changes.

Table 1: Morphology and clinical features of patients at diagnosis.

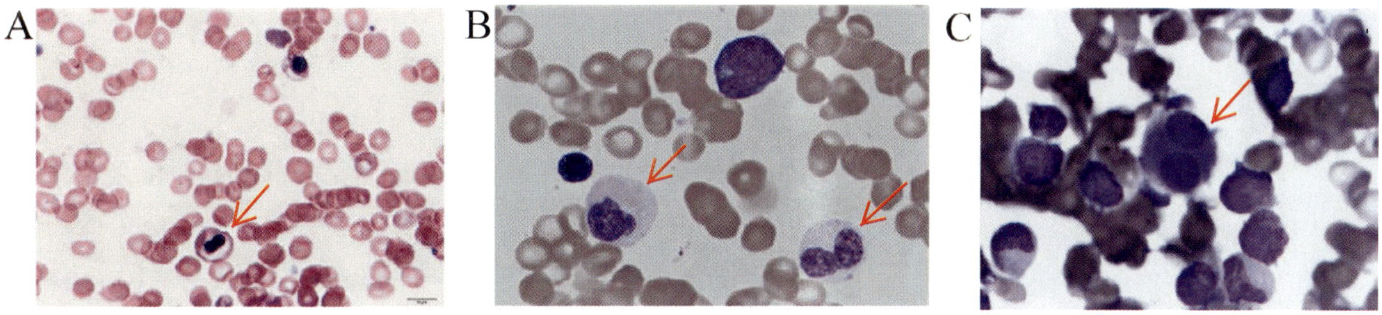

Figure 1: Characteristic cytologic changes of AML or MDS associated with t(3;12)(q26.2;p13) (red arrows)
A: Erythroid dysplasia: a normoblast shows irregular nucleus, case 3
B: Myeloid dysplasia: two myeloid elements show abormal nuclei and cytoplasmic granulation, case 7
C: A dysplastic hypolobated megakaryocyte with two lobes, case 7

case#	diagnosis	Karyotype	*ETV6/EVI1* FISH
1	AML, M1	45,XY,t(3;12)(q26.2;p13),-7[19]	*ETV6*
2	AML, M5a	46,XY,t(3;12)(q26.2;p13), del(11)(q23.1)[20]	*ETV6, EVI1*
3	AML arising from MDS	46,XY,t(3;12)(q26.2;p13),add(7)(q11.2)[18], 46,XY[2]	ND
4	AML arising from MDS	46,XY,t(3;12)(q26.2;p13),del(10)(q22q24)[19], 46,XY[1]	*ETV6*
5	Recurrent AML	46,XX,t(3;12)(q26;p13)[20]	ND
6	RAEB-1	46,XX,t(3;12)(q26.2;p13)[20]	ND
7	RAEB-2	46,XX,t(3;12)(q26;p13) [18] 46,XX[2]	ND
8	t-MDS	46,XY,t(3;12)(q26.2;p13),r(7)[17], 45,XY,t(3;12)(q26.2;p13),-7[3]	*EVI1*

AML: acute myeloid leukemia; M5a: acute monocytic leukemia; MDS: myelodysplastic syndrome; ND: Not Done; t-MDS: therapy related myelodysplastic syndrome; RAEB-2: refractory anemia with excess blasts -2;

Table 2: Cytogenetic Data at Initial Dectection of t(3;12)(q26.2;p13).

megakaryocytes were observed in 7/7 cases (Figure 1). Blasts ranged from 1% to 18% in cases of MDS and 35 % to 91% in case of AML.

The 8 cases were classified as follows. Two *de novo* AML: one was AML without maturation (case 1) and the other acute monoblastic leukemia (case 2). Two were AML that evolved from MDS diagnosed 7 and 11 months earlier and were classified as AML with myelodysplasia-related changes (case 3 and 4). One case of AML was diagnosed at time of relapse (case 5). Two cases of MDS were classified as refractory anemia with excess blasts (RAEB-1 and RAEB-2) (cases 6 and 7) and 1 patient had therapy-related MDS following therapy for 8 months (case 8).

Immunophenotypic findings

Flow cytometric immunophenotypic analysis of BM aspirate specimens from the 5 AML cases showed that the blasts were of myeloid origin. Blasts were positive for CD13, CD33, CD34, CD117, and HLA-DR in all cases. They were also positive for CD5 (partial, 1/3, 33%), CD7 (partial, 2/4, 50%), CD14 (1/2, 50%), CD15 (3/3, 100%), CD38 (2/3, 67%), and CD64 (2/3, 67%).

Cytogenetic findings

All 8 cases carried the t(3;12)(q26.2;p13). Three (37%) cases (cases 5-7) had t(3;12)(q26.2;p13) as the sole abnormality at the time of first detection (Table 2). The other 5 cases (63%) showed additional chromosomal abnormalities, including monosomy 7 (case 1), del(11)(q23.1) (case 2), and add(7)(q11.2) (case 3), del10(q22q24) (case 4), r(7) and monosomy 7 (case 8). In case 5, t(3;12) was not identified in the leukemic blasts at initial diagnosis of AML, but was detected 9 months later at time of relapse. In the whole cohort (n=8), the median number of additional chromosomal abnormalities was 1 (range, 0-2). All 4 patients with available initial karyotypes had other cytogenetic abnormalities prior to detection of t(3;12): add 7 (case 3), monosomy 7 (case 8), t(10;12)(q24;p13) (case 4) and 46,X, t(X;19)(p11.2;p13.1) (case 5) preceded that of t(3;12) by approximately 11, 12, 6 and 10 months, respectively, suggesting that t(3;12) evolved as a secondary event. In cases 1, 2 and 6, the initial karyotype was unknown. There was no cytogenetic follow up for case 7.

Fluorescence *in situ* hybridization was performed in a subset of cases. *ETV6* rearrangements were seen in all 3 cases assessed and *EVI1* rearrangements were detected in both cases assessed (Figure 2).

Molecular findings

FLT3-ITD was identified in 3 of 5 cases assessed (cases 1, 2 and 4). *KRAS* mutation was detected in 2 of 5 cases (G12D in case 4 and G12A in case 8). *NRAS* mutation (1/3, G13D in case 4) and *KIT D816V* mutation (1/3, in case 3) were also identified.

Clinical Outcome

Clinical follow-up was available for 7 patients. All patients received multi-agent chemotherapy. Three also underwent stem cell transplantation (cases 1, 2 and 8). At last follow-up, 5 patients had died and 2 were alive. For the 3 patients who underwent transplantation, the OS was 12, 17 and 58 months, respectively. The median OS for the 4 patients who did not undergo transplantation was 7 months (range, 7-11 months). There was no significant difference in OS between patients who did or did not undergo transplantation. Of the two cases of MDS that had follow up data (cases 6 and 8), the disease evolved to AML within 2

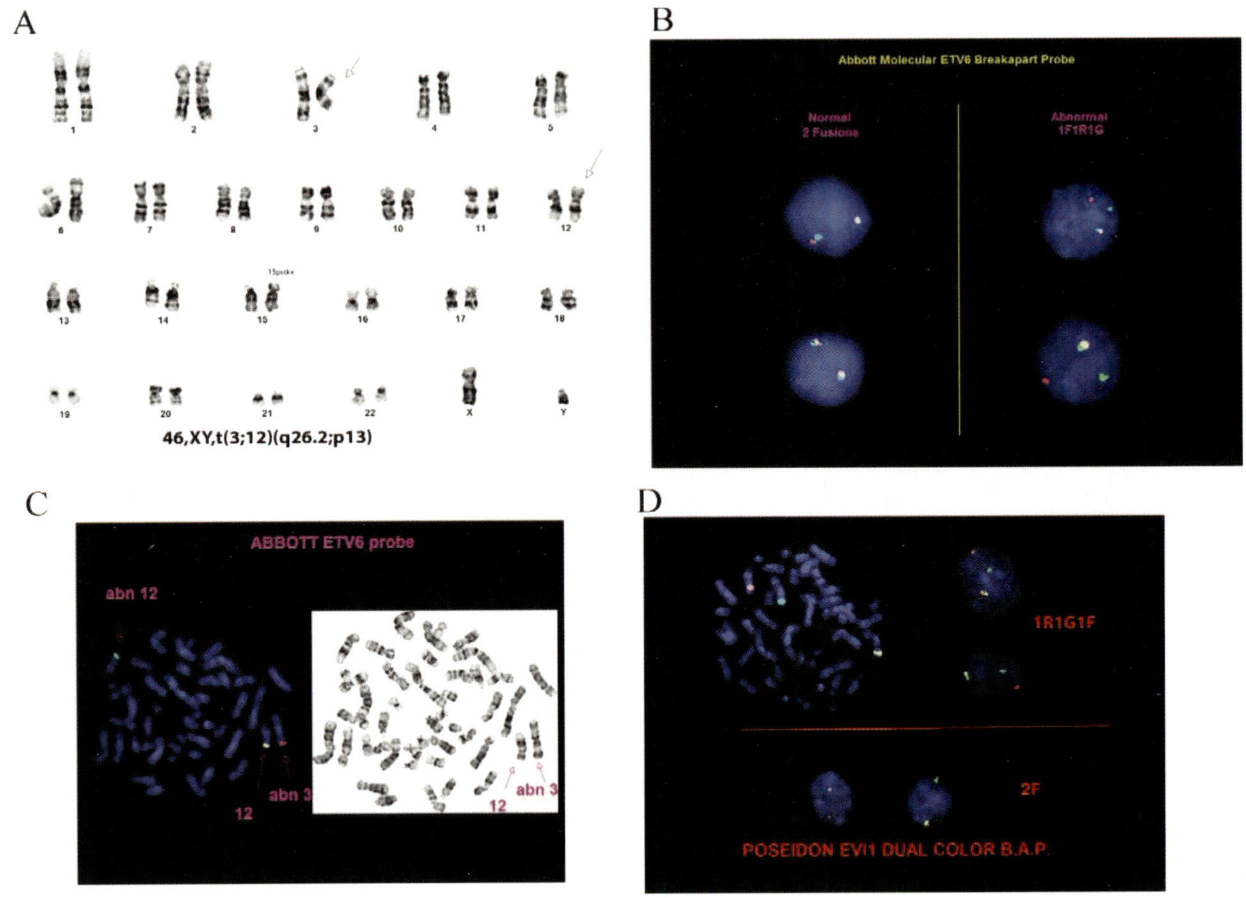

Figure 2: A. Karyotype from a metaphase cell of a patient by G-banding analysis showing the t(3;12)(q26.2;p13). The arrowheads indicate the abnormal chromosomes 3 and 12. There is an increase in length of the stalk on the short arm of chromosome 15 (15pstk+).
B. FISH analysis using LSI *ETV6* break apart probe showing two normal interphase cells (2 fusion signals) on the left and 2 abnormal cells with t(3;12)(q26.2;p13)(3'ETV6+;5'ETV6+) (1F1R1G).
C. The LSI *ETV6* probe on the metaphase shows *ETV6* rearrangement.
D. The Dual-Color *EVI1* break apart probe hybridized to the metaphase showing a rearrangement involving the *EVI1* gene region at 3q26.
The green *EVI1* signal remained on the abnormal chromosome 3 while the *EVI1* red signal was translocated to the abnormal chromosome 12.
The normal (2 fusion signals) and abnormal signal (1R1G1F) patterns are also shown in two interphases, respectively.

and 6 months, respectively, after detection of t(3;12), with the BM blast count rising from 8% to 71%, and from 2 to 25%, respectively .

Discussion

The t(3;12)(q26.2;p13) was first reported by Secker-Walker et al. in 3 patients as part of a larger series of 66 myeloid neoplasms with chromosomal abnormalities in the 3q26.2 region [12]. To date, 42 patients have been recorded in the Mitelman database, including AML (n=35), CML (n=4), and MDS (n=3) [13]. However, data regarding these cases are limited (Table 3) [1,14]. Our study is the largest series to date and provided both conventional cytogenetic as well as molecular genetic findings that were missing in many of the previous case reports.

In this study, we show that myeloid neoplasms associated with t(3;12) are mostly adults who usually presented with anemia and had poor clinical outcome. Multilineage dysplasia was consistently observed in all patients with frequent small hypolobated megakaryocytes. Karyotypic abnormalities in addition to t(3;12) were common, with monosomy 7 occurring in approximately half of the cases. Furthermore, the t(3;12) was preceded by other karyotypic aberrations in 4 patients whose initial cytogenetic data were available, indicating that the t(3;12) was likely a secondary event or existed as a small subclone initially in these patients. The frequent association with chromosome 7 abnormalities is in accordance with the others reported in Mitelman database (Table 2). The t(3;12)(q26.2;p13) was the sole abnormality in 21 of 38 (55%) cases [12,13]. Nine (24%) cases had additional chromosome 7 abnormalities, with loss of part or all of chromosome 7 (8/9, 89%) being the most common. We also showed *FLT3-ITD* mutations in over half of the cases assessed, a frequency that appears to be higher than the reported overall frequency of 20% to 30% in AML patients [14] and a reported frequency of 18% in balanced t(3q26;v) AML [1].

The *EVI1* proto-oncogene is located on human chromosome 3q26. Its transcriptional activation is relatively common in myeloid malignancies and has been reported in up to 10% of AML, blast phase of CML and MDS. [15] The EVI1 protein is a transcriptional regulator with DNA-binding zinc finger domains. Overexpression of EVI1 is an indicator of poor prognosis in myeloid malignancies. The major cellular effects are promoting proliferation, interfering with myeloid differentiation and preventing cellular apoptosis. In retrovirally-transduced marrow cell recipient mice, coexpression of EVI1 and Trib1 accelerates leukemogenesis [16]. EVI1 binds CCAAT/enhancer binding

Age /Sex	Cytogenetics	Diagnosis	Survival
NA	46,X?,t(3;12)(q26;p13)	AML, NOS (RAEB-T)	NA
29 y/m	46,XY,t(3;12)(q26;p13)	AML, NOS	NA
43 y/m	46,XY,t(3;12)(q26;p13)/46,idem,i(14)(q10)	MDS	NA
61 y/M	46,XY,t(3;12)(q26.2;p13)[20]	AML (FAB-M2)	NA
37 y/M	46,XY,t(3;12)(q26.2;p13)[19]/46,idem,der(9)t(1;9)(q10;p10)[2]	AML (FAB-M0)	NA
53 y/F	46,XX,t(3;12)(q26.2;p13)[20]	AML, NOS	NA
74 y/m	46,XY,t(3;12)(q26;p13)	AML, NOS (de novo)	NA
27 y/m	46,XY,t(3;12)(q26;p13)	AML, NOS (de novo)	NA
61y/f	46,XX,t(3;12)(q26;p13),del(5)(q14q34)	s-AML	NA
77y/f	46,XX,t(3;12)(q26;p13),del(5)(q14q34)	s-AML	NA
67y/f	46,XX,t(3;12)(q26;p13)	s-AML	NA
50y/m	45,XY,t(3;12)(q26;p13),-7	AML, NOS (de novo)	NA
48y/m	45,XY,t(3;12)(q26;p13),-7	t-AML	NA
57y/m	46,XY,t(3;12)(q26;p13)	MDS	NA
64y/m	46,XY,t(3;12)(q26;p13),del(7)(q12)	MDS	NA
13y/F	45,XX,t(3;12)(q26;p13),-7	AML (FAB-M2) (de novo)	10 mon
46y/m	46,XY,t(3;12)(q26;p13)	AML (FAB-M4)	6 mon
NA	46,XY,t(3;12)(q26;p13)	AML, NOS	NA
NA	46,XX,t(3;12)(q26;p13)	AML, NOS	NA
NA	46,XX,t(3;12)(q26;p13)	AML, NOS	NA
NA	46,XY,t(3;12)(q27;p13),add(9)(p24)	AML, NOS	NA
NA	46,XY,t(3;12)(q26;p13)	AML, NOS	NA
NA	46,XY,t(3;12)(q26;p13)/47,idem,+18	AML, NOS	NA
NA	46,XX,t(3;12)(q26;p12)	AML, NOS	NA
NA	46,XX,t(3;12)(q26;p13)	AML, NOS	NA
NA	46,XX,t(3;12)(q26;p13)	AML, NOS	NA
6mon/m	45,XY,-7,del(12)(p11p12)/45,XY,t(3;12)(q26;p12),-7	s-AML	9 mon
79y/f	46,XX,t(3;12)(q26;p13),add(7)(q11)	AML (FAB-M0)	270 mon
52y/m	46,XY,t(3;12)(q26;p13),-7,+r	s-AML (FAB type M2)	NA
60y/m	46,XY,t(3;12)(q26;p13),del(7)(q21q35)	s-AML (FAB type M2)	7 mon
87y/m	46,XY,t(3;12)(q26;p13),del(7)(q21q34)	s-AML (FAB type M2)	10 mon
57y/?	46,XY,t(3;12)(q26;p13)	AML (FAB-M0) (de novo)	15 mon
21y/f	46,XX,t(3;12)(q26;p13)	AML (FAB type M2)	39 mon
24y/m	46,XY,del(1)(p3?2p3?4),t(3;12)(q26;p13)	AML, NOS	NA
59y/f	46,XX,t(3;12)(q26;p13)	s-AML (FAB type M4)	5 mon
70y/m	46,XY,t(3;12)(q26;p13)	s-AML	18 mon
36y/f	46,XX,t(3;12)(q26;p13)	s-AML (RAEB-T)	44 mon
45y/m	46,XY,t(3;12)(q26;p13),t(7;12)(p15;p13)/46,idem,t(2;10)(p23;q22)	AML-MRC (de novo)	9 mon

FAB type M0: Acute myeloblastic leukemia with minimal differentiation FAB type M2: Acute myeloblastic leukemia with maturation FAB type M4: Acute myelomonocytic leukemia; AML, NOS: Acute myeoid leukemia not otherwise specified
MDS: Myelodysplastic syndrome; MRC: Myelodysplasia-related changes; RAEB-T: Refractory anemia with excess blasts in transformation
s: secondary; t: therapy related; NA: not available

Table 3: Characteristics of 38 AML and MDS Cases Associated With t(3;12) From the Mitelman Database.

protein-ε (C/EBP-ε) and deregulates terminal differentiation of granulocytes [17]. Kurokawa et al. demonstrated that EVI1 inhibits c-Jun N-terminal kinase (JNK) to suppress stress induced apoptosis [18].

A number of inversions and translocations have been described in human AML and MDS marrow cells involving chromosome 3q26, where the human gene is located. The most common *EVI1* chromosomal rearrangements include inv(3), t(3;3), t(3;12) and t(3;21). The t(3;12)(q26;p13) results in a fusion protein involving *ETV6* (also termed *TEL*), an ETS family transcription factor required for normal hematopoiesis. The prototype of AML/MDS with *EVI1* disruption is inv(3)/t(3;3)/*EVI1-GATA1*, which is recognized as a distinct entity in the current World Health Organization (WHO) classification. These patients often present de novo or arise from prior MDS, with frequent concurrent chromosomal 7 aberrations and have a short overall survival [1,19]. BM typically shows increased small hypolobated megakaryocytes and multilineage dysplasia. It is unclear if cases in which 3q26.2/*EVI1* partners with genes other than *GATA1* behave similarly to those with inv(3)/t(3;3) in clinical presentation and outcome. The t(3;12) is thought to juxtapose *ETV6* upstream of *EVI1* gene resulting in *EVI1* overexpression. We have demonstrated here that these cases are similar to those of AML/MDS with inv(3)/t(3;3) in many of the features described above and justify their classification in the same subgroup as AML with inv(3)/t(3;3). As inv(3)/t(3;3) is identified following -7 in some cases, we also observed that t(3;12) may emerge several months after other cytogenetic aberrations or during relapsed AML. Interestingly, the emergence of t(3;12) was accompanied by rapid evolution to AML, within 6 months, in the MDS cases. These observations suggest that the t(3;12) may signify a general genetic instability and is a secondary event in many cases that contributes to disease progression. Based on rapid progression to AML, we also believed that the cases with a blast count in the range of MDS be still considered as AML in a similar approach as that of AML with t(8;21) or inv(16).

In summary, we have described 8 cases of AML or MDS with t(3;12)(q26.2;p13). Similar to cases with inv(3)q21q26.2) or t(3;3)(q21;q26.2), they usually show dysplasia, associated with abnormalities of chromosome 7 and a short survival despite multi-agent chemotherapy and bone marrow transplantation. However, unlike cases with inv(3)(q21q26.2) or t(3;3)(q21;q26.2), these cases are frequently associated with thrombocytopenia, megakaryocytic hypoplasia and *FLT3-ITD* mutation. The t(3;12) also occurred following other cytogenetic aberrations, suggesting it existed as a small subclone initially or emerged a secondary event in some cases. Overall, the findings suggest that this group of patients should be classified in the same subgroup as AML with inv3/t(3;3).

References

1. Lugthart S, Groschel S, Beverloo HB, Kayser S, Valk PJ, et al. (2010) Clinical, molecular, and prognostic significance of WHO type (3)(q21q26.2)/t(3;3)(q21;q26.2) and various other 3q abnormalities in acute myeloid leukemia. Journal of clinical oncology 28: 3890-3898.

2. Raynaud SD, Baens M, Grosgeorge J, Rodgers K, Reid CD et al. (1996) Fluorescence in situ hybridization analysis of t(3;12)(q26;p13): a recurring chromosomal abnormality involving the TEL gene (ETV6) in myelodysplastic syndromes. Blood 88: 682-689.

3. Voutsadakis IA, Maillard N (2003) Acute myelogenous leukemia with the t(3;12)(q26;p13) translocation: case report and review of the literature. Am J Hematol 72: 135-137.

4. Haferlach C, Bacher U, Schnittger S, Alpermann T, Zenger M, et al. (2012) ETV6 rearrangements are recurrent in myeloid malignancies and are frequently associated with other genetic events. Genes Chromosomes Cancer 51: 328-337.

5. Yin CC, Lin P, Carney DA, Handy BC, Rassidakis GZ, et al. (2005) Chronic lymphocytic leukemia/small lymphocytic lymphoma associated with IgM paraprotein. Am J Clin Pathol 123: 594-602.

6. Onciu M, Schlette E, Medeiros LJ, Abruzzo LV, Keating M, et al. (2001) Cytogenetic findings in mantle cell lymphoma cases with a high level of peripheral blood involvement have a distinct pattern of abnormalities. Am J Clin Pathol 116: 886-892.

7. ISCN (2013): An International System for Human Cytogenetic Nomenclature, L.G. Shaffer, McGowan-Jordan J, Schmid M S. Karger, Basel.

8. Lin P, Jones D, Medeiros LJ, Chen W, Vega-Vazquez F, et al. (2006) Activating FLT3 mutations are detectable in chronic and blast phase of chronic myeloproliferative disorders other than chronic myeloid leukemia. American journal of clinical pathology 126: 530-533.

9. Zuo Z, Chen SS, Chandra PK, Galbincea JM, Soape M, et al. (2009) Application of COLD-PCR for improved detection of KRAS mutations in clinical samples. Mod Pathol 22: 1023-1031.

10. Barakat FH, Luthra R, Yin CC, Barkoh BA, Hai S et al. (2011). Detection of nucleophosmin 1 mutations by quantitative real-time polymerase chain reaction versus capillary electrophoresis: a comparative study. Archives of pathology & laboratory medicine 135: 994-1000.

11. Lasa A, Carricondo MT, Carnicer MJ, Perea G, Aventín A, et al. (2006) A new D816 c-KIT gene mutation in refractory AML1-ETO leukemia. Haematologica 91: 1283-1284.

12. Secker-Walker LM, Fitchett M (1995) Constitutional and acquired trisomy 8. Leuk Res 19: 737-740.

13. Mitelman F JB, Mertens F (2013) Mitelman Database of Chromosome Aberrations and Gene Fusions in Cancer.

14. Barjesteh van Waalwijk van Doorn-Khosrovani S, Erpelinck C, van Putten WL, Valk PJ, van der Poel-van de Luytgaarde S, et al. (2003) High EVI1 expression predicts poor survival in acute myeloid leukemia: a study of 319 de novo AML patients. Blood 101: 837-845.

15. Nucifora G (1997) The EVI gene in myeloid leukemia. Leukemia 11: 2022-2031.

16. Jin G, Yamazaki Y, Takuwa M, Takahara T, Kaneko K, et al. (2007) Trib1 and Evil cooperate with Hoxa and Meisl in myeloid leukemogenesis. Blood 109: 3998-4005.

17. Akagi T, Thoennissen NH, George A, Crooks G, Song JH, et al. (2010) In vivo deficiency of both C/EBPÎ² and C/EBPÎµ results in highly defective myeloid differentiation and lack of cytokine response. PLoS One 5: e15419.

18. Kurokawa M, Mitani K, Yamagata T, Takahashi T, Izutsu K, et al. (2000) The evi-1 oncoprotein inhibits c-Jun N-terminal kinase and prevents stress-induced cell death. EMBO J 19: 2958-2968.

19. Testoni N, Borsaru G, Martinelli G, Carboni C, Ruggeri D, et al. (1999) 3q21 and 3q26 cytogenetic abnormalities in acute myeloblastic leukemia: biological and clinical features. Haematologica 84: 690-694.

3

Burden of Tyrosine Kinase Inhibitor Failure in Patients with Chronic Myeloid Leukemia

Patricia Kropf[1], Gisoo Barnes[2*], Boxiong Tang[2], Ashutosh Pathak[2] and Jean-Pierre Issa[3]

[1]*Fox Chase Cancer Center, Philadelphia, PA, USA*
[2]*Global Health Economics & Outcomes Research, Teva Pharmaceuticals, Frazer, PA, USA*
[3]*Fels Institute for Cancer Research, Temple University School of Medicine, Philadelphia, PA, USA*

Abstract

Tyrosine kinase inhibitors (TKIs) have been extremely effective at inducing remissions and slowing down the progression of chronic myeloid leukemia (CML) resulting in a significant reduction in morbidity and mortality. Most patients with CML must remain on TKIs indefinitely and many experience resistance or intolerance to TKIs requiring a switch to a second-line TKI, third-line TKI or more. The purpose of the current review is to examine the underlying factors and subsequent economic and quality of life burdens associated with TKI failure. We discuss the definitions and rates of TKI failure in CML and the extent to which mutations and non-adherence are associated with TKI failure. We also review the few studies that have examined economic and patient outcomes associated with TKI failure and we suggest avenues for future research examining the consequences of TKI failure.

Keywords: Tyrosine kinase inhibitors; Chronic myeloid leukemia; Resistance; Burden

Introduction

In 2012, chronic myeloid leukemia (CML) accounted for 15% to 20% of newly diagnosed cases of adult leukemia in the U.S. [1]. In 2014, there will be an estimated incidence of 5,980 new cases (men=3,130; women=2,850) and a total of 810 deaths (men=550; women=260) due to CML [2]. Tyrosine kinase inhibitors (TKIs), the primary therapy used to manage CML, has the following treatment goals: (1) to induce complete clinical remissions; (2) to prevent the progression from chronic phase (CP) to any other phase (e.g., accelerated or blast); (3) to reduce the risk of death from disease; and (4) to increase the quality of life (QoL) of CML patients [3]. TKI therapy has resulted in a 2% annual all-cause mortality rate among CML patients, a major decrease from the historical rate of 10% to 20% [2]; the estimated 10-year survival rate has increased from 20% to 80% [4]. These gains in survival are only realized if CML patients remain on TKIs long-term. However, over the course of therapy, many patients experience resistance or intolerance to TKIs, requiring a switch to a second- or third-line TKI. TKI failure is expected to be associated with a substantial economic and humanistic burden of illness. In the current paper, we review the underlying factors and subsequent economic, and QoL burden of TKI failure.

TKI Failure: Definitions and Rates

Failure is often used to mean that continuing a specific treatment is no longer appropriate because a favorable outcome is unlikely and includes both resistance and intolerance. Although several definitions of resistance to TKIs have been used, the 2014 National Comprehensive Cancer Network (NCCN) guidelines [5] define primary resistance as the failure to achieve a response by a specific time point. Primary hematologic resistance to TKIs is defined as the failure to achieve hematologic remission within 3 to 6 months of treatment initiation. Primary cytogenetic resistance to imatinibis defined as the failure to achieve any level of cytogenetic response (CyR) at 6 months, major cytogenetic response (MCyR) at 12 months, or complete cytogenetic response (CCyR) at 18 months [5]. The 2013 European LeukemiaNet (ELN) guidelines define failure as less than CyR at 3 months, MCyR at 6 months, and CCyR from 12 months onwards [6]. Secondary resistance refers to a loss of therapeutic effect and disease progression while continuing on a TKI regimen that had previously been effective. The 2014 NCCN [5] and 2013 European LeukemiaNet guidelines [6] both stress the percentage of *BCR-ABL1* transcript as a marker of treatment response. Treatment could be reevaluated if *BCR-ABL1* transcript levels are greater than 10% at 3 and 6 months.

Despite the effectiveness of imatinib, the most common TKI used in first-line therapy, up to 40% of patients with CP CML will become resistant to imatinib [7-9]. For example, in the pivotal International Randomized Study of Interferon versus STI571 (IRIS) trial, approximately 30% of CML patients did not achieve CCyR after 12 months [10,11]; at 18 months, 24% of patients had primary resistance [11]. Long-term follow-up analysis of the IRIS trial reported that secondary resistance occurred in 24% of patients after 5 years [12]. Results from additional studies suggest that the failure rate of imatinib could be as high as 45% at 24 months [13] or 26% after a median follow-up of 38 months [9]. Rates of resistance to first-line therapy with nilotinib and dasatinib are lower than that of imatinib, but are still substantial [14,15]. At 12 months, the rates of resistance to nilotinib and dasatinib are 16% and 18%, respectively [14,15]. At 24 months, the rates increase to 23% for nilotinib and 26% for dasatinib [16]. With second-line therapy, 37% to 52% of patients failed to have a response to therapy [17-19]. Many patients who were not initially resistant lost their response by 2 years [17,19].

Intolerance to TKI therapy, another type of failure, is one of the most common reasons for discontinuation. However, reported rates of intolerance are not consistent across studies, possibly because there is currently not an agreed upon definition of intolerance. Data from

***Corresponding author:** Gisoo Barnes, Ph.D., GHEOR/EBM - Medical Affairs, 41 Moores Rd., Frazer PA 19355, 1E-169C, USA,
E-mail: Gisoo.Barnes@tevapharm.com

clinical trials have suggested that intolerance to TKI therapy occurs in less than 5% of patients taking imatinib [20,21]. However, a real-world study found imatinib intolerance in 30% of patients [22]. With long-term therapies like TKIs, a patient's QoL may be a better tool to gauge therapy intolerance.

Factors associated with TKI failure

Mutations: Several mechanisms have been associated with TKI resistance, but the best-characterized are the BCR-ABL1 kinase domain (BCR-ABL1 KD) mutations [23]. Mutations are rare in newly diagnosed patients in CP and become significantly more prevalent in CP disease that develops resistance, as well as advanced-phase disease [24-26]. Twelve to 63% of patients who develop resistance to imatinib have the BCR-ABL1 KD mutation [27]. Most patients with secondary resistance developed mutations during imatinib treatment [28]. Patients with existing mutations are more likely to develop additional mutations. Sequential treatment with different TKIs is associated with the emergence of new mutations [29]. During second-line TKI treatment (dasatinib or nilotinib), approximately 14% to 33% of patients develop new BCR-ABL1 mutations [28]. The appearance of multiple mutations is associated with poorer prognosis [23]. Up to 40% of patients resistant to second-line TKIs involves the T315I mutation [30,31], which is resistant to all TKIs except ponatinib [32]. The reported median survival of patients with the T315I mutation is approximately 22 months after the mutation is detected [33].

Medication non-adherence: Approximately 30% of CML patients taking TKIs are non-adherent [34,35]. This is not surprising as adherence to oral anticancer therapy has been reported as ranging from 16% to 100% [36]. TKI non-adherence is related to an increased risk of suboptimal response, disease progression, higher healthcare costs, and increased mortality [34,37,38]. Marin et al. found that imatinib adherence was one of only two variables that uniquely predicted whether patients achieved a major molecular response [38]. A follow-up to this study found that imatinib's adherence rate was an independent predictor for loss of CCyR and the discontinuation of imatinib therapy [37]. Patients with adherence rates of 85% or less were significantly more likely to lose CCyR at 2 years and less likely to remain on imatinib than patients with an adherence rate greater than 85%. A retrospective cohort study conducted in Taiwan found that better long-term adherence to imatinib was associated with better clinical outcomes [39].

With respect to second-generation TKIs, one study found patients treated with nilotinib had significantly higher adherence rates compared to patients treated with dasatinib, regardless of dasatinib dose (100 mg/day and 140 mg/day) [40]. Adherence was found to be worse in dasatinib patients compared to nilotinib patients [41], perhaps because adverse events (AE) are more common with dasatinib than nilotinib. However, another retrospective claims database study reported that patients taking second-line nilotinib were almost two times more likely to have poor adherence than patients taking second-line dasatinib at 100 mg/day [42]. This difference between the two studies could be due to their methodology; the former stratified by dasatinib dosage, the latter by age.

Given the substantial impact of non-adherence, a number of studies have identified covariates associated with non-adherence to TKIs. Adherence has been found to be worse as the number of medications increased, worse among women, worse in patients receiving a higher initial dose of imatinib, and worse in patients with high cancer complexity [43]. Non-adherence has also been linked to the treating physicians' experience, practice patterns, and practice environment [34]. Furthermore, an attitudinal study of CML patients found that the most common reasons for non-adherence were simply forgetting to take the dose and to avoid experiencing side effects [44].

Suboptimal response: A suboptimal response, referred to as a warning response by the 2013 European Leukemia Net guidelines [6], is defined as one that does not meet the criteria for failure (resistance) or for an adequate response [5]. Patients with a suboptimal response have a greater risk of disease progression compared with optimal responders [12,45,46]. Studies have found that a suboptimal response at the beginning of therapy is more prognostic than a suboptimal response later in treatment. For instance, patients with a suboptimal response at 6 months have similar outcomes including overall survival (OS), progression-free survival (PFS) and event-free survival (EFS) as patients who experienced TKI failure. In contrast, there were no significant differences between patients with a suboptimal response at 18 months and those with an optimal response [47,48].

Lack of early response: Studies have found that achieving CCyR at 12 months after the start of TKI therapy is significantly related to better patient outcomes [9,49]. CyR at 3 months significantly predicts 3-year OS, regardless of the first-line therapy regimen that patients had received [50]. Patients with a poor molecular response early in first-line therapy are more likely to experience significantly shorter duration of PFS [51], worse OS [52], and greater probability of TKI resistance [53]. Marin et al. found molecular response at 3, 6, or 12 months from the start of imatinib therapy was significantly associated with OS, PFS, and CyR 8 years later [52]. The values at month 3 were the strongest predictors of patient outcomes [52]. Similarly, Jain et al. found that patients with a better molecular response at 3 months had longer EFS, failure-free survival, and OS, regardless of whether the first-line treatment was imatinib, nolotinib, or dastinib [50]. Consequently, patients' cytogenetic and molecular response to first-line therapy during the first year, particularly at month 3, is significantly related to long-term outcomes. Patients with poor responses are more likely to fail first-line therapy. It is critical that patients are routinely tested and monitored per guidelines to insure the detection of resistance or suboptimal response to first-line therapy.

First-line resistance leads to subsequent resistance: There are a number of factors associated with how well a patient responds to a second-line TKI. The first prognostic factor is the initial response to the first-line imatinib therapy. Jabbour et al. found that better survival rates were observed in patients who had experienced cytogenetic relapse or had been intolerant to imatinib therapy compared to patients who had hematologic relapse or resistance to imatinib [49]. Furthermore, patients who had experienced previous CyR to imatinib therapy had significantly better MCyR rates during second-line therapy. Patients with poor performance status and no previous CyR to imatinib therapy had a low probability of responding to second-generation TKI with poor EFS and could be offered additional treatment options [49].

Another predictive factor is early response to the second-line therapy. Tam et al. found that CyR to second-line dastinib or nilotinib at 3 and 6 months was strongly predictive of achievement of MCyR at 12 months [54]. In fact, 90% of patients showing no CyR at 3 to 6 months did not attain the target of MCyR at 12 months. A lower BCR-ABL1 transcript level at 3 months in patients taking second-line TKI was the most salient predictor of outcomes following second-line therapy [6].

Economic and patient burden of TKI failure: Relatively few studies have examined the economic and humanistic impact of TKI failure. This is somewhat surprising because resistance or intolerance to TKIs is expected to be associated with a substantial burden to both healthcare systems and patients, including costs and lower quality of life and mortality. Studies show that most of the related health care costs are associated with patient's non-adherence rates and side effects. As well, these patients have lower quality of life (QoL).

Healthcare costs associated with non-adherence: A retrospective analysis of medical claims data reported that the medication possession ratio (MPR) for imatinib patients was 77.7% and 31% of these patients experienced an interruption in their TKI therapy [43]. MPR is calculated as the number of days of medication supplied within the refill interval divided by the numbers of days in the refill interval as a proportion ranging between 0% and 100%, a lower MPR is associated with less adherence to therapy. The same study found that with every 10% decrease in MPR, there was a 14% increase in healthcare costs and a 15% difference in medical costs (excluding the cost of imatinib). Darkow et al. reported that patients with adherence below 50% experienced healthcare costs three times higher than patients with an MPR of 95% or higher [43]. In another retrospective claims database analysis, patients with low adherence to imatinib had significantly more all-cause inpatient visits and days than patients with high adherence to imatinib [35]. The low-adherence group experienced a 283% increase in healthcare costs compared to high-adherence patients.

Healthcare costs associated with side effects: Little published research has examined healthcare costs associated with TKI side effects and this work has focused on a few specific adverse events (AEs). Pleural effusion (PE) is a side effect that occurs very infrequently during imatinib treatment (0% to 2%) [55] and nilotinib treatment (1%) [56], but it is a relatively common side effect during dasatinib therapy (14% to 30%) [57]. In a retrospective study using claims data from 1999 through 2009, patients treated with TKIs who experienced PE had more inpatient days, hospitalization, outpatient visits, and emergency room visits than CML patients taking TKIs who did not experience PE [58]. The all-cause medical cost for PE patients ($88,526) was significantly greater than for PE-free patients ($30,434). PE patients also incurred higher CML-related medical costs compared to PE-free patients. Another cost-of-treatment analysis was based on resource utilization data for 48 patients with dasatinib-related PE at a large US cancer center. Sixty percent of PEs were managed medically, costing $750 per episode. Forty percent of PEs were more significant, with half of those requiring invasive procedures. The average cost of treating a PE was $2,062 to $2,700 for all severity levels and $6,400 to $9,000 for invasive procedures. This economic analysis using observed treatment patterns suggests that managing PE-adverse events in CML patients could be costly [59].

A small retrospective cohort study used patient records of 91 adults with CP CML who were treated at a university medical center in the Netherlands to estimate the cost of grade III/IV hematological AEs. Patients were included irrespective of the type of CML pharmacological treatment received. Overall, treatment costs per AE episode varied considerably, but the mean cost of an episode of anemia was €1,572, of thrombocytopenia €2,955, of neutropenia €1,152, and of febrile neutropenia €2,462 [60].

Quality of life: Many CML patients who receive TKI therapy remain in CP for years. Some patients experience few symptoms and an overall improvement in QoL after 6 months of imatinib treatment was reported in a study of tertiary care patients in Pakistan [61]. However, a significant number consistently experience moderate-to-severe levels of symptoms, including pain, fatigue, drowsiness, disturbed sleep, muscle soreness and cramping, and difficulty remembering. Many of these symptoms are probably treatment-related because they occur in patients with complete or major molecular remission [62]. The most severe symptoms (including edema, musculoskeletal pain, muscle cramps, and fatigue) identified in 25% to 30% of CML patients receiving imatinib remained consistently problematic over time and may occur with all TKIs [63]. The stability and chronicity of these symptoms is especially troubling from a patient-centric perspective, as even a mild symptom that persists for years can become problematic. Moderate-to-severe symptoms that are present for years can profoundly affect patients' functional status and QoL. This may lead patients to be non-compliant with therapy or abandon treatment entirely.

The QoL of individuals resistant to TKI treatment has rarely been examined. It is unclear whether aspects of QoL are unaffected by treatment or by becoming resistant or intolerant to first-line therapy. After first-line failure, CML patients' QoL suffers and is potentially improved with second-line therapy. One study reported that CP CML patients resistant or intolerant to imatinib had little impairment on most facets of QoL based on the Functional Assessment of Cancer Therapy - Leukemia (FACT-Leukemia) prior to beginning second-line treatment with bosutinib [64]. The FACT-Leukemia results observed at baseline were similar to the samples of individuals used to validate the measure. Specifically, patients' Physical Well-Being and Functional Well-Being subscales measuring lack of energy, presence of pain, ability to work, and ability to enjoy life showed little impairment. Patients also reported few symptoms of leukemia, despite being intolerant or resistant to imatinib treatment [64]. However, these data were collected within the context of a clinical trial; baseline QoL was assessed just prior to starting second-line treatment with bosutinib, rather than longitudinally during first-line TKI failure. An earlier clinical trial reported a trend of lower QoL scores in the imatinib arm among those who discontinued treatment [65].

Trask et al. examined QoL based on the FACT-Leukemia in CP CML patients prior to first, second, and third lines of TKI therapy from Phase II and III clinical trials as well as in advanced (both accelerated and blast phase) CML patients [66]. The results showed that QoL scores (across a variety of subscales and summary scores) worsened as the number of treatments increased and as the CML phase progressed, although these changes were not statistically significant across increasing numbers of treatments [66].

Suggestions for Future Research and Conclusions

Real-world research that examines resource utilization and healthcare costs associated with the use of first-, second-, and third-line TKI therapy and the associated failure will be useful in making treatment decisions. Descriptive treatment pattern studies that examine percentage of patients who switch TKIs from first and second line, as well as stop therapy altogether could clarify the actual rates of TKIs failure. It will also be valuable to identify and contrast indirect costs such as loss of productivity among patients during the period directly before they fail (i.e., switch) TKI therapy compared to a prior TKI period.

Only a few studies have examined costs of treatment for specific side effects associated with TKI therapy in CML patients. Additional analyses of a broader range of more serious side effects associated with TKI use, such as pulmonary arterial hypertension and vascular thrombosis [67], would help further identify the true cost of these therapies. Although a fair amount of work has examined QoL and patient-reported outcomes, there is very little research specifically looking at QoL associated with TKI failure. Since TKIs can have significant side effects, it is likely that intolerance to TKIs may result in decreased QoL and an associated humanistic burden. The majority of work reviewed in this paper was conducted in the U.S. and E.U.; however, research that examines resistance and intolerance to TKIs and the subsequent burden of TKI failure in other countries or regions would provide a valuable addition to the literature.

TKIs have revolutionized the treatment of CML and have generally been found to be cost-effective as first-line therapy [68,69]. As long as CP-CML patients receive appropriate TKIs and adhere to treatment, they live close to normal lifespans [4]. However, not much is known about the burden of continuous TKI treatment. Over time, the patient's risk of TKI resistance or intolerance is likely to increase. Consequently, a greater understanding of antecedents and consequences of TKI failure is needed to make better treatment decisions. Of note, 2 new TKIs received FDA approval in 2012: ponatinib for adult patients with T315I-positive CML and bosutinib for adult patients with resistance or intolerance to prior CML therapy. Furthermore, omacetaxine, a protein translation inhibitor with a different mechanism of action than that of TKIs, also received FDA approval in 2012 for the treatment of CML with resistance or intolerance to two or more TKIs [70,71]. Future research is needed to determine the impact on healthcare costs and patients' QoL of switching to another therapy after first and second-line TKI failure, including these newer agents. TKI therapy alone does not cure the majority of patients with CML, additional therapeutic strategies should be considered to try to achieve a cure before intolerance and mutations occur.

Acknowledgements

This study was sponsored by Teva Pharmaceuticals, Frazer, PA, USA. Editorial assistance in the preparation of this manuscript was provided by Dr. Jason Allaire, PhD of Generativity Solutions Group, Cary, NC, USA. Support for this assistance was funded by Teva Pharmaceuticals, Frazer, PA, USA.

Authorship

Contribution: P.K., G.B., J.P.I., A.P, and B.T. were responsible for the evaluation and critique of previous research and all contributed equally to the writing of the paper. G.B. and A.P. were responsible for the conceptualization of the paper.

References

1. Chen Y, Wang H, Kantarjian H, Cortes J (2013) Trends in chronic myeloid leukemia incidence and survival in the United States from 1975 to 2009. Leuk Lymphoma 54: 1411-1417.

2. Siegel R, Ma J, Zou Z, Jemal A (2014) Cancer statistics, 2014. CA Cancer J Clin 64: 9-29.

3. Baccarani M, Castagnetti F, Gugliotta G, Palandri F, Rosti G (2014) Treatment recommendations for chronic myeloid leukemia. Mediterr J Hematol Infect Dis 6: e2014005.

4. Gambacorti-Passerini C, Antolini L, Mahon FX, Guilhot F, Deininger M, et al. (2011) Multicenter independent assessment of outcomes in chronic myeloid leukemia patients treated with imatinib. J Natl Cancer Inst 103: 553-561.

5. O'Brien S, Radich JP, Abboud CN (2014) Clinical Practice Guidelines: Chronic Myelogenous Leukemia, Version 2.2014, National Comprehensive Cancer Network (NCCN). Journal of the National Comprehensive Cancer Network.

6. Baccarani M, Deininger MW, Rosti G, Hochhaus A, Soverini S, et al. (2013) European LeukemiaNet recommendations for the management of chronic myeloid leukemia: 2013. Blood 122: 872-884.

7. Quintás-Cardama A, Cortes JE, O'Brien S, Ravandi F, Borthakur G, et al. (2009) Dasatinib early intervention after cytogenetic or hematologic resistance to imatinib in patients with chronic myeloid leukemia. Cancer 115: 2912-2921.

8. O'Brien S, Tefferi A, Valent P (2004) Chronic myelogenous leukemia and myeloproliferative disease. Hematology Am Soc Hematol Educ Program .

9. de Lavallade H, Apperley JF, Khorashad JS, Milojkovic D, Reid AG, et al. (2008) Imatinib for newly diagnosed patients with chronic myeloid leukemia: incidence of sustained responses in an intention-to-treat analysis. J Clin Oncol 26: 3358-3363.

10. Shah NP, Tran C, Lee FY, Chen P, Norris D, et al. (2004) Overriding imatinib resistance with a novel ABL kinase inhibitor. Science 305: 399-401.

11. O'Brien SG, Guilhot F, Larson RA, Gathmann I, Baccarani M, et al. (2003) Imatinib compared with interferon and low-dose cytarabine for newly diagnosed chronic-phase chronic myeloid leukemia. N Engl J Med 348: 994-1004.

12. Druker BJ, Guilhot F, O'Brien SG, Gathmann I, Kantarjian H, et al. (2006) Five-year follow-up of patients receiving imatinib for chronic myeloid leukemia. N Engl J Med 355: 2408-2417.

13. Lucas CM, Wang L, Austin GM, Knight K, Watmough SJ, et al. (2008) A population study of imatinib in chronic myeloid leukaemia demonstrates lower efficacy than in clinical trials. Leukemia 22: 1963-1966.

14. Kantarjian H, Shah NP, Hochhaus A, Cortes J, Shah S, et al. (2010) Dasatinib versus imatinib in newly diagnosed chronic-phase chronic myeloid leukemia. N Engl J Med 362: 2260-2270.

15. Saglio G, Kim DW, Issaragrisil S, le Coutre P, Etienne G, et al. (2010) Nilotinib versus imatinib for newly diagnosed chronic myeloid leukemia. N Engl J Med 362: 2251-2259.

16. Kantarjian HM, Shah NP, Cortes JE, Baccarani M, Agarwal MB, et al. (2012) Dasatinib or imatinib in newly diagnosed chronic-phase chronic myeloid leukemia: 2-year follow-up from a randomized phase 3 trial (DASISION). Blood 119: 1123-1129.

17. Cortes JE, Kantarjian HM, Brümmendorf TH, Kim DW, Turkina AG, et al. (2011) Safety and efficacy of bosutinib (SKI-606) in chronic phase Philadelphia chromosome-positive chronic myeloid leukemia patients with resistance or intolerance to imatinib. Blood 118: 4567-4576.

18. Kantarjian HM, Giles F, Gattermann N, Bhalla K, Alimena G, et al. (2007) Nilotinib (formerly AMN107), a highly selective BCR-ABL tyrosine kinase inhibitor, is effective in patients with Philadelphia chromosome-positive chronic myelogenous leukemia in chronic phase following imatinib resistance and intolerance. Blood 110: 3540-3546.

19. Shah NP, Kantarjian HM, Kim DW, Rea D, Dorlhiac-Llacer PE, et al. (2008) Intermittent target inhibition with dasatinib 100 mg once daily preserves efficacy and improves tolerability in imatinib-resistant and -intolerant chronic-phase chronic myeloid leukemia. J Clin Oncol 26: 3204-3212.

20. Mauro MJ (2006) Defining and managing imatinib resistance. Hematology Am Soc Hematol Educ Program .

21. Garg RJ, Kantarjian H, O'Brien S, Quintás-Cardama A, Faderl S, et al. (2009) The use of nilotinib or dasatinib after failure to 2 prior tyrosine kinase inhibitors: long-term follow-up. Blood 114: 4361-4368.

22. Michallet M, Tulliez M, Corm S, Gardembas M, Huguet F, et al. (2010) Management of chronic myeloid leukaemia in clinical practice in France: results of the French subset of patients from the UNIC study. Curr Med Res Opin 26: 307-317.

23. Parker WT, Ho M, Scott HS, Hughes TP, Branford S (2012) Poor response to second-line kinase inhibitors in chronic myeloid leukemia patients with multiple low-level mutations, irrespective of their resistance profile. Blood 119: 2234-2238.

24. Khorashad JS, de Lavallade H, Apperley JF, Milojkovic D, Reid AG, et al. (2008) Finding of kinase domain mutations in patients with chronic phase chronic myeloid leukemia responding to imatinib may identify those at high risk of disease progression. J Clin Oncol 26: 4806-4813.

25. Soverini S, Martinelli G, Rosti G, Bassi S, Amabile M, et al. (2005) ABL mutations in late chronic phase chronic myeloid leukemia patients with up-front cytogenetic resistance to imatinib are associated with a greater likelihood

of progression to blast crisis and shorter survival: a study by the GIMEMA Working Party on Chronic Myeloid Leukemia. J Clin Oncol 23: 4100-4109.

26. Branford S, Rudzki Z, Walsh S, Parkinson I, Grigg A, et al. (2003) Detection of BCR-ABL mutations in patients with CML treated with imatinib is virtually always accompanied by clinical resistance, and mutations in the ATP phosphate-binding loop (P-loop) are associated with a poor prognosis. Blood 102: 276-283.

27. Soverini S, Hochhaus A, Nicolini FE, Gruber F, Lange T, et al. (2011) BCR-ABL kinase domain mutation analysis in chronic myeloid leukemia patients treated with tyrosine kinase inhibitors: recommendations from an expert panel on behalf of European LeukemiaNet. Blood 118: 1208-1215.

28. Soverini S, Branford S, Nicolini FE, Talpaz M, Deininger MW, et al. (2014) Implications of BCR-ABL1 kinase domain-mediated resistance in chronic myeloid leukemia. Leuk Res 38: 10-20.

29. Soverini S, Gnani A, Colarossi S, Castagnetti F, Abruzzese E, et al. (2009) Philadelphia-positive patients who already harbor imatinib-resistant Bcr-Abl kinase domain mutations have a higher likelihood of developing additional mutations associated with resistance to second- or third-line tyrosine kinase inhibitors. Blood 114: 2168-2171.

30. Hughes T, Saglio G, Branford S, Soverini S, Kim DW, et al. (2009) Impact of baseline BCR-ABL mutations on response to nilotinib in patients with chronic myeloid leukemia in chronic phase. J Clin Oncol 27: 4204-4210.

31. Soverini S, Colarossi S, Gnani A, Castagnetti F, Rosti G, et al. (2007) Resistance to dasatinib in Philadelphia-positive leukemia patients and the presence or the selection of mutations at residues 315 and 317 in the BCR-ABL kinase domain. Haematologica 92: 401-404.

32. O'Hare T, Shakespeare WC, Zhu X, Eide CA, Rivera VM, et al. (2009) AP24534, a pan-BCR-ABL inhibitor for chronic myeloid leukemia, potently inhibits the T315I mutant and overcomes mutation-based resistance. Cancer Cell 16: 401-412.

33. Nicolini FE, Mauro MJ, Martinelli G, Kim DW, Soverini S, et al. (2009) Epidemiologic study on survival of chronic myeloid leukemia and Ph(+) acute lymphoblastic leukemia patients with BCR-ABL T315I mutation. Blood 114: 5271-5278.

34. Noens L, van Lierde MA, De Bock R, Verhoef G, Zachée P, et al. (2009) Prevalence, determinants, and outcomes of nonadherence to imatinib therapy in patients with chronic myeloid leukemia: the ADAGIO study. Blood 113: 5401-5411.

35. Wu EQ, Johnson S, Beaulieu N, Arana M, Bollu V, et al. (2010) Healthcare resource utilization and costs associated with non-adherence to imatinib treatment in chronic myeloid leukemia patients. Curr Med Res Opin 26: 61-69.

36. Ruddy K, Mayer E, Partridge A (2009) Patient adherence and persistence with oral anticancer treatment. CA Cancer J Clin 59: 56-66.

37. Ibrahim AR, Eliasson L, Apperley JF, Milojkovic D, Bua M, et al. (2011) Poor adherence is the main reason for loss of CCyR and imatinib failure for chronic myeloid leukemia patients on long-term therapy. Blood 117: 3733-3736.

38. Marin D, Bazeos A, Mahon FX, Eliasson L, Milojkovic D, et al. (2010) Adherence is the critical factor for achieving molecular responses in patients with chronic myeloid leukemia who achieve complete cytogenetic responses on imatinib. J Clin Oncol 28: 2381-2388.

39. Chen TC, Chen LC, Huang YB, Chang CS (2014) Imatinib adherence associated clinical outcomes of chronic myeloid leukaemia treatment in Taiwan. Int J Clin Pharm 36: 172-181.

40. Guerin A, Chen L, Wu EQ, Ponce de Leon D, Griffin JD (2012) A retrospective analysis of therapy adherence in imatinib resistant or intolerant patients with chronic myeloid leukemia receiving nilotinib or dasatinib in a real-world setting. Curr Med Res Opin 28: 1155-1162.

41. Wu EQ, Guerin A, Yu AP, Bollu VK, Guo A, et al. (2010) Retrospective real-world comparison of medical visits, costs, and adherence between nilotinib and dasatinib in chronic myeloid leukemia. Curr Med Res Opin 26: 2861-2869.

42. Yood MU, Oliveria SA, Cziraky M, Hirji I, Hamdan M, et al. (2012) Adherence to treatment with second-line therapies, dasatinib and nilotinib, in patients with chronic myeloid leukemia. Curr Med Res Opin 28: 213-219.

43. Darkow T, Henk HJ, Thomas SK, Feng W, Baladi JF, et al. (2007) Treatment interruptions and non-adherence with imatinib and associated healthcare costs: a retrospective analysis among managed care patients with chronic myelogenous leukaemia. Pharmacoeconomics 25: 481-496.

44. Eliasson L, Clifford S, Barber N, Marin D (2011) Exploring chronic myeloid leukemia patients' reasons for not adhering to the oral anticancer drug imatinib as prescribed. Leuk Res 35: 626-630.

45. Hochhaus A, Baccarani M, Deininger M, Apperley JF, Lipton JH, et al. (2008) Dasatinib induces durable cytogenetic responses in patients with chronic myelogenous leukemia in chronic phase with resistance or intolerance to imatinib. Leukemia 22: 1200-1206.

46. Hochhaus A, Druker B, Sawyers C, Guilhot F, Schiffer CA, et al. (2008) Favorable long-term follow-up results over 6 years for response, survival, and safety with imatinibmesylate therapy in chronic-phase chronic myeloid leukemia after failure of interferon-alpha treatment. Blood 111: 1039-1043.

47. Hughes TP, Kaeda J, Branford S, Rudzki Z, Hochhaus A, et al. (2003) Frequency of major molecular responses to imatinib or interferon alfa plus cytarabine in newly diagnosed chronic myeloid leukemia.N Engl J Med 349: 1423-1432.

48. Marin D, Goldman JM, Olavarria E, Apperley JF (2003) Transient benefit only from increasing the imatinib dose in CML patients who do not achieve complete cytogenetic remissions on conventional doses. Blood 102: 2702-2703.

49. Jabbour E, Kantarjian H, O'Brien S, Shan J, Garcia-Manero G, et al. (2011) Predictive factors for outcome and response in patients treated with second-generation tyrosine kinase inhibitors for chronic myeloid leukemia in chronic phase after imatinib failure. Blood 117: 1822-1827.

50. Jain P, Kantarjian H, Nazha A, O'Brien S, Jabbour E, et al. (2013) Early responses predict better outcomes in patients with newly diagnosed chronic myeloid leukemia: results with four tyrosine kinase inhibitor modalities. Blood 121: 4867-4874.

51. Press RD, Love Z, Tronnes AA, Yang R, Tran T, et al. (2006) BCR-ABL mRNA levels at and after the time of a complete cytogenetic response (CCR) predict the duration of CCR in imatinib mesylate-treated patients with CML. Blood 107: 4250-4256.

52. Marin D, Ibrahim AR, Lucas C, Gerrard G, Wang L, et al. (2012) Assessment of BCR-ABL1 transcript levels at 3 months is the only requirement for predicting outcome for patients with chronic myeloid leukemia treated with tyrosine kinase inhibitors. J Clin Oncol 30: 232-238.

53. Hughes T, Branford S (2006) Molecular monitoring of BCR-ABL as a guide to clinical management in chronic myeloid leukaemia. Blood Rev 20: 29-41.

54. Tam CS, Kantarjian H, Garcia-Manero G, Borthakur G, O'Brien S, et al. (2008) Failure to achieve a major cytogenetic response by 12 months defines inadequate response in patients receiving nilotinib or dasatinib as second or subsequent line therapy for chronic myeloid leukemia. Blood 112: 516-518.

55. Kelly K, Swords R, Mahalingam D, Padmanabhan S, Giles FJ (2009) Serosal inflammation (pleural and pericardial effusions) related to tyrosine kinase inhibitors. Target Oncol 4: 99-105.

56. Masiello D, Gorospe G 3rd, Yang AS (2009) The occurrence and management of fluid retention associated with TKI therapy in CML, with a focus on dasatinib. J Hematol Oncol 2: 46.

57. Breccia M, Alimena G (2010) Pleural/pericardic effusions during dasatinib treatment: incidence, management and risk factors associated to their development. Expert Opin Drug Saf 9: 713-721.

58. Guérin A, Wu EQ, Bollu VK, Williams D, Guo A, et al. (2013) The economic burden of pleural effusions in patients with chronic myeloid leukemia treated with tyrosine kinase inhibitors. J Med Econ 16: 125-133.

59. Stephens J, Carpiuc KT, Botteman M (2010) The burden of managing pleural effusions in patients with chronic myelogenous leukemia post-imatinib failure: A literature-based economic analysis. Int J Gen Med 3: 31-36.

60. Bouwmans C, Janssen J, Huijgens P, Uyl-de Groot C (2009) Costs of haematological adverse events in chronic myeloid leukaemia patients: a retrospective cost analysis of the treatment of anaemia, neutropenia and thrombocytopenia in patients with chronic myeloid leukaemia. J Med Econ 12: 164-169.

61. Aziz Z, Iqbal J, Aaqib M, Akram M, Saeed A (2011) Assessment of quality of life with imatinib mesylate as first-line treatment in chronic phase-chronic myeloid leukemia. Leuk Lymphoma 52: 1017-1023.

62. Williams LA, Garcia Gonzalez AG, Ault P, Mendoza TR, Sailors ML, et al. (2013) Measuring the symptom burden associated with the treatment of chronic myeloid leukemia. Blood 122: 641-647.

63. Efficace F, Baccarani M, Breccia M, Alimena G, Rosti G, et al. (2011) Health-related quality of life in chronic myeloid leukemia patients receiving long-term therapy with imatinib compared with the general population. Blood 118: 4554-4560.

64. Trask PC, Cella D, Besson N, Kelly V, Masszi T, et al. (2012) Health-related quality of life of bosutinib (SKI-606) in imatinib-resistant or imatinib-intolerant chronic phase chronic myeloid leukemia. Leuk Res 36: 438-442.

65. Hahn EA, Glendenning GA, Sorensen MV, Hudgens SA, Druker BJ, et al. (2003) Quality of life in patients with newly diagnosed chronic phase chronic myeloid leukemia on imatinib versus interferon alfa plus low-dose cytarabine: results from the IRIS Study. J Clin Oncol 21: 2138-2146.

66. Trask PC, Cella D, Powell C, Reisman A, Whiteley J, et al. (2013) Health-related quality of life in chronic myeloid leukemia. Leuk Res 37: 9-13.

67. Aichberger KJ, Herndlhofer S, Schernthaner GH, Schillinger M, Mitterbauer-Hohendanner G, et al. (2011) Progressive peripheral arterial occlusive disease and other vascular events during nilotinib therapy in CML. Am J Hematol 86: 533-539.

68. Reed SD, Anstrom KJ, Li Y, Schulman KA (2008) Updated estimates of survival and cost effectiveness for imatinib versus interferon-alpha plus low-dose cytarabine for newly diagnosed chronic-phase chronic myeloid leukaemia. Pharmacoeconomics 26: 435-446.

69. Pavey T, Hoyle M, Ciani O, Crathorne L, Jones-Hughes T, et al. (2012) Dasatinib, nilotinib and standard-dose imatinib for the first-line treatment of chronic myeloid leukaemia: systematic reviews and economic analyses. Health Technol Assess 16: 1-277.

70. Cortes JE, Nicolini FE, Wetzler M, Lipton JH, Akard L, et al. (2013) Subcutaneous omacetaxine mepesuccinate in patients with chronic-phase chronic myeloid leukemia previously treated with 2 or more tyrosine kinase inhibitors including imatinib. Clin Lymphoma Myeloma Leuk 13: 584-591.

71. Nicolini FE, Khoury HJ, Akard L, Rea D, Kantarjian H, et al. (2013) Omacetaxinemepesuccinate for patients with accelerated phase chronic myeloid leukemia with resistance or intolerance to two or more tyrosine kinase inhibitors. Haematologica 98: e78-9.

Membranous Expression of pan CD66, CD66a, CD66b, and CD66c and their Clinical Impact in Acute Leukemia: Cross Sectional Longitudinal Cohort Study

Manar M. Ismail[1,2*], Amal Zaghloul[3,4], Abdulateef Nahla AB[2,5] and Morsi Heba K[1,6]

[1]Laboratory Medicine Department, Faculty of Applied Medical Science, Umm Al Qura University, KSA,
[2]Clinical Pathology Department, National Cancer Institute, Cairo University, Egypt,
[3]Hematology and Immunology Department, Faculty of Medicine, Umm Al Qura University, KSA,
[4]Clinical Pathology Department, Faculty of Medicine, Ain Shams University, Egypt,
[5]Laboratory and Blood Bank Department, KAMC, Makkah, KSA,
[6]Medical Biochemistry Department, Faculty of Medicine, Mansoura University, Egypt

Abstract

CD66 and its isoforms modulate several physiologic processes and have a role in aggressiveness of malignancies. We aimed at investigating pan CD66, CD66 a, b, and c expression and their clinical implication in acute leukemia. This study included 85 cases, 50 AML, 33 ALL and 2 mixed lineage leukemia from King Abdullah Medical City, Saudi Arabia. Pan CD66, CD66a, CD66b and CD66c were detected by flow cytometry at diagnosis and pan CD66 was reanalyzed at day28. Pan CD66 and CD66c expression rate was 51.8% in B-ALL and significantly correlated with BCR/ABL gene, P-value 0.037. CD66a was detected in 11.1% and significantly associated with shorter overall survival (OS), P-value 0.045. In AML, the expression rates were 40%, 28% and 32% for pan CD66, CD66b and CD66c respectively. CD66b was significantly correlated with favorable cytogenetic and prolonged OS, P-value 0.001 and 0.025 respectively. CD66c was correlated with CD25 positivity, P-value 0.003. The expression of pan CD66 at diagnosis and day 28, were significantly correlated, P-value <0.0001. Accordingly, pan CD66 could be added to the panel for MRD. Our data were encouraging to our center to follow other centers that already included CD66c in their panel for MRD detection. CD66c may be tried as a target for monoclonal antibody therapy in CD66c positive acute leukemia. Large-scale studies are needed to verify the association of CD66b expression with cytogenetics and survival in AML.

Keywords: AML; ALL; Adhesion molecules; Pan CD66; CD66a; CD66b; CD66c; MRD

Introduction

CD66 refers to a family of heavily glycosylated glycoproteins (CD66a to CD66f) that can be [1]. Members of this family are critical modulators of several key physiologic processes, including cell adhesion, motility, and regulation of immune processes [1,2]. Additionally, they play a significant role in other cellular processes, including the inhibition of differentiation [3], inhibition of apoptosis in colon cells [4], and disruption of cell polarization and tissue architecture [3]. Carcinoembryonic antigen (CEA) regulates these activities by activating integrin signaling pathways [5].

In normal haematopoiesis, CD66a, CD66b, CD66c and CD66d are strongly expressed in the myeloid lineage on the surface of myelocytes, metamyelocytes and neutrophilic and eosinophilic granulocytes [6]. A low expression of CD66 is found on normal promyelocytes and no expression has been described for myeloblasts. For the lymphoid lineage, strong expression has been described for CD66a and CD66c on precursor B-cells and for CD66a on T-cell precursors [7].

CD66 antigens are frequently upregulated in diverse cancers, and their overexpression is often associated with poor clinical outcome and reduced survival [6]. In haematologic malignancies, CD66 is expressed on myeloid cells at different stages of maturation and in acute [8] and chronic leukaemia [9].

CD66a is the most widely distributed protein within the CEA family, is expressed on macrophages, B- cells, IL-2 activated T- cells, NK-cell, and platelets [10], is dimly expressed on promyelocytes and mature neutrophils [11] and is overexpressed in lung and gastric cancers [12]. In tumour tissue, the expression of CD66a is reduced in the early phases of many cancers including colon, prostate, liver, and breast cancers, and it is thought to be a tumour suppressor protein [13]. However, CECAM1-L, CD66a isoforms is overexpressed in other types of aggressive cancers, such as melanoma, gastric, thyroid, bladder cancers [14] and metastatic colon cancer [15], thus demonstrating its role in metastasis [14].

CD66b is highly expressed on the surface of peripheral blood eosinophils [16]. It is expressed by promyelocytes and early myelocytes, reaches maximal expression at the late myelocyte and metamyelocyte stages and then decreases at the band and segmented neutrophil stages [11].

CD66c is expressed on granulocytes and their precursors [16]. In contrast to CD66b, CD66c expression is highest at the promyelocyte stage and progressively declines during maturation [11]. It inhibits anoikis, a form of programmed cell death [17], and modulating its expression alters the malignant phenotype of cancer cells. Its deregulation was first noticed in chronic myeloid leukaemia [9] and childhood B- acute lymphoblastic leukaemia [18]. CD66c might be the most specific marker for some aggressive cancers [13].

***Corresponding author:** Manar Ismail, Faculty of Applied Medical Science Laboratory Medicine, Umm Al Qura University, Saudi Arabia;
E-mail: manarismail4@yahoo.com

Acute leukaemia is an aggressive disease that involves lymphoid and myeloid progenitor cells. Leukaemic cells usually have genetic lesions that lead to altered protein expression patterns that may include changes in normal adhesion molecule expression. CD66c expression represents an example of this association where a strong correlation was found between CD66c expression in childhood and adult ALL and nonrandom genetic changes, including BCR/ABL positivity, hyperdiploidy and absence of TEL/AML1 [19]. This altered expression of adhesion molecules may affect the patient's response to treatment, overall survival or disease recurrence because they alter the adhesive qualities and survival of leukaemia stem cells in the supporting bone marrow microenvironment with a subsequent change in the sensitivity of the blasts to chemotherapy [20].

Objectives

To detect the Expression of pan CD66, CD66a, CD66b, and CD66c on the surface of malignant cell population in acute leukemia and study the relation of their expression with the initial laboratory investigation, clinical data and disease outcome, and to identify the validity of their usage in investigating minimal residual disease (MRD) or as targets for immunotherapy.

Subjects and Methods

Subjects

This study included 85 newly diagnosed cases of acute leukaemia of both sexes selected from King Abdullah Medical City, Makkah, Saudi Arabia from May 2014 to May 2016. The diagnosis was based on WHO criteria. The cases included 50 acute myeloid leukaemia (AML), 33 acute lymphoblastic leukaemia (ALL) and two mixed lineage leukaemia (MLL) cases. Secondary leukaemia and relapsed cases were excluded from the study. This study was approved by the ethics committee of Umm Al Qura University, Saudi Arabia. An informed written consent was obtained from each participant. The study conformed to the Code of Ethics of the World Medical Association (Declaration of Helsinki).

The treatment protocol of all patients followed the previously mentioned National Comprehensive Cancer Network (NCCN) guidelines [21- 23].

Samples

All cases had representative bone marrow (BM) aspiration together with trephine core biopsy specimens for evaluation of BM cellularity. EDTA peripheral blood (PB) and BM aspirate specimens were prepared for fowcytometry analysis of surface, cytoplasmic markers, and the studied adhesion molecules. Heparinised BM samples were obtained for cytogenetic and molecular studies. A four ml blood sample was collected; 2ml was placed in an EDTA tube for complete blood count, and 2 ml was placed in a plain tube for biochemical studies after serum separation

Methods

All patients were subjected to a full medical history, clinical examination, routine laboratory investigations included complete blood count and determination of liver enzymes and routine leukemia work up that included:

- Examination of stained PB and BM films together with biopsy specimen.

- Immunophenotyping was performed using the BD-FACS-Canto II System (BD- Bio Science- San Jose, CA, USA).) and reagent system (BD- FACS Setup) as previously described [24] using an extended panel of monoclonal antibodies (MoAbs) that included B cell lineage markers (CD10, CD19, CD20, CD22, cyt CD79a, Kappa and Lambda light chains, surface and cyt IgM); T cell lineage markers (CD2, surface and cyt CD3, CD5, CD7, CD4, CD8, CD1a, CD25), myelomonocytic markers (CD13, CD14, CD15, CD33, CD64, CD68, CD117, CD11c, cyto MPO) and miscellaneous markers (CD56, CD38, HLA-DR, TdT). CD45 was included in each tube to allow the identification of abnormal cell populations from the normal hematopoietic population. CD34 is used to identify early progenitors or blasts, together with weak positivity for CD45, confirm the hematopoietic origin of the tumor cells [25]. Cell populations were designated as positive for a particular surface antigen if expressed in $\geq$ 20% and for the intracellular antigen if $\geq$ 10% of blast events stained beyond an appropriate isotype cut-off. - Cytogenetic analysis: Conventional karyotype analysis was performed on metaphase cells using standard culturing and banding techniques. The results were reported according to the International System for Human Cytogenetics Nomenclature [26].

- Fluorescence in situ hybridization (FISH) was used as a complement to conventional karyotyping to detect or confirm gene rearrangements.

- Detection of *BCR/ABL* fusion gene by qualitative RT-PCR methods

Expression of pan CD66, CD66a, CD66b and CD66c by flow cytometry: Monoclonal antibodies directly labeled with fluorescent dye: Pan CD66 labelled with FITC (BD cat #551479), CD66a labelled with PE (R&D cat # FAB2244p), CD66b labelled with FITC (BD cat # 555724), and CD66c labelled with PE (BD cat # 551478) were used. A series of dilutions were tried to find the highest dilution that gave the strongest stain for the detection system. Similar to other studies, the antigen was considered positive when $\geq$ 20% cells in the blast region expressed the antigen [7].

Flow cytometry analysis of pan CD66 at day 28: The stability of pan CD66 expression at diagnosis was evaluated in morphologic CR specimens obtained for MRD monitoring at the end of induction therapy. Based on immunophenotypes at diagnosis, phenotypic abnormalities (co-expression patterns and aberrant expressions) were defined and used in the investigations of follow-up samples using tailored MoAb combination. Live-gate analysis was used where a total of 100-500$\times 10^3$ cells were analyzed cells. In most cases CD34/SSC or CD117/SSC gates were applied [27].

Statistical analysis

The data were analysed using SPSS program version 20. Quantitative data were presented as the mean ± SD or median (min - max) and range as appropriate. Categorical data were presented as frequency and percentage. Comparison between two groups was conducted using Student's t-test, and nonparametric Mann–Whitney U and Kruskal–Wallis tests were used for the data that were not normally distributed. Comparison between more than 2 groups was made by using the ANOVA test. The Wilcoxon signed rank test was used for comparison between pan CD66 expression at diagnosis and after induction for the same patients. A chi-square or Fisher's exact test was used for comparisons between qualitative data as appropriate. The Kaplan-Meier method was used for survival studies. For all comparisons, a two-sided alpha value was set at 0.05. Probability (P-value) < 0.05 and <0.001 were considered significant and highly significant, respectively.

Results

This study included 85 patients with acute leukaemia. They included 50 AML cases, 27 B-ALL cases, 6 T-ALL and 2 MLL cases. According to WHO classifications, 11/50 AML cases has recurrent genetic abnormalities including (4= t(8;21), 6= t(15;17) and 1= (9;11)), and 39/50 not otherwise specified . The morphological classification was M1 = 13, M2 = 17, M3=6, M4 = 4 and M5= 10. 11/27 B-ALL cases have recurrent genetic abnormalities including (4= hyperdiploidy and 7 = t (9;22)) and 16/27 not otherwise specified, and their immunophenotypic distribution was pro-B-ALL = 9, common ALL = 14 and pre-B ALL = 4. Demographic and initial laboratory investigations of the studied patients are presented in (Table1).

Expression of pan CD66 and its isoforms in the studied group

The marker expression levels in AML, B-ALL and T- ALL are presented as the mean ± SD and median (min - max) in (Table 2 and Figure 1).

In B-ALL cases, 14/27(58.1%) were positive (≥20%) for both pan CD66 and CD66c expression.

Parameters studied	AML (n=50)	ALL (n=33)
Age (years)*	44.5 (15.0-81.0)	20.0 (12.0 - 64.0)
Sex: Male (n & %)	29.0(58%)	19.0 (57.6%)
Female (n & %)	21.0(42%)	14.0 (42.4%)
Clinical presentation		
Organomegaly	3(6%)	6(18.8%)
Anaemia	20(40%)	15(46.9%)
Bleeding tendency	17(34%)	7(21.9%)
Fever	15 (30%)	16(50%)
TLC (x10^9/L)*	20.6 (0.8-381.7)	9.8(0.8-250.0)
Hemoglobin (g/dl)*	8.0(3.8-12.7)	8.6(4.6-13.6)
Platelets (x10^9/L)*	46.0(6.0-374.0)	53.0(6.0-306.0)
Peripheral blood blast %*	39.5(0.0-92.0)	45.0(1.0-96.0)
Bone marrow blast %*	63.0(21.0-94.0)	89.5(21.0-96.0)
LDH(U/l)*	481.0(131.0-1597.0)	416.0(153.0-5658.0)
s GOT (U/l)*	24.5(5.6- 1075.0)	27.0(11.0-132.0)
s GPT (U/l)*	30(8.0-220.0)	36.5(15.0- 153.0)

*Data are presented as median (min-max).TLC: Total leukocytic count. sGOT: Serum glutamic oxaloacetic transaminase. sGPT: Serum glutamic pyruvic transaminase. LDH: Lactate dehydrogenase.

Table 1: Demographic and initial haematological and chemical investigation of the studied patients.

Parameters studied	AML (n=50)	B-ALL (n=27)	T-ALL (n=6)	P-value^
Pan CD66 Mean ± SD Median (min-max)	23.7 ± 27.9 9.5(0.3-99.0) a &b	36.7 ± 35.5 24 (0.0-97.0) a	0.9 ± 1.5 0.8(0.0-4.0) b	0.023*
CD66a Mean ± SD Median (min-max)	6.0 ± 7.2 2.5(0.1-25.0)	8.7 ± 17.2 1.9 (0.0-62.0)	3.9 ± 8.4 3.8(0.0-14.0)	0.593
CD66b Mean ± SD Median (min-max)	20.5 ± 29.5 4.5(0.0-98.0) a	2.2 ± 2.7 1.0(0.0-10.0) b	0.2 ± 0.2 0.2(0.0-1.0) a &b	0.004*
CD66c Mean ± SD Median (min-max)	19.2 ± 23.3 7.0(0.0-98.0) a &b	31.1 ± 32.8 23 (0.0-93.0) a	2.5 ± 5.1 0.2(0.0-13.0) b	0.037

Groups sharing the same letter indicate that no statistically significant difference exists between them.
^ P-values were used to compare the mean values
* Significant

Table 2: Expression levels of pan CD66 and its isoforms among different studied groups.

The number of positive cases in relation to different phenotypes was as follows: pan CD66 and CD66c were positive in 4/9 of pre-B, 7/14 of common and 3/4 of pro-B. CD66a was positive in 2 cases of common and one case of pro-B phenotype with no significant difference between them, P-value >0.05.

All studied T-ALL cases failed to express pan CD66 or any of its studied isoforms beyond the cut-off, and only one case showed a partial expression (17%) of pan CD66 and CD66a.

According to morphological examination of AML cases, there was a significant higher expression level of pan CD66 and CD66b in M3 morphology compared to myeloid and monocytic morphology , P-value <0.001 and 0.003 respectively. The level of the studied marker expression is represented in (Figure 2).

There was no significant difference between the rate of positive expression per the cut-off (≥20%) of pan CD66, CD66a or CD66c in AML versus B- ALL. CD66b showed a significantly higher expression rate in AML as it failed to be expressed in any of the studied B-ALL cases, P- value 0.002. There was no significance difference in positive expression rate between the FAB subgroups of AML. The data are shown in (Table 3).

One of the two MLL cases expressed pan CD66 and CD66c.This patient had myeloid and B-cell lineage differentiations, whereas the other patient had myeloid/T cell markers and failed to express any of them.

Clinical presentation and initial laboratory investigations

The only difference observed was a significantly higher peripheral blood blast count in the CD66a+ AML group compared to the negative group (85.0±7 versus 37. 95±31.2), P-value 0.049. Otherwise, no significant difference was detected in terms of the clinical presentation, laboratory investigation or demographic data in B-ALL or AML.

Expression of pan CD66 and its isoforms in different cytogenetic classes

Cytogenetic analysis in AML cases revealed that 10/48(20.8%) cases had favourable profiles [t(8;21), t(15;17),and inv 16], 30/49 (62.5 %) had intermediate profiles [normal karyotype, +8,+4, +11q23, t(9;11),and t(1;9;22)], and 8/48(16.7%) were unfavourable [complex abnormality, inv 17, t (7;11), monosomy 7, hypodiploidy and t(9;22)]. Two AML cases failed karyotyping due to failed metaphase and no recurrent translocations detected by FISH. Cytogenetic analysis of B-ALL cases revealed that 3/27 (11.1%) had a favourable profile [hyperdiploidy], 13/27(48.1%) had an unfavourable profile [near tridiploidy, t (9; 22), t (17; 19), 17p- and 14q-], and 11/27 (40.7%) with an unknown prognostic category [normal karyotype, 9p21- and -12p13] [28].

In the AML group, there were significantly higher levels of the mean value of pan CD66 and CD66c expression in the favourable group compared to the intermediate group. Additionally, the mean values of CD66b expression were significantly higher in the favourable group compared to both the intermediate and unfavourable groups. The data are shown in Table 4. There was no significant difference in the number of cases that expressed the markers ≥ 20% and the cytogenetic classes (P-value > 0.05). There was no significant difference in the different cytogenetic classes in B-ALL in either the percentage of expression or the number of positive cases (P-value >0.05).

Pan CD66 and its isoforms and *BCR/ABL* gene rearrangement in B-ALL

In the B-ALL group, the *BCR/ABL* fusion gene was detected

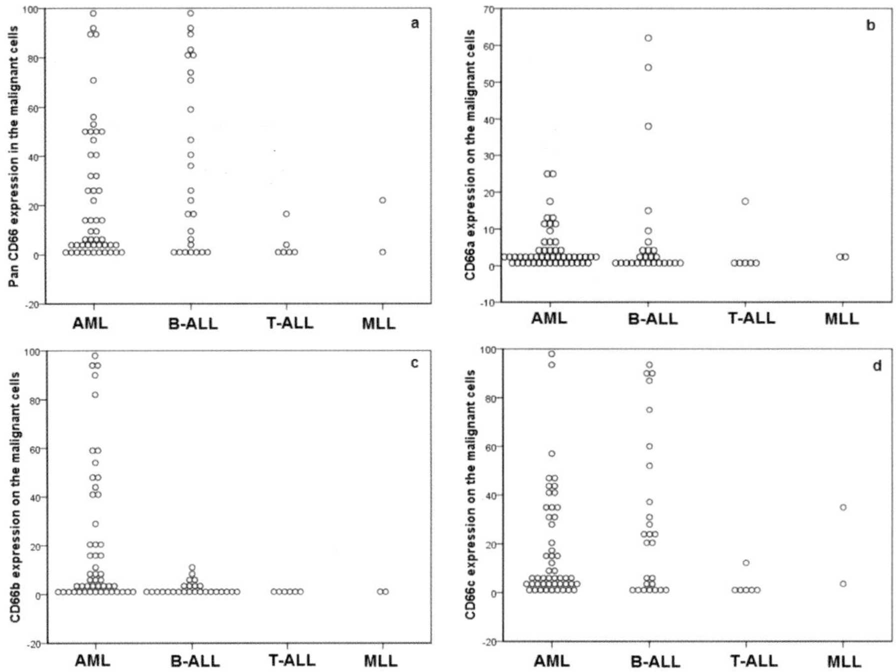

Figure 1: The expression levels of pan CD66 and its studied isoforms in the malignant cell population in acute myeloid leukaemia (AML), B- acute lymphoblastic leukaemia (B-ALL), T- acute lymphoblastic leukaemia (T-ALL), and mixed lineage leukaemia (MLL). **(a)** Pan CD66 expression is at very low levels in T-ALL compared to B-ALL. **(b)** CD66a expression shows no significant difference between the different categories. **(c)** CD66b expression revealed higher levels of expression in AML cases **(d)** CD66c expression revealed low levels of expression in T-ALL compared to B-ALL.

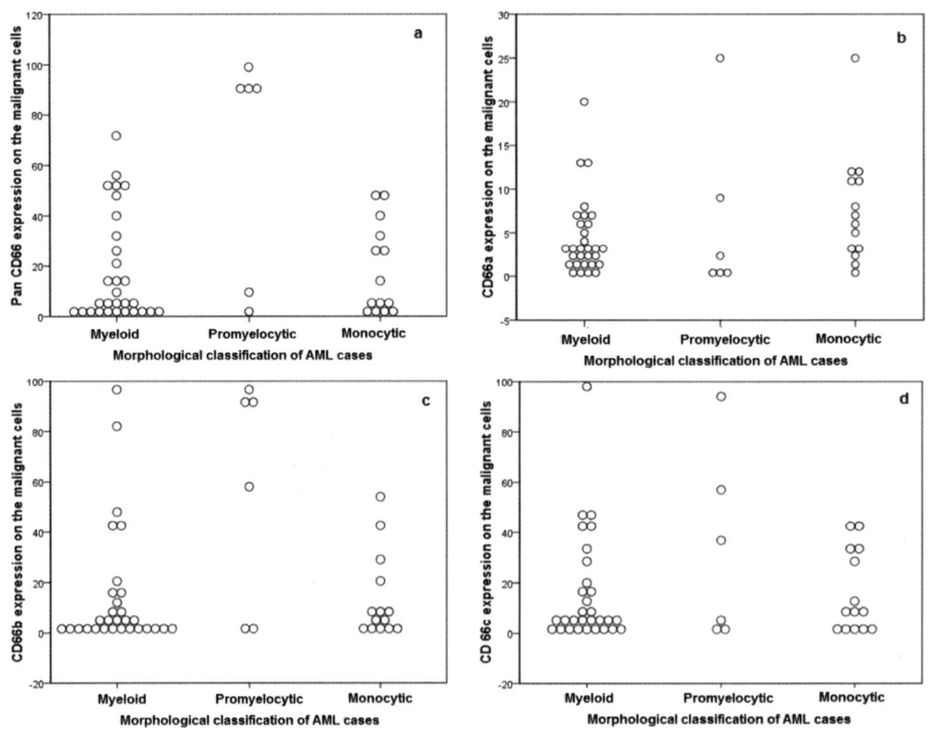

Figure 2: The expression levels of pan CD66 and its studied isoforms on the malignant cell population in acute myeloid leukemia morphological subtypes. (a) Pan CD66 expression shows significantly higher levels in promyelocytic leukemia (P-value<0.001). (b) CD66a expression shows no significant difference between the different subtypes. (c) CD66b expression was higher in promyelocytic leukemia (P-value 0.003) (d) CD66c expression shows no significant difference between the different subtypes.

Parameters studied	AML morphological subtypes #				B-ALL (n=27)	P- value^
	Myeloid (n=30)	Promyelocytic (n=6)	Monocytic (n=14)	Total (n=50)		
Pan CD66	10 (33.3%)	4(66.7%)	6(42.9%)	20 (40%)	14 (51.8%)	0.196
CD66a	1(6.7%)	1(16.7%)	1(12.5%)	3 (6%)	3(11.1%)	0.697
CD66b	6(22.2%)	4 (66.7%)	4(30.8%)	14 (28%)	0 (0%)	0.002*
CD66c	8(29.6%)	3(50.0%)	5(61.5%)	16 (32%)	14 (51.8%)	0.053

#AML-morphological subtypes: Myeloid cases included M1 and M2, promyelocytic referred to M3 morphology and Monocytic cases included M4 and M5.
^P-value between the whole AML and B-ALL groups.
* Significant

Table 3: The rate of positive expression of pan CD66 and its isoforms in the studied AML and B-ALL according to the standard cutoff for surface marker expression.

Studied parameter	Favourable N=10	Intermediate N=30	Unfavourable N=8	P- value^
Pan CD66 Mean ± SD Median(min-max)	51.4 ± 39.8 54.5 (2-99) a	14.9 ± 18.5 4.5(0-72) b	27.4 ± 21.7 26.5 (2-51) a &b	0.001*
CD66a Mean ± SD Median(min-max)	7.0 ± 10.1 3(0-25)	6.5 ± 7.4 3(0-25)	3.4 ± 2.6 4(0-7)	0.629
CD66b Mean ± SD Median(min-max)	55.5 ± 44.9 32(2-98) a	13.1 ± 20.0 3.5(0-82) b	15.6 ± 18.3 8.7(0-48) b	0.001*
CD66c Mean ± SD Median(min-max)	42.8 ± 38.7 21(1-98) a	12.1 ± 13.4 4(0-44) b	24.4 ± 19.4 23.2(3-48) a &b	0.002*

* Significance
^ P-values were used to compare the mean values
Groups sharing the same letter indicate that no statistically significant difference exists.

Table 4: Expression levels of pan CD66 and its isoforms in AML group in relation to the cytogenetic profile.

in 7/27 (25.9%) cases. Of the 14 cases that expressed pan CD66 and CD66c, 6 cases had a *BCR/ABL* gene rearrangement, with a significant correlation, P-value 0.037.

Pan CD66 and its isoforms and CD25 expression

In B-ALL, only 2 cases expressed CD25 (7.4%): one of them expressed pan CD66 and CD66c, but the other one did not, and both were *BCR/ABL* fusion gene positive.

In AML, CD25 was expressed in 5/50 (10%) cases and showed a significant positive correlation with pan CD66 and CD66c expression, P-value 0.008 and 0.003, respectively.

Pan CD66 expression at day 28

Evaluation of pan CD66 in 34(20 AML and 14 B-ALL) paired diagnosis/morphological CR specimens revealed no significant difference between the mean value of pan CD66 expression at diagnosis and day 28 in the both AML and B-ALL studied groups denoting a constant stable expression with no antigen loss (P-value >0.05).

Regarding the positive expression (≥20%) of pan CD66 in B-ALL at day 28, 13/14 cases that expressed the marker at diagnosis were still expressing it (≥20%) and the expression in the remaining case was 6% at day 28 with highly significant correlation, P-value <0.0001.

In AML cases, 14/20 cases that expressed the marker at diagnosis were still expressing it at day 28, and 5/20 showed partial expression of pan CD66 (from 10-19%), with a highly significant correlation, P-value <0.0001. The data are shown in (Figure 3).

Complete remission (CR)

The remission rate in B-ALL cases was 76.9%: 20/26 cases achieved CR, one case was missed, 3 cases died before completion of the induction therapy, and 3 cases were refractory to induction therapy. The remission rate in AML cases was 60%: 30/50 cases achieved CR, 6 cases were refractory to induction therapy, and the remaining cases died early during induction therapy. No significant difference could be detected between the patients who achieved CR and the others with respect to the expression of the studied markers in B-ALL and AML, P-value >0.05.

Overall Survival (OS)

The median (min - max) follow-up period for B-ALL cases was 31.8 (0.0-190) weeks. At the end of this period, 5/26 (19.2%) patients were dead. The median OS for the whole group was 48.6 weeks. CD66a positive cases had a shorter OS, means ± SE 26.4 ±14.1 weeks and one year OS 0.0% versus 57.6 ± 10.8 and 60.0 % in the CD66a negative with a significant difference, P- value 0.045. Otherwise, no significant differences were detected. Figure 4 represents OS curves.

The median (min - max) follow-up period of AML cases was 20.8(0-88) weeks. At the end of this period, 12 (24 %) patients were dead. The median OS for the whole group was 64.6 weeks. There was no impact of pan CD66, CD66a or CD66c positive expression on survival, P-value >0.05. The CD66b positive group had a significantly longer OS, mean ± SE 76.0 ± 7.4 weeks and one year OS of 85.7% versus 44.8 ± 4.7 and 68.4% in the CD66b negative group, P- value 0.025. Figure 5 represents OS curves.

Discussion

A proper diagnosis of acute leukaemia is essential to start efficient chemotherapy but the subsequent monitoring of MRD to detect early recurrence is equally important and is currently recommended by many guidelines [29]. In acute leukaemia, the occurrence of aberrant

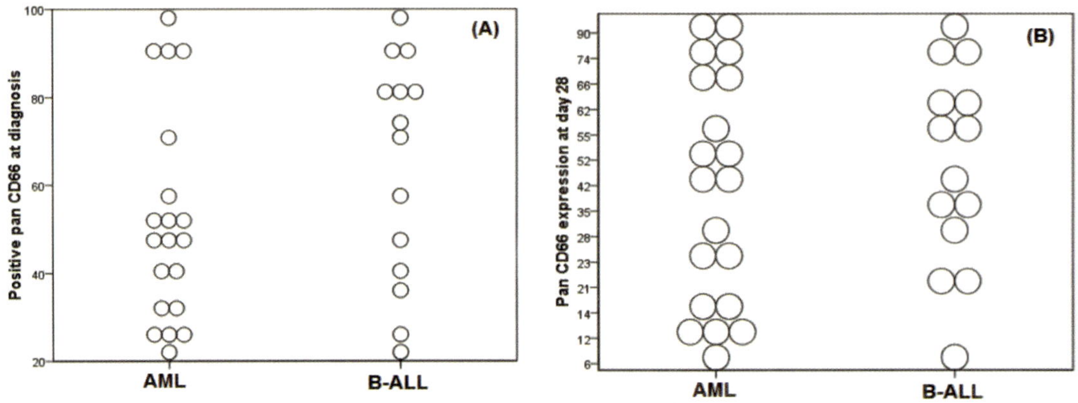

Figure 3: The expression levels of the positive pan CD66 cases in AML and B-ALL. (a) Represents the positive cases that expressed pan CD66 ≥ 20% at presentation. (b) Represents follow up of the previously positive cases at day 28. There was a highly significant correlation between the expression at presentation and at day 28 (P-value<0.0001).

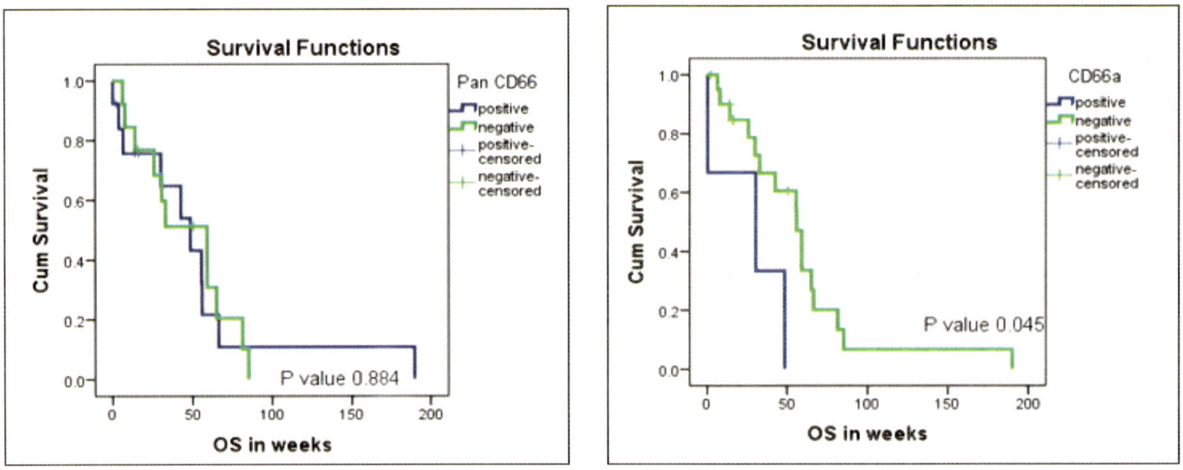

Figure 4: Impact of pan CD66 and CD66a on overall survival (OS) in B-ALL cases studied by the Kaplan-Meier method. (a) Impact of pan CD66 on OS and the same for CD66c. (b) Impact of CD66a on OS. NB. CD66b is not expressed in B-ALL.

antigen expression has been reported with varying frequency [30]. One aspect of the clinical importance of aberrant antigen expression is the ability to use them as a marker of MRD. Comparably, abnormal overexpression or downregulation of some antigens have equal clinical importance. CD66 family members are candidates for both aberrancy and overexpression in ALL and AML.

The currently studied B-ALL cases showed that the rate of pan CD66 and CD66c expression was 51.8%. Both are aberrant myeloid antigens, and they have the most frequent aberrant antigen expression compared to other myeloid antigens, such as CD13, CD33, CD117, CD14, CD15, and CD64 (data are not shown), in agreement with previous reports [9,29-32].

CD66a showed a low expression rate (11.1%), in agreement with Skubitz et al. [33].This low rate is explained by the downregulation of CD66a in early phases of many cancers, as it is suggested to be a tumour suppressor protein [13]. Comparable to the findings of previous authors, the expression of pan CD66, CD 66a, and CD66c was not restricted to certain B-ALL phenotypes and the studied markers never reached the cut-off in T-ALL cases [7].

In AML, the rate of pan CD66 expression was 40%, with the heterogeneous expression of the studied isoforms. Our results are comparable to those of Ratei et al. [7].

We reported a more frequent expression of pan CD66 in B-ALL than AML that did not reach the level of significance that was in contrast to Carrasco et al. [34] who detected a significant higher frequency in B-ALL. In agreement with a previous study, we could not detect any significant difference between the rate of positive expression of CD66a or CD66c in AML compared with B-ALL [7].

In this study, all cases that expressed pan CD66 at diagnosis were reanalysed after morphological CR. This analysis revealed a highly significant correlation between pan CD66 expression at these two different time points in both AML and B-ALL cases, indicating the stability of the marker after induction chemotherapy. We studied pan CD66 in 2 relapsed AML cases that revealed preserved stability of the marker (data are not shown). Our initial data makes pan CD66 suitable for use in the follow-up and detection of MRD in combination with the already used monoclonals.

CD66c is expressed in B-ALL cases at the same percentage of pan

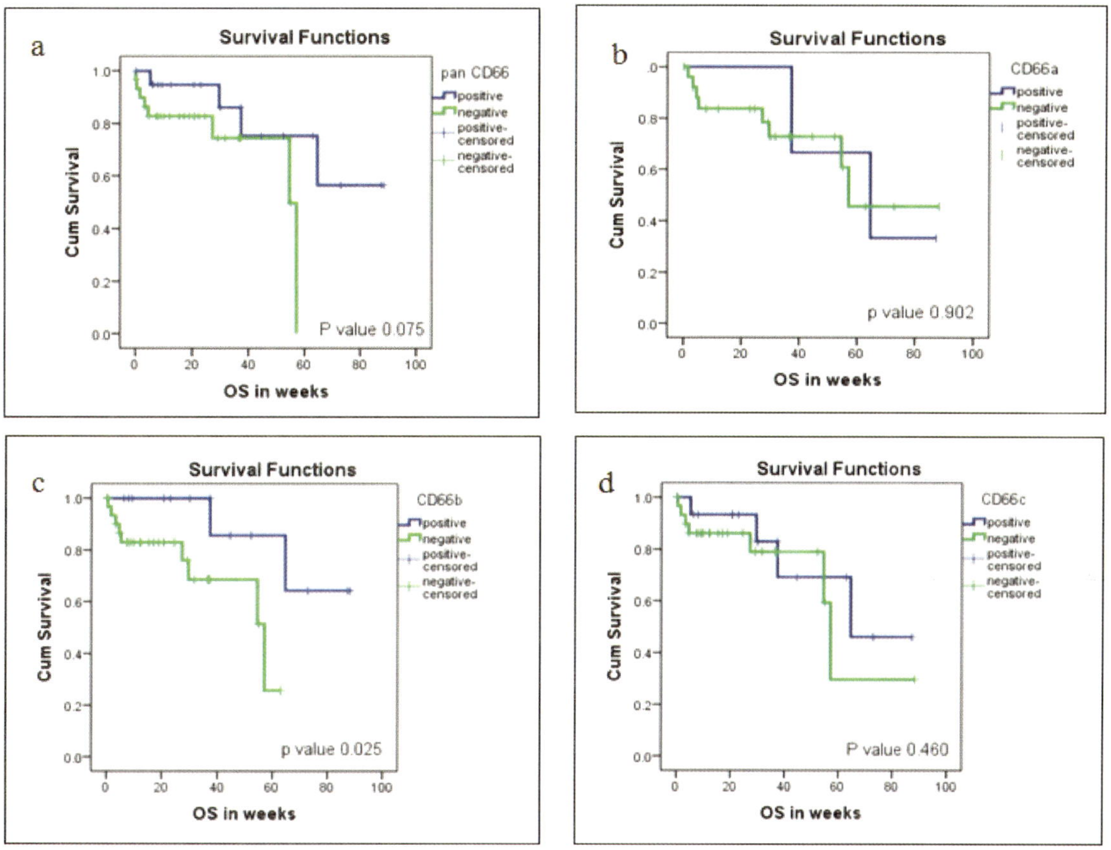

Figure 5: Impact of pan CD66 and its studied isoforms on overall survival (OS) in AML cases studied by the Kaplan-Meier method. (a) Impact of pan CD66 on OS. (b) Impact of CD66a on OS. (c) Impact of CD66b on OS (d) Impact of CD66c on OS.

CD66 but we did not examine its stability after induction therapy. However, Tang et al confirmed the stable expression pattern of CD66c and recommended its use in the recognition of abnormal leukemia cells at primary diagnosis and in monitoring of MRD during the treatment [29]. Our data were encouraging to our center to follow the EuroFlow panel for detection of MRD that included CD66c as a discrimination marker between malignant B-ALL and the normal B-cell precursors [35].

A good target for monoclonal antibody therapy should be expressed at a higher percentage and not shed during therapy to be available for treatment [36]. On the basis of our results, we can consider pan CD66 good candidate for immunotherapy in B-ALL and AML due to its high frequency of expression and molecular stability after induction therapy. However, anti-CD66 radioimmunotherapy may not be the optimal radioimmunoconjugate as its mechanism is indirect with no direct fixation on the leukemic blasts as it was tried earlier [37].

For more specific therapy, CD66c is suggested rather than pan CD66 in B-ALL. Dysregulated over-expression of CD66c plays a role in several of the hallmarks of cancer, including uncontrolled proliferation, anoikis resistance, neoangiogenesis, immune evasion, invasion and metastasis [38]. Silencing CD66c promotes anoikis with down regulation of cell survival pathway [39]. The efficacy of antibody-drug conjugate targeting CD66c was investigated in animal models where marked diminish in tumor size was reported. The only noticed adverse effect was dose- dependent reversible neutropenia because CD66c shows low level of expression in the earliest myeloid lineage (CD34+/ CD38+/ CD33+) [40]. Accordingly, targeting of CD66c may be a promising immunotherapy in B-ALL.

In the studied B-ALL, a significant correlation between CD66c expression and BCR-ABL gene rearrangement was detected, in agreement with other authors [31,32,41].This significant association enables the use of CD66c as a predictor for the *BCR/ABL* rearrangement as reported earlier [29].It is noteworthy that in our study, the expression of CD66c was not restricted to cases harbouring the *BCR/ABL* fusion gene, in agreement with Tang et al. [29]. Therefore, a lack of CD66c expression might indicate the absence of the BCR/ABL rearrangement but the vice is not verse [33]. CD66c is considered a marker for some aggressive cancers [13] that may add to the aggressiveness of Ph+ B-ALL [41].

The correlations between CD66c and BCR/ABL fusion genes prove its expression on the malignant clone. This result, together with the high frequency of CD66c positivity in B-ALL cases, strongly supports the inclusion of CD66c for MRD detection.

In AML cases, there were significantly higher levels of pan CD66 and CD66c in the favourable cytogenetic group compared to the intermediate group. CD66b showed significantly higher levels in the favourable group compared to both the intermediate and unfavourable groups, thus making CD66b a superior isoform in predicting favourable cytogenetic profiles. However, a large-scale study is needed to verify this finding.

CD25, high affinity interlukin2 receptor α chain (IL-2RA), was expressed in 10% (5/50) of AML cases. These cases had a unique phenotype as they expressed HLA-DR, pan CD66, CD66c, CD11c (in all cases) and CD64 (in 4/5 cases), which give the AML blasts a dendritic cell-like phenotype [43,44] that enables them to interact with T-helper cells and deviate their differentiation towards T-regulatory cells. The biological role of IL-2RA was studied in lymphoma, wherein the interaction between IL-2 and IL-2RA can promote differentiation of T-cells into regulatory T-cells, leading to immune escape status [44].Therefore, a similar situation may be generated in the BM microenvironment of CD25+ AML cells. Because this issue may be fundamentally important, further investigations are needed.

CD66a expression in B-ALL had a negative impact on patient prognosis with significantly shorter overall survival. To our knowledge, no comparable results were detected in acute leukaemia. However, in the same context, pan CD66 and CD66a expression were linked to short OS in cervical and pancreatic cancer [45,46]. Short OS could be explained by the anti-apoptotic effect of CD66a [47], which make the tumour more aggressive. In AML cases, no such impact of CD66a expression was detected on OS, but it was linked to another poor prognostic factor: high peripheral blood blast, which may reflects its role in regulating cell migration [48].

CD66b expression was significantly associated with prolonged survival in AML. Interestingly, CD66b was not correlated with any of the poor prognostic factors, CD25 or CD34 expression, high total leukocyte count or blast count, but it was highly expressed with favourable cytogenetics. These findings are taken together with the results of previous authors who measured CD66b in the immature compartment of myeloblast in MDS and stated that CD66b is an independent prognostic factor associated with longer OS irrespective of CD34 or CD117 expression. However, further investigations are needed to clarify similar results in AML [49].

Conclusions

Pan CD66 and CD66c were expressed in 51.8% of B-ALL cases, and their expression was linked to one of the poor prognostic factors, the *BCR/ABL* fusion gene. In AML, pan CD66 was expressed in 40% of AML cases with a predominance of both CD66b and CD66c. The clinical significance of CD66 isoform expression in AML was heterogeneous. Whereas CD66a expression is correlated with high PB blast count, CD66b is associated with favourable cytogenetics and prolonged OS, and CD66c is correlated with CD25 expression.

Recommendations

Our initial results regarding CD66c expression in B-ALL are encouraging for our center to follow the Euro Flow panel for MRD detection. Also, CD66c could be a monoclonal antibody therapy research area in B-ALL; especially it is correlated with the poor prognosis factors: *BCR/ABL* fusion gene. Further investigations are needed to study the stability of CD66c expression after morphological CR and during relapse and to evaluate its biological value as a target molecule for immunotherapy.

Acknowledgements

The authors would like to thank Institute of Scientific Research and Revival of Islamic Heritage at Umm Al-Qura University, Kingdom of Saudi Arabia (project# 43309033) for the financial support.

The authors would like to acknowledge Mrs. / Nawal Hennawi, and Ms. / Alaa Bannani, laboratory specialist at the haematology unit, KAMC for their technical support in sample preparation and the fowcytometry technique.

Author Contributions

MMI: Designed the study, shared in clinical selection of cases, performed the laboratory investigations, shared in statistical analysis, preparing tables, and figures and critically reviewed the manuscript. **AZ**: Shared in the study design, and performed statistical analysis, writing the first draft of the main manuscript text, tables and figures. **NABA:** Was involved in the clinical selection of cases, the performance of laboratory investigations and collection of patient data. **HKM**: Shared in study design and study plans, performance of laboratory investigations and preparation of the master tables including patient data and collected the scientific materials. All authors researched literature, shared in manuscript writing, revised, edited, and approved the final version of the manuscript.

References

1. Hauck CR, Agerer F, Muenzner P, Schmitter T (2006) Cellular adhesion molecules as targets for bacterial infection. Eur J Cell Biol 85: 235-242.
2. Eades-Perner AM, van der Putten H, Hirth A, Thompson J, Neumaier M, et al. (1994) Mice transgenic for the human carcinoembryonic antigen gene maintain its spatiotemporal expression pattern. Cancer Res 54: 4169-4176.
3. Ilantzis C, De Marte L, Screaton RA, Stanners CP (2002) Deregulated expression of the human tumor marker CEA and CEA family member CEACAM6 disrupts tissue architecture and blocks colonocyte differentiation. Neoplasia 4: 151-163.
4. Ordonez C, Screaton RA, Ilantzis C, Stanners CP (2000) Human carcinoembryonic antigen functions as a general inhibitor of anoikis. Cancer Res 60: 3419-3424.
5. Camacho-Leal P, Zhai AB, Stanners CP (2007) A co-clustering model involving alpha 5 beta1 integrin for the biological effects of GPI-anchored human carcinoembryonic antigen (CEA). J Cell Physiol 211: 791-811.
6. Chan CH, Stanners CP (2007) Recent advances in the tumour biology of the GPI-anchored Carcinoembryonic antigen family members CEACAM5 and CEACAM6. Curr Oncol 14: 70-73.
7. Ratei R, Karawajew L, Schabath R, Ehrfeldt A, Grunert F, et al. (2008) Differential expression of the carcinoembryonic antigen-related cell adhesion molecules pan CD66, CD66a, CD66c and sialyl-Lewis x (CD15s) on blast cells of acute leukemia. Int J Hematol 87: 137-136.
8. Lasa A, Serrano E, Carricondo M, Carnicer MJ, Brunet S, et al. (2008) High expression of CEACAM6 and CEACAM8 mRNA in acute lymphoblastic leukemias. Ann Hematol 87: 205-211.
9. Berling B, Kolbinger F, Grunert F, Thompson JA, Brombacher F, et al. (1990) Cloning of a carcinoembryonic antigen gene family member expressed in leukocytes of chronic myeloid leukemia patients and bone marrow. Cancer Res 50: 6534-6535.
10. Thirion G, Feliu AA, Coutelier JP (2008) CD66a (CECAM1) expression by mouse natural killer cells. Immunology 125: 535-540.
11. Carey JL, Philip Mc-Coy J, Keren DF (2007) Flow Cytometry in Clinical Diagnosis. Chicago press: USA.
12. Thom I, Schult-Kronefeld O, Burkholder I (2009) Expression of CECAM-1 in pulmonary adenocarcinomas and their metastases. Anticancer Res 29: 249-254.
13. Beauchemin N, Arabzadeh A (2013) Carcinoembryonic antigen-related cell adhesion molecules (CEACAMs) in cancer progression and metastasis. Cancer Metastasis Rev 32: 643-648.
14. Fiori V, Magnani M, Cianfriglia M (2010) The expression and modulation of CEACAM1 and tumor cell transformation. Annali dell'Intituto Superiore di Sanita 48: 161-170.
15. Ieda J, Yokoyama S, Tamura K, Takifuji K, Hotta T, et al. (2011) Reexpression of CEACAM1 long cytoplasmic domain isoform is associated with invasion and migration of colorectal cancer. Int J Cancer 129: 1351-1360.
16. Yoon J, Terada A, Kita H (2007) CD66b regulates adhesion and activation of human eosinophils. J Immunol 179: 8454-8458.
17. Blumenthal RD, Hansen JH, Goldenberg DM (2005) Inhibition of adhesion, invasion, and metastasis by antibodies targeting CEACAM6 (NCA-90) and CEACAM5 (carcinoembryonic antigen). Cancer Res 65: 8809-8817.
18. Hanenberg H, Baumann M, Quentin I, Nagel G, Grosse-Wilde H, et al. (1994)

Expression of the CEA gene family members NCA-50/90 and NCA-160 (CD66) in childhood acute lymphoblastic leukemias (ALLs) and in cell lines of B-cell origin. Leukemia 8: 2127-2133.

19. Hrusak O, Mac-Donald AP (2002) Antigen expression patterns reflecting genotype of acute leukemia. Leukemia 16: 1233-1258.

20. Ana Sofia C, Daniela S, Dias Sérgio (2012) Bone marrow malignancies as paradigms of dysfunctional cell adhesion mechanisms. Journal of Hematological Malignancies 2: 19-36.

21. Wiernik PH, Banks PL, Case DC Jr, Arlin ZA, Periman PO, et al. (1992) Cytarabine plus idarubicin or daunorubicin as induction and consolidation therapy for previously untreated adult patients with acute myeloid leukemia. Blood 79: 313-319.

22. National Comprehensive Cancer Network (NCCN) (2015) Guidelines for acute myeloid leukemia treatment.

23. National Comprehensive Cancer Network (NCCN) (2014) Guidelines for acute lymphoblastic leukemia treatment.

24. Ludwig W, Rieder H, Bartram C (1998) Immunophenotypic and genotypic features, clinical characteristics, and treatment outcome of adult pro-B acute lymphoblastic leukemia: results of the German multicenter trials GMALL 03/87 and 04/89. Blood 92: 1898-1901.

25. Wood BL, Arroz M, Barnett D, Di Giuseppe J, Greig B, et al. (2007) Bethesda International Consensus recommendations on the immunophenotypic analysis of hematolymphoid neoplasia by flow cytometry: Optimal reagents and reporting for the flow cytometric diagnosis of hematopoietic neoplasia. Cytometry B Clin Cytom 72: 14-22.

26. No authors (1985) An international system of human cytogenetic nomenclature. Report of the Standing Committee on Human Cytogenetic Nomenclature. Birth Defects Origi Artic Ser 21: 1-117.

27. Laane E, Derolf AR, Björklund E, Mazur J, Everaus H, et al. (2006) The effect of allogeneic stem cell transplantation on outcome in younger acute myeloid leukemia patients with minimal residual disease detected by flow cytometry at the end of post-remission chemotherapy. Haematologica 91: 833-836.

28. Swerdlow SH, Campo E, Harris NL, Jaffe ES, Pileri SA, et al. (2008) WHO Classification of Tumours of Hematopoietic and Lymphoid Tissue. (4thedn), Lyon, France, International Agency for Research on Cancer (IARC).

29. Tang G, Wu J, Liu M, Chen H, Gong S, et al. (2015) BCR-ABL1 and CD66c exhibit high concordance in minimal residual disease detection of adult B-acute lymphoblastic leukemia. Am J Transl Res 7: 632-637.

30. Bhushan B, Chauhan P S, Saluja S (2010) Aberrant phenotypes in childhood and adult acute leukemia and its association with adverse prognostic factors and clinical outcome. Clin Exp Med 10: 33-37.

31. Kiyokawa N, Iijima K, Tomita O, Miharu M, Hasegawa D, et al. (2014) Significance of CD66c expression in childhood acute lymphoblastic leukemia. Leuk Res 38: 42-46.

32. Guillaume N, Penther D, Vaida I, Gruson B, Harrivel V, et al. (2011) CD66c expression in B-cell acute lymphoblastic leukemia: strength and weakness. Int J Lab Hematol 33: 92-94.

33. Kishimoto T, Kikutani H (1998) Leucocyte typing VI. New York: Garland.

34. Carrasco M, Munoz L, Bellido M, Bernat S, Rubiol E, et al. (2000) CD66 expression in acute leukaemia. Ann Hematol 79: 299-294.

35. Theunissen P, Mejstrikova E , Sedek L, van der Sluijs-Gelling A, et al. (2017) Standardized flow cytometry for highly sensitive MRD measurements in B-cell acute lymphoblastic leukemia. Blood 129: 347-357.

36. Pagel JM, Boerman OC, Breitz HB, Meredith RF (2003) Targeted radionuclide therapy of cancer; in: Dilman RO, Oldham RK (editors), Principles of Cancer Biotherapy, Springers.

37. Bodet-Milin C, Kraeber-Bodéré F, Eugène T, Guérard F, Gaschet J, et al. (2016) Radioimmunotherapy for Treatment of Acute Leukemia. Semin Nucl Med 46: 135-146.

38. Johnson B, Mahadevan D (2015) Emerging Role and Targeting of Carcinoembryonic Antigen-related Cell Adhesion Molecule 6 (CEACAM6) in Human Malignancies. Clin Cancer Drugs 2: 100-111.

39. Duxbury MS, Ito H, Zinner MJ, Ashley SW, Whang EE (2004) CEACAM6 gene silencing impairs anoikis resistance and in vivo metastatic ability of pancreatic adenocarcinoma cells. Oncogene 23: 465-473.

40. Strickland L A, Ross J, Williams S, Ross S, Romero M, et al. (2009) Preclinical evaluation of carcinoembryonic cell adhesion molecule (CEACAM) 6 as potential therapy target for pancreatic adenocarcinoma. J Pathol 218: 380-390.

41. Owaidah TM, Rawas FI, Al khayatt MF, Elkumb NB (2008) Expression of CD66c and CD25 in acute lymphoblastic leukemia as a predictor of the presence of BCR/ABL rearrangement. Hematol Oncol Stem Cell Ther 1: 34-37.

42. Riaz W, Zhang L, Horna P, Sokol L (2014) Blastic plasmacytoid dendritic cell neoplasm: update on molecular biology, diagnosis, and therapy. Cancer Control 21: 279-210.

43. Derolf AR, Laane E, Bjorklund E, Saft L, Bjorkholm M, et al. (2014) Dendritic cells in bone marrow at diagnosis and after chemotherapy in adult patients with acute myeloid leukemia. Scand J Immunol 80: 424-431.

44. Yang ZZ, Grote DM, Ziesmer SC, Manske MK, Witzig TE, et al. (2011) Soluble IL-2Rα facilitates IL-2-mediated immune responses and predicts reduced survival in follicular B-cell non-Hodgkin lymphoma. Blood 118: 2809-2811.

45. Ammothumkandy A, Maliekal T, Bose M, Rajkumar T, Shirley S, et al. (2016) CD66 and CD49f expressing cells are associated with distinct neoplastic phenotypes and progression in human cervical cancer. Eur J Cancer 60: 166-172.

46. Gebauer F, Wicklein D, Horst J, Sundermann P, Maar M, et al. (2014) Carcinoembryonic Antigen-Related Cell Adhesion Molecules (CEACAM) 1, 5 and 6 as Biomarkers in Pancreatic Cancer. PLOS ONE 9: e113023.

47. Ozeki M, Shively J (2008) Differential cell fates induced by all-trans retinoic acid-treated HL-60 human leukemia cells. J Leukoc Biol 84: 769-770.

48. Klaile E, Muller MM, Kannicht C, Singer BB, Lucka L (2005) CEACAM1 functionally interacts with filamin A and exerts a dual role in the regulation of cell migration. J Cell Sci 118: 5513-5521.

49. Falco P, Levis A, Stacchini A, Ciriello MM, Geuna M, et al. (2011) Prognostic relevance of cytometric quantitative assessment in patients with myelodysplastic syndromes. Eur J Haematol 87: 409-419.

Oral Hygiene Status and Selected Saliva Biomarkers in Children with Acute Lymphoblastic Leukaemia During Anticancer Therapy

Elżbieta Pels*

Department of Paedodontics, Medical University of Lublin, Poland

Abstract

Altered secretion of saliva and its changed composition in patients undergoing chemotherapy often results in oral mucosa pathologies. The aim of this study was to assess the impact of oral hygiene and the concentration of calcium, phosphate and magnesium ions in the saliva on developing oral mucositis in children with acute lymphoblastic leukaemia (ALL) during anticancer therapy. The study included 78 children, aged from 2 to 18 yrs suffering from ALL on anticancer therapy. The results of biochemical scores found that the concentrations of calcium, phosphate and magnesium ions in the saliva of children with ALL were affected. Oral hygiene condition and lower concentrations of selected biomarkers in the saliva in children with ALL during chemotherapy may affect the intensity of the pathological changes in the oral mucosa.

Keywords: Oral mucositis; Saliva biomarkers; Acute lymphoblastic leukemia; Children

Introduction

Under normal conditions the saliva is saturated with calcium, magnesium and phosphorus ions that promote maintaining the integrity of the teeth and oral mucosa. The relationship between micronutrient ions in the saliva is particularly important to maintain proper functioning of the oral mucosa. The abnormalities in the secretion of saliva and changes in its composition in patients undergoing chemotherapy are often observed. This leads to pathological changes in the oral mucosa - mucositis. Oral mucositis is a common and difficult to treat complication during high-dose chemotherapy and radiotherapy followed by hematopoietic stem-cell support (HSCT) [1-4]. At present the condition is often referred to as mucosal barrier injury – MBI.

The aim of this study was to assess the impact of oral hygiene and the concentration of calcium, phosphate and magnesium ions in the saliva on oral mucositis in children with acute lymphoblastic leukaemia during anticancer therapy.

Material and Methods

The study included 78 children aged from 2 to 18 yrs suffering from acute lymphoblastic leukaemia (ALL). In the study group, 5 children had leukaemia recurrence confirmed by the cerebrospinal fluid tests, 2 children had recurrence of leukaemia in the bone marrow, in 7 children the CNS was affected and 3 children had Down's syndrome. The children with acute lymphoblastic leukaemia were examined in three stages: examination 1 – prior to chemotherapy; examination 2 – after the initiation of chemotherapy up to five months of treatment; examination 3 – from 6mths to 1.5 year of anti-cancer treatment. The children were treated according to the ALLIC BFM 2002 program.

Clinical dental examination was conducted by a dentist using basic diagnostic tools in artificial lightning.

Oral hygiene status was assessed using the Oral Hygiene Simplified Index (OHI-S Index), according to Greene and Vermillion, with the use of the Plaque Test.

In the group of patients with ALL, oral mucosa conditions were assessed clinically according to five-grade WHO classification of oral mucositis. Changes in the oral mucosa were monitored every day.

In the group of children examined unstimulated saliva was collected in the morning two hours after a meal to determine the concentration of calcium, phosphorus and magnesium ions. The samples of collected saliva were centrifuged for 15 min at 5,000 rot/min. The centrifuged saliva samples were frozen at -80°C, until the time of biochemical scores.

The concentration of calcium ions was determined by the colorimetric method of Arsenazo III at neutral pH, the complex was read at 660nm wavelength with the use of reagent kit Konelab™ CALCIUM, Thermo Electron Corporation.

The concentration of phosphorus ions was determined calorimetrically by the direct method without deproteinization by measuring UV absorption of the resulting phosphorus-molybdenum complex formed in the acidic environment/absorption at 340 nm wavelength is proportional to the concentration of phosphate ions in the material tested. The measurement was done using reagent kit Phosphorus UV BioMerieux.

The concentrations of magnesium ions were determined by colorimetric method without deproteinization, using calmagite as chromogen and the reagent kit Mg-Kit, BioMérieux.

Microelements were determined on a biochemical analyzer Konelab Kone Pro.

The results were analyzed statistically. The measurable parameters were presented as mean, Median, minimum and maximum values and standard deviation. Mann-Whitney U test was used to compare 2 independent groups, Spearman's Rank Order Correlation test was used to analyze the relationship between two quantitative parameters;

***Corresponding author:** Elżbieta Pels, Chair and Department of Paedodontics, Medical University of Lublin, Poland, Karmelicka 7 St. , 20-081 Lublin, Poland, E-mail: elzbieta.pels@umlub.pl

$p<0.05$ was assumed as statistically significant. The database and the statistical analyses were performed using STATISTICA 8.0 software (StatSoft, Poland).

Results

Table 1 shows oral health status of children with acute lymphoblastic leukemia and generally healthy children (expressed as OHI-S index).

In the group of children with acute lymphoblastic leukemia, the value of OHI-S index determined in examination 1 was 0.64 ± 0.85, in examination 2 it was 0.68 ± 0.74 and in examination 3 it was the lowest 0.49 ± 0.69. However, in healthy children the value of OHI-S index was the highest 0.98 ± 0.70. The comparison of OHI-S values found statistically significantly lower values in the children with acute lymphoblastic leukaemia compared to healthy controls, indicating better oral health in the group of children with acute lymphoblastic leukaemia. In the group of patients, oral hygiene status was worse in examination 2, however it was still better than in the group of healthy controls (Table 1).

Our results found lesions of the mucositis type in the children with acute lymphoblastic leukaemia which were detected after 48 hours to 6 months of chemotherapy; those were of varied intensity with periods without any pathological changes, which was related to the intensity of chemotherapy. Mucosal opacity followed by redness usually occurred within 2-4 days from the Methotrexate infusion. Most intensive oral mucosal lesions developed over the first month of chemotherapy. Changes in the oral mucosa were of different severity. The following pathologies were observed: localized erythema of the mucosa (Grade 1) in 35% children, pseudomembraneous mucosa (Grade 2) in 18% children, ulcers with extensive erythema (Grade 3) in 40% children, massive mucosal ulcers and tissue necrosis (Grade 4) in 4% patients. Wounds and difficult to heal ulcers were related to poor blood parameters. It was observed that healing was faster, especially with regard to oral mucosa ulceration, when blood morphological parameters improved. The lesions of mucositis type were neutropenia-dependent. Each child with neutropenia had fungal complications in the oral mucosa. Generally, no lesions were observed in the periods between subsequent protocols. After 6 months of chemotherapy, oral mucosa lesions were less intense and were observed in 3.17% of the children examined. Redness and erosions were the most frequent. No ulcers in the oral cavity were observed.

Tables 2-4 present the concentrations of calcium, phosphorus and magnesium ions in the saliva of children with acute lymphoblastic leukaemia and the control group.

Biochemical studies found that the concentration of calcium ions in the saliva of patients with acute lymphoblastic leukemia decreased during anticancer therapy. The mean value of the calcium ion concentration in the saliva of children with acute lymphoblastic leukaemia in examination 1 was 1.7 ± 1.99 mmol/l, in examination 2 it was reduced to the value of 1.4 ± 0.78 mmol/l, and the lowest value was observed in examination 3 - 1.3 ± 0.75 mmol/l The average concentration of calcium in the saliva of children with acute lymphoblastic leukaemia in examination 3 was lower compared with healthy children, and the difference was close to statistical significance ($p=0.0676$) (Table 2).

The results of biochemical tests showed that the concentration of phosphorus ions in the saliva of patients with acute lymphoblastic leukemia before chemotherapy was significantly lower compared to the controls ($p < 0.0001$, Table 3). In examinations 2 the concentration of phosphorus ions in the saliva of children with acute lymphoblastic leukaemia was increased, but compared to otherwise healthy children the values were still significantly lower ($p < 0.005$) (Table 3).

The analysis of examination 1 results revealed that worsened oral

Children	index	N	X	Me	SD	Mann-Whitney U Test (Z)	Significance level (p)
ALL examination 1		78	0.64	0.4	0.85	3.42736	0.00061*
ALL Examination 2		54	0.68	0.5	0.74	2.65201	0.00800*
ALL examination 3	OHI-S	63	0.49	0.0	0.69	4.36259	0.00001*
healthy		78	0.98	1.0	0.70	Test results compared to generally healthy children	

Table 1: Oral hygiene index (OHI-S) in children with acute lymphoblastic leukemia and in healthy children.

Children	Ca^{2+} $\bar{x}$	Me	Min.	Max	SD	Mann-Whitney U Test (Z)	Significance level (p)
ALL examination 1	1.7	1.2	0.59	9.94	1.99	-0.0144	0.9885
ALL examination 2	1.4	1.2	0.62	5.77	0.78	-0.0792	0.9369
ALL examination 3	1.3	1.0	0.56	4.06	0.75	1.8279	0.0676
Healthy	1.4	1.2	0.33	4.25	0.75	Test results compared to generally healthy children	

Table 2: The concentration of calcium ions in the saliva of children with acute lymphoblastic leukemia and in healthy children (mmol/l).

Children	P^{3+} $\bar{x}$	Me	Min.	Max	SD	Mann-Whitney U Test (Z)	Significance level (p)
ALL examination 1	7.6	3.8	1.66	31.28	7.78	3.3617	0.0008*
ALL Examination 2	11.7	4.4	2.00	38.40	11.07	1.6391	0.1012
ALL examination 3	10.4	3.8	0.58	38.88	11.19	3.0167	0.0025*
Healthy	14.4	18.6	2.01	35.32	9.61	Test results compared to generally healthy children	

Table 3: The concentration of phosphorus ions in the saliva of children with acute lymphoblastic leukemia and in healthy children (mmol/l).

Children	Mg^{2+} $\bar{x}$	Me	Min.	Max	SD	Mann-Whitney U Test (Z)	Significance level (p)
ALL examination 1	0.2	0.2	0.02	1.00	0.17	-1.2662	0.2054
ALL examination 2	0.3	0.2	0.01	1.87	0.34	-2.3409	0.0192*
ALL examination 3	0.2	0.2	0.02	1.07	0.23	-1.5888	0.1121
Healthy	0.2	0.1	0.03	0.97	0.16	Test results compared to generally healthy children	

Table 4: The concentration of magnesium ions in the saliva of children with acute lymphoblastic leukemia and in healthy children (in mmol/l).

hygiene was related to decreased concentration of phosphorus ions in the saliva of children with acute lymphoblastic leukaemia (Spearman rank correlations R=-0.303; t=-1.93, p=0.06; Figure 1).

Biochemical the research showed that the concentration of magnesium ions in the saliva of patients with acute lymphoblastic leukemia in the period from 1 to 5 months of chemotherapy was significantly higher compared to the control group (p = 0.0192, Table 4).

Discussion

In recent years, the saliva has been more and more often used to evaluate biomarkers in different and sometimes serious diseases. Due to non-invasive character of the method to obtain material for study, saliva tests have become a good method to diagnose various oral 5 pathologies as they enable the evaluation of the effects of treatment, and monitoring of patients after treatment with minimal discomfort for both patient and doctor [5,6].

Abnormal secretion of saliva is often observed in the patients on chemo-and radiotherapy. In case of salivary gland dysfunction, the majority of protective properties of the saliva disappear. However, the researchers agree that the saliva saturated with calcium and phosphorus ions promotes remineralization of the tooth enamel [7]. Ca^{2+} ions are involved in changes of cell membrane potential which affects the enzymatic pathways of many metabolic processes that lead to the production of fibrin [8,9]. Moreover, Ca^{2+} ions play a very important role in tissue repair and regulation mechanisms by being an essential part of the intracellular signal transduction system that brings about cell growth and metabolism [10].

The most common complaints of patients who suffer from damage to the mucosal barrier include burning and dryness of the mouth, difficulty speaking and eating food, and altered taste. Using an oral solution containing supersaturated calcium phosphate, e.g. Caphosol, is an option to treat or alleviate such symptoms, as it can reduce the frequency, severity and duration of oral mucositis [11-13]. Supersaturated calcium phosphate reduces the frequency, intensity and duration of oral mucositis in patients undergoing HSCT [12]. It might be related to leveling serum Ca^{2+} ions and phosphate ions in the saliva of patients undergoing chemotherapy, which needs further examination though.

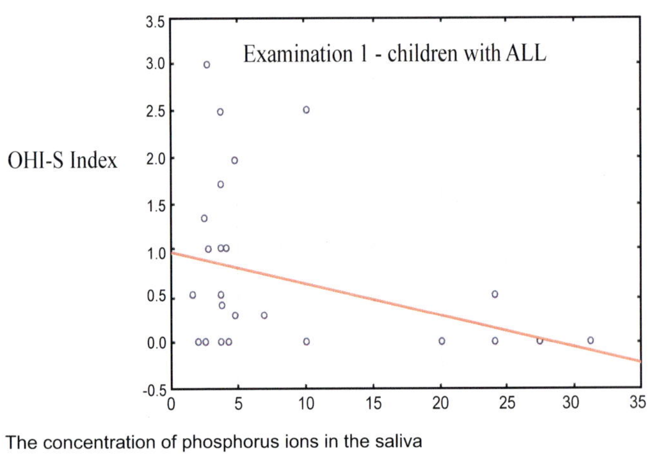

Figure 1: Oral hygiene and the concentration of phosphorus ions in the saliva in examination 1 in children with ALL.

Moreover, the scientists who studied various microelement concentrations in the saliva in other diseases, observed oral pathologies too. Błoniarz et al. [14] found higher concentrations of calcium, magnesium and sodium in the saliva of patients with oral carcinoma planoepitheliale spinocellulare [14]. Brik et al. [15] demonstrated that patients with oligoarticular inflammations had mean concentration of calcium and phosphate in the saliva by 25% lower compared to the patients with systemic inflammation of polyarthritis and control patients. The concentrations of Mg ions, total protein and α-amylase in the saliva in the patients with oligoarticular inflammations were lowered in comparison to the patients in the control group [15].

Inadequate oral hygiene may lead to oral mucosal inflammations. They pose significant problems in patients undergoing chemotherapy as oral lesions are painful, cause ulcerations and eventually result in poor nutrition, underhydration, and may create life threat eventually. Complications that develop within the oral cavity are likely to prolong treatment time and increase its costs too [3,16-20].

Patients on chemotherapy are recommended to change their oral hygiene habits, which are often improper, to maintain good oral hygiene. Doctors agree that regular tooth brushing, two times daily at the least, the application of oral rinses and effective motivating patient to thoroughly brush all tooth surfaces and clean the soft tissues surrounding them are of utmost importance to lower the risk of developing complications within the oral cavity. Adequate oral hygiene helps avoid many adverse side effects, particularly in patients with lowered immunity and patients undergoing anticancer treatment certainly belong to the group of high risk [4,21-25].

Conclusion

Oral hygiene status and lowered concentrations of calcium, phosphate and magnesium ions in the saliva in children with ALL during chemotherapy may affect the intensity the pathological changes in the oral mucosa in that group of patients.

References

1. Thomaz EB, Mouchrek JC Jr, Silva AQ, Guerra RN, Libério SA, et al. (2013) Longitudinal assessment of immunological and oral clinical conditions in patients undergoing anticancer treatment for leukemia. Int J Pediatr Otorhinolaryngol 77: 1088-1093.
2. Lalla RV, Sonis ST, Peterson DE (2008) Management of oral mucositis in patients who have cancer. Dent Clin North Am 52: 61-77, viii.
3. Epstein JB, Schubert MM (2004) Managing pain in mucositis. Semin Oncol Nurs 20: 30-37.
4. Keefe DM, Schubert MM, Elting LS, Sonis ST, Epstein JB, et al. (2007) Updated clinical practice guidelines for the prevention and treatment of mucositis. Cancer 109: 820-831.
5. Shankar AA, Routray S (2012) Trends in salivary diagnostics - a 5-year review of oral oncology (2007-2011). Oral Oncol 48: e22-23.
6. Wu JY, Yi C, Chung HR, Wang DJ, Chang WC, et al. (2010) Potential biomarkers in saliva for oral squamous cell carcinoma. Oral Oncol 46: 226-231.
7. Carl W (1995) Oral complications of local and systemic cancer treatment. Curr Opin Oncol 7: 320-324.
8. Bick RL, Murano G (1994) Physiology of hemostasis. Clin Lab Med 14: 677-707.
9. Berridge MJ (2008) Smooth muscle cell calcium activation mechanisms. J Physiol 586: 5047-5061.
10. Berridge MJ, Lipp P, Bootman MD (2000) The versatility and universality of calcium signaling. Nat Rev Mol Cell Biol 1: 11-21.
11. Wasko-Grabowska A, Rzepecki P, Oborska S, Barzal J, Gawronski K, et al. (2011) Efficiency of supersaturated calcium phosphate mouth rinse treatment

in patients receiving high-dose melphalan or BEAM prior to autologous blood stem cell transplantation: a single-center experience. Transplant Proc 43: 3111-3113.

12. Papas AS, Clark RE, Martuscelli G, O'Loughlin KT, Johansen E, et al. (2003) A prospective, randomized trial for the prevention of mucositis in patients undergoing hematopoietic stem cell transplantation. Bone Marrow Transplant 31: 705-712.

13. Markiewicz M, Dzierzak-Mietla M, Frankiewicz A, Zielinska P, Koclega A, et al. (2012) Treating oral mucositis with a supersaturated calcium phosphate rinse: comparison with control in patients undergoing allogeneic hematopoietic stem cell transplantation. Support Care Cancer 20: 2223-2229.

14. Bloniarz J, Rahnama M, Zareba S (2003) Influence of carcinogenesis in the oral cavity on the level of some bioelements in the saliva. Rocz Panstw Zakl Hig 54: 295-300.

15. Brik R, Livnat G, Pollack S, Catz R, Nagler R (2006) Salivary gland involvement and oxidative stress in juvenile idiopathic arthritis: novel observation in oligoarticular-type patients. J Rheumatol 33: 2532-2537.

16. Sonis ST, Elting LS, Keefe D, Peterson DE, Schubert M, et al. (2004) Perspectives on cancer therapy-induced mucosal injury: pathogenesis, measurement, epidemiology, and consequences for patients. Cancer 100: 1995-2025.

17. Herrstedt J (2000) Prevention and management of mucositis in patients with cancer. Int J Antimicrob Agents 16: 161-163.

18. Karolewska E, Konopka T, Pupek M, Chaber R (2007) Mucositis in Children with Leukemia and Salivary Defense Factors. Dent Med Probl 44: 30–36.

19. Karolewska E, Konopka T (2006) Preventive-therapeutic dental care protocol in children with leukemia. Czas Stomatol 59: 245-252.

20. Peterson DE (2006) New strategies for management of oral mucositis in cancer patients. J Support Oncol 4: 9-13.

21. Bonnaure-Mallet M, Bunetel L, Tricot-Doleux S, Guérin J, Bergeron C, et al. (1998) Oral complications during treatment of malignant diseases in childhood: effects of tooth brushing. Eur J Cancer 34: 1588-1591.

22. Cheng KK, Chang AM, Yuen MP (2004) Prevention of oral mucositis in paediatric patients treated with chemotherapy; a randomised crossover trial comparing two protocols of oral care. Eur J Cancer 40: 1208-1216.

23. Cheng KK (2004) Children's acceptance and tolerance of chlorhexidine and benzydamine oral rinses in the treatment of chemotherapy-induced oropharyngeal mucositis. Eur J Oncol Nurs 8: 341-349.

24. Harris DJ, Eilers J, Harriman A, Cashavelly BJ, Maxwell C (2008) Putting evidence into practice: evidence-based interventions for the management of oral mucositis. Clin J Oncol Nurs 12: 141-152.

25. de Koning BA, Philipsen-Geerling B, Hoijer M, Hählen K, Büller HA, et al. (2007) Protection against chemotherapy induced mucositis by TGF-beta(2) in childhood cancer patients: results from a randomized cross-over study. Pediatr Blood Cancer 48: 532-539.

6

The Time-Dependent Morphological Alteration and Enucleation Process during the Differentiation of Mammalian Erythroid Cells

Zuli Yang, Yajuan Zheng, Fan Hu, Zhang Zhang, Fukun Zhao and Shifu Zhang*

College of Life Sciences, Zhejiang Sci-Tech University, Hangzhou, China

Abstract

One characteristic of the erythroid terminal differentiation is hemoglobin expression and enucleation. In the present study, by using real-time cultured Friend Virus Anemia-inducing (FVA) cells, scanning electron microscopy (SEM), immunofluorescence combined with laser scanning confocal microscopy (LSCM), the FVA cells induced by Erythropoietin (EPO) for were used for: 1) to study the shape and proportion of cells at different differentiating stages, enucleation process, the formation of blood islands, and engulfment of nuclei by macrophages in real time, 2) to quantitatively analyze erythroid cell surface markers including CD71 and Ter119, and cytoskeletal-associated proteins (stathmin, septin8 and RBBP4). The results of real-time monitoring of enucleation indicated that it took about 7 to 8 hours to extrude the nuclei from karyopyknosis (polychromatic erythroblasts). It further showed that the macrophages engulfed the expelled erythroid nuclei. SEM showed a variety of shapes of the nascent reticulocytes. In the process of erythroid differentiation, expressions of both the transferring receptors CD71 and Ter119 were higher than that of adult blood cells, whereas, cytoskeletal-associated proteins (stathmin, septin8 and RBBP4) decreased gradually. Therefore, systematic observation of the process of differentiation and enucleation will provide a deeper understanding of cellular and molecular mechanisms for erythroid differentiation and carcinogenesis.

Keywords: Erythroid differentiation; Enucleation; Real-time cultured cell monitoring; Morphology; LSCM; Occurrence of Leukemia

Introduction

Erythroid differentiation is a complex process, and the terminally differentiated cells are characterized by shrinkage of the cells, karyopyknosis, enucleation, and ultimately differentiating into mature red blood cells. Mice were injected with FVA, and the erythroid cells from their spleen were synchronized as proerythroblast and retained the differentiation characteristics of Colony Forming Unit-Erythroid (CFU-E) cells [1-3]. Therefore, the medium was supplemented with EPO in the culture, the cells mainly generated basophilic erythroblasts at 12 h to 24 h, polychromatic erythroblasts at 36 h, dominantly orthochromatic erythroblasts and reticulocytes at 48 h to 60 h [4]. There were many changes in the cell morphology, haemoglobin accumulation, the expelled nuclei were wrapped by small amount of cytoplasm and plasma membrane, and then formed reticulocytes [5,6] in the process of differentiation.

In the early stages of erythroid differentiation, the macrophage functions as a "nurse" cell for forming blood islands [7-9], the direct contact of macrophages and erythroid cells improves the proliferation of erythroid cells [10-13], and provides conditions for erythrocyte formation [14], the nuclei are engulfed by macrophages through related molecules on the nucleus that interact with macrophages [15].

Recently, there are a few reports regarding to the erythroid differentiation and enucleation [14,16]. However, there is still a lack of systematic study about cell morphology at various differentiation stages, surface markers, changes in cell number, the time needed for enucleation and polymorphism of the nascent reticulocytes.

This research has systematically studied the morphology and enucleation at various differentiation stages of the FVA cells. It took about 7 to 8 hours from polychromatic erythroblasts to the exclusion of nuclei and showed a variety of shapes of the nascent reticulocytes.

Materials and Methods

Animal and virus Six to eight-weeks old mature BALB/c female mice (20 -25 g) were purchased from Hangzhou Normal University (Hangzhou, China). Friend virus anemia-inducing (FVA) was purchased from ATCC (American Tissue Culture Collection, Rockville, USA).

Reagents

IMDM medium (Gibco, Grand Island, USA), fetal bovine serum (HyClone, Logan, USA), 4% paraformaldehyde (Sigma-Aldrich, steinheim, Germany), antibodies for stathmin, Ter-119, CD68, and CD71 (Abcam, Cambridge, UK), antibodies for septin8 (Santa, Dallas, USA), antibodies for RBBP4 (Epitomics, Burlingame, USA), EPO, FITC-conjugate goat anti-mouse IgG and Cy3-conjugate goat anti-rabbit IgG (Invitrogen, Eugene, USA).

FVA cells isolation and culture

Mice were injected with FVA via tail vein. Spleens from these mice were harvested two weeks later. Single cell suspension of the spleens was prepared, and cultured in IMDM medium containing 30% FBS, 0.1% bovine serum albumin (Sigma-Aldrich, St.Louis, USA), 10^{-4} mol/L 1-Thioglycerol (Sigma-Aldrich, St. Louis, USA), and 2 mmol/L L-glutamine (Gibco, Grand Island, USA). 1×10^{6}/mL FVA cells were seeded in the culture flask with 2×10^{-4} IU/L EPO, and were grown in the incubator in 5% CO_2 at 37°C for 2 h, 12 h, 24 h, 36 h, 48 h, 60 h, 72 h.

Benzidine and Wright's staining for the morphology of erythroid cells

Benzidine staining: FVA cells were collected and then centrifuged at 1000 rpm for 3 min, stained with 100 μL of 0.02% benzidine dye

***Corresponding author:** Shifu Zhang, College of Life Sciences, Zhejiang Sci-Tech University, 928 the 2nd Ave, Xiasha Hi-Tech Park, Hangzhou 310018, People's Republic of China; E-mail: cklzhang@163.com

(Yuanhang, Shanghai, China) premixed with 30% H_2O_2, and then examined. Wright's stain: FVA cells were fixed with 4% paraformaldehyde for 20 min., and stained according to the established procedure [17] described elsewhere, and then examined with Nikon ECLIPSE TE2000-U microscope.

The sizes of FVA cells

Count Star Automated Cell Counter was used to study the statistics of the size of FVA cells after cultured with EPO for 0 h, 2 h, 12 h, 24 h, 36 h, 48 h, 60 h and 72 h.

Scanning electron microscopy for morphology of FVA cells

FVA cells were washed twice with PBS (GN, Hangzhou, China), fixed with 1 mL 3% glutaraldehyde (SH, Shanghai, China) solution at 4°C for 2 h and washed 3 times with PBS. They were then fixed with 1 mL of 1% osmium tetroxide at 4°C for 2 h, washed 3 times with PBS for 10 min each time. The cells were then dehydrated in graded ethanol (50%, 70%, 80%, 90%, 100%; Changzheng, Hangzhou, China) every 5 min, replaced with acetonitrile (50%, 70%, 80%, 90%, 100%; Tedia, USA) every 15 min until dry. Then the slice was plated platinum and detected with Hitachi s-4800 scanning electron microscopy.

Morphology of macrophages during erythroid differentiation

MurineErythroLeukemia (MEL) cells, mouse peritoneal macrophages, and FVA cells were fixed with 4% paraformaldehyde for 20 min, washed 3 times with PBS, and stained with 500 μL DAPI (1 mg/L, KeyGEN, Nanjing, China) working solution at 37°C for 15 min. The cells were then rinsed with methanol (Changzheng, Hangzhou, China), washed 3 times with PBS, and blocked with 1% BSA for 30 min. Furthermore, the cells were incubated with anti-CD68 primary antibody (1:200) at 4°C overnight. After incubation, they were washed 3 times with PBST (Phosphate buffer solution with Tween 20), incubated with Cy3-conjugate goat anti-rabbit IgG (1:10,000) for 1 h, rinsed with PBST. Anti-fade mounting medium was then added and observed with Nikon C1SI LSCM.

Real-time cultured cell monitoring for enucleation

FVA cells were seeded at a concentration of 1×10^6/mL, EPO (2×10^{-4} IU/L) was added and the cells were grown in 5% CO_2 at 37°C in miniature incubator for real-time cultured cell monitoring. These cells in the same position were imaged one frame per minute for 48 h.

Quantitative analysis of Ter119 and CD71 in erythroid cells and adult blood cells

FVA cells, mouse bone marrow cells, mouse blood cells, MEL cells and NIH3T3 cells were fixed with 4% paraformaldehyde for 20 min, washed 3 times with PBS, and blocked with 1% BSA for 30 min. The samples were then incubated with CD71 (1:3,000) or Ter119 (1:6,000) antibodies at 4°C overnight and then washed 3 times with PBST, incubated with Cy3-conjugate secondary antibody (goat anti-rabbit) IgG (1:10,000) and FITC-conjugate secondary antibody (goat anti-mouse) IgG (1:10,000) for 1 h. They were then rinsed with PBST and anti-fading agent was added, and then observed with LSCM. Results were quantified using the EZ-C1 3.20 software for CD71 and TER119. All data were expressed as means ± SD of three independent experiments.

The expression of stathmin, RBBP4, and septin8 in erythroid cells

Immunofluorescence was combined with LSCM to detect the expression of the three cytoskeletal-associated proteins, i.e. stathmin, RBBP4, and septin8.

Statistical analysis

Quantitative experimental data were expressed as mean ± SD and analyzed using IBM SPSS Statistics 21.0 software with t-test. The difference with $P < 0.05$ was regarded as statistically significant.

Results

As shown in Figure 1, the weight of the normal adult mouse spleen was about 0.1 g, that increased to 1~1.5 g due to the cells being synchronized as proerythroblasts after transfection with FVA that increased the blood volume of spleen.

Change in the sizes of FVA Cells

Benzidine (Figure 2a-e) was used to detect the differentiation process of cells, while Wright's staining (Figure 2f-j) could observed the cell morphology, the cells could be divided into: mostly proerythroblast with diameter of 12 μm at 2h, basophilic erythroblast with diameter of 10 μm after 12h, mainly polychromatic and orthochromatic erythroblasts with diameter from 10 μm to 8 μm at 36 h. Most of the cells were differentiated into reticulocytes with diameter of 8 μm at 48 h, and almost all of the erythroblast was differentiated into reticulocytes after 60 h. And 14 μm represented small cell clusters (Table 1). The results showed that the ratio of cells with 12 μm in diameter was decreased from about 43% at 2 h to below 10% at 72 h, while the number of cells with a diameter of 8 μm gradually increased from 15% at 2 h to 85% at 72 h (Figure 3).

The result of SEM showed that (Figure 4), the cellular volume gradually decreased. The volume of minimal cell was orthochromatic Erythroblasts (Figure 4e). Further, the cellular volume was slightly increased and the reticulocytes formed biconcave discoid structures.

Enucleation process of Erythroblast

The SEM results of the whole process of enucleation are shown in Figure 5. Before enucleation, the nucleus deviated and then the cytoplasm extended into a gourd shape. During the process, the nuclear was extruded from the cell and the entire nuclear and cytoplasm was separated. The nascent reticulocytes formed irregular shapes after enucleation (Figure 6).

Real-Time cultured cell monitoring of enucleation

Figure 7a-f show that it spent about 7-8 hours from the karyopyknosis to enucleation, and ultimately the formation of reticulocytes. During

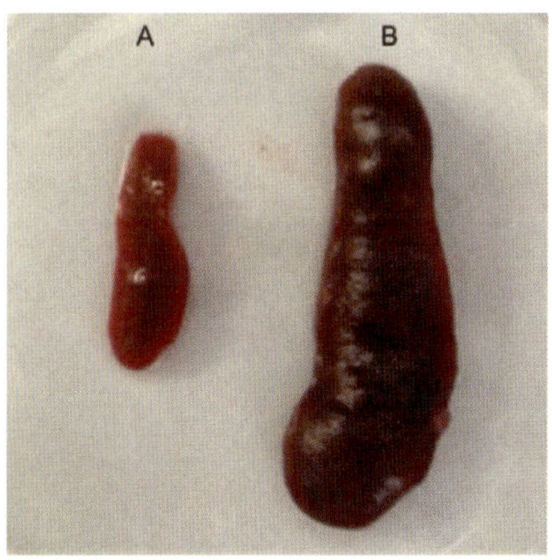

Figure 1: The spleen from normal adult mouse and the spleen after FVA transfection. (a): Spleen from normal adult mouse; (b): Spleen from normal adult mouse after FVA transfection

differentiation, the cellular volumes were gradually decreased, and the cells eventually changed from the original round nucleated cells to enucleated reticulocytes.

Morphologic changes of the macrophages during erythroid differentiation

As shown in Figure 8a-b, erythroid cells gathered around macrophages and the number was gradually increased, then the macrophages became large gradually due to engulfment of nuclei (Figure 8c-d). Fetal liver cells from E14.5 d fetal mouse cultured *in vitro* had similar results (Figure 9). Furthermore, the macrophage-specific cell surface marker CD68 confirmed that it was macrophage. The volumes of the macrophages increased tremendously due to the endocytosis of naked nuclei. After 72 h, macrophages expanded into oval shapes, and their volumes were decreased with the intracellular naked nuclei being gradually digested (Figure 10).

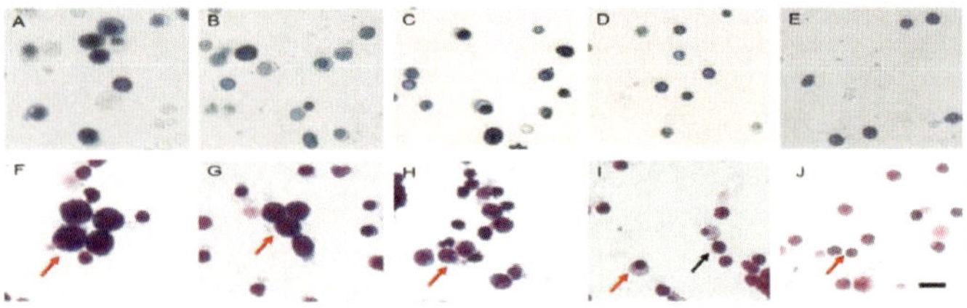

Figure 2: Benzidine staining of FVA cells cultured after 2 h-60 h (a-e): 2 h; (b) 24 h; (c) 36 h; (d) 48 h; (e) 60 h; Wright's staining of FVA cells cultured after 2 h-60 h (f-j): (f) 2 h, Proerythroblasts. Red arrow; (g) 24 h, Basophilic Erythroblast, Red arrow; (h) 36 h, polychromatic Erythroblast, Red arrow; (i) 48 h, orthochromatic erythroblast, red arrow; reticulocytes, black arrow; (j) 60 h, nucleus, red arrow. Bar =10 μm.

FVA cells	8 μm cells	10 μm cells	12 μm cells	14 μm cells
0h	3183 ± 176	4018 ± 207	5067 ± 265	799 ± 59
2h	277 ± 23	621 ± 39	775 ± 31	98 ± 14
12h	633 ± 41	319 ± 32	148 ± 17	35 ± 12
24h	887 ± 23	264 ± 22	123 ± 10	30 ± 15
36h	534 ± 24	242 ± 13	89 ± 12	9 ± 5
48h	2426 ± 213	954 ± 70	556 ± 19	58 ± 20
60h	4004 ± 124	548 ± 25	330 ± 17	27 ± 7
72h	3055 ± 190	321 ± 10	168 ± 3	14 ± 6

Table 1: The sizes of cells at induced different times the number of 8 μm, 10 μm, 12 μm, and 14 μm diameters cells.

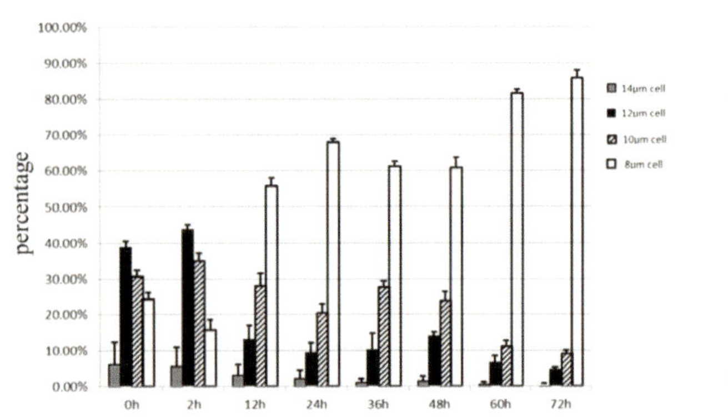

Figure 3: Trends of cells with diameters of 8 μm, 10 μm, 12 μm, 14 μm. 14 μm cells represented small cell clusters, 12 μm cells were Proerythroblasts, 10 μm cells represented basophilic and polychromatic erythroblasts, and 8 μm cells were orthochromatic Erythroblasts and reticulocytes.

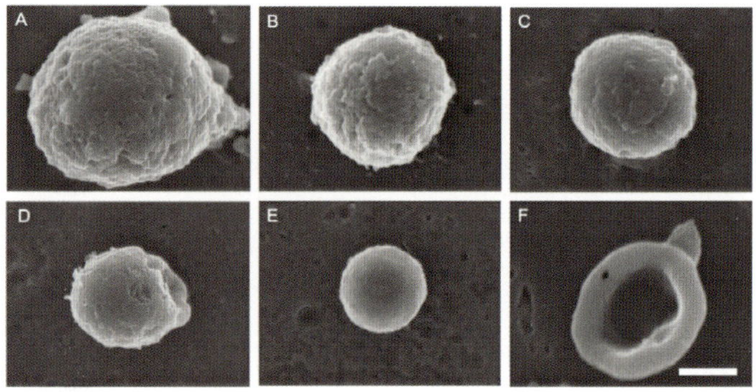

Figure 4: The SEM results of FVA cells cultured after 2h-48h. (a-c) nucleated cells, (d-e) Cellular volume gradually reduced; (f) Nascent reticulocytes after enucleation.
Bar =2 μm.

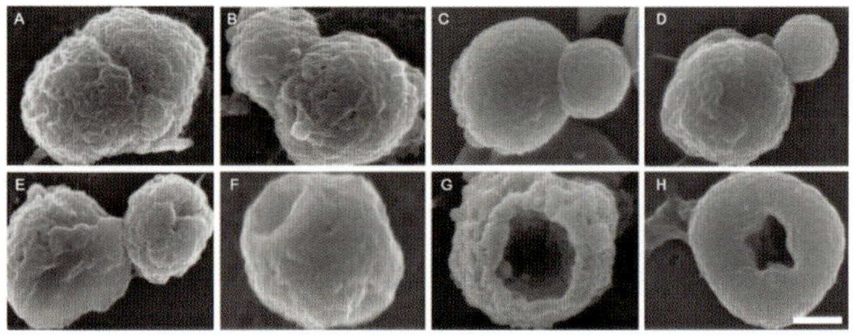

Figure 5: The SEM results of FVA cells cultured after 2 h-48 h. (a-e) Enucleating cell; (f-h) Cell after enucleation. Bar =1 μm.

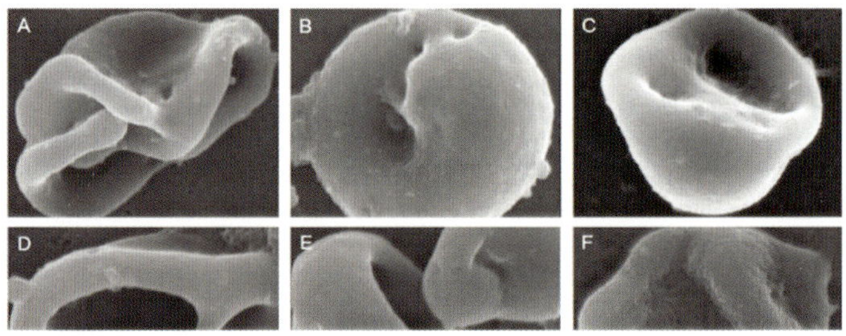

Figure 6: Distinct shapes of nascent reticulocytes after enucleation. Bar =2 μm..

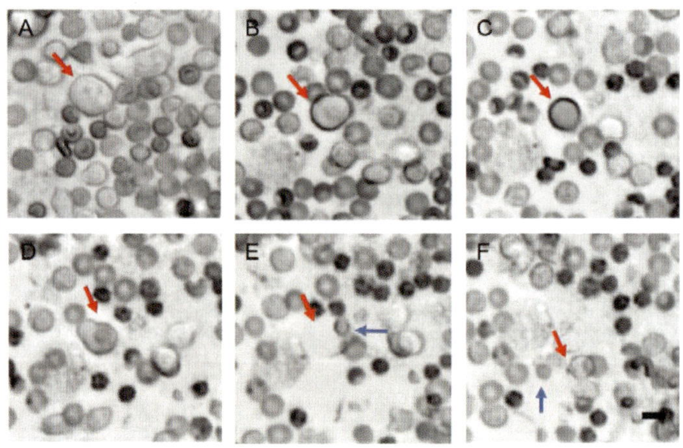

Figure 7: Real-time cultured of cells at Bright field. The red arrows indicate continuous change of the same cell from nuclear karyopyknosis to enucleation, and the blue arrows indicate extruded nucleus. Bar =5 μm.

Expression of erythroblast specific surface markers

Transferrin receptor (CD71) was involved in the absorption of iron and essential proteins that regulate the cell growth [18]. Presence of Ter119 was a sign of nucleated red blood cells. The expression of both markers could be used to determine the differentiation capability of erythroid cells. FVA cells cultured for 12 h, mouse bone marrow cells, mouse peripheral blood cells, MEL cells and NIH3T3 cells were tested. The results showed a decrease in CD71 and Ter119 expression from erythroid cells to NIH3T3 cells (Figure 11). The expression of both the proteins (CD71 and Ter119) in FVA cells cultured for 12 h were significantly higher than that of bone marrow cells and peripheral blood cells (Table 2).

Expression of the three cytoskeletal-associated proteins in eythroblast

The expression of three cytoskeletal-associated proteins (stathmin, RBBP4, and septin8) was decreased in the order of proerythroblasts, basophilic, polychromatic, and orthochromatic erythroblasts (Figure 12).

Discussion

Enucleation in the terminal differentiation of erythroblast is a multi-step complex process in which the nucleus, membrane, and cytoskeletal system are all involved. In this study, FVA cells were used for systematically studying the processes of differentiation and enucleation. By the stimulation of EPO, FVA cells proliferated and synergetically differentiated into basophilic, polychromatic, and orthochromatic erythroblasts. SEM results showed karyopyknosis, nuclear deviation, enucleation, and then generation of reticulocytes.

Real-time monitoring results showed it took about 7~8 hours from karyopyknosis to enucleation. During differentiation, immature nucleated cells gradually gathered around macrophages. Macrophages then engulfed the extruded nuclei, resulting in increased volumes at first and narrowed volumes later because the nuclei were digested in the latter phase.

Quantitative analysis of erythroid-specific marker proteins (CD71 and Ter119) showed that the expressions of both were higher than adult blood cells. All the results indicate that the differentiation of erythroid cells requires the synthesis of hemoglobin in abundance, so the transferrin receptor CD71 is highly expressed. When erythroid differentiation was induced in the constant presence of EPO in an *in vitro* differentiation system, CD71 expression was maintained during all stages of erythroid differentiation [19]. When EPO was removed from the culture medium, erythroid differentiation was better coupled with down-regulation of CD71 expression [20].

The microtubule depolymerization protein stathmin is a member of the protein family, which regulates the microtubule cytoskeleton. It also regulates microtubule polymerization via promoting microtubule depolymerization and preventing tubulin heterodimers [21]. Septin8 is a member of class conserved cytoskeletal GTP-binding proteins. It plays an important role in cell division, cell polarization, vesicle trafficking, membrane remodeling and many other important physiological processes [22]. Histone-binding protein RBBP4 is a component of

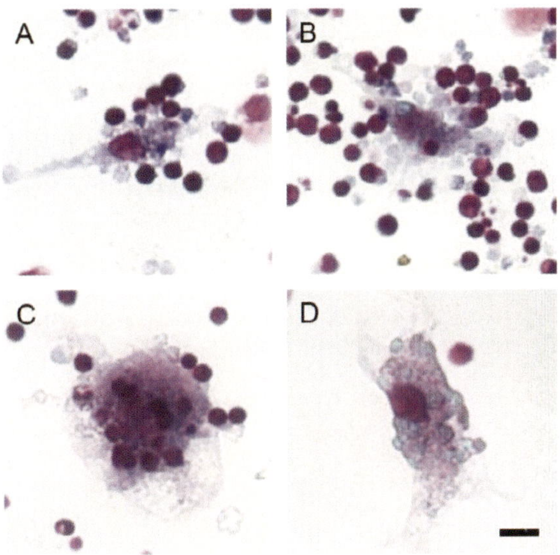

Figure 8: Wright's staining results of blood islands during Erythroid differentiation. (a-c) Engulfing nuclei by macrophage, (d) The shrunken cells due to the digestion of the nuclei. Bar =10 μm.

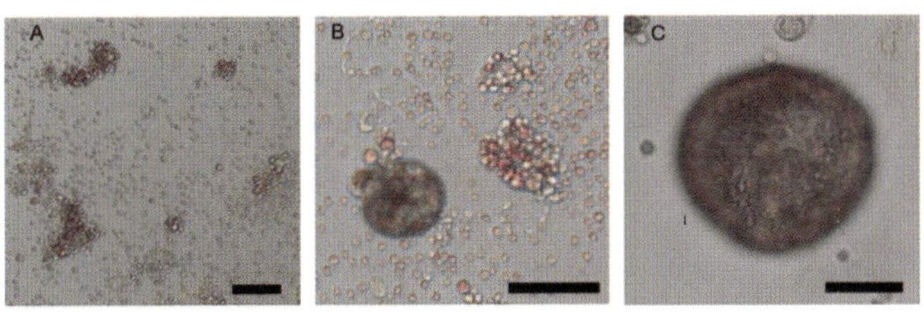

Figure 9: Bright field results of Fetal liver cells from E14.5 d fetal mouse after being induced by EPO for 24 h, 48 h, and 60 h in vitro. (a) Formation of blood islands at 24 h; (b) Increase in blood islands at 48 h (c) engulfment of nuclei at 60 h. Bar= 20 μm.

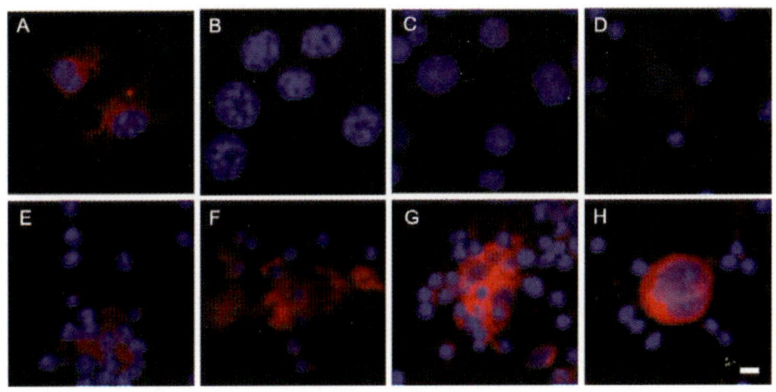

Figure 10: LSCM results of macrophage specific cell surface marker CD68 (red) and DAPI (blue). (a) Macrophages, CD68 positive control; (b) MEL cells, CD68 negative control; (c-h) CD68 and DAPI co-staining results of FVA cells in vitro after 12 h, 24 h, 36 h, 48 h, 60 h, 72 h. Bar =5 μm.

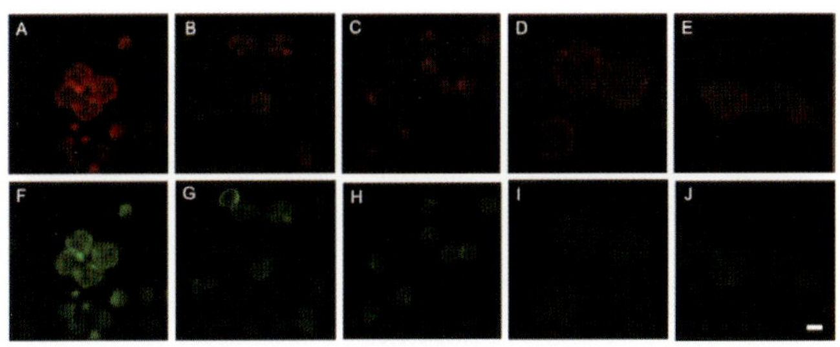

Figure 11: (a-e): The CD71 immunofluorescence staining results (red) of FVA 12 h cells, bone marrow cells, peripheral blood cells, MEL cells, and NIH3T3 cells, respectively. (f-j): The Ter119 (green) of FVA 12 h cells, bone marrow cells, peripheral blood cells, MEL cells, and NIH3T3 cells. Bar =5 μm.

Surface markers	FVA 12h cells	Bone marrow cells	Peripheral blood cells	MEL cells	NIH3T3 cells
CD71	1204.01 ± 25.02	374.56 ± 32.00*	425.48 ± 17.25*	258.16 ± 15.54*	222.43 ± 6.56*
Ter119	694.85 ± 23.43	230.46 ± 15.03*	214.48 ± 4.29*	100.31 ± 5.38*	67.76 ± 5.31*

P<0.05

Table 2: Fluorescence intensity of CD71 and Ter119 in five kinds of cells The fluorescence intensities of CD71 and Ter119 in FVA cells were significantly different from those of the other four cells (P <0.05)

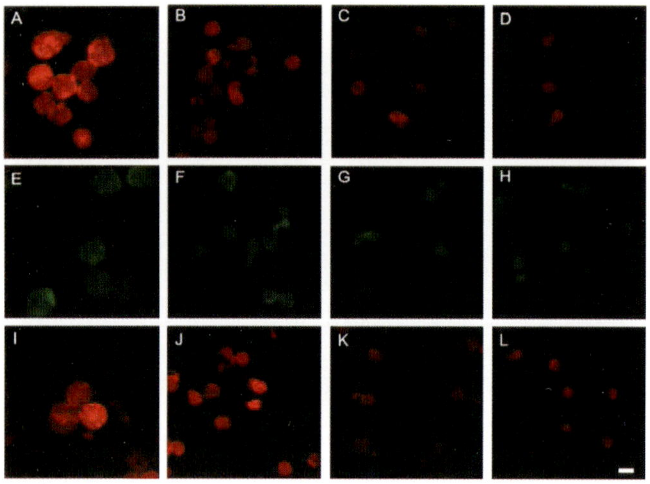

Figure 12: Immunofluorescence staining results of stathmin, septin8, RBBP4 in FVA cells after 2 h, 24 h, 36 h and 48 h. (a-d) Stathmin; (e-h) Septin8; (i-l) RBBP4. Bar =5 μm.

ATP-dependent chromosomal rearrangements complex, such as the nuclear chromatin remodeling and histone deacetylase complexes Sin3, and regulates the functions of the Sin3 [23]. The contents of the three cytoskeletal-associated proteins (stathmin, septin8, and RBBP4) decrease gradually during differentiation.

During the development and differentiation of mammalian erythroid cells, the changes in cell morphology and gene expression are showed regularity [24]. Enucleation is regulated by microtubules and PI3K signaling in a manner mechanistically similar to directed cell locomotion [25]. However, most molecular events in enucleation remain unclear, which gene regulates this process is not clear. Functions of cytoskeletal proteins, gene regulation and the mechanism of Erythroid differentiation need to be clarified by further studies.

References

1. Wendling F, Moreau-Gachelin F, Tambourin P (1981) Emergence of tumorigenic cells during the course of Friend virus leukemias. Proc Natl Acad Sci USA 78: 3614-3618.
2. Tambourin PE, Gallien-Lartigue O, Wendling F, Huaulme D (1973) Erythrocyte production in mice infected by the polycythaemia-inducing Friend virus or by the anaemia-inducing Friedn virus. Br J Haematol 24: 511-524.
3. Troxler DH, Ruscetti SK, Linemeyer DL, Scolnick ME (1980) Helper-independent and replication-defective erythroblastosis-inducing viruses contained within anemia-inducing friend virus complex (fv-a). Virology 102: 28-45.
4. Xue S, Zhang S, Du Q, Sun H, Xin J, et al. (1997) The role of cytoskeletal elements in the two-phase denucleation process of mammalian erythroblasts in vitro observed by laser confocal scanning microscope. Cell Mol Biol (Noisy-le-grand) 43: 851-860.
5. Koury ST, Koury MJ, Bondurant MC (1988) Morphological changes in erythroblasts during erythropoietin-induced terminal differentiation in vitro. Exp Hematol 16: 758-763.
6. Koury ST, Koury MJ, Bondurant MC (1989) Cytoskeletal distribution and function during the maturation and enucleation of mammalian erythroblasts. J Cell Biol 109: 3005-3013.
7. Bessis MC, Breton-Gorius J (1962) Iron metabolism in the bone marrow as seen by electron microscopy: a critical review. Blood 19: 635-663.
8. Seki M, Shirasawa H (1965) Role of the reticular cells during maturation process of the erythroblast. 3. The fate of phagocytized nucleus. Acta Pathol Jpn 15: 387-405.
9. Skutelsky E, Danon D (1972) On the expulsion of the erythroid nucleus and its phagocytosis. Anat Rec 173: 123-126.
10. Hanspal M, Hanspal JS (1994) The association of erythroblasts with macrophages promotes erythroid proliferation and maturation: a 30-kD heparin-binding protein is involved in this contact. Blood 84: 3494-3504.
11. Sadahira Y, Mori M (1999) Role of the macrophage in erythropoiesis. Pathol Int 49: 841-848.
12. Yokoyama T, Kitagawa H, Takeuchi T, Tsukahara S, Kannan Y (2002) No apoptotic cell death of erythroid cells of erythroblastic islands in bone marrow of healthy rats. J Vet Med Sci 64: 913-919.
13. Rhodes MM, Kopsombut P, Bondurant MC, Price JO, Koury MJ (2008) Adherence to macrophages in erythroblastic islands enhances erythroblast proliferation and increases erythrocyte production by a different mechanism than erythropoietin. Blood 111: 1700-1708.
14. Ramos P, Casu C, Gardenghi S, Breda L, Crielaard BJ, et al. (2013) Macrophages support pathological erythropoiesis in polycythemia vera and β-thalassemia. Nat Med 19: 437-445.
15. Lee JC, Gimm JA, Lo AJ, Koury MJ, Krauss SW, et al. (2004) Mechanism of protein sorting during erythroblast enucleation: role of cytoskeletal connectivity. Blood 103: 1912-1919.
16. Dzierzak E, Philipsen S (2013) Erythropoiesis: development and differentiation. Cold Spring Harb Perspect Med 3: a011601.
17. Paape M, Hafs H, Snyder W (1963) Variation of estimated numbers of milk somatic cells stained with wright's stain or pyronin yâ€"methyl green stain. Journal of Dairy Science 46: 1211-1216.
18. Daniels TR, Delgado T, Rodriguez JA, Helguera G, Penichet ML (2006) The transferrin receptor part I: Biology and targeting with cytotoxic antibodies for the treatment of cancer. Clin Immunol 121: 144-158.
19. Sposi NM, Cianetti L, Tritarelli E, Pelosi E, Militi S, et al. (2000) Mechanisms of differential transferrin receptor expression in normal hematopoiesis. Eur J Biochem 267: 6762-6774.
20. Zhang J, Socolovsky M, Gross AW, Lodish HF (2003) Role of Ras signaling in erythroid differentiation of mouse fetal liver cells: functional analysis by a flow cytometry-based novel culture system. Blood 102: 3938-3946.
21. Rubin CI, Atweh GF (2004) The role of stathmin in the regulation of the cell cycle. J Cell Biochem 93: 242-250.
22. Saarikangas J, Barral Y (2011) The emerging functions of septins in metazoans. EMBO Rep 12: 1118-1126.
23. Dobrzycka KM, Townson SM, Jiang S, Oesterreich S (2003) Estrogen receptor corepressors -- a role in human breast cancer? Endocr Relat Cancer 10: 517-536.
24. Lu SJ, Feng Q, Park JS, Vida L, Lee BS, et al. (2008) Biologic properties and enucleation of red blood cells from human embryonic stem cells. Blood 112: 4475-4484.
25. Wang J, Ramirez T, Ji P, Jayapal SR, Lodish HF, et al. (2012) Mammalian erythroblast enucleation requires PI3K-dependent cell polarization. J Cell Sci 125: 340-349.

7

Clinical Significance of Wt1 mRNA Levels in Japanese Acute Lymphoblastic Leukemia Patients

Yoshiko Hashii[1, 29]*, Yoshiyuki Kosaka[2], Kenichiro Watanabe[3], Koji Kato[4], Masue Imaizumi[5], Takashi Kaneko[6], Shosuke Sunami[7], Arata Watanabe[8], Hidefumi Hiramatsu[9], Yuhki Koga[10], Masahiro Hirayama[11], Takafumi Nakao[12], Tomoko Hata[13], Naoyuki Uchida[14], Ken Ishiyama[15], Kinuko Mitani[16], Michihiro Hidaka[17], Kunio Kitamura[18], Hiroko Tsunemine[19], Yasunori Ueda[20], Atsuko Mugitani[21], Kensuke Usuki[22], Yoshinobu Kanda[23], Yoshihide Miyazaki[24], Kiyotoshi Imai[25], Tomoki Naoe[26], Katsuyoshi Koh[27], Haruo Sugiyama[28] and Keizo Horibe[29]

[1]*Department of Pediatrics, Osaka University Graduate School of Medicine, Osaka, Japan*
[2]*Department of Hematology and Oncology, Children's Cancer Center, Hyogo Prefectural Kobe Children's Hospital, Hyogo, Japan*
[3]*Department of Hematology and Oncology, Shizuoka Children's Hospital, Shizuoka, Japan*
[4]*Department of Pediatrics, Japanese Red Cross Nagoya Daiichi Hospital, Aichi, Japan*
[5]*Department of Hematology and Oncology, Miyagi Children's Hospital, Miyagi, Japan*
[6]*Department of Hematology/Oncology, Tokyo Metropolitan Children's Medical Center, Tokyo, Japan*
[7]*Department of Pediatrics, Japanese Red Cross Narita Hospital, Chiba, Japan*
[8]*Department of Pediatrics, Nakadori General Hospital, Akita, Japan*
[9]*Department of Pediatrics, Graduate School of Medicine, Kyoto University, Kyoto, Japan*
[10]*Department of Pediatrics, Graduate School of Medical Sciences, Kyushu University, Fukuoka, Japan*
[11]*Department of Pediatrics, Mie University Graduate School of Medicine, Mie, Japan*
[12]*Department of Hematology, Osaka City General Hospital, Osaka, Japan*
[13]*Department of Hematology, Atomic Bomb Disease Institute, Nagasaki University, Nagasaki, Japan*
[14]*Department of Hematology, Toranomon Hospital, Tokyo, Japan*
[15]*Department of Hematology, Kanazawa University Hospital, Ishikawa, Japan*
[16]*Department of Hematology and Oncology, Dokkyo Medical University, School of Medicine, Tochigi, Japan*
[17]*Department of Hematology, National Hospital Organization Kumamoto Medical Center, Kumamoto, Japan*
[18]*Division of Hematology, Ichinomiya Municipal Hospital, Aichi, Japan*
[19]*Department of Hematology, Shinko Hospital, Hyogo, Japan*
[20]*Department of Haematology/Oncology, Transfusion and Haemapheresis Center, Kurashiki Central Hospital, Okayama, Japan*
[21]*Department of Hematology, Seichokai Fuchu Hospital, Osaka, Japan*
[22]*Department of Hematology, NTT Medical Center, Tokyo, Japan*
[23]*Division of Hematology, Department of Medicine, Jichi Medical University, Tochigi, Japan*
[24]*Diagnostic Division, Otsuka Pharmaceutical Co., Ltd., Tokushima, Japan*
[25]*Department of Hematology, Sapporo Hokuyu Hospital, Sapporo, Japan*
[26]*National Hospital Organization Nagoya Medical Center, Aichi, Japan*
[27]*Department of Hematology/Oncology, Saitama Children's Medical Center, Saitama, Japan*
[28]*Department of Cancer Immunotherapy, Osaka University Graduate School of Medicine, Osaka, Japan*
[29]*Clinical Research Center, National Hospital Organization Nagoya Medical Center, Aichi, Japan*

Abstract

This study enrolled 49 patients with *de novo* childhood acute lymphoblastic leukemia (ALL) and 19 adult patients with ALL. WT1 mRNA showed high positive expression rates of 90% or more in ALL patients, and fusion gene transcripts were detected in 22.4% of childhood ALL cases prior to treatment. During follow-up at 4-6 months, WT1 mRNA levels in childhood ALL cases were observed to be lower in patients undergoing hematological remission after treatment when compared to the initial stages. We also assessed hematological remission via ROC analysis. The upper cut-off values were calculated to be 220 and 1,820 copies/μg-RNA in the peripheral blood (PB) and bone marrow (BM) samples, respectively. Since 50 copies/μg-RNA was determined to be both, the limit of detection (LOD) and minimal residual disease (MRD) threshold, WT1 mRNA regions below the upper cut-off values indicated remission depth. The detection of high WT1 mRNA levels, even in patients without fusion gene transcripts, reflected the treatment effects and remission depth, demonstrating its capacity to be a useful MRD monitoring marker in ALL.

Keywords: WT1 mRNA; Reverse transcription-polymerase chain reaction (RT-PCR); Acute lymphoblastic leukemia (ALL); Minimal residual disease (MRD)

Introduction

Acute lymphoblastic leukemia (ALL), a hematologic malignancy characterized by tumorigenic changes in the juvenile lymphoid cell and the bone marrow infiltration, has an annual incidence of approximately 1.7 in 100,000 children and adult per year [1]. ALL accounts for 70% of leukemia/malignant lymphoma in children, and it is estimated to be newly diagnosed in 550–600 children annually in Japan [2].

When selecting a treatment strategy to induce the remission of ALL/Lymphoblastic Lymphoma (LBL), the presence of the Philadelphia (Ph) chromosome is initially used for classification purposes. While a positive Ph chromosome results in priority treatments with tyrosine kinase inhibitors such as imatinib, a pediatric protocol (Programa Español de Tratamiento en Hematología ALL-96) [3] has been recommended for adolescent or young adult patients (below 30 years of age) presenting as Ph chromosome-negative. In Europe and America, more than 2,000

***Corresponding author:** Yoshiko Hashii, MD, PhD, Department of Pediatrics, Osaka University Graduate School of Medicine, 2-2 Yamadaoka, Suita, Osaka 565-0871, Japan, E-mail: yhashii@ped.med.osaka-u.ac.jp patients included in the Berlin-Frankfurt-Münster, Medical Research Council or Children's Oncology Group clinical studies have shown improved treatment outcomes via appropriate stratification [4].

Currently, treatment optimization has been attempted by quantifying and using minimal residual disease (MRD) for stratification. In the Japan Pediatric Leukemia Lymphoma Study Group (JPLSG), which was started in 2012, MRD has been used for stratification under the ALL-B12 protocol throughout Japan.

Monitoring MRD is important in predicting a patient's disease relapse and optimizing the treatment strategy. While morphological examination can reveal a decrease in lymphoblasts in the bone marrow (BM) or peripheral blood (PB), indicating hematological remission, MRD cannot be detected by this method and therefore, molecular methods are employed. MRD in ALL patients has been measured and assessed using several techniques such as quantification of fusion gene transcripts [5-8], immunoreceptor (immunoglobulin/T-cell receptor (*Ig/TCR*)) gene rearrangements [9-12], and flow cytometry [8,13-15]. However, fusion gene transcripts are expressed in approximately 25% of adult ALL patients and 3% of childhood ALL patients, even in minor *BCR/ABL*, which is thought to have the highest expression frequency [16]. Even when other fusion gene transcripts are combined, fusion gene transcripts as an MRD monitoring marker can only be used in a small number of patients. MRD quantification via flow cytometry [8,17] requires professional skills and experience and is only used in medical (research) institutions. MRD quantification via *Ig/TCR* gene rearrangements requires a primer setting specific to the clone. Although the sensitivity of the technique is high, the associated cost is also high, and the proliferation needs to occur in the same clone. Recently, a next-generation sequencer identified cancerous cells to have multiple clones rather than just one. Based on this theory, relapse is thought to occur via the subclones tolerant to chemotherapy. This sequencer detects relapse with different gene rearrangements [18]. MRD detection and the use of bone marrow has also been investigated with this next-generation sequencer, but the associated cost was high [19].

Wilms' tumor 1 (WT1) is expressed in high frequency in the PB and BM of many patients with acute myeloid leukemia (AML) [20,21]. The development of *in vitro* WT1 messenger RNA (mRNA) diagnostics has resulted in its wide use in clinical practice as an MRD monitoring marker. Interestingly, WT1 mRNA is also expressed in ALL patients as noted in the following reports. In adult ALL patients, immature B-ALL cases expressed higher levels of WT1 mRNA than B-ALL cases [22], and T-ALL cases expressed higher levels of WT1 mRNA than B-ALL cases [23]. Furthermore, WT1 mRNA levels in a positive group of myeloid markers (CD13, CD33, CD15, and CD65) were higher than those in a negative group [22]. Patients with high expressions of WT1 mRNA exhibited shorter overall survival and disease-free survival periods, and the increase in the WT1 mRNA level in the BM related to the significantly increased risk of relapse. Therefore, WT1 mRNA has been reported to be a useful indicator in predicting prognosis [23-25].

Based on the above findings, we investigated the clinical significance of WT1 mRNA as an MRD monitoring marker in ALL patients by measuring the PB and BM WT1 mRNA levels in childhood and adult ALL patients.

Materials and Methods

Patients and samples

Between December 2014 and December 2015, BM and PB samples from 49 children and 19 adult patients with *de novo* ALL were collected by the investigators from their respective medical institutions as shown in Table 1. PB and BM samples from each patient were collected on the same day and used for WT1 mRNA measurement. The experimental protocol was reviewed and approved by the appropriate local ethics committees.

Among the pediatric patients, 43 patients were diagnosed with B-precursor ALL, 5 with pre-B-ALL, and 1 with T-ALL according to the immunophenotypic analysis. Among the adult ALL patients, 15 were diagnosed with B-precursor ALL and 3 were diagnosed with pre-B-ALL. The subclass for 1 remaining adult ALL patients could not be determined due to the lack of the flow cytometry measurement.

Out of the 49 childhood ALL patients who underwent induction therapy, 1 patient was transferred and hence, follow up was not possible. The remaining 48 childhood ALL patients achieved hematological remission after induction therapy.

All childhood ALL patients followed the JPLSG ALL-B12 protocol, which consisted of a prophase therapy (prednisolone across all risks), an induction therapy (prednisolone, daunorubicin, L-asparaginase, intrathecal injection of prednisolone + methotrexate + cytarabine), and an early consolidation therapy (cyclophosphamide, cytarabine, 6-mercaptopurine for intermediate risk, randomization of vincristine + L-asparaginase for high risk, intrathecal injection of prednisolone + methotrexate + cytarabine) followed by a consolidation therapy and a maintenance therapy. We classified the follow-up period as 4–6 months after the start of the treatment and collected the BM and PB samples from childhood ALL patients at the following time points: 1) before treatment, 2) after induction therapy, 3) after early consolidation therapy, and 4) later stage of the early consolidation therapy. BM and PB samples from adult ALL patients were collected prior to the treatment. Informed consent was obtained from all patients above 20 years of age, or from a legal representative for patients 16 years and above but less than 20 years, or from the guardians of patients under the age of 16 years.

WT1 mRNA level

We used the following calculation method elucidated by Kitamura et al. [26] to measure the expression of WT1 mRNA: total RNA was extracted from the patient PB or BM samples using the QIAamp RNA Blood Mini kit (Qiagen, Valencia, CA, USA), and WT1 mRNA was determined using the WT1 mRNA OneStep Assay Kit (Otsuka Pharmaceutical Co., Ltd., Tokyo, Japan) based on a one-step reverse transcription quantitative polymerase chain reaction (RT-qPCR). The PCR primer and TaqMan probe from this kit assigned to exon 6–7, and glyceraldehyde-3-phosphate dehydrogenase (GAPDH) was used as a comparative control [26,27]. The WT1 mRNA expression levels were calculated by multiplying the value obtained after dividing the measured WT1 mRNA with the measured value of GAPDH mRNA

Classification for the immunophenotypic groups		No. of patients		
		Childhood	Adult	Total
B-lineage ALL	B-precursor ALL	43	15	58
	pre-B ALL	5	3	8
	mature B ALL	0	0	0
T-lineage ALL		1	0	1
Unknown		0	1	1
Total		49*	19	68

ALL adult acute lymphoblastic leukemia
* In one out of 49 children, peripheral blood samples could not be collected before treatment.
a. WT1 mRNA expression levels in PB

Table 1: Immunophenotypic profile of 68 de novo cases of childhood and adult acute lymphoblastic leukemia by flow cytometric analysis in JPLSG.

(number of WT1 mRNA copies per copy of GAPDH mRNA) with the mean GAPDH mRNA measurement value per 1 μg of RNA (2.7×10^7 copies/μg-RNA) based on independent tests in healthy adults [20]. The unit for WT1 mRNA expression was prescribed as copies/μg-RNA. The method to calculate WT1 mRNA expression is shown below:

$$WT1\ mRNA\ expression = (copies / \mu g - RNA)\frac{Measured\ value\ of\ WT1\ mRNA\ (copies/mL)}{Measured\ value\ of\ GAPDH\ mRNA\ (copies/mL)} \times 2.7 \times 10^7\ (copies / \mu g - RNA)^*$$

*2.7×10^7 (copies/μg-RNA): Mean GAPDH mRNA measurement value per 1 μg of RNA in a PB sample of a healthy adult.

Fusion gene transcripts

At the initial diagnosis, we screened for fusion gene transcripts. In this test, total RNA was extracted from the patient PB or BM samples and the following nine fusion gene transcripts were measured by RT-qPCR: major *BCR-ABL*, minor *BCR-ABL*, *E2A-PBX1*, *ETV6-AML1*, *MLL-AF4*, *MLL-AF6*, *MLL-AF9*, *MLL-ENL*, and *SIL-TAL1* [28]. Upon detection, we assayed the fusion gene transcripts and measured the WT1 mRNA levels [29,30].

Ig/TCR gene rearrangements

For the analysis of the rearranged immunoglobulin (Ig) and T-cell receptor (*TCR*) genes, qPCR was performed using standardized allele-specific oligonucleotide (ASO) primer/probe sets for the junctional regions of IgH, Igκ, TCRδ, TCRγ, TCRβ, or TAL1 [10]. Genomic DNA was isolated from the PB or BM samples using the QIAamp DNA Mini kit (Qiagen, Valencia, CA, USA), and a 10-μL aliquot of the isolated DNA was subjected to qPCR involving 50 cycles with 0.25 μL of each ASO primer using a StepOnePlus Real-Time PCR system (Thermo Fisher Scientific, Waltham, MA, USA). Each PCR cycle included denaturation at 95°C for 15 s and primer annealing and extension at 60°C for 1 min, after pretreatment at 50°C for 2 min and 95°C for 10 min. MRD was identified by screening by multiplex PCR with allele-specific oligonucleotide primers. Then, the quantitative value of Ig/TCR gene rearrangements was corrected using the albumin gene, which was simultaneously quantified as the internal control. The quantitative limit of the MRD targets in qPCR was 10^{-5} for the *Ig/TCR* gene rearrangements.

Flow cytometry

Ficoll-Hypaque-enriched blasts were stained by five-color immunofluorescence staining. The fluorophores phycoerythrin (PE), fluorescein isothiocyanate (FITC), phycoerythrin-cyanin 7 (PC7), or allophycocyanin (APC) were used in conjugation with the following antigens: CD1a, CD2, CD3, CD4, CD5, CD7, CD8, CD10, CD11b, CD13, CD14, CD15, CD19, CD20, CD21, CD22, CD24, CD33, CD34, CD36, CD38, CD41, CD42b, CD45, CD56, CD58, CD61, CD64, CD65, CD66c, CD99, CD117, Glycophorin-A (CD235a), HLA-DR, Immunoglobulin κ and λ light chains, T-cell receptor (TCR-α/β and TCR-γ/δ), cytoplasmic μ chain, cytoplasmic CD3, cytoplasmic CD22, cytoplasmic CD79a, cytoplasmic MPO, cytoplasmic TdT, and CRLF2. An isotype-matched immunoglobulin was used as the negative control. The analysis gate was set using CD45, for which low-blast gates were stained using various combinations of monoclonal antibodies. These antibody combinations used in this study were modified from those used in the study by Iwamoto et al. [31].

Classification of pediatric and adult ALL patients

The ALL patients were classified into immunophenotypic groups from the results obtained via flow cytometry according to the immunological diagnostic criteria of the JPLSG [31]. Definition of the four risk groups are as follows: B-precursor ALL (positive for 2 or more of CD19, CD20, CD22, or CD79a, and negative throughout the intracytoplasmic μ-chain, Igκ, and Igλ); pre-B ALL (positive for 2 or more of CD19, CD20, CD22, or CD79a, positive intracytoplasmic μ-chain, and negative Igκ and Igλ); mature B-ALL (positive for 2 or more of CD19, CD20, CD22, or CD79a, and positive Igκ or positive Igλ); and T-ALL (T-cell line).

Statistical analysis

For group comparison, logarithmic transformed values of WT1 mRNA levels (copies/μg-RNA) were used for the Student's *t*-test, Fisher's exact test, two-way factorial analysis of variance, and Dunnett test or Tukey-Kramer honestly significant difference (HSD) test. Differences with $p<0.05$ were considered to be significant.

For the WT1 mRNA level, mean ± standard deviation was calculated with logarithmic transformed values of WT1 mRNA (copies/μg-RNA) and the mean was considered to be the value (back-transformed mean). Measured values below 50 copies/μg-RNA of WT1 mRNA were all treated as 49 copies/μg-RNA. Additionally, the Pearson's correlation coefficient was also calculated and evaluated.

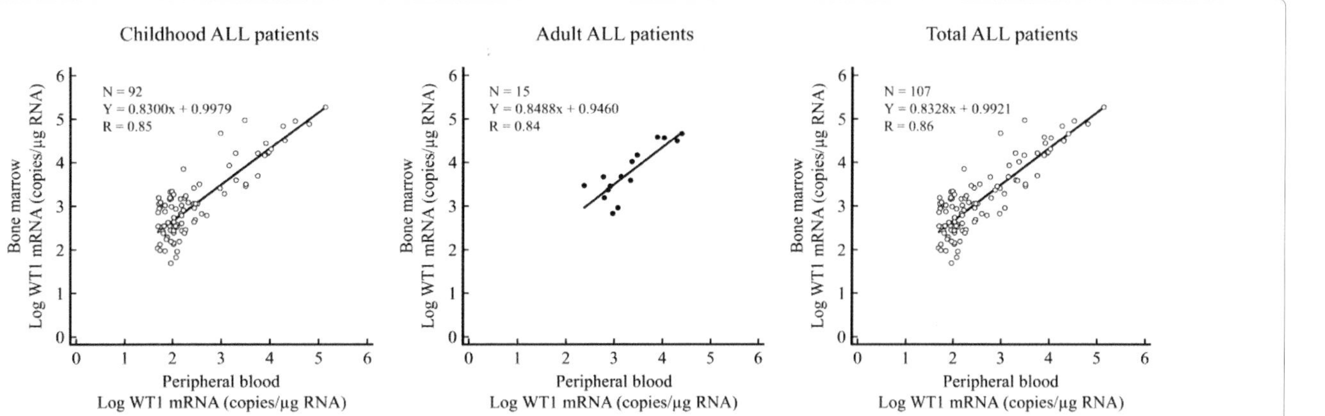

Figure 1: Correlation of WT1 mRNA expression in peripheral blood (PB) and Wilms' tumor 1 (WT1) mRNA expression in bone marrow (BM) from childhood acute lymphoblastic leukemia (ALL) patients, adult ALL patients, and total ALL patients.

Results

Correlation between the PB and BM WT1 mRNA levels

Figure 1 shows the correlation between the PB and BM WT1 mRNA levels from all the measured samples. Samples from both, childhood ALL and adult ALL, demonstrated good correlation of WT1 mRNA values between BM and PB (correlation coefficient: r=0.85 and 0.84, respectively) and the regression lines were similar. The limit of detection (LOD) in PB was 50 copies/μg-RNA, which was used as a threshold for MRD. Therefore, 260 copies/μg-RNA of BM, which was obtained by substituting the LOD of PB into the correlation regression line equation, was considered to be the cut-off value to indicate BM abnormality. Subsequently, it was also specified as the cut-off value for WT1 mRNA positivity in the BM samples of ALL patients.

WT1 mRNA level and the positive rate in de novo ALL patients

Table 2 shows the WT1 mRNA levels and positive rates with respect to subtypes (B-precursor ALL and pre-B ALL) in the PB and BM samples of *de novo* ALL patients. The cut-off values for WT1 positive/negative were determined as 50 copies/μg-RNA for PB and 260 copies/μg-RNA for BM. In *de novo* childhood ALL patients, WT1 mRNA positivity was detected in the PB of 45 out of 48 patients (excluding one patient whose PB sample was not collected at diagnosis; 93.8%) and the BM of 39 out of 43 patients who were able to provide samples (90.7%). In *de novo* adult ALL patients, the positivity rate was 89.5% (17 out of 19 patients) for PB samples and 94.1% (16 out of 17 patients) for BM samples. The PB and BM sample from both, childhood and adult ALL patients, showed a high rate of positivity. With respect to the subtypes, PB samples from B-precursor ALL showed higher mean values than those from pre-B ALL in both, childhood and adult ALL patients (Figure 2a). The BM samples from B-precursor ALL also showed higher mean values than those from pre-B ALL (Figure 2b). Among the entire ALL subtype, the mean values of the PB samples from the B-precursor ALL was significantly higher than those from the pre-B ALL ($p<0.05$; Figure 2a).

Changes in the WT1 mRNA levels during follow-up

Figure 3 shows the changes in the WT1 mRNA levels in the PB and BM samples from 48 childhood ALL patients during follow-up, except for the one transferred patient. All 48 patients were in the hematological remission phase at all blood collection points after treatment. WT1 mRNA levels were observed to decrease (in 40 out of 48 PB samples (83.3%) and in 35 out of 42 BM samples (83.3%); $p < 0.01$; Dunnett test) at all points of blood collection after treatment when compared to any point prior to treatment.

WT1 mRNA and fusion gene transcripts

Screening for fusion gene transcripts in childhood ALL patients was performed prior to treatment and 7 patients with *ETV6-AML1*, 2 patients with *E2A-PBX1*, 1 patient with minor *BCR-ABL*, and 1 patient with major *BCR-ABL* was detected. The detection rate was observed to be 22.4% (11 out of 49 samples), which was significantly lower than that of WT1 mRNA (93.8% in PB and 90.7% in BM, $p<0.01$; Fisher's exact test). Figure 4 shows the changes in expression during follow-up in 11 patients with fusion gene transcripts. Moreover, the WT1 mRNA expression level in the BM and PB of all the patients tended to decrease to that of the fusion gene transcripts.

WT1 mRNA levels by hematological phases

Except for one patient who transferred during the follow-up, the other 48 childhood ALL patients were in the hematological remission phase at blood collection points after starting treatment. Therefore, we compared the WT1 mRNA levels at all blood collection points during the untreated and remission phases (Figure 5). As a result, WT1 mRNA levels during the remission phase were significantly lower than those during the untreated phase in both, PB and BM samples ($p<0.01$; Student's t-test). To assess remission in terms of WT1 mRNA levels, we calculated the cut-off values of WT1 mRNA in both groups to

Group		B-precursor ALL	pre-B ALL	T ALL	unknown	Total
Childhood ALL	No. of patients	42	5	1	-	48
	Mean (range) (copies/μg RNA)	1,100 (<50-140,000)	270 (<50-3,300)	91		910 (<50-140,000)
	Positive rate (%)	95.2 (40/42)	80.0 (4/5)	100 (1/1)		93.8 (45/48)
Adult ALL	No. of patients	15	3	-	1	19
	Mean (range) (copies/μg RNA)	2,090 (<50-25,000)	330 (<50-3,000)		1,100	1,480 (<50-25,000)
	Positive rate (%)	93.3 (14/15)	66.7 (2/3)		100 (1/1)	89.5 (17/19)
Total ALL	No. of patients	57	8	1	1	67
	Mean (range) (copies/μg RNA)	1,290 (<50-140,000)	290 (<50-3,300)	91	1,100	1,050 (<50-140,000)
	Positive rate (%)	94.7 (54/57)	75.0 (6/8)	100 (1/1)	100 (1/1)	92.5 (62/67)
	b. WT1 mRNA expression in BM					
Group		B-precursor ALL	pre-B ALL	T ALL	unknown	Total
Childhood ALL	No. of patients	38	4	1	-	43
	Mean (range) (copies/μg RNA)	3,890 (90-180,000)	800 (320-3,100)	1,500		3,240 (90-180,000)
	Positive rate (%)	89.5 (34/38)	100 (4/4)	100 (1/1)		90.7 (39/43)
Adult ALL	No. of patients	14	3	-	-	17
	Mean (range) (copies/μg RNA)	5,620 (650-45,000)	1,260 (<50-14,000)			4,270 (<50-45,000)
	Positive rate (%)	100 (14/14)	66.7 (2/3)			94.1 (16/17)
Total ALL	No. of patients	52	7	1	-	60
	Mean (range) (copies/μg RNA)	4,270 (90-180,000)	960 (<50-14,000)	1,500		3,310 (<50-180,000)
	Positive rate (%)	92.3 (54/57)	85.7 (6/7)	100 (1/1)		91.7 (55/60)

Numbers in parentheses indicate number of patients

Table 2: WT1 mRNA expression levels and WT1 mRNA-positive rate in PB and BM on initial untreated ALL patients.

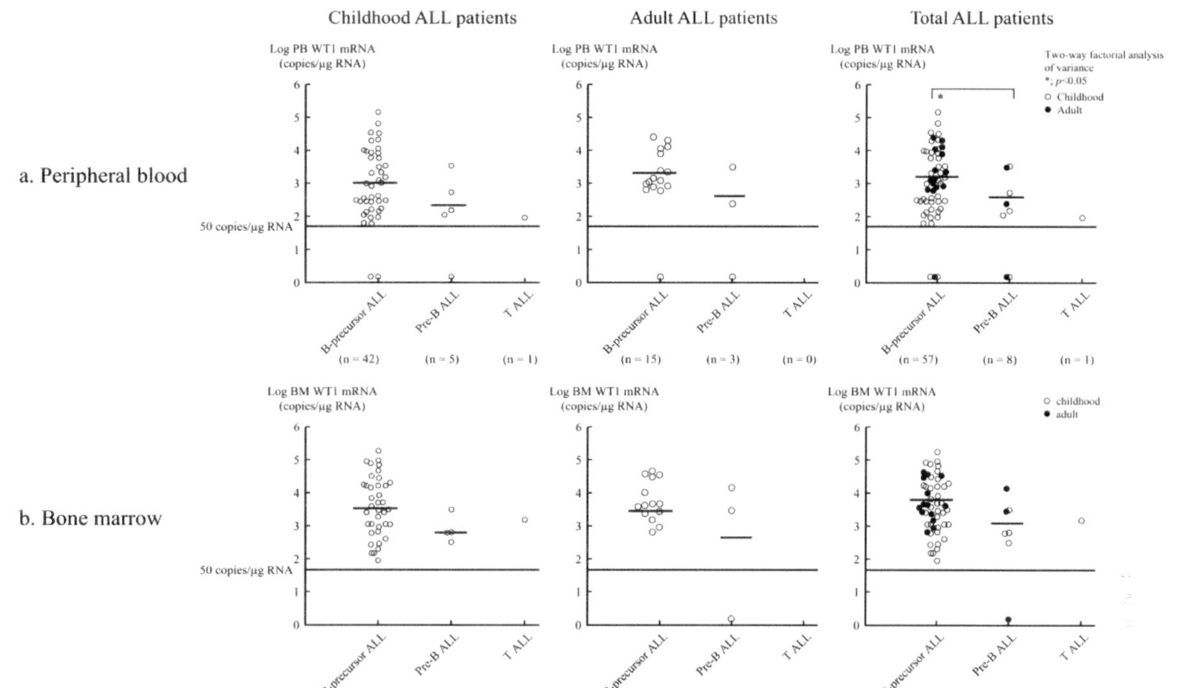

Figure 2: Comparison among ALL immunophenotypes by Wilms' tumor 1 (WT1) mRNA expression from childhood acute lymphoblastic leukemia (ALL) patients, adult ALL patients, and total ALL patients. a. peripheral blood; b. Bone marrow. Bold lines represent mean WT1 mRNA expression after log transformation. Fine line represents minimum limit of detection of WT1 mRNA (50 copies/µg-RNA).

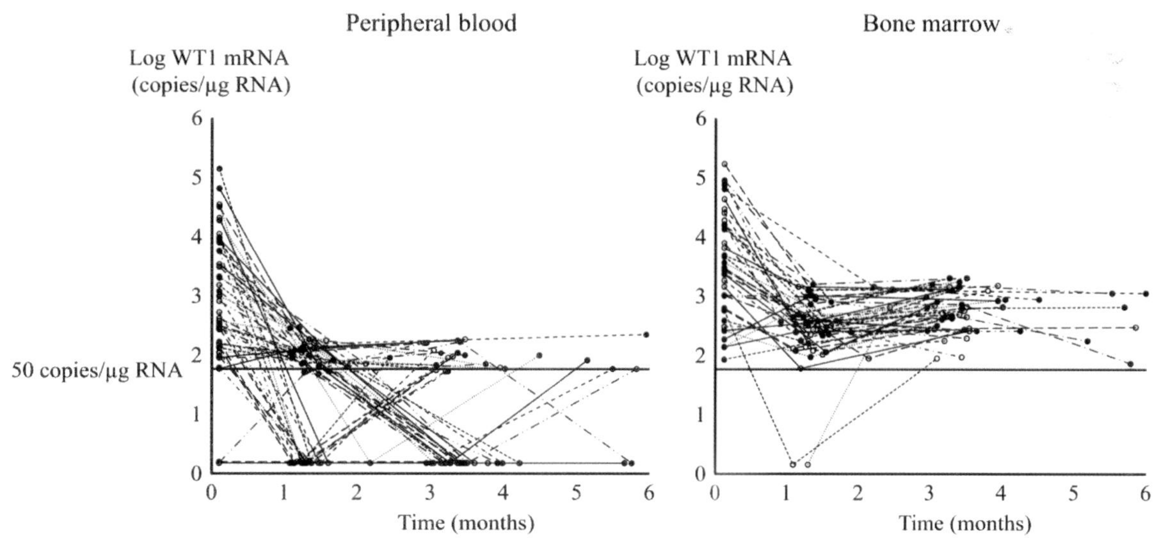

Figure 3: Changes in Wilms' tumor 1 (WT1) mRNA expression levels in peripheral blood (PB) and bone marrow (BM) samples on 48 follow-up cases. Fine line represents minimum limit of detection of WT1 mRNA (50 copies/µg-RNA).

differentiate the remission phase via receiver operating characteristic (ROC) analysis. Figure 6 shows the results of the analysis. The cutoff values obtained to determine remission were 220 copies/µg-RNA for PB and 1,820 copies/µg-RNA for BM. The -sensitivity and specificity for PB were determined to be 68.8% (33 out of 48 samples) and 98.0% (99 out of 101 samples) respectively, whereas the sensitivity and specificity for BM were determined to be 58.1% (25 out of 43 samples) and 98.0% (97 out of 99 samples) respectively.

WT1 mRNA and Ig/TCR gene rearrangements

The analysis of Ig/TCR gene rearrangements was performed using BM from five child patients with B-precursor ALL and one with Pre-B ALL at different time points before treatment, after induction, and after early consolidation. The gene rearrangements were detected in the BM of all six patients at the time point before treatment, and in four patients after induction. After early consolidation, the gene rearrangements

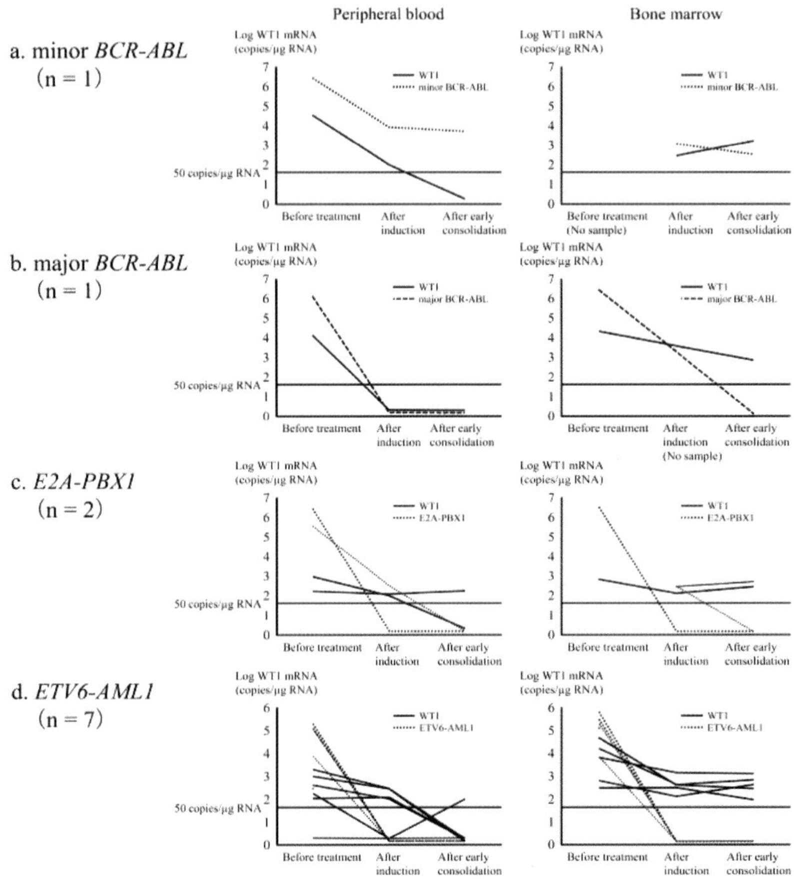

Figure 4: Transition between fusion gene transcript and Wilms' tumor 1 (WT1) mRNA expression levels. a. minor *BCR-ABL* (n=1); b. major *BCR-ABL* (n=1; c. E2A/PBX1 (n=2); and d. ETV6-AML1 (n=7). Fine line represents minimum limit of detection of WT1 mRNA (50 copies/μg-RNA). Changes in expression levels of fusion gene transcript in PB on the left side and BM on the right side were indicated by dotted lines for each detected type of fusion gene transcript, the transition of WT1 mRNA expression in the same patient was superimposed by solid line.

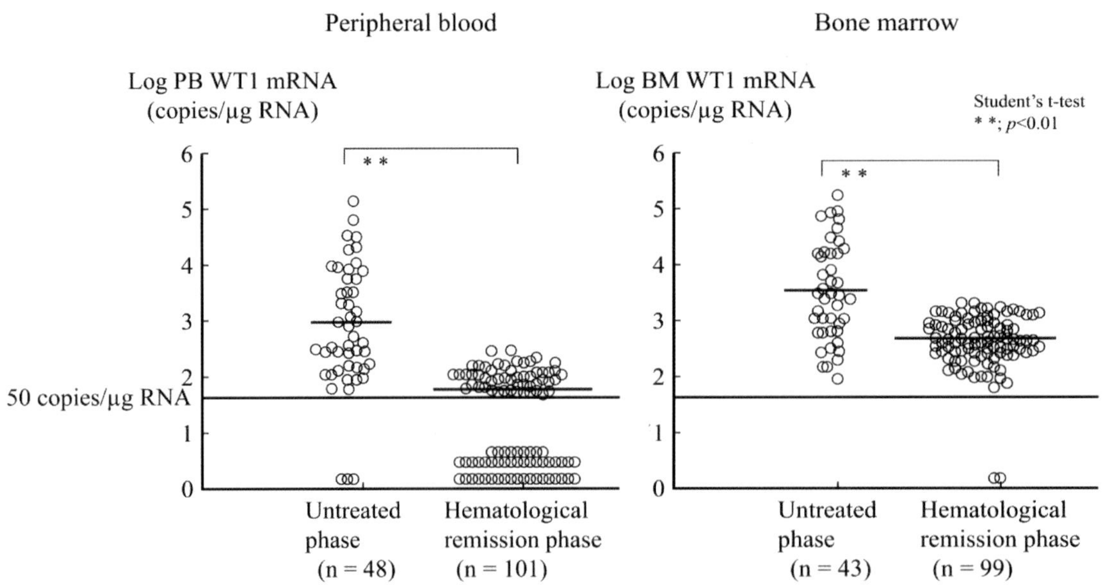

Figure 5: Comparison of Wilms' tumor 1 (WT1) mRNA expression levels in PB and BM between hematological remission phase and untreated phase. Fine line represent minimum limit of detection of WT1 mRNA (50 copies/μg-RNA).

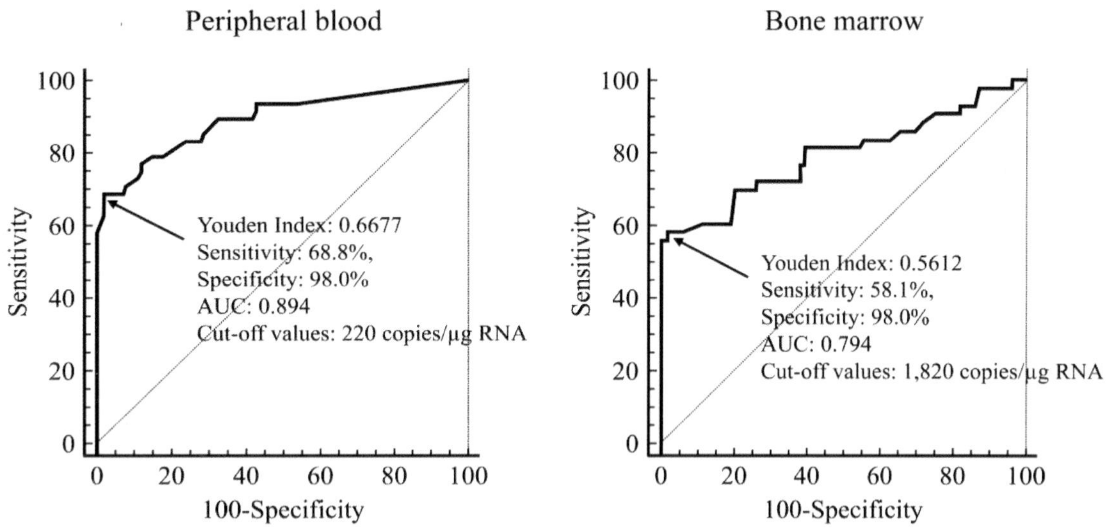

Figure 6: Receiver operating characteristic (ROC) analysis by Wilms' tumor 1 (WT1) mRNA expression as an indicator to differentiate between hematological remission phase and untreated phase.

Patient No.	Analysis method for MRD	Sample	Time point for sample collection		
			Before treatment	After induction	After early consolidation
No.02-001 (B-precursor ALL)	WT1 mRNA	BM	280	370	1,500
		PB	60	130	180
	Ig/TCR gene Rearrangement	BM	1	negative	negative
No.02-004 (B-precursor ALL)	WT1 mRNA	BM	31,000	330	1,300
		PB	21,000	<50	<50
	Ig/TCR gene rearrangement	BM	1	1.90×10^{-4}	positive, outside QR
No.05-001 (B-precursor ALL)	WT1 mRNA	BM	76,000	230	490
		PB	64,000	66	<50
	Ig/TCR gene rearrangement	BM	1	9.20×10^{-5}	negative
No.07-001 (Pre-B ALL)	WT1 mRNA	BM	640	130	270
		PB	150	110	160
	Ig/TCR gene rearrangement	BM	1	positive, outside QR	negative
No.07-003 (B-precursor ALL)	WT1 mRNA	BM	no sample	290	1,500
		PB	32,000	100	<50
	Ig/TCR gene rearrangement	BM	1	1.60×10^{-4}	positive, outside QR
No.07-004 (B-precursor ALL)	WT1 mRNA	BM	16,000	1,700	2,100
		PB	5,800	190	100
	Ig/TCR gene rearrangement	BM	1	negative	negative

Abbreviations: ALL, acute lymphoblastic leukemia; Ig, immunoglobulin; MRD, minimal residual disease; TCR, T-cell receptor; Positive, outside QR, Positive, outside quantitative range; BM, bone marrow; PB, peripheral blood. WT1 mRNA level was expressed as the copy number in a microgram of RNA; contrastingly, the quantitative value of *Ig/TCR* gene rearrangements was a value relative to the value when the patient visited the hospital at first, and was expressed as a power of 10 ($\times10^{-n}$). MRD targets with quantitative limits of $<10^{-5}$ for qPCR for *Ig/TCR* gene rearrangements and <50 copies/μg RNA for RT-qPCR for WT1 mRNA.

Table 3: Correlation between WT1 mRNA expression levels and Ig/TCR gene rearrangements.

were shown to be "positive, outside quantitative range" in two patients; however, the other four showed negative (Table 3).

WT1 mRNA levels in the BM of all six patients after induction were determined to be lower than 1,820 copies/μg RNA, which was determined as the cut-off value in BM for remission, as described above. WT1 mRNA levels in the PB of all six patients at all time points were determined to be lower than 220 copies/μg RNA, which was determined as the cut-off value in PB for remission, as described above.

Discussion

ALL is the most common childhood malignancy representing nearly one-third of pediatric cancers [32]. Several studies reported the increase in WT1 mRNA to be one of risk factors resulting in relapse in AML [33-35]. Moreover, overexpression of WT1 mRNA was frequently detected in *de novo* childhood ALL [23,36,37]. We showed high positive rates of WT1 mRNA expression (approximately 90%) in the PB and BM samples of *de novo* childhood and adult ALL patients. They were also expressed at a high frequency.

In this study, it is considered that there is no difference in WT1 mRNA expression level and positive rate between childhood ALL and adult ALL before treatment, so it is speculated that the kinetics of WT1 mRNA expression level after treatment will show the same trend for both childhood ALL and adult ALL. From the literature of the authors [38-41], WT1 mRNA expression level in adult ALL reflects the therapeutic effect and has been shown to be useful as a monitoring marker.

In Japan, the incidence of ALL by subtype has been reported as 70.5% for B-precursor ALL, 14.0% for pre-B ALL, 2.5% for mature B-ALL, and 13.0% for T-ALL [31]; a similar distribution was also demonstrated in this study. Furthermore, subtype B-precursor ALL showed higher mean values of WT1 mRNA levels than pre-B ALL. This suggests higher levels of WT1 mRNA expression in undifferentiated hematopoietic cells, which is consistent with previous studies that reported higher WT1 mRNA levels in B-precursor ALL than in other subtypes [22,42]. Moreover, intracellular WT1 mRNA levels decreased when K562 cells (a CML-derived cell strain) differentiated into erythroids or megakaryocytes, and when HL60 cells (a promyelocytic leukemia-derived cell strain) differentiated into granulocytes, monocytes, and macrophages via various inducers of differentiation [43,44].

The correlation of WT1 mRNA expression in both, PB and BM, was evaluated in this study, which demonstrated a good correlation with a correlation coefficient (r) of 0.85 in childhood ALL and 0.84 in adult ALL. This result was also reported in myelodysplastic syndrome (MDS) and AML [26,45]. PB and/or BM were chosen for clinical monitoring, depending on the patient's condition and treatment strategy. Measurement of PB was preferred owing to its convenience and lower burden on the patient.

Fusion gene transcripts were detected in 11 of 49 (22.4%) *de novo* childhood ALL patients, and the detection rate was similar to that reported in a previous study [16]. Contrastingly, the rate of positivity for WT1 mRNA was 93.8%. Since the levels of the fusion gene transcript and WT1 mRNA correlated well, WT1 mRNA was selected as a monitoring marker instead of the fusion gene transcripts owing to the childhood ALL patient cases that did not express the fusion gene transcripts. The significance was considerable.

Now that a next-generation sequencer has identified cancerous cells to also have multiple clones rather than just one, relapse is thought to occur via subclones that are tolerant to chemotherapy [18].

During the study, a total of 48 childhood ALL patients underwent a follow-up procedure (with the exception of one patient that was transferred), and were assessed to be in remission after starting treatment. During the post-treatment remission phase, WT1 mRNA positivity rates were observed to be 83.3% in both PB and BM, and significantly lower than the rates before treatment ($p<0.01$; Student's *t*-test). To assess hematological remission via ROC analysis, we calculated the cut-off values of WT1 mRNA expression to be 220 copies/μg-RNA for PB and 1,820 copies/μg-RNA for BM. Although the decrease in WT1 mRNA level after treatment was previously reported in AML and ALL [26,36,46], this study was the first to attempt to obtain the upper cut-off values of WT1 mRNA expression indicating the remission phase. Miyawaki et al. reported that relapse in AML patients was possible if WT1 mRNA levels rose above 200 copies/μg-RNA in PB from the remission phase [20]. Since this value was similar to the PB upper cut-off value obtained in the present study, it seemed appropriate to use it as the reference value for early relapse in ALL. MRD after induction therapy is useful for stratification of the treatment [13]. Optimization of treatment using stratification results in improved prognosis of ALL treatment. Measurement of WT1 mRNA is useful for stratification, which is thought to contribute to the improvement of treatment outcome. Common MRD targets include recurrent cytogenetic abnormalities and mutations in important hematological genes. Unfortunately, well-characterized targets are lacking in many ALL patients. WT1 is expressed in leukemic stem cells and in most cases of AML and ALL.

In this study we performed PCR to detect *Ig/TCR* gene rearrangements in 6 patients considered to represent severe cases. The results showed that 4 patients were positive and 2 were negative after induction, and the 2 negative patients remained negative after consolidation. In 2 of the 4 positive patients, *Ig/TCR* gene rearrangement values decreased to 10^{-4} or less after induction, and became negative after consolidation. For the 2 patients, whose values were 10^{-4} or more after induction, the values became positive within quantitative range. A clinical study by the AIEOP-BFM group assessing the usefulness of MRD quantification based on Ig/TCR gene rearrangements evaluated by PCR reported that the presence of MRD equal to or greater than 10^{-3} at time points after consolidation indicates poor prognosis in the patients for whom allogeneic SCT is recommended [11]. This report suggested that our 6 patients also have poor prognosis, which demonstrates the clinical usefulness of the *Ig/TCR* gene rearrangement evaluation. Meanwhile, the WT1 mRNA levels in the PB of the 6 patients mentioned above were 220 copies/μg RNA or less at all time points, suggesting that the patients achieved remission. Recently the methods of MRD evaluation and interpretation of the evaluation results have been strictly standardized for multiregional clinical trials in Europe, including those for *Ig/TCR* gene rearrangements [8], which were highly sensitive and useful. As with the *Ig/TCR* gene rearrangements, the WT1 mRNA levels, also indicating remission, were observed to be reduced. Furthermore, the WT1 mRNA levels indicated remission for not only BM, but also PB, confirming the usefulness of the measurement.

Although 24 out of 48 pediatric patients (50.0%) still expressed ≥ 50 copies/μg-RNA of WT1 mRNA in the PB samples after treatment and during the remission phase, the expression levels were observed to have decreased. In these cases, the presence of MRD, which was undetectable in hematological remission, was suspected. Detection is considered difficult when the blast cell is only available in minimum amounts of MRD during microscopic examination. The depth of remission was assumed to be shallower in these cases than in cases that showed a decreased level in PB (below LOD) after treatment. The WT1 mRNA levels increased when the disease stage progressed from the remission to the relapse phase in ALL patients [23,36,38-41,46-48], and the depth of remission proved to be much shallower when the expression levels surpassed the upper cut-off values for remission (i.e., 220 copies/μg-RNA for PB and 1,820 copies/μg-RNA for BM).

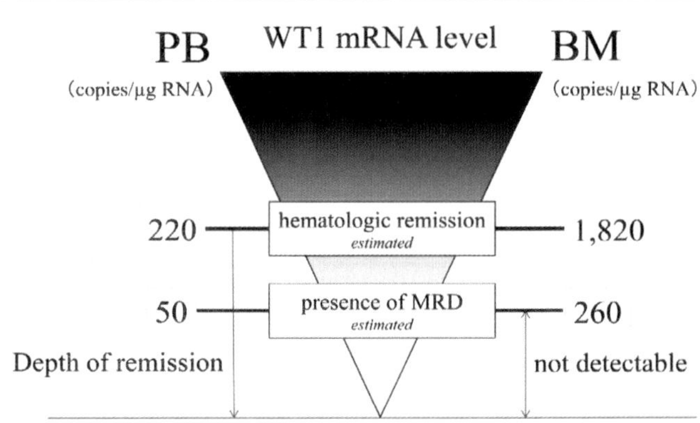

Figure 7: The depth of remission in Wilms' tumor 1 (WT1) expression levels.

This type of result suggests relapse and needs to be noted for treatment (Figure 7). Moreover, the WT1 mRNA levels after transplantation also predict recurrence. The level of WT1 mRNA in PB is also useful for immunization after transplantation (e.g., induction of GVL), thereby alleviating the load on the patient [49].

Conclusion

WT1 mRNA detected in high frequency, even in *de novo* ALL patients exhibiting evidence of fusion gene transcripts, reflected the treatment effects and depth of remission in ALL patients. Therefore, WT1 mRNA may possibly be a useful monitoring marker of MRD in ALL patients.

Competing Interests

This study was funded by Otsuka Pharmaceutical Co., Ltd., Tokyo, Japan. Y.H., Y.Kosaka, K.W., K.Kato, M.I., T.K., S.S., A.W., H.H., Y.Koga, M.Hirayama, T.Nakao, T.H., N.U., K.Ishiyama, K.M., M.Hidaka, K.Kitamura, T.T., Y.U., A.M., K.U., Y.Kanda, K.Koh, and K.H. received research funding from Otsuka to conduct this study. Moreover, T.Naoe and H.S. also received personal fees from Otsuka to conduct this study. Y.M. is employee of Otsuka. K.Imai declares no conflict of interest.

Acknowledgments

We thank all the participating institutions and physicians, including the authors and their principal investigators, for their support during the study. Furthermore, we thank Ms. Tokuko Okuda for performing the flow cytometry analysis.

References

1. Sugiura I (2016) Philadelphia chromosome-positive acute lymphoblastic leukemia. Nippon Rinsho 74: S151-155.
2. Horibe K (2012) Treatment strategy for childhood acute lymphoblastic leukemia. Rinsho Ketsueki 53: 1538-1548.
3. Ribera JM, Oriol A, Sanz MA, Tormo M, Fernández-Abellán P, et al. (2008) Comparison of the results of the treatment of adolescents and young adults with standard-risk acute lymphoblastic leukemia with the Programa Español de Tratamiento en Hematología pediatric-based protocol ALL-96. J Clin Oncol 26: 1843-1849.
4. Pui CH, Yang JJ, Hunger SP, Pieters R, Schrappe M, et al. (2015) Childhood acute lymphoblastic leukemia: progress through collaboration. J Clin Oncol 33: 2938-2948.
5. Fronkova E, Madzo J, Zuna J, Reznickova L, Muzikova K, et al. (2005) TEL/AML1 real-time quantitative reverse transcriptase PCR can complement minimal residual disease assessment in childhood ALL. Leukemia 19: 1296-1297.
6. Pane F, Cimino G, Izzo B, Camera A, Vitale A, et al. (2005) Significant reduction of the hybrid BCR/ABL transcripts after induction and consolidation therapy is a powerful predictor of treatment response in adult Philadelphia-positive acute lymphoblastic leukemia. Leukemia 19: 628-635.
7. Zaliova M, Fronkova E, Krejcikova K, Muzikova K, Mejstrikova E, et al. (2009) Quantification of fusion transcript reveals a subgroup with distinct biological properties and predicts relapse in BCR/ABL-positive ALL: implications for residual disease monitoring. Leukemia 23: 944-951.
8. Brüggemann M, Schrauder A, Raff T, Pfeifer H, Dworzak M, et al. (2010) Standardized MRD quantification in European ALL trials: proceedings of the Second International Symposium on MRD assessment in Kiel, Germany, 18-20 September 2008. Leukemia 24: 521-535.
9. van Dongen JJ, Langerak AW, Brüggemann M, Evans PA, Hummel M, et al. (2003) Design and standardization of PCR primers and protocols for detection of clonal immunoglobulin and T-cell receptor gene recombinations in suspect lymphoproliferations: report of the BIOMED-2 Concerted Action BMH4-CT98-3936. Leukemia 17: 2257-2317.
10. van der Velden VH, Cazzaniga G, Schrauder A, Hancock J, Bader P, et al. (2007) Analysis of minimal residual disease by Ig/TCR gene rearrangements: guidelines for interpretation of real-time quantitative PCR data. Leukemia 21: 604-611.
11. Flohr T, Schrauder A, Cazzaniga G, Panzer-Grümayer R, van der Velden V, et al. (2008) Minimal residual disease-directed risk stratification using real-time quantitative PCR analysis of immunoglobulin and T-cell receptor gene rearrangements in the international multicenter trial AIEOP-BFM ALL 2000 for childhood acute lymphoblastic leukemia. Leukemia 22: 771-782.
12. Yamaji K, Okamoto T, Yokota S, Watanabe A, Horikoshi Y, et al. (2010) Minimal residual disease-based augmented therapy in childhood acute lymphoblastic leukemia: a report from the Japanese Childhood Cancer and Leukemia Study Group. Pediatr Blood Cancer 55: 1287-1295.
13. Borowitz MJ, Devidas M, Hunger SP, Bowman WP, Carroll AJ, et al. (2008) Clinical significance of minimal residual disease in childhood acute lymphoblastic leukemia and its relationship to other prognostic factors: a Children's Oncology Group study. Blood 111: 5477-5485.
14. Pui CH, Campana D, Pei D, Bowman WP, Sandlund JT, et al. (2009) Treating childhood acute lymphoblastic leukemia without cranial irradiation. N Engl J Med 360: 2730-2741.
15. Campana D (2010) Minimal residual disease in acute lymphoblastic leukemia. Hematology Am Soc Hematol Educ Program 2010: 7-12.
16. Pui CH, Relling MV, Downing JR (2004) Acute lymphoblastic leukemia. N Engl J Med 350: 1535-1548.
17. Teachey DT, Hunger SP (2013) Predicting relapse risk in childhood acute lymphoblastic leukemia. Br J Haematol 162: 606-620.
18. Ding L, Ley TJ, Larson DE, Miller CA, Koboldt DC, et al. (2012) Clonal evolution in relapsed acute myeloid leukemia revealed by whole-genome sequencing. Nature 481: 506-510.
19. Kotrova M, Muzikova K, Mejstrikova E, Novakova M, Bakardjieva-Mihaylova V, et al. (2015) The predictive strength of next-generation sequencing MRD detection for relapse compared with current methods in childhood ALL. Blood 126: 1045-1047.
20. Miyawaki S, Emi N, Mitani K, Oyashiki K, Kitamura K, et al. (2005) Clinical course of the disease and the level of WT1 mRNA in 191 patients with acute myeloid leukemia (AML): joint research by 23 institutions in Japan. Rinsho Ketsueki 46: 1279-1287.
21. Miyawaki S, Hatsumi N, Tamaki T, Naoe T, Ozawa K, et al. (2010) Prognostic potential of detection of WT1 mRNA level in peripheral blood in adult acute myeloid leukemia. Leuk Lymphoma 51: 1855-1861.
22. Busse A, Gökbuget N, Siehl JM, Hoelzer D, Schwartz S, et al. (2009) Wilms' tumor gene 1 (WT1) expression in subtypes of acute lymphoblastic leukemia (ALL) of adults and impact on clinical outcome. Ann Hematol 88: 1199-1205.
23. Boublikova L, Kalinova M, Ryan J, Quinn F, O'Marcaigh A, et al. (2006) Wilms' tumor gene 1 (WT1) expression in childhood acute lymphoblastic leukemia: a wide range of WT1 expression levels, its impact on prognosis and minimal residual disease monitoring. Leukemia 20: 254-263.
24. Chiusa L, Francia di Celle P, Campisi P, Ceretto C, Marmont F, et al. (2006) Prognostic value of quantitative analysis of WT1 gene transcripts in adult acute lymphoblastic leukemia. Haematologica 91: 270-271.
25. Xu B, Song X, Yip NC, Xiao P, Zhang Y, et al. (2010) Simultaneous detection of MDR1 and WT1 gene expression to predict the prognosis of adult acute lymphoblastic leukemia. Hematology 15: 74-80.
26. Kitamura K, Nishiyama T, Ishiyama K, Miyawaki S, Miyazaki K, et al. (2016) Clinical usefulness of WT1 mRNA expression in bone marrow detected by a new WT1 mRNA assay kit for monitoring acute myeloid leukemia: a comparison with expression of WT1 mRNA in peripheral blood. Int J Hematol 103: 53-62.
27. Shimada A, Taki T, Koga D, Tabuchi K, Tawa A, et al. (2012) High WT1 mRNA expression after induction chemotherapy and FLT3-ITD have prognostic impact in pediatric acute myeloid leukemia: a study of the Japanese Childhood AML Cooperative Study Group. Int J Hematol 96: 469-476.
28. Elia L, Mancini M, Moleti L, Meloni G, Buffolino S, et al. (2003) A multiplex reverse transcriptase-polymerase chain reaction strategy for the diagnostic molecular screening of chimeric genes: a clinical evaluation on 170 patients with acute lymphoblastic leukemia. Haematologica 88: 275-279.

29. Osumi K, Fukui T, Kiyoi H, Kasai M, Kodera Y, et al. (2002) Rapid screening of leukemia fusion transcripts in acute leukemia by real-time PCR. Leuk Lymphoma 43: 2291-2299.

30. Elia L, Grammatico S, Paoloni F, Vignetti M, Rago A, et al. (2011) Clinical outcome and monitoring of minimal residual disease in patients with acute lymphoblastic leukemia expressing the MLL/ENL fusion gene. Am J Hematol 86: 993-997.

31. Iwamoto S, Deguchi T, Ohta H, Kiyokawa N, Tsurusawa M, et al. (2011) Flow cytometric analysis of de novo acute lymphoblastic leukemia in childhood: report from the Japanese Pediatric Leukemia/Lymphoma Study Group. Int J Hematol 94: 185-192.

32. Ribera JM, Ribera J, Genescà E (2014) Treatment of adolescent and young adults with acute lymphoblastic leukemia. Mediterr J Hematol Infect Dis 6: e2014052.

33. Østergaard M, Olesen LH, Hasle H, Kjeldsen E, Hokland P (2004) WT1 gene expression: an excellent tool for monitoring minimal residual disease in 70% of acute myeloid leukaemia patients - results from a single-centre study. Br J Haematol 125: 590-600.

34. Weisser M, Kern W, Rauhut S, Schoch C, Hiddemann W, et al. (2005) Prognostic impact of RT-PCR-based quantification of WT1 gene expression during MRD monitoring of acute myeloid leukemia. Leukemia 19: 1416-1423.

35. Cilloni D, Messa F, Arruga F, Defilippi I, Gottardi E, et al. (2008) Early prediction of treatment outcome in acute myeloid leukemia by measurement of WT1 transcript levels in peripheral blood samples collected after chemotherapy. Haematologica 93: 921-924.

36. Kletzel M, Olzewski M, Huang W, Chou PM (2002) Utility of WT1 as a reliable tool for the detection of minimal residual disease in children with leukemia. Pediatr Dev Pathol 5: 269-275.

37. Magyarosy E, Varga N, Timár J, Rásó E (2003) Follow-up of minimal residual disease in acute childhood lymphoblastic leukemia by WT1 gene expression in the peripheral blood: the Hungarian experience. Pediatr Hematol Oncol 20: 65-74.

38. Sakatani T, Hirai H, Okano M, Hatsuse M, Okamoto R, et al. (2001) Early relapse after high-dose chemotherapy rescued by tumor-free autologous peripheral blood stem cells in acute lymphoblastic leukemia: Importance of monitoring for WT1-mRNA quantitatively. Leuk Lymphoma 42:225-229.

39. Tamaki H, Mishima M, Kawakami M, Tsuboi A, Kim EH, et al. (2003) Monitoring Minimal Residual Disease in Leukemia using real-time quantitative polymerase chain reaction for Wilms Tumor Gene (WT1). Int J Hematol 78:349-356.

40. He ZY, Liang Z, Wu MR, Wen Q, Deng L, et al. (2015) Overexpression of EPS58 is associated with poor prognosis in patients with acute lymphoblastic leukemia. Leuk Res 39: 575-581.

41. Maeda T, Hosen N, Fukushima K, Tsuboi A, Morimoto S, et al. (2013) Maintenance of complete remission after allogeneic stem cell transplantation in leukemia patients treated with Wilms tumor 1 peptide vaccine. Blood Cancer Journal 3: e130.

42. Shabani M, Asgarian-Omran H, Vossough P, Sharifian RA, Faranoush M, et al. (2008) Expression profile of orphan receptor tyrosine kinase (ROR1) and Wilms' tumor gene 1 (WT1) in different subsets of B-cell acute lymphoblastic leukemia. Leuk Lymphoma 49: 1360-1367.

43. Phelan SA, Lindberg C, Call KM (1994) Wilms' tumor gene, WT1, mRNA is down-regulated during induction of erythroid and megakaryocytic differentiation of K562 cells. Cell Growth Differ 5: 677-686.

44. Sekiya M, Adachi M, Hinoda Y, Imai K, Yachi A (1994) Downregulation of Wilms' tumor gene (wt1) during myelomonocytic differentiation in HL60 cells. Blood 83: 1876-1882.

45. Ueda Y, Mizutani C, Nannya Y, Kurokawa M, Kobayashi S, et al. (2013) Clinical evaluation of WT1 mRNA expression levels in peripheral blood and bone marrow in patients with myelodysplastic syndromes. Leuk Lymphoma 54: 1450-1458.

46. Hu SY, Gu WY, Chen ZX, Wang XL, Cen JN, et al. (2010) The significance of detecting WT1 expression in childhood acute leukemias. Pediatr Hematol Oncol 27: 581-591.

47. Sakamoto K, Imamura T, Tomoyasu C, Yano M, Goto S, et al. (2016) Prognostic analysis of relapsed acute leukemia following first allogeneic hematopoietic stem cell transplantation. Jpn J Pediatr Hematol Oncol 53: 105-111.

48. Chen JS, Hsiao CC, Sheen JM, Cheng CN (2007) Comparison of minimal residual disease (MRD) estimated by flow cytometry and by real-time quantitative PCR of Wilms tumor gene 1 (WT1) transcript expression in children with acute lymphoblastic leukemia. Leuk Res 31: 1351-1357.

49. Ishikawa T, Fujii N, Imada M, Aoe M, Meguri Y, et al. (2017) Graft-versus-leukemia effect with a WT1-specificT-cell response induced by azacitidine and donor lymphocyte infusions after allogeneic hematopoietic stem cell transplantation. Cytotherapy 19: 514-520.

Changes in Antigen Expression in a Follow-up of Chronic Lymphocytic Leukemia/Small Lymphocytic Lymphoma

Jiehao Zhou, Anupama Tewari, Mehdi Nassiri and Magdalena Czader*

Department of Pathology and Laboratory Medicine, Indiana University, Indianapolis, IN 46202, USA

Abstract

Objectives: Diagnosis of chronic lymphocytic leukemia/small lymphocytic lymphoma (CLL/SLL) depends on specific immunophenotype of select antigens and their characteristic density. However, reports detailing how the expression of specific antigen changes over time of disease course are sparse.

Methods: We identified 37 CLL/SLL with initial and follow-up samples studied by flow cytometry. Expression levels of a panel of antigens were compared between initial and follow-up samples from the same patients.

Results: There is a significant decrease in the CD23 density and in the percentage of CD23 positive cells, and a decrease in the density of CD5 in the follow-up samples. In contrast, a significant increase in the density of HLA-DR antigen was observed in the follow-up.

Conclusion: The expression of selected antigen changes in the course of CLL/SLL. These alterations do not impact the diagnosis of CLL/SLL based on the immunophenotype of follow-up samples and should not influence the ability to determine minimal residual disease by flow cytometry. However, they can potentially influence the responsiveness to the monoclonal antibody therapy and should be further systematically evaluated.

Keywords: Flow cytometry; CLL; Immunophenotyping

Introduction

According to the World Health Organization, the diagnosis of chronic lymphocytic leukemia/small lymphocytic lymphoma (CLL/SLL) is based on the combination of morphologic, immunophenotypic, laboratory and clinical features [1]. Flow cytometry plays a paramount role in the diagnosis by establishing the characteristic immunophenotype and, in cases of primarily leukemic presentation, by defining the diagnostic threshold of peripheral blood lymphocytosis [2]. Typical CLL/SLL is characterized by the expression of B-cell markers including CD19, low-density CD20 antigen, and the positivity for CD5, CD23, CD43 and low density surface immunoglobulin light chain. The FMC7 is typically negative. These markers allow for a confident diagnosis of CLL/SLL and have been a cornerstone of the CLL/SLL scoring system [3,4]. They are also included in the automated pattern-guided principal component analysis classification of B-cell lymphoproliferative disorders [5]. Even though the majority of CLL/SLL patients present with a typical immunophenotype, cases with atypical immuno phenotypic features are not infrequently encountered. Similar to CLL/SLL with typical immunophenotype, some of these cases are also associated with presence of genetic abnormalities [6]. These cases may be challenging to diagnose since they are also more frequently associated with atypical morphological and/or clinical presentation. Due to the expansion of therapeutic options and more widespread clinical trials, patients with CLL/SLL are increasingly immunophenotyped at various time points after initial presentation either for the confirmation of the original diagnosis or to monitor residual disease. Flow cytometric immunophenotyping may also be relevant for the therapeutic decision making as the efficacy of the immunotherapy may be dependent on the level of expression of the target antigen as it has been demonstrated for rituximab and CD20 antigen [7-9].

Extensive literature describes the CLL/SLL immunophenotype at the time of initial diagnosis. However, the data on the modulation of antigen expression during the natural course of CLL/SLL and following chemotherapy/immunotherapy are sparse. In a limited case series, Kusenda et al. compared the antigen expression of 13 CLL/SLL cases at the time of initial diagnosis with 10 unrelated patients with CLL/SLL following treatment [10]. Even though differences in the expression levels of select antigens were seen, small study sample size and potential variations among individuals did not allow for definitive conclusions. In the current study, we have evaluated the antigen expression in paired samples from 37 patients with CLL/SLL at the time of initial diagnosis and in the follow-up samples.

Material and Methods

Patients and samples

The review of the archives of Clinical Flow Cytometry Laboratory at Indiana University between years 2005-2011 showed more than 400 samples with the diagnosis of CLL/SLL and a detailed immunophenotypic analysis. The immunophenotypes at the time of initial diagnosis and at the follow-up of the disease were available for 37 individuals. There were 24 males and 13 females with a median age of 64 years (age range 46-84 years). The samples included 30 bone marrows (BM), 32 peripheral blood specimens (PB), 10 lymph nodes (LN), and 2 spleens. The follow-up samples were collected at least one month apart from the initial sampling (1 month to 3 year intervals). All the patients met the criteria for CLL/SLL diagnosis according to 2008 WHO classification including diagnostic threshold of $\geq 5.0\times10^9$/L

***Corresponding author:** Dr. Magdalena Czader, Department of Pathology and Laboratory Medicine, 350 W.11th Street, Room 5034, Indianapolis, IN 46202-5200, USA; E-mail: mczader@iupui.edu monoclonal lymphocytes and/or evidence of lymph node involvement. Most patients showed either lymphocytosis or lymphadenopathy at the time of initial diagnosis. The diagnosis was reviewed independently by two hematopathologists. A subset of patients was tested for cytogenetic abnormalities and 75% of tested patients showed cytogenetic alterations. A significant portion of patients (23 out of 37) were treated with chemotherapy after initial diagnosis. Seven patients did not receive any treatment. The treatment status of seven patients remains unknown after careful review of available clinical charts. When comparing the follow-up vs. initial presentation, approximately 74% of patients showed a reduction in WBC count whereas lymphadenopathy appeared to persist. The detailed clinical information is listed in Table 1.

Flow cytometric immunophenotyping

Patient samples were analyzed using four-color flow cytometry. Dependent on the sample type, the red blood cell depletion with ammonium chloride was performed. Total cell count was determined and the sample viability was analyzed with 7-AAD staining. The antibodies were directly conjugated with fluorescein isothiocyanate (FITC), phycoerythrin (PE), PE-Cy5 (PC5) or PE-Texas Red (ECD). The following antibodies were analyzed: CD45-ECD, HLA-DR-PC5, CD38-PC5, CD71-FITC, CD33-PE, CD3-ECD, CD5-FITC, CD7-PE, CD4-FITC, CD8-PC5, CD56-PC5, CD19-FITC (or PE), CD20-PE (or PC5), CD10-PC5, CD22-PE, CD23-ECD, FMC7-FITC, kappa-FITC and lambda light chains-PE. When comparing geometric mean of fluorescence intensity (GMFI) of specific antigen expression, the antibody conjugated with same fluorochrome was used. All antibodies were purchased from BD Biosciences (San Jose, CA) except for kappa and lambda light chain antibodies which were obtained from DAKO (Houston, TX).

Data acquisition was performed using Coulter EPICS XL or Coulter FC-500 flow cytometers using the Expo System II or CXP software, respectively. At least 100,000 events/cells were acquired in each sample. Data was analyzed using EXPO32 and CXP software (Beckman Coulter, Miami, FL, USA). The cellular debris was excluded before the analysis. Depending on the primary antibody combination, the cells of interest were gated on right angle light scatter vs forward scatter, or on right angle light scatter vs. CD45 display. Antigen expression was assessed quantitatively in relation to available controls. Briefly, the antigen was considered positive when the majority of cells expressed a given marker. Partial expression represented the presence of separate positive and negative populations. Heterogeneous distribution indicated variable fluorescence intensity from negative to bright positive cells. Percentages of cells positive for given antigen and/or GMFI were obtained and compared between the diagnostic and follow-up samples from the same patients. Isotype controls were used as negative controls. Frozen stock mononuclear cells with known antigen expression level were used as positive controls to ensure the consistency of antigen GMFI measurement. These controls showed no systematic bias in the antigen expression levels that could influence obtained results (data not shown). The typical CLL/SLL immunophenotype was defined as positive for CD19, CD5, CD23, CD22, low density expression of CD20, and low density expression of immunoglobin surface light chain [3,4]. CD10 and FMC7 were typically negative. The atypical immunophenotypic features included expression of FMC7, absence of CD5 or CD23 antigen expression as well as moderate to bright CD20 and/or surface immunoglobin light chain. In patient 4 and patient 8, immunohistochemical study of cyclin D1 was performed and it was negative, excluding the possibility of mantle cell lymphoma.

Statistical analysis

For all variables, their means and standard deviations were calculated. To establish the statistical significance, the paired *t* test was used. A p value less than 0.05 was defined as statistically significant.

Pt #	Gender	Age at Dx	Sample	Initial Ly # (k/ul)	FU Ly # (k/ul)	Initial Lymphadenopathy	FU Lymphadenopathy	Treatment	Atypical Immunophenotype	ZAP-70/ CD38	Cytogenetics
1	F	55	BM, BM	5.3	2.6	Yes	Yes	FCR	No	20% / 4%	46,XX
2	F	61	PB, BM	3.1	1.5	Yes	N/A	RCHOP	No	N/A / 12%	N/A
3	F	62	PB, BM	26.2	20	Yes	Yes	N/A	No	N/A / 1%	46,XX
4	F	59	LN, BM	5.4	0.8	Yes	Yes	RCHOP	Negative CD5	16% / 42%	47,XX,+12
5	F	67	BM, PB	215	149	Yes	Yes	FCR	No	N/A / N/A	46,XX,del(13)(q12q14)
6	M	57	PB, Spleen	73.2	1.9	No	Yes	FCR	No	94% / 73%	N/A
7	M	62	PB, BM	39.9	2.4	No	No	FCR	No	N/A / N/A	N/A
8	F	62	BM, PB	N/A	N/A	Yes	Yes	FCR	Bright CD20 and FMC7+	2% / 23%	Del(11)(q13q23)
9	M	54	PB, BM	6.3	2.3	N/A	N/A	Chlorambucil and Rituxan	No	1% / 1%	N/A
10	M	55	PB, PB	195	41.3	N/A	N/A	Fludarabine	No	6% / 96%	Del11q22.3/ Del13q14.3
11	M	56	BM, BM	18.4	1.6	Yes	Yes	Bendamustine	No	40% / 80%	N/A
12	M	84	PB, PB	N/A	5.8	N/A	N/A	N/A	No	70% / 21%	N/A
13	M	56	LN, BM	2.4	39.8	Yes	Yes	RCVP	No	N/A / N/A	Complex cytogenetics
14	M	70	PB, PB	10.7	10.2	No	No	No	No	36% / 85%	Del(11)(?q13q23),+12
15	M	64	BM, BM	31.8	14.2	No	Yes	FCR	No	N/A / N/A	Complex cytogenetics
16	F	48	LN, LN	145.7	0.1	Yes	Yes	RCHOP	No	N/A / 69%	N/A
17	M	72	PB, LN	72.6	N/A	No	Yes	No	No	N/A / 21%	N/A
18	M	67	LN, LN	N/A	N/A	Yes	Yes	FCR	Moderate light chain	N/A / 85%	N/A
19	M	64	PB, PB	3.7	2.2	Yes	Yes	FCR	No	N/A / 35%	N/A

20	M	66	BM, BM	31	1.7	N/A	N/A	FCR	Moderate light chain	61% / 38%	47,XY Trisomy 12
21	M	52	PB, BM	74.5	248	N/A	N/A	N/A	Moderate light chain	N/A / N/A	N/A
22	M	80	LN, BM	N/A	0.5	Yes	N/A	Fludarabine	No	44% / 77%	47,XY,+12
23	M	64	PB, PB	71	62	N/A	N/A	N/A	No	1% / 1%	N/A
24	M	68	PB, PB	20.6	3.8	No	Yes	No	No	N/A / 81%	N/A
25	M	81	BM, PB	5.2	N/A	N/A	N/A	No	No	2% / 9%	46, XY.
26	M	63	BM, Spleen	42.7	0.2	Yes	Yes	FCR	Moderate light chain	64% / 14%	47,XY,t(6;7) (p23;p22),+12
27	M	50	PB, BM	20.1	304	No	Yes	No	No	3% / 3%	13q14 deletion
28	F	77	PB, BM	21	3	Yes	Yes	RCVP	No	N/A / 60%	46,XX
29	F	81	PB, BM	5.8	2.3	No	No	No	No	N/A / 78%	Complex cytogenetics
30	F	73	BM, BM	14	1.7	Yes	Yes	RCVP	No	1% /59%	46,XX
31	M	71	LN, BM	5.5	29	Yes	Yes	N/A	No	6% / 9%	N/A
32	M	78	PB, LN	24	N/A	Yes	Yes	N/A	No	1% / 1%	N/A
33	F	77	BM, PB	29	24	Yes	Yes	FCR	No	80% / 78%	47,XX,t(2;14) (p15;q32) +12
34	M	49	BM, BM	3.4	1.2	Yes	Yes	FCR and stem cell transplant	No	N/A / N/A	Complex cytogenetics
35	M	62	BM, PB	145.7	1.1	No	Yes	FCR	No	35% / 7%	Complex cytogenetics
36	F	73	PB, BM	47	260	Yes	Yes	No	No	22% / 14%	47,XX,+12
37	F	46	PB, PB	8.4	4.1	Yes	Yes	N/A	No	54% / 2%	N/A

FCR: fludarabine, cyclophosphamide, and rituximab
RCHOP: rituximab, cyclophosphamide, doxorubicin, vincristine and prednisone
RCVP: rituximab, cyclophosphamide, vincristine and prednisone

Table 1: Patient's characteristics.

Results

Immunophenotype of initial samples

The majority of the samples demonstrated a typical CLL/SLL immunophenotype: positive for CD19, CD20 (dim), CD22, HLA-DR, CD5, CD23, surface immunoglobulin light chain (dim), and negative for CD10 and FMC7 (Figure 1). Among all antigens tested, CD19 and HLA-DR demonstrated a uniformly bright expression pattern in the majority of neoplastic cells. The CD5 expression by CLL/SLL cells was evident in the majority of cases showing the CD5 expression levels slightly lower than those of CD3-positive T cells. The expression of CD22 antigen detected by flow cytometry was distinct but relatively dim compared to normal B cell population. In our study, neoplastic B cells demonstrated a dim to moderate CD23 antigen expression. In addition, there were considerable variations among individual patients in regards to the expression levels of the following antigens: CD19, CD20, CD22, CD5, CD23, HLA-DR, and immunoglobulin light chains. Although the majority of cases showed a typical CLL/SLL immunophenotype, there were 6 cases with one or more atypical immunophenotypic features. The most common atypical finding was brighter than expected expression of immunoglobin light chains seen in 4 cases (~10% studies cases). One case was negative for CD5 antigen. One case showed simultaneous positive FMC7 and bright CD20 expression. Other markers characteristic for non-CLL type B cell lymphoproliferative disorder such as CD10 were not identified in these atypical CLL cases. Therefore, despite some atypical immunophenotypic features, the overall morphology, immunophenotypic and cytogenetics features of these cases were most compatible with CLL/SLL. These atypical immunophenotypic features remained unchanged in the follow up samples (Table 1). For example, an absence of CD5 antigen was seen in both initial and follow-up samples of patient 4.

Few patients had concurrent samples from multiple sites including 5 patients with concurrent samples from peripheral blood and bone marrow, 1 patient with concurrent samples from peripheral blood and lymph node, and 1 patient with concurrent samples from bone marrow and lymph node. The surface antigen expression pattern and expression density were compared between different anatomic sites and showed no overt differences. However, the number of the cases was too low for a statistical analysis.

Comparison of the immunophenotype of initial and follow-up samples

When comparing initial and follow-up samples, statistically significant differences were identified in the expression of CD23, HLA-DR and CD5 antigens. The expression of CD23 antigen was found to be decreased in the follow-up samples. The decrease in the percentages of CD23 positive B cells and the decrease in the density of CD23 antigen were both seen. Seventy-eight percent of patients showed a decrease in the percentage of CD23 positive B cells in the follow-up samples (Figure 2A, $p<0.01$). The extent of decrease varied among patients. The mean percentage of CD23 positive B cells decreased from 81% in initial samples to 72% in the follow up samples with the greatest reduction of approximately 33% (from 98% in the initial sample to 66% in the follow-up specimen). In addition, when comparing the initial and follow-up samples of the same patients, 72% of patients showed an average 19% decrease in CD23 antigen density in CD23-positive B cells as defined by changes in GMFI (from initial 4.6 to follow-up 3.7) (Figure 2B). Despite the variation in antigen expression among different patients, the decrease in CD23 antigen density in CD23-positive B cells was statistically significant ($p<0.01$). Approximately 55% of patients showed both decrease in frequency of CD23-positive B cells and decreased CD23 antigen density as illustrated in Figure 2C.

Seventy seven percent of patients showed decreased CD5 antigen expression in the follow-up samples as depicted by GMFI (initial

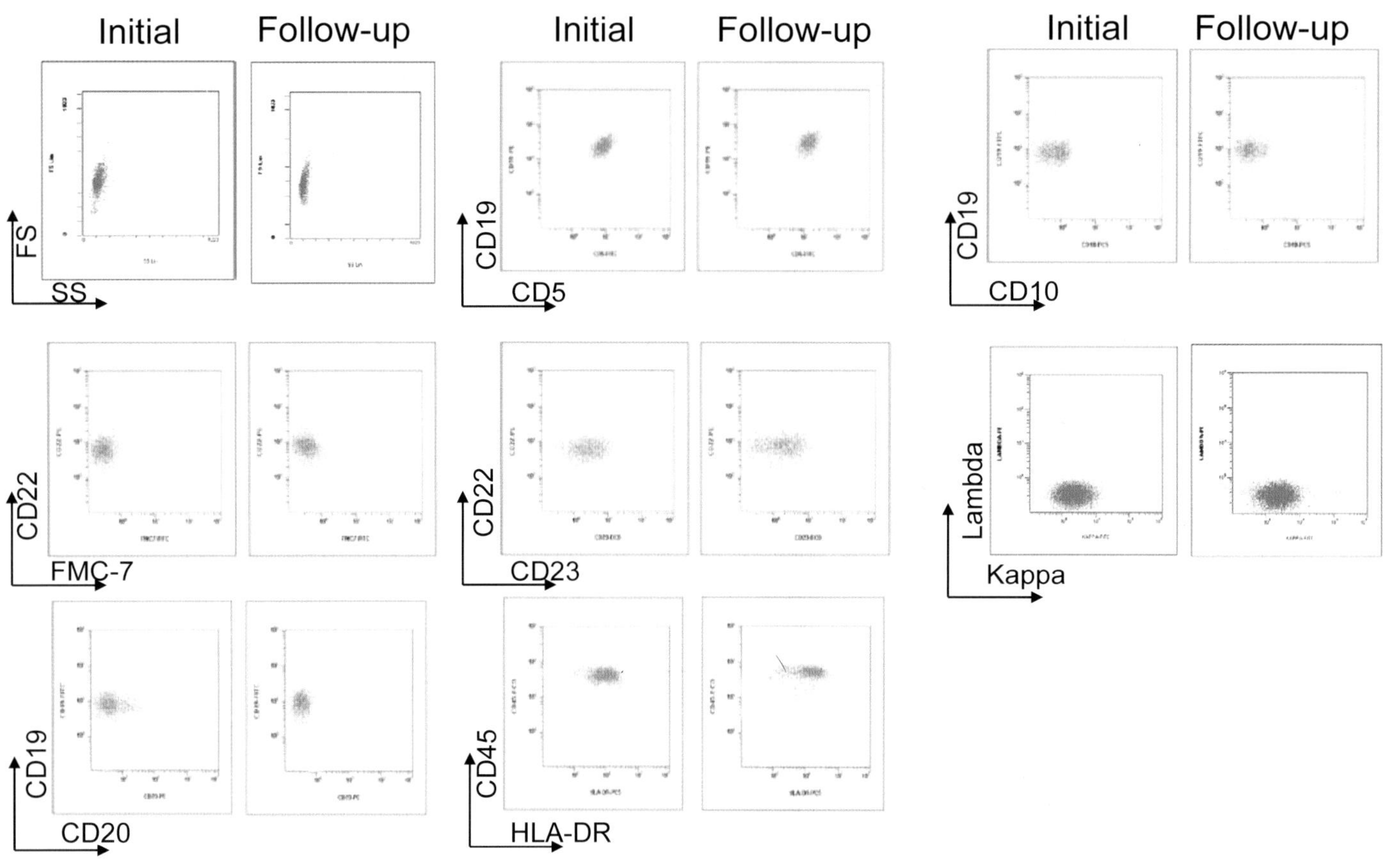

Figure 1: Typical CLL/SLL immunophenotype of initial and follow-up samples. Representative flow cytometric scattergram showing CLL/SLL cells positive for CD19, CD20(dim), CD22,CD5, CD23 and surface immunoglobulin light chain (dim), and negative for FMC7 and CD10.The scattergrams are gated on B cells.

10.6, follow-up 8.9) (Figures 3A and B). This change represented a 16% reduction in CD5 antigen expression levels and was statistically significant by paired t-test ($p<0.05$). In contrast, the percentages of CD5-positive cells remained stable when comparing follow-up samples and initial samples (follow-up 88% vs. initial 87%). The patient with atypical CLL/SLL immunophenotype showing negative to very dim CD5 was excluded from this analysis.

On the contrary, 81% of follow-up samples showed increased HLA-DR expression. This change was statistically significant with an average of 54% increase in GMFI (from initial 16.2 to follow-up 25.0, $p<0.01$, Figures 4A and B). There was no difference in the percentages of HLA-DR-positive cells as this antigen was uniformly expressed in the CLL/SLL cells from the initial and follow-up samples (follow-up 94% vs. initial 94%).

To confirm the above discussed differences in antigen expression, we have performed a separate statistical analysis in treated and untreated patients. Twenty three patients were treated with various regimens after initial diagnosis, 7 patients received no treatment and 7 patients' treatment status was unknown. The differences in the expression of CD5, CD23 and HLA-DR remained statistically significant in patients who received chemotherapy. Similar trends were seen in untreated patients. A statistical significance was achieved when comparing CD5 expression between diagnostic and follow-up samples ($p=0.04$). The expression of HLA-DR ($p=0.19$) and of CD23 ($p=0.07$) were not significantly different, however the numbers of untreated patients may be too low for an adequate statistical analysis.

There was no statistically significant difference between initial and follow-up samples in respect to the percentage of cells and GMFI of CD19, CD22 and surface immunoglobulin light chain. The analysis of the percentages of CD20 positive cells and GMFI for CD20 was not performed due to a significant subset of patients treated with anti-CD20 therapy.

Discussion

Typical CLL/SLL is diagnosed by a combination of clinical, laboratory and morphological features as well as characteristic flow cytometric immunophenotype: positive for CD19, CD20 (dim), CD22, CD5, CD23, HLA-DR, sIg(dim), and negative for CD10 and FMC7. The clinical course of CLL/SLL is highly heterogeneous and the patients are either treated at time of diagnosis or simply monitored depending on the severity of clinical symptoms and disease stage [11-13]. Repeated flow cytometry is sometimes performed for disease follow-up [14]. Our data demonstrated that in CLL/SLL the follow-up samples show immunophenotype similar to those seen in the initial diagnostic material, and thus allow a pathologist to render a confident diagnosis of CLL/SLL based on the follow-up specimens. Nevertheless, for select antigens significant differences occurred in the percentages of positive neoplastic cells and/or in the antigen density. The most prominent differences were seen in the expression of CD23, CD5 and HLA-DR.

CD23 is a trans-membrane glycoprotein typically present on activated mature B-lymphocytes. It functions as a B cell growth and activation factor, promoting rescue of germinal center cells and

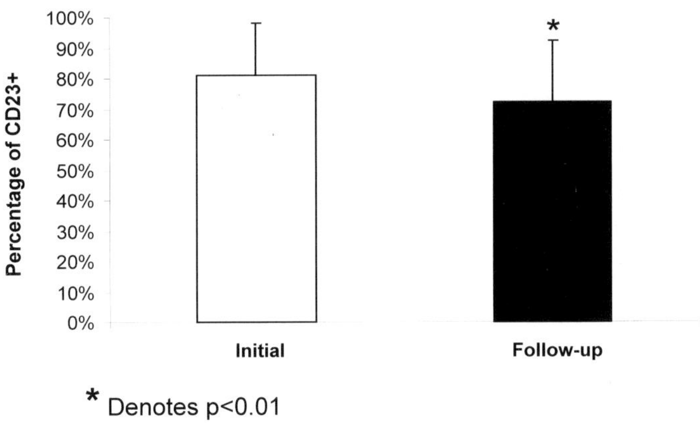

Figure 2A: Down-regulation of CD23 in the follow-up samples. A. Decrease in the frequency of CD23-positive B cells in the follow-up sample. The percentages of CD23-positive B cells in the initial and follow-up samples from the same patients were compared (n=36, paired t-test p<0.01).

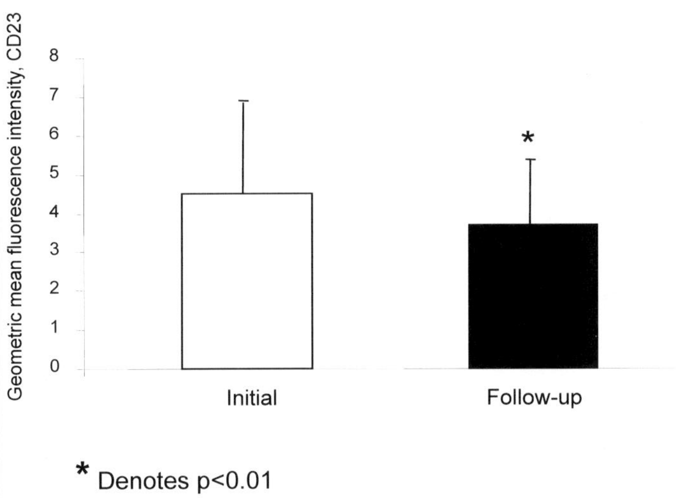

Figure 2B: Decrease in the CD23 antigen density in CD23-positive B cells. Surface CD23 expression levels denoted by GMFI were compared in the initial and follow-up samples from the same subjects (n=36, paired t-test p<0.01).

differentiation into plasma cells. Typical CLL/SLL cells express CD23 antigen, however, Juristic et al. [15] reported that the percentage of CD23 positive cells and CD23 antigen expression level is highly variable among CLL/SLL patients. In Juristic's study, the higher percentage of CD23 positive cells was associated with longer survival and lower percentages of CD23 positive cells were seen in the advanced stages of the disease and in patients with high lymphocyte counts. Our study shows a significant decrease in percentage of CD23-positive cells and a decrease in CD23 antigen density in CLL/SLL cells in the follow-up samples. It is conceivable that the low CD23 expression seen in the advanced stages of the disease reported by Jurisic et al. is due to diagnosing these patients later in the course of the disease. In the current study, the lower CD23 expression in the follow-up CLL/SLL was not associated with increased leukocyte count as reported in Juristic's article (Table 1), which might be due to the fact that a significant portion of patients were treated. Furthermore, the changes in CD23 expression reported in our study may also have implications for therapy decision making. The humanized anti-CD23 has been developed and used in clinical trials [16]. A phase I/II clinical trial showed that the addition of anti-CD23 to fludarabine, cyclophosphamide, and rituximab (FCR) in previously treated CLL/SLL patients resulted in a higher complete response rate, and did not appear to enhance toxicity, indicating that anti-CD23 synergistically enhances antitumor activity of FCR [17]. The investigation of the relation between the levels of CD23 expression and clinical response may be beneficial to achieve the best therapeutic effect without inadvertent addition of toxicity.

CD5 is typically considered as T cell associated antigen which acts as a co-receptor in the stimulation of T cell growth [18]. The upregulation/expression of CD5 antigen in B cells is observed in a variety of B-cell lymphoproliferative disorders including CLL/SLL, mantle cell lymphoma and a subset of diffuse large B cells lymphomas. The CD5 antigen and other markers including CD23, FMC7, surface immunoglobin light chain and CD22/CD79b have also been used in the immunophenotyping scoring system to distinguish CLL/SLL from other chronic B-cell malignancies with acceptable sensitivity and specificity [19,20]. Previous studies have indicated that the

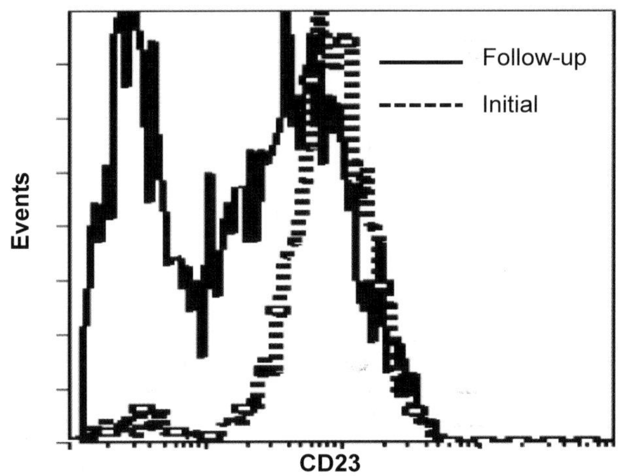

Figure 2C: Representative flow cytometry histogram of CD23 expression demonstrating a concurrent decrease in the frequency of CD23-positive B cells and decreased CD23 antigen density in the follow-up CLL/SLL samples.

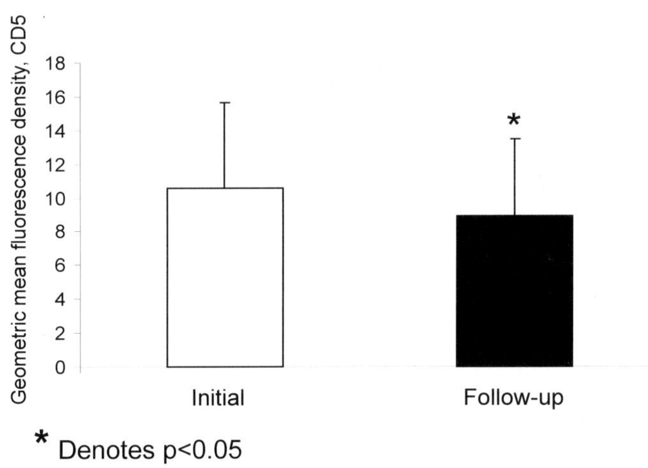

Figure 3A: Downregulation of CD5 antigen expression in the follow-up CLL/SLL. **A.** Surface CD5 expression levels denoted by GFMI were compared between initial and follow-up samples from the same subjects (n=35, paired t-test p<0.05).

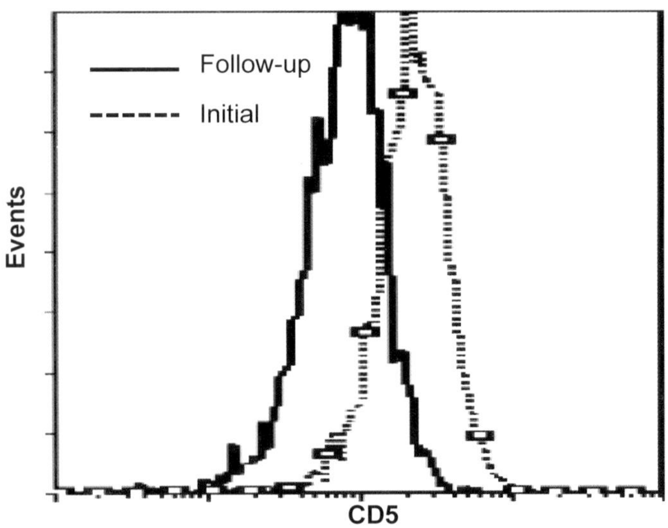

Figure 3B: Representative flow cytometry histogram of CD5 expression demonstrating a decrease of antigen density in the follow-up CLL/SLL samples.

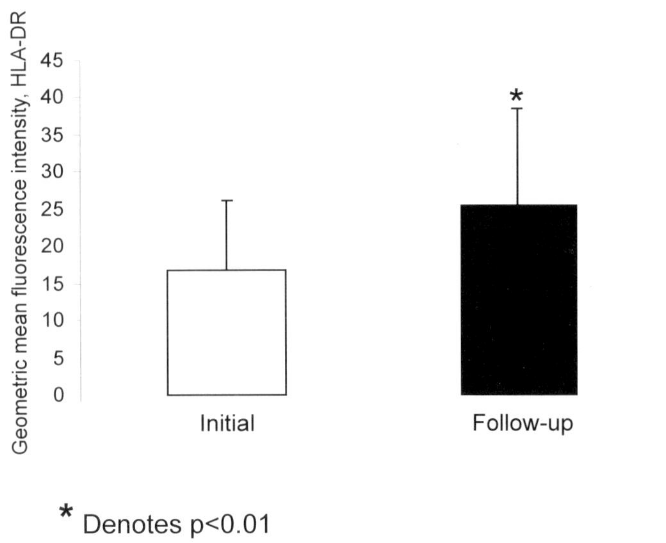

Figure 4A: Upregulation of HLA-DR antigen expression in the follow-up CLL/SLL samples. **A.** HLA-DR expression levels denoted by GMFI were compared between initial and follow-up samples from the same subjects (n=37, paired t-test p<0.01).

expression of CD5 in CLL/SLL is associated with chronic activation of B cell receptors, anergy and a survival of malignant B cells [21,22]. Our current study shows a statistically significant decrease in CD5 antigen density in the follow-up as compared to the initial diagnostic samples. The biological significance of this finding is not clear. The decrease in CD5 can be related to treatment since a significant portion of the patients in our study have been treated. Kusenda et al. reported a slight increase in CD5 antigen expression in CLL/SLL patients after treatment [10]. However, this previous study did not include paired, pre- and post-treatment samples and was limited by a low number of cases.

HLA-DR is a part of class II major histocompatibility complex, normally seen on the surface of antigen presenting cells including macrophages, dendritic cells and B lymphocytes. The primary function of HLA-DR is to present peptide antigens to the immune system for the purpose of eliciting or suppressing T helper cell responses leading to the production of antibodies against the same peptide antigen. Apolizumab, a humanized anti-HLA-DR monoclonal antibody, was initially tested to treat relapsed CLL/SLL. Due to the toxicity and lack of response, the trial was discontinued [23]. Most recently, another monoclonal Ab, IMMU-114 was used in a CLL/SLL clinical trial. The IMMU-114 is a humanized IgG4 form of the murine anti–human HLA-DR. Unlike most of other therapeutic monoclonal Ab (mAbs), which exert the in vivo effects largely through immunologic effector mechanisms dependent on intact immunologic function, IMMU-114 acts through direct cytotoxicity, independent of recipient's own immunologic status. Most of mature B cell lymphomas express HLA-DR antigen, making it a potential target for anti-HLA-DR immunotherapy [24,25]. Our current study shows that CLL/SLL express bright HLA-DR and more interestingly that the HLA-DR antigen levels increase over the time of disease course. The HLA-DR expression pattern and kinetics make the anti-HLA-DR mAb a promising reagent to treat CLL/SLL at the time of initial diagnosis and later in the course of the disease.

To evaluate whether the above discussed differences in antigen expression are seen in both treated and untreated patients, we have performed a separate statistical analysis in these patient groups. The treated cohort included 23 patients. There were only 7 untreated patients. The differences in the expression of CD5, CD23 and HLA-DR antigens remained statistically significant in patients who received chemotherapy. Similar trends were seen in untreated patients, however the differences in the expression of HLA-DR and CD23 did not reach statistical significance. The low number of patients in the untreated group is a significant drawback in this analysis and the results should be confirmed in a larger cohort of untreated patients.

In conclusion, to our knowledge, this study is the first flow cytometric evaluation of changes in antigen expression during the course of CLL/SLL in paired diagnostic and follow-up samples from the same patients. Statistically significant decrease in the expression of CD23 and CD5, as

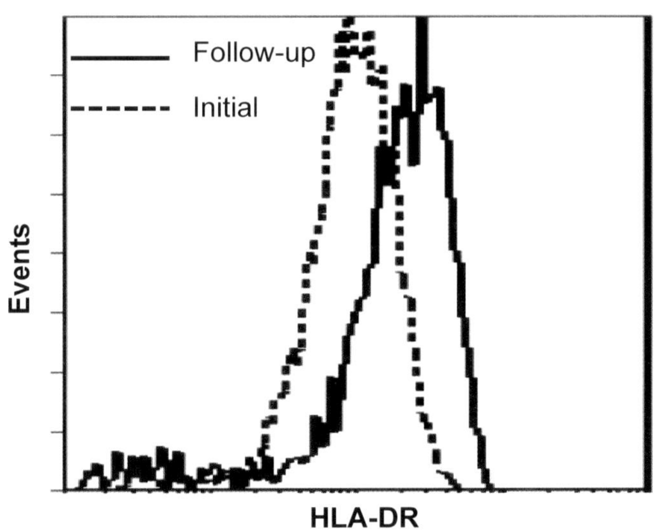

Figure 4B: Representative flow cytometry histogram of HLA-DR expression demonstrating an increase in antigen density in the follow-up CLL/SLL sample.

well as increase in HLA-DR expression was identified. These alterations can potentially influence the responsiveness of the disease to the monoclonal antibody therapy and should be further systematically evaluated. Despite the significant changes in antigen expression seen in the follow-up samples in the majority of cases, the diagnosis of CLL/SLL can still be rendered based on the follow-up immunophenotype.

References

1. Muller-Hermelink HK (2008) Chronic lymphocytic leukaemia/small lymphocytic lymhoma, in WHO Classification of Tumours of Haematopoietic and lymphoid Tissues. S. Swerdlow IARC: Lyon. 180-182.
2. DiGiuseppe JA, Borowitz MJ (1998) Clinical utility of flow cytometry in the chronic lymphoid leukemias. Semin Oncol 25: 6-10.
3. Matutes E, Attygalle A, Wotherspoon A, Catovsky D (2010) Diagnostic issues in chronic lymphocytic leukaemia (CLL). Best Pract Res Clin Haematol 23: 3-20.
4. Matutes E, Wotherspoon A, Catovsky D (2007) Differential diagnosis in chronic lymphocytic leukaemia. Best Pract Res Clin Haematol 20: 367-384.
5. Costa ES, Pedreira CE, Barrena S, Lecrevisse Q, Flores J, et al. (2010) Automated pattern-guided principal component analysis vs expert-based immunophenotypic classification of B-cell chronic lymphoproliferative disorders: a step forward in the standardization of clinical immunophenotyping. Leukemia 11: 1927-1933.
6. Quijano S, López A, Rasillo A, Sayagués JM, Barrena S, et al. (2008) Impact of trisomy 12, del(13q), del(17p), and del(11q) on the immunophenotype, DNA ploidy status, and proliferative rate of leukemic B-cells in chronic lymphocytic leukemia. Cytometry B Clin Cytom 74: 139-149.
7. Mavromatis B, Cheson BD (2003) Monoclonal antibody therapy of chronic lymphocytic leukemia. J Clin Oncol 21: 1874-1881.
8. Jilani I, O'Brien S, Manshuri T, Thomas DA, Thomazy VA, et al. (2003) Transient down-modulation of CD20 by rituximab in patients with chronic lymphocytic leukemia. Blood 102: 3514-3520.
9. Jaglowski SM, Byrd JC (2010) Rituximab in chronic lymphocytic leukemia. Semin Hematol 47: 156-169.
10. Kusenda J, Babusíková O (2004) Antigen modulation followed by quantitative flow cytometry of B-chronic lymphocytic leukemia cells after treatment. Neoplasma 51: 97-102.
11. Riches JC, Ramsay AG, Gribben JG (2011) Chronic lymphocytic leukemia: an update on biology and treatment. Curr Oncol Rep 13: 379-385.
12. Gribben JG, Hosing C, Maloney DG (2011) Stem cell transplantation for indolent lymphoma and chronic lymphocytic leukemia. Biol Blood Marrow Transplant 17: S63-70.
13. Gribben JG, O'Brien S (2011) Update on therapy of chronic lymphocytic leukemia. J Clin Oncol 29: 544-550.
14. Eichhorst B, Dreyling M, Robak T, Montserrat E, Hallek M; ESMO Guidelines Working Group (2011) Chronic lymphocytic leukemia: ESMO Clinical Practice Guidelines for diagnosis, treatment and follow-up. Ann Oncol 22 Suppl 6: vi50-54.
15. Jurisic V, Colovic N, Kraguljac N, Atkinson HD, Colovic M (2008) Analysis of CD23 antigen expression in B-chronic lymphocytic leukaemia and its correlation with clinical parameters. Med Oncol 25: 315-322.
16. Christian BA, Lin TS (2008) Antibody therapy for chronic lymphocytic leukemia. Semin Hematol 45: 95-103.
17. Byrd JC, Kipps TJ, Flinn IW, Castro J, Lin TS, et al. (2010) Phase 1/2 study of lumiliximab combined with fludarabine, cyclophosphamide, and rituximab in patients with relapsed or refractory chronic lymphocytic leukemia. Blood 115: 489-495.
18. Raab M, Yamamoto M, Rudd CE (1994) The T-cell antigen CD5 acts as a receptor and substrate for the protein-tyrosine kinase p56lck. Mol Cell Biol 14: 2862-2870.
19. Matutes E, Owusu-Ankomah K, Morilla R, Garcia Marco J, Houlihan A, et al. (1994) The immunological profile of B-cell disorders and proposal of a scoring system for the diagnosis of CLL. Leukemia 8: 1640-1645.
20. Moreau EJ, Matutes E, A'Hern RP, Morilla AM, Morilla RM, et al. (1997) Improvement of the chronic lymphocytic leukemia scoring system with the monoclonal antibody SN8 (CD79b). Am J Clin Pathol 108: 378-382.
21. Gary-Gouy H, Sainz-Perez A, Marteau JB, Marfaing-Koka A, Delic J, et al. (2007) Natural phosphorylation of CD5 in chronic lymphocytic leukemia B cells and analysis of CD5-regulated genes in a B cell line suggest a role for CD5 in malignant phenotype. J Immunol 179: 4335-4344.
22. Hippen KL, Tze LE, Behrens TW (2000) CD5 maintains tolerance in anergic B cells. J Exp Med 191: 883-890.
23. Lin TS, Stock W, Xu H, Phelps MA, Lucas MS, et al. (2009) A phase I/II dose escalation study of apolizumab (Hu1D10) using a stepped-up dosing schedule in patients with chronic lymphocytic leukemia and acute leukemia. Leuk Lymphoma 50: 1958-1963.
24. Park KH, Sawada T, Murakami T, Ishii Y, Yasuo M, et al. (2012) Anti-class II -DR humanized monoclonal antibody, IMMU-114, blocks allogeneic immune response. Am J Surg 204: 527-534.
25. Stein R, Gupta P, Chen X, Cardillo TM, Furman RR, et al. (2010) Therapy of B-cell malignancies by anti-HLA-DR humanized monoclonal antibody, IMMU-114, is mediated through hyperactivation of ERK and JNK MAP kinase signaling pathways. Blood 115: 5180-5190.

9

Dissecting the *In Vivo* Leukemogenic Potency of Bclxl

Kumar Saurabh[1], Michael T Scherzer[1,4], Amy Song[1], Kenneth W Yip[5,6], John C Reed[5,7], Chi Li[1-3], Levi J Beverly*[1,2,3]

[1]James Graham Brown Cancer Center, University of Louisville, Louisville, KY 40202, USA
[2]Department of Medicine, Division of Hematology and Oncology, University of Louisville, School of Medicine, Louisville, KY 40202, USA
[3]Department of Pharmacology and Toxicology, University of Louisville School of Medicine, Louisville, KY 40202, USA
[4]Department of Bioengineering, University of Louisville, Louisville, KY 40292, USA
[5]Sanford-Burnham Medical Research Institute, La Jolla, CA, 92037, USA
[6]Ontario Cancer Institute, Princess Margaret Cancer Centre, University of Toronto, Toronto, Ontario M5G 2M9, Canada

Abstract

Overexpression of anti-apoptotic members of the BCL2 family has been found in all types of cancer. A member of the family, BCLxl (B-cell lymphoma extra-large), is known to be associated with the progression of leukemogenesis. In the present study, we focused on understanding the domains of BCLxl responsible for *in vivo* oncogenic potency. To this end, we utilized engineered BCLxl proteins with alternative transmembrane domains or chimeric BCLxl proteins containing domains from a less potent BCL2-like protein, BCLb. As expected, mice receiving MYC-only expressing bone marrow develop leukemia by 100 days, whereas co-expression of MYC with wild type BCLxl led to aggressive myeloid leukemia with an average latency of ~25 days. Interestingly, mice injected with bone marrow co-expressing MYC and BCLxl targeted specifically to either mitochondria or ER also succumbed to leukemia with an average latency of ~25 days. Further, our study was extended to examine the role of the BH4 domain in driving potent leukemogenesis. Mice injected with bone marrow coexpressing MYC and BCLb succumb to leukemia in an average of ~55 days, but interestingly a BCLxl protein containing only the loop region of BCLb drove MYC-induced leukemogenesis with the same latency as wild-type BCLxl. These data suggest that the localization of exogenous BCLxl to either mitochondria or ER is not a steadfast dictator of *in vivo* oncogenic potency. Further, our findings suggest that the loop domain of BCLb and BCLxl is not responsible for dictating the *in vivo* leukemogeneic potency. This study provides further mechanistic details into the biochemical functions of BCLxl.

Keywords: Apoptosis; Leukemia; MYC; BH4; BCL2L1; BCL2L10

Introduction

The B-cell lymphoma 2 (BCL2) family of proteins plays a fundamental role in deciding the fate of cells when challenged with death stimuli by regulating Mitochondrial Outer Membrane Permeabilization (MOMP). The family can be divided into pro-apoptotic proteins like BAX, BAK, which potentiate MOMP, cytochrome *c* release and cell death, and anti-apoptotic proteins like BCL2, BCLxl, BCLw which inhibit MOMP to allow cell survival [1-4]. One remarkable feature of BCL2 family members is that they differentially interact with each other to control apoptosis [1,3,5,6]. Modulating the ability of cells to undergo apoptosis is a key approach in the development of therapies for many diseases, including cancer [7-9]. Therefore, many studies have been previously directed to explore the role of BCL2 family members in driving tumorigenesis and to develop candidate molecules that inhibit anti-apoptotic BCL2-like proteins to be used as therapeutics against hematologic malignancies and solid cancers [3,8-10]. Previous work from our laboratory directly determined the comparative *in vivo* oncogenic potency of all six anti-apoptotic proteins; BCL2, BCLxl/BCL2L1, BCLw/BCL2L2, BFL1/BCL2A1, MCL1 and BCLb/BCL2L10 [2]. Of importance, this work also demonstrated that although each anti-apoptotic BCL2-like gene can drive MYC-induced leukemogenesis, there were significant differences in the oncogenic potencies of each family member [2].

Individual anti-apoptotic BCL2 family members are characterized as having four conserved BCL2 Homology (BH) domains known as BH1, BH2, BH3 and BH4 and a c-terminal α-helix Transmembrane Domain (TM) that is imperative for its localization to the mitochondrial outer membranes, Endoplasmic Reticulum (ER) membranes, and nuclear membranes. The variations in the domains present on each of the members is likely responsible for the structural and functional activity of these proteins. For example, the BH1, BH2 and BH3 domains of all six anti-apoptotic BCL2-like proteins are extremely conserved while, the n-terminal BH4 domain is less conserved. The lack of conservation within the BH4 domain would suggest that this domain could be a significant factor in determining how potently each individual BCL2-like gene can drive leukemogenesis [1,3,4,7,9-12].

There are numerous studies providing evidence that BCL2 family members are localized not only on mitochondrial outer membranes, but also Endoplasmic Reticulum (ER) or nuclear membranes [3,6,13]. Localization at the mitochondrial outer membranes has been shown to be important for inhibiting apoptosis, whereas localization to the ER may be important for regulating ER homeostasis and calcium storage [6,13,14]. The *in vivo* significance of targeting BCLxl to individual sub-cellular compartments has not been examined.

Overexpression of BCLxl has been found in many human cancers. Increased level of BCLxl results in decreased overall patient survival and is a marker for tumor progression [2,15-18]. In addition, the increased level of BCLxl protein causes tumor cells to gain resistance to chemotherapeutic drugs and inhibit Tumor Necrosis Factor (TNF) related or p53 mediated apoptosis [15,19]. Studies suggest that inhibition of antiapoptotic BCL2-like proteins with BH3-mimetics is

***Corresponding author:** Levi J.- Beverly, Department of Medicine, University of Louisville , 505 S. Hancock Street, CTRB rm 204,Louisville, KY 40202, USA, E-mail: Levi.Beverly@Louisville.edu

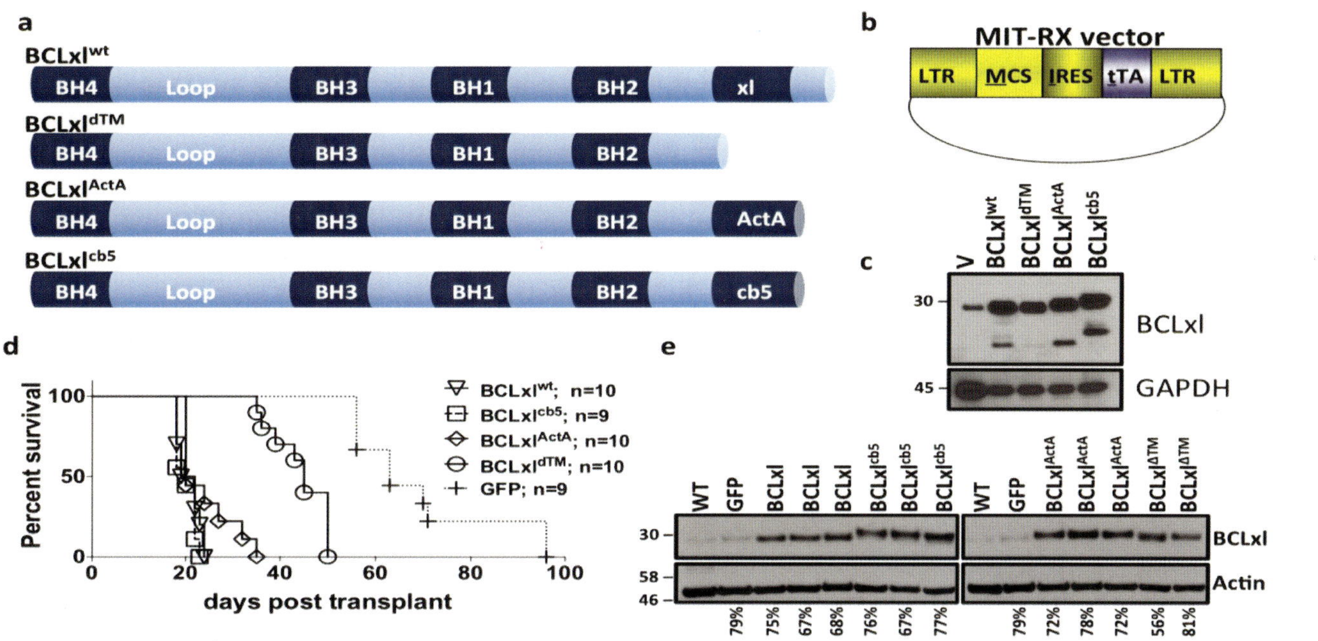

Figure 1: Targeting BCLxl to mitochondria or ER does not alter *in vivo* oncogenic potency.
a). Schematic of BCLxl constructs ($BCLxl^{wt}$, $BCLxl^{dTM}$, $BCLxl^{ActA}$ and $BCLxl^{cb5}$) used in the study.
b). Schematic of MIT-RX retroviral plasmid used in the studies.
c). Western blot of lysates expressing BCLxl constructs.
d). Kaplan-Meier survival curve of mice receiving Tet-O-MYC bone marrow infected with the indicated retrovirus.
Mantel-Cox Log-rank test was used to determine statistical significance, compared to $BCLxl^{wt}$ survival ($BCLxl^{dTM}$, p=<0.0001; $BCLxl^{ActA}$, p=0.063; $BCLxl^{cb5}$: p=0.324; GFP: p=<0.0001).
e). Western blot of splenocytes from leukemic mice.

a potential therapeutic approach. For example, inhibiting BCL2, BCLxl and BCLw with ABT-737 or ABT-263 sensitizes many different cancer cell lines to apoptosis [20-22]. These findings support the importance of exploring the detailed biochemical mechanisms by which anti-apoptotic BCL2-like family members drive leukemogenisis.

To date, most studies examining the anti-apoptotic ability of mutants of BCL2-like members have been exclusively performed in cell culture with defined apoptotic stimuli. The contribution of the different domains *in vivo* in the regulation of apoptosis is largely unknown. Therefore, in the present study we wanted to explore the contribution of the loop domain of BCLb and subcellular localization of BCLxl on *in vivo* oncogenic potency. Using our previously published MYC-induced leukemogenesis assay [23], we demonstrate that while the BH4 domain of BCLxl is critical for determining full oncogenic potency, the intracellular localization of BCLxl does not impact oncogenic potency. Taken together these studies suggest that understanding the biochemical details of how individual BCL2-like family members regulate apoptosis and tumorigenesis will provide insight into mechanisms that regulate apoptosis.

Results and Discussion

Targeting BCLxl only to mitochondria or ER does not alter *in vivo* oncogenic potency

Previous studies have shown that targeting exogenous BCLxl to the mitochondria or the ER does not alter the apoptotic response to toxic stimuli of Mouse Embryonic Fibroblasts (MEF) cells expressing endogenous BCLxl [6]. In the same study, researchers targeted BCLxl to the mitochondria or ER in MEFs deficient for endogenous BCLxl. These studies demonstrated that endogenous BCLxl was required for the ability of ER targeted $BCLxl^{cb5}$ to block apoptosis, whereas endogenous BCLxl was dispensable for mitochondrially targeted $BCLxl^{ActA}$ to inhibit cell death [6,24]. Herein, we wanted to determine the oncogenic potency of these BCLxl mutants in an *in vivo* MYC-induced model of leukemogenesis. We subcloned the described BCLxl constructs ($BCLxl^{WT}$, $BCLxl^{dTM}$, $BCLxl^{ActA}$, and $BCLxl^{cb5}$) into a retroviral plasmid expressing the tetracycline transactivator (tTA) (Figure 1a and 1b). To confirm construct overexpression, HEK293T cells were transfected and western blot analysis was performed (Figure 1c). Retroviruses expressing tTA and BCLxl constructs or GFP were used to infect bone marrow harvested from mice harboring a tetracycline transactivator (tTA)-dependent MYC allele (TET-O-MYC). The MIT-BCLxl retrovirus allows for constitutive co-expression of MYC and the individual BCLxl constructs. After infection of the bone marrow and transplantation into syngeneic recipients, mice were monitored for disease progression and then euthanized for further analysis and their survival noted on a Kaplan-Meier curve (Figure 1d). Previous studies have shown that $BCLxl^{WT}$ and MYC co-expression causes lethal myeloid leukemia in less than 30 days [2]. Mice expressing only MYC usually develop myeloid leukemia with a long latency, but in some instances mice will develop CD4+ T-cell leukemia, judged by a large abberant population of T-cells in the bone marrow, as we have shown previously [2,23,25]. In this study, mice that received cells co-expressing MYC and BCLxl constructs accelerated leukemogenesis compared to mice that received cells coexpressing MYC and GFP (Figure 1d). All BCLxl constructs accelerated disease in the mice, when compared to GFP, suggesting that oncogenic potency is not affected by BCL localization, *in vivo*. These data are consistent with previous *in vitro* biochemical

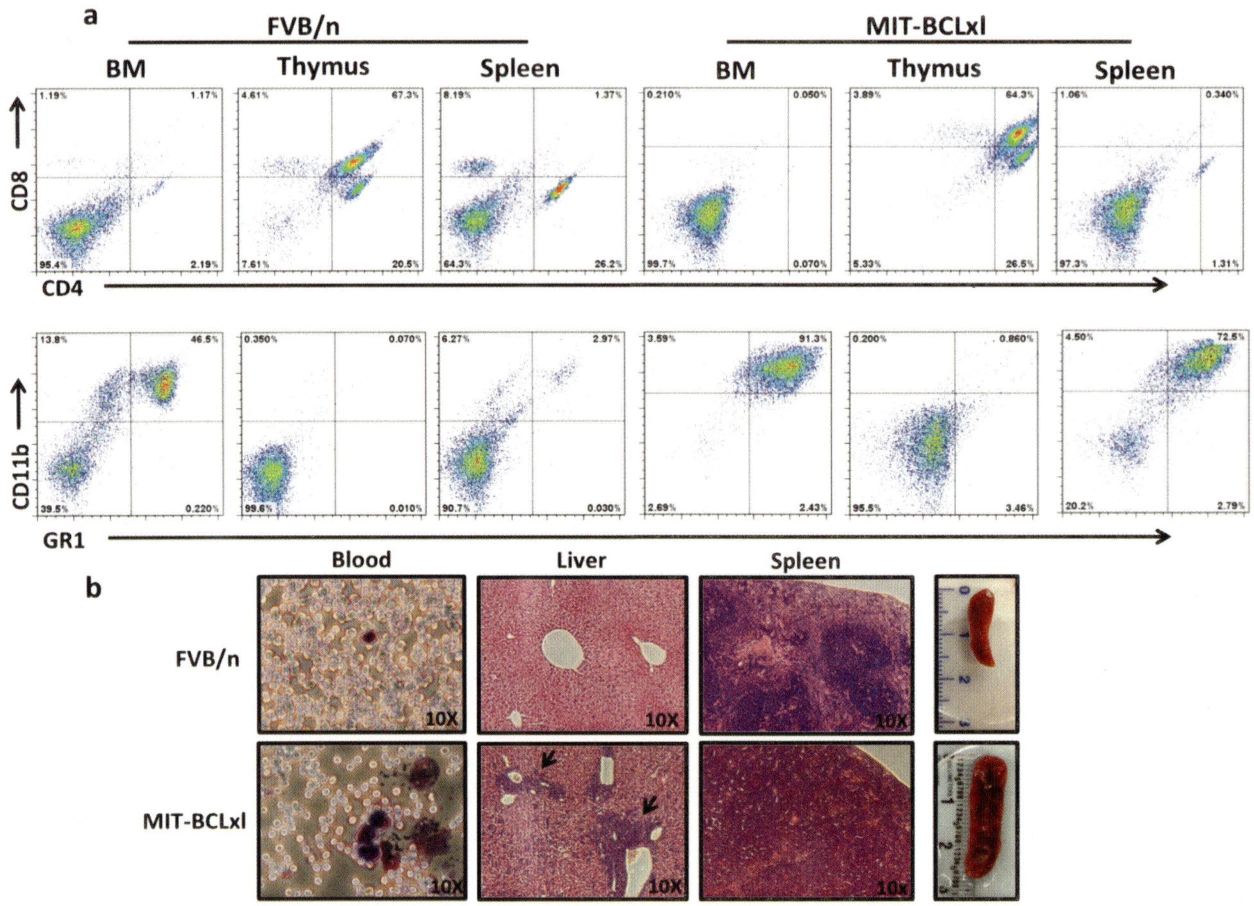

Figure 2: Characterization of leukemias that arise in mice receiving Tet-O-MYC bone marrow infected with MIT-BCLxl retroviruses.
a). Flow cytometry of Bone Marrow (BM), thymus and splenocytes from a non-manipulated 12 week old FVB/n mouse or a representative MIT-BCLxl leukemic mouse. Percentages indicate the percent of GR1/CD11b and CD4/CD8 cells in each sample, as determined by FACS analysis.
b). Histological analysis from a non-manipulated 12 week old FVB/n mouse or a representative MIT-BCLxl leukemic mouse.

studies using the same constructs [6]. Interestingly, BCLxl confined to the cytosol only ($BCLxl^{dTM}$), accelerated leukemogenesis compared to GFP, but subjects showed a longer survival (~60 days) compared to the mitochondrial or ER targeted constructs. To demonstrate that all BCLxl constructs were expressed at similar levels in the leukemias, spleen samples were examined by western blot analysis (Figure 1e). All leukemic spleens showed a comparable increase in the presence of BCLxl compared to ahealthy spleen or a spleen from a leukemic spleen expressing MYC and GFP. The leukemia that developed in all mice was consistent with our previous observations. The mice developed an Acute Myeloid Leukeima (AML) defined by an increase in cells with the myeloid cell markers GR-1 and CD11b in the spleen and bone marrow (Figure 2a), an enlarged spleen and leukemic infiltration of the blood, liver, and spleen also confirm the cancerous disease (Figure 2b).

The result that oncogenic potency is not modified when BCLxl is targeted to different organelles may be somewhat expected based on our previous observations in MEF cells [6]. However, it is interesting to note that there is a correlation between apoptotic sensitivity *in vitro* and oncogenic potency *in vivo*. This correlation could be further investigated by implementing the exogenous BCLxl constructs into $BCLxl^{WT}$ deficient hematopoietic progenitor cells.

Oncogenic role of the loop domain of BCLb

If BCLxl localization to ER or mitochondria does not alter oncogenic potency, then what does? It has been shown previously that a BH4 domain peptide is sufficient for anti-apoptotic activity in mouse models [26] but the role of the loop domain of BCL2-like proteins in oncogenic transformation is unknown. We therefore wanted to determine the role that the BCLb loop domain plays in dictating *in vivo* oncogenic potency of BCLxl. We developed a novel chimeric gene that has the loop domain from the less oncogenically potent BCLb engineered onto BCLxl. BCLb has been shown in previous studies, that although its expression is up regulated in some leukemic tumors, it is a less potent oncogene than BCLxl, in the same TET-O-MYC mouse model [2]. The n-terminal loop domain (loop) from BCLb was engineered to replace the corresponding domain of BCLxl (Figure 3a). To investigate if the stability of the BCLxl/b construct is altered *in vitro*, we treated cells expressing either wild-type BCLxl or the BCLxl/b chimera with MG132 (a proteasome inhibitor) or cycloheximide (CH; a protein biosynthesis inhibitor) (Figures 3b and 3c). No obvious differences were observed after either treatment, suggesting that the loop domain of BCLb is not responsible for dictating the half-life of the protein. Next, we determined the oncogenic potency of chimera *in vivo*, using the same TET-O-MYC mouse model of leukemia described above. The

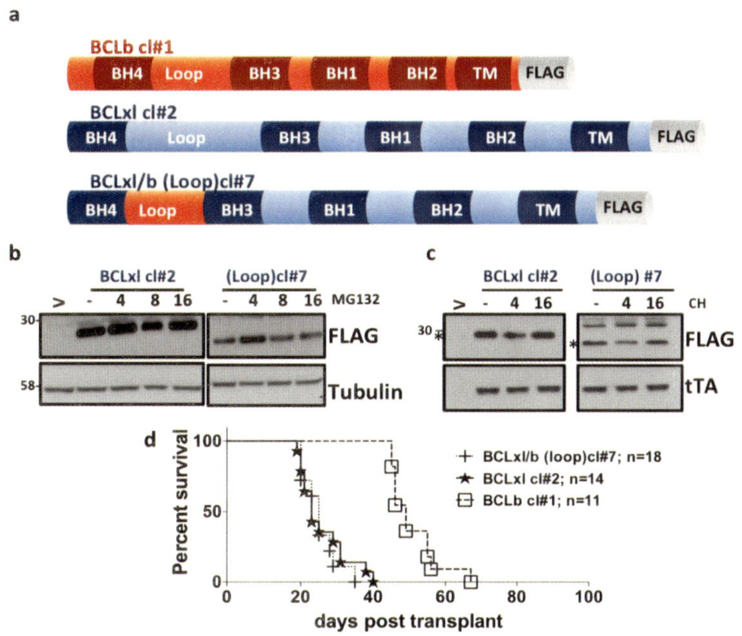

Figure 3: Oncogenic potency of loop domain of BCLb.
a) Schematic of BCLb cl#1-wild-type BCLb; BCLxl cl#2- wild-type BCLxl; BCLxl/b (BH4/loop) and cl#7- BCLxl engineered to harbor the loop domain of BCLb, constructs.
b) Western blot of lysates expressing indicated BCLxl constructs followed by treatment with MG132 at 25 μM for the indicated times.
c) Western blot of indicated BCLxl constructs after treatment with Cycloheximide (CH) at 20 μM for the indicated times Whereas (V) is empty vector.
d) Kaplan-Meier survival curve of mice receiving Tet-O-MYC bone marrow infected with the indicated MIT-RX containing retroviruses. Mantel-Cox Log rank test was used to determine statistical significance, compared to BCLxl^{WT} (#1: p=<0.0001; #7: p=0.568).

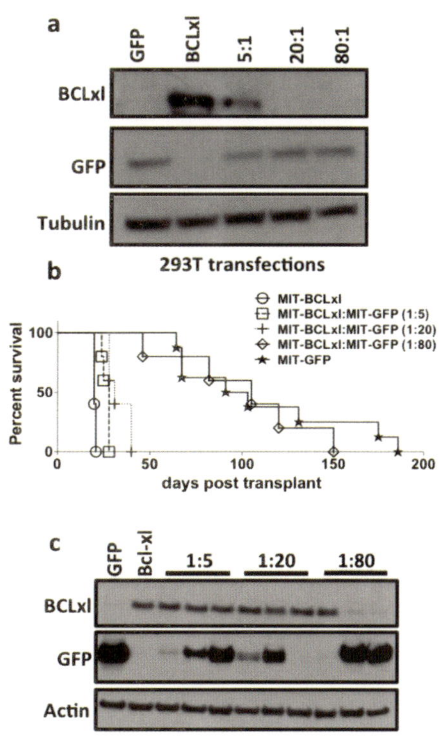

Figure 4: Determining the correlation between amount of BCLxl and oncogenic potency.
a) Western blot of HEK293T cells transfected with the indicated ratios of MIT-GFP and MIT-BCLxl.
b) Kaplan-Meier survival curve of mice receiving Tet-O-MYC bone marrow infected with equal amounts of the indicated retroviral supernatant containing decreasing amounts of MIT-BCLxl virus. Five mice received bone marrow infected with each viral supernatant.
c) Western blot of splenocytes from leukemic mice were performed as indicated above.

oncogenic potency of the BCLb loop domain construct was equivalent to wild type BCLxl (20-30 day survival) (Figure 3d). This data suggests that loop domain of BCLb does not change the survival span of mice in comparison to wild type BCLxl.

To support the notion that the observed results are due to intrinsic differences in biochemical properties of the tested BCLxl constructs and not simply due to alterations in the number of cells infected, a simple viral dilution experiment was carried out. Different ratios of non-potent MIT-GFP plasmids to potent MIT-BCLxl plasmids (5:1,20:1,80:1) were transfected into HEK293T cells and confirmed by western blot (Figure 4a). These viruses were then used to infect TET-O-MYC mouse bone marrow and monitored for the expected leukemic symptoms, as noted previously. It is clear that simply decreasing the amount of potent BCLxl plasmid up to 20 times less does not significantly alter *in vivo* disease onset (Figure 4b). In fact, a mouse that was transplanted with 20:1 GFP to BCLxl virus infected cells expressed similar amounts of BCLxl in leukemic splenocytes, indicating the strong selective pressure for cells expressing BCLxl even when there is 20 times less BCLxl virus present (Figure 4c). It is also interesting that at lower dilutions although all leukemias are clearly driven by infection with the tTA and BCLxl expressing virus some leukemias also express GFP. This represents the co-infection of the cells which become the leukemic are carrying both viruses. However at the larger dilution, the leukemia is either driven by tTA and BCLxl or only by the tTA and GFP expressing virus. This experiment reinforces the idea that it may be intrinsic biochemical properties of individual BCL2-like proteins, such as expression levels, can dictate oncogenic potential.

The results herein demonstrate the importance of moving experiments done in cell culture into *in vivo* assays. Critically, it is always of significance to determine if the ability of BCL2-like proteins to inhibit apoptosis induced by selected stimuli translates into the ability to more potently cause disease in a model system. Since leukemias generated in this model are readily transplantable, future experiments can be directed at understanding if decreased initiation of leukemogenesis, by certain BCLxl constructs, also means that these leukemias will respond better to cytotoxic therapeutics. These studies will increase our general knowledge of the biochemical mechanisms required for BCL2-like proteins to drive tumorigenesis and therapeutic responses.

Methods

Plasmids

All constructs (BCLxl^{WT} - wildtype BCLxl; BCLxld^{TM} - BCLxl lacking the cterminal transmembrane domain; BCLxl^{ActA} - BCLxl engineered to have the mitochondrial targeted transmembrane domain from Listeria ActA protein; BCLxl^{cb5} -BCLxl engineered to have the ER targeted transmembrane domain from cytochrome b5) were produced in Li laboratory, Departments of Medicine, Pharmacology, and Toxicology, University of Louisville, Louisville and epitope tagged BCLb cl#1 - wild-typeBCLb; BCLxl cl#2 - wildtype BCLxl; BCLxl/b (BH4/loop); cl#7- BCLxl engineered to harbor the loop domain of BCLb were produced in our laboratory and sub-cloned into MIT-RX; a murine retroviral vector, as described in our earlier study [27]. Where, LTR -long terminal repeats; MCS- multiple cloning sites; IRES- internal ribosomal entry sequence; tTA- tetracycline transactivator. Details of BCLxl constructs have also been previously characterized [6]. Clones were then transformed into 5-α competent strain of E. coli cells (NEB, Ipswich, MA, USA, #C2987H) and DNA was isolated using eZNA kit as per the manufacturer's protocol (Omega, Norcross, GA, USA, #D6924).

Cell culture and transfection

Human embryonic kidney 293T cells (HEK293T) were procured from American Type Culture Collection (ATCC, Rockville, MD, USA) and cultured in DMEM medium (Hyclone, Logan, UT, USA, #SH30243) supplemented with 10% fetal bovine serum (Hyclone, Logan, UT, USA, #SH30070) and 1% antibiotic/antimycotic (Hyclone, Logan, UT, USA, #SV30010). DNA transfections were done with BCLxl constructs using polyethylenimine (Polysciences, Warrington, PA, USA, #23966-2) in HEK293T cells and viruses were collected as described [23].

Bone marrow transplantation, Western Blots and flow cytometry

In vivo experiments were done as described previously [2,23,27]. Briefly, bone marrow was flushed from untreated donor mice that carried the Tet-O-MYC transgene. Red blood cells were lysed and viral infections were then carried out in the presence of polybrene (Millipore, Danvers, MA, USA, #TR-1003-G) using retroviral BCLxl construct. After infection, cells were immediately transplanted into the tail vein of lethally irradiated FVB/n recipients acquired from Taconic. Spleens from leukemic mice were snap frozen in liquid nitrogen and pulverized with mortar and pestle. Cells were lysed in with 1% CHAPS lysis buffer and protein was estimated as described in our previous study [28].

Western blots were performed in Bolt Bis-Tris gels (Life Technologies, Grand island, NY, USA, #BG4120BOX) as per manufacturers protocol using anti-BCLxl (Cell Signaling Technology, Danvers, MA, # 2764) or anti-Actin (Sigma, St. Louis, MO, #A2228). Spleen, bone marrow and thymus were analyzed by flow cytometer. In brief, single cells were isolated from indicated organ; red blood cells were lysed and blocked for 10 mins at room temperature with Fc Block (BD Biosciences, Miami, FL, USA, #553142). Afterward, FACS analysis were performed by standard techniques using anti-PE Ly-6G & Ly-6C (BD, San Jose, CA, # 553128) and anti-PE-Cy7 CD11b (BD, #552850) on Becton Dickinson FACScan with FlowJo.

Histology and biochemical analysis

For histological staining peripheral blood from the indicated mice was smeared on a glass slide and stained with Hema 3 (Fisher, Hampton, NH, # 22-122-911) as indicated by manufacturer's protocol. Liver and spleen were fixed in neutral buffered formalin and embedded in paraffin. Sections were stained with Hematoxylin and Eosin (H&E) using standard techniques and photographed at 10X or 20X. For biochemical analysis, MIT-BCLxl (cl#1, cl#2 & cl#7) or empty vector (V) were transfected into HEK293T cells and 36 hrs after transfection, the cells were treated with MG132 at 25 μM for the 4, 8 & 16 hrs followed by western blot with the anti-epitope tagged antibodies (FLAG and Tubulin, Sigma, # F1804). The same constructs were also transfected into HEK293T cells and 36 hrs later cells were treated with Cycloheximide (CH) at 20 μM for the 4 and 16 hrs followed by western blot with FLAG and anti-tTA (Clontech, Mountain View, CA, # 631108). To determine the correlation between amount of BCLxl and oncogenic potency, HEK293T cells were transfected with the ratios of the MIT-GFP and MIT-BCLxl (3 μg of MIT-GFP; BCLxl, 3 μg of MIT-BCLxl; 1:5, 2.4 μg of MIT-GFP and 0.6 μg of MIT-BCLxl; 1:20, 2.85 μg of MIT-GFP and 0.15 μg of MIT-BCLxl; 1:80, 2.9625 μg of MIT-GFP and 0.0375 μg of MIT-BCLxl), virus were produced, infected in bone marrow and transplanted as described above. Western blot of splenocytes from leukemic mice were also performed using anti-BCLxl, GFP and actin.

Acknowledgement

We would like to thank members of the Beverly laboratory for technical support, especially Lavona Casson. Portions of this work were performed in the laboratory of Harold Varmus at MSKCC, we extend our gratitude for his generosity and support. This work was supported by start-up funds from James Graham Brown Cancer Center to LJB, The Kosair Pediatric Cancer Research Program, Molecular Targets COBRE 8P20GM103482-10 from NIH, a Wendy Will Case Cancer Fund grant to LJB, R25-CA-134283 from the National Cancer Institute to AS.

References

1. Gross A, McDonnell JM, Korsmeyer SJ (1999) BCL-2 family members and the mitochondria in apoptosis. Genes Dev 13: 1899-1911.
2. Beverly LJ, Varmus HE (2009) MYC-induced myeloid leukemogenesis is accelerated by all six members of the antiapoptotic BCL family. Oncogene 28: 1274-1279.
3. Kvansakul M, Hinds MG (2013) Structural biology of the Bcl-2 family and its mimicry by viral proteins. Cell Death Dis 4: e909.
4. Shamas-Din A, Kale J, Leber B, Andrews DW (2013) Mechanisms of action of Bcl-2 family proteins. Cold Spring Harb Perspect Biol 5: a008714.
5. Reed JC, Jurgensmeier JM, Matsuyama S (1998) Bcl-2 family proteins and mitochondria. Biochim Biophys Acta 1366: 127-137.
6. Eno CO, Eckenrode EF, Olberding KE, Zhao G, White C, et al. (2012) Distinct roles of mitochondria- and ER-localized Bcl-xL in apoptosis resistance and Ca2+ homeostasis. Mol Biol Cell 23: 2605-2618.
7. Fischer U, Schulze-Osthoff K (2005) New approaches and therapeutics targeting apoptosis in disease. Pharmacol Rev 57: 187-215.
8. Gerl R, Vaux DL (2005) Apoptosis in the development and treatment of cancer. Carcinogenesis 26: 263-270.
9. Yip KW, Reed JC (2008) Bcl-2 family proteins and cancer. Oncogene 27: 6398-6406.
10. Elkholi R, Floros KV, Chipuk JE (2011) The Role of BH3-Only Proteins in Tumor Cell Development, Signaling, and Treatment. Genes Cancer 2: 523-537.
11. Strasser A, O'Connor L, Dixit VM (2000) Apoptosis signaling. Annu Rev Biochem 69: 217-245.
12. Frenzel A, Grespi F, Chmelewskij W, Villunger A (2009) Bcl2 family proteins in carcinogenesis and the treatment of cancer. Apoptosis 14: 584-596.
13. Scorrano L, Oakes SA, Opferman JT, Cheng EH, Sorcinelli MD, et al. (2003) BAX and BAK regulation of endoplasmic reticulum Ca2+: a control point for apoptosis. Science 300: 135-139.
14. Thomenius MJ, Distelhorst CW (2003) Bcl-2 on the endoplasmic reticulum: protecting the mitochondria from a distance. J Cell Sci 116: 4493-4499.
15. Schott AF, Apel IJ, Nuñez G, Clarke MF (1995) Bcl-XL protects cancer cells from p53-mediated apoptosis. Oncogene 11: 1389-1394.
16. Olopade OI, Adeyanju MO, Safa AR, Hagos F, Mick R, et al. (1997) Overexpression of BCL-x protein in primary breast cancer is associated with high tumor grade and nodal metastases. Cancer J Sci Am 3: 230-237.
17. Zhuang L, Lee CS, Scolyer RA, McCarthy SW, Zhang XD, et al. (2007) Mcl-1, Bcl-XL and Stat3 expression are associated with progression of melanoma whereas Bcl-2, AP-2 and MITF levels decrease during progression of melanoma. Mod Pathol 20: 416-426.
18. Cao X, Yap JL, Newell-Rogers MK, Peddaboina C, Jiang W, et al. (2013) The novel BH3 Î±-helix mimetic JY-1-106 induces apoptosis in a subset of cancer cells (lung cancer, colon cancer and mesothelioma) by disrupting Bcl-xL and Mcl-1 protein-protein interactions with Bak. Mol Cancer 12: 42.
19. Walczak H, Bouchon A, Stahl H, Krammer PH (2000) Tumor necrosis factor-related apoptosis-inducing ligand retains its apoptosis-inducing capacity on Bcl-2- or Bcl-xL-overexpressing chemotherapy-resistant tumor cells. Cancer Res 60: 3051-3057.
20. Chauhan D, Velankar M, Brahmandam M, Hideshima T, Podar K, et al. (2007) A novel Bcl-2/Bcl-X(L)/Bcl-w inhibitor ABT-737 as therapy in multiple myeloma. Oncogene 26: 2374-2380.
21. Lin X, Morgan-Lappe S, Huang X, Li L, Zakula DM, et al. (2007) 'Seed' analysis of off-target siRNAs reveals an essential role of Mcl-1 in resistance to the small-molecule Bcl-2/Bcl-XL inhibitor ABT-737. Oncogene 26: 3972-3979.
22. Casson L, Howell L, Mathews LA, Ferrer M, Southall N, et al. (2013) Inhibition of ceramide metabolism sensitizes human leukemia cells to inhibition of BCL2-like proteins. PLoS One 8: e54525.
23. Beverly LJ (2013) Oncogenic driver supersedes BM preparation as the critical determinant of leukemic outcome: a one day protocol for BM harvest, infection and transplantation. Bone Marrow Transplant 48: 1003-1005.
24. Zhu W, Cowie A, Wasfy GW, Penn LZ, Leber B, et al. (1996) Bcl-2 mutants with restricted subcellular location reveal spatially distinct pathways for apoptosis in different cell types. EMBO J 15: 4130-4141.
25. Saurabh K, Scherzer MT, Shah PP, Mims AS, Lockwood WW5, et al. (2014) The PIM family of oncoproteins: small kinases with huge implications in myeloid leukemogenesis and as therapeutic targets. Oncotarget .
26. Sugioka R, Shimizu S, Funatsu T, Tamagawa H, Sawa Y, et al. (2003) BH4-domain peptide from Bcl-xL exerts anti-apoptotic activity *in vivo*. Oncogene 22: 8432-8440.
27. Beverly LJ, Lockwood WW, Shah PP, Erdjument-Bromage H, Varmus H (2012) Ubiquitination, localization, and stability of an anti-apoptotic BCL2-like protein, BCL2L10/BCLb, are regulated by Ubiquilin1. Proceedings of the National Academy of Sciences of the United States of America 109: E119-126.
28. Shah PP, Lockwood WW, Saurabh K, Kurlawala Z, Shannon SP, et al. (2014) Ubiquilin1 represses migration and epithelial-to-mesenchymal transition of human non-small cell lung cancer cells. Oncogene .

Can we Reduce the Toxicity of the Mediastinal Irradiation Using New Highly Conformal Techniques?

Victor Pernin, Sofia Zefkili, Dominique Peurien, Alain Fourquet and Youlia M Kirova*

Department of Radiation Oncology, Institute Curie, Paris, France

Abstract

Objectives: Three-Dimensional Conformal Radiotherapy (3DCRT) has been successfully used to treat Hodgkin's Lymphoma (HL) but treatment delivery is often complex and requires large fields that may result in significant exposure of normal tissues to ionizing radiation. The present study was undertaken to compare the dosimetry of Involved Field (IF) 3DCRT to HT in female patients treated for HL.

Materials/Methods: A total of 10 young female patients affected with early stage mediastinal HL and treated with IF radiotherapy after chemotherapy were selected from our database. For each patient, 3DCRT and HT plans were designed to deliver 30 Gy to the target volume and 36 Gy in case of residual masses. HT planning solutions were optimized by inverse planning with specific dose-volume constraints on OAR (breasts, lungs, heart). Dose-Volume Histograms (DVHs) were calculated and then compared, both for target and OAR by a statistical analysis (Wilcoxon's Test).

Results: Mean doses to the PTV were almost identical for all plans. Conformity index was better with HT and homogeneity index didn't differ. Mean dose to the breasts were increased with HT compared to 33DCRT (right breast: 3.28 vs 2.19, $p<0.05$; left breast: 3.76 vs 2.81, $p<0.05$) whereas no difference in mean doses appeared for heart, coronary arteries, lungs, thyroid and normal tissue. Maximal doses were reduced with HT for breasts (right breast: 19.9 vs 28.87, $p<0.05$; left breast: 24.76 vs 30.29, $p<0.05$) and spinal cord (20.87 vs 33.88, $p<0.05$). Volume exposed to high doses was smaller with HT whereas volume exposed to low doses was smaller with 3DCRT. Pronounced benefits of HT in terms of heart sparing were observed for patients with lymph nodes anterior to the heart.

Conclusions: Although high dose to organ at risk was reduced with HT, increasing low dose especially to the breasts must be taken into account for IF HT. HT may be considered for large PTV especially when the anterior mediastinum is involved.

Keywords: Radiotherapy; Lymphoma; Toxicity; Second malignancies; Lung and Heart sparing

Introduction

Hodgkin lymphoma belongs to the group of malignancies with a high curability rate, as the 5-year relative survival is close to 84% for all forms of Hodgkin lymphoma combined, as a result of treatment based on chemotherapy and radiotherapy [1]. Progress in the management of Hodgkin lymphoma is related to the development of combination chemotherapy regimens and progress in radiotherapy techniques. However, these treatments are accompanied by late adverse effects such as cardiac toxicity and a risk of second cancers such as lung cancer and breast cancer for women [2-8]. The benefit-risk balance of the various treatment regimens must therefore be carefully assessed in order to achieve optimal disease control without increasing the risk of long-term sequelae.

The toxicity of radiotherapy can be decreased in three ways: reduce the dose, reduce treatment volumes and use innovative radiotherapy techniques such as Intensity-Modulated Radiotherapy (IMRT) [8]. The classical dose of 44 Gy has been reduced to 30-36 Gy. Similarly, treatment volumes have been reduced by replacing subtotal lymphoid irradiation by "involved-field" (IF) radiotherapy, which only includes lymph node territories initially invaded, then "involved-node" radiotherapy, only including invaded lymph nodes, which is currently at the stage of clinical evaluation [9]. In contrast, the respective roles of the various radiotherapy techniques in the treatment of Hodgkin's lymphoma differ from one radiotherapy centre to another and no consensus has been reached on this subject.

Several comparative dosimetric studies have demonstrated improved coverage of target volumes and better sparing of certain organs at risk when IF radiotherapy is delivered by classical IMRT compared to three-dimensional conformal radiotherapy (3DCRT) for patients with supradiaphragmatic Hodgkin lymphoma, which could result in a reduction of late radiation-induced toxicity [10-12].

Few data are currently available concerning the use of tomotherapy in this indication [13]. The objective of this dosimetric study was to compare 3DCRT treatment plans and tomotherapy treatment plans in women treated by IF radiotherapy at a dose of 30 Gy and at a dose of 30 Gy plus 6 Gy for Hodgkin lymphoma in order to determine the place of tomotherapy in this indication.

Materials and Methods

Patient selection

This dosimetric study was based on 14 female patients with a

***Corresponding author:** Youlia M. Kirova, Radiation Oncology, Institute Curie 26, Rue d'Ulm 75005 Paris, France; Email: youlia.kirova@curie.fr

Characteristics	
Age	
- median	23 years [16-45]
Women	14 (100%)
Histology : - sclero-nodular	14 (100%)
Ann Arbor classification- stage II	14 (100%)
Chemotherapy :	
- 3 ABVD	4 (29%)
- 4 ABVD	7 (50%)
- 2 BEACOPP + 2 ABVD	3 (21%)
Irradiation at the dose of 30 Gy :	7 (50%)
- volume of PTV 30 Gy in 3D-CRT (median)	620 cm^3 [272-1536]
- médiastinal invasion alone	2 (14%)
- mediastinal and pericardial invasion	1 (7%)
- mediastinal and cervical invasion	3 (22%)
- mediastinal, cervical and axillary invasion	1 (7%)
Irradiation at the dose of 30 Gy + 6 Gy on the residual tumor :	7 (50%)
- volume of PTV 30 Gy in 3D-CRT (median)	506 [341-898]
- médiastinal invasion alone	3 (22%)
- mediastinal and pericardial invasion	2 (14%)
- mediastinal and cervical invasion	1 (7%)
- mediastinal, cervical and axillary invasion	1 (7%)

Table 1: Patient characteristics (n=14).

Parameters	Objectives
PTV	
- $V_{95\,Gy}$	95 %
Lungs	$V_{20\,Gy}$ < 35% $V_{30\,Gy}$ < 20 %
Heart	$V_{30\,Gy}$ < 40 % Mean dose < 20 Gy
Left and right parotid (if high cervical irradiation)	$V_{26\,Gy} \leq 50$ %
Canal médullaire	Maximum dose < 30 Gy

Dmax: maximum dose
An order of priority of OAR dose constraints was used for tomotherapy planning: in the case of a lateralised lesion, contralateral lung to the lesion > ipsilateral lung to the lesion > heart > ipsilateral breast > contralateral breast > parotid gland > spinal canal; in the case of a central lesion: left lung > right lung > heart > left breast > right breast > parotid gland > spinal canal.

Table 2: Dose constraints to target volumes and organs at risk.

median age of 23 years (range: 16-45 years) treated at Institute Curie for histologically documented stage II supradiaphragmatic Hodgkin lymphoma treated by a sequential combination of chemotherapy and radiotherapy. All patients were assessed by FDG PET before and after chemotherapy. All patients received ABVD and/or BEACOPP chemotherapy followed by "involved-field" radiotherapy to a total dose of 30 Gy with a 6 Gy boost to the residual tumour for 7 patients. Patient characteristics are shown in (Table 1).

Radiotherapy simulation

Simulation in the treatment position was based on two CT scans with a slice thickness of 3 mm about two weeks before starting radiotherapy: unenhanced CT followed by contrast-enhanced CT. Patients were positioned in the supine position with their arms above the head. A personalized immobilization mask was created for each patient. CT acquisition was performed under free breathing conditions.

Definition of radiotherapy volumes

CT and FDG PET performed before chemotherapy were fused with CT performed during radiotherapy simulation. Contouring was performed with Eclipse software (Varian Medical Systems, Palo Alto, USA) for all treatment plans. The Clinical Target Volume (CTV) was determined by the same radiation oncologist. Clinical target volumes treated at the total dose of 30 Gy corresponded to initially invaded lymph nodes according to the "involved-field" modality with the following modifications: cervical lymph nodes situated above the larynx were irradiated only when they were initially invaded; right and left supraclavicular lymph nodes were irradiated only when the mediastinum was initially invaded; the lower limit of the mediastinal field did not extend beyond the level of the initially invaded lymph nodes [14]. In the case of residual tumour on contrast-enhanced CT and/or FDG PET, a clinical target volume was determined to continue irradiation to a dose of 6 Gy. For the Planning Target Volume (PTV), a 10 mm margin was added to the CTV. The following organs at risk were delineated: spinal canal, heart, left and right lung, oesophagus, trachea, thyroid, left and right breasts. The origins of the left and right coronary arteries were contoured according to the anatomical atlas. The dose to healthy tissues was also studied by measuring the doses delivered to the external contour (extending 5 cm on either side of the PTV) without the PTV.

Treatment plans

Dosimetries were calculated by Eclipse software (Varian Medical Systems, Palo Alto, CA, USA) and Tomotherapy software (Tomotherapy Incorporated, Madison, WI, USA) for tomotherapy plans. Dose constraints are presented in (Table 2).

3DCRT treatment plan

3DCRT ballistics are based on 6 MV or 20 MV beams using a multi-leaf collimator.

- In the absence of residual tumour after chemotherapy, a total dose of 30 Gy in 15 fractions (2 Gy per fraction) was prescribed to the isocentre of the 30 Gy PTV.
- In the presence of residual tumour after chemotherapy, an initial treatment plan delivering a dose of 30 Gy in 15 fractions (2 Gy per fraction) to the isocentre of the 30 Gy PTV was prescribed followed by a second plan delivering a dose of 6 Gy in 3 fractions (2 Gy per fraction) to the isocentre of the 36 Gy PTV.

To improve dosimetry, a field-in-field technique was used for treatment plans, when necessary. Dosimetries were calculated with Eclipse software using a convolution-superposition dose calculation algorithm in order to take into account the heterogeneities for a Varian Clinac accelerator.

Tomotherapy treatment plan: Tomotherapy treatment plans were elaborated for each patient using the same simulation CT scan as 3DCRT treatment plans. The same PTV and the same organs at risk were therefore used for 3DCRT and tomotherapy treatment plans. Tomotherapy treatment plans presented the following parameters: field width: 2.5 cm, pitch: 0.287 and modulation factor: 3. Dose constraints to target volumes and organs at risk were identical to those used for 3DCRT.

- In the absence of residual tumour after chemotherapy, a total dose of 30 Gy in 15 fractions (2 Gy per fraction) was prescribed to the 30 Gy PTV.
- In the presence of residual tumour after chemotherapy, simultaneous integrated boost (SIB) tomotherapy was

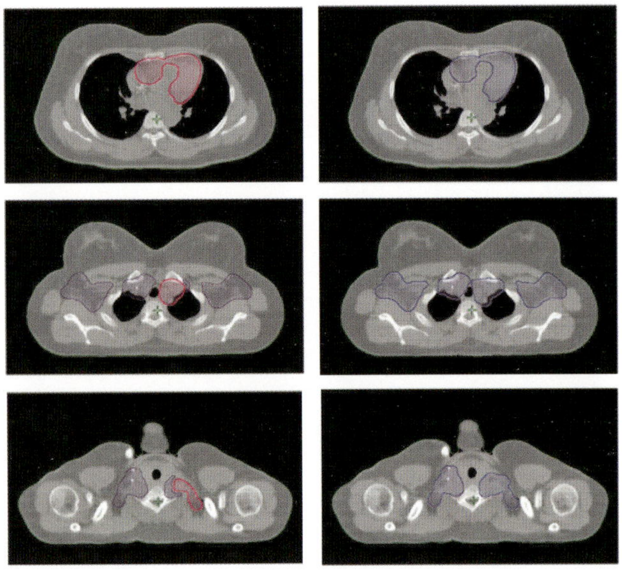

Figure 1: Tomotherapy plan (left) and 3DCRT plan (right): PTV_{tomo} 30 Gy (blue on left) with tomotherapy corresponds to PTV 30 Gy (blue on right) with 3DCRT minus PTV 36 Gy (magenta) with a 5 mm margin between PTV_{tomo} 30 Gy and PTV 36 Gy.

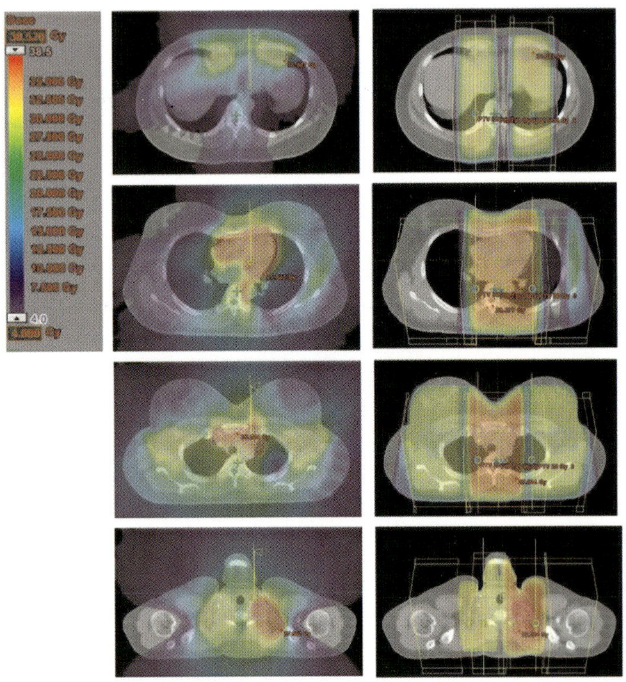

Figure 2: Comparison of isodoses from 4 Gy to 38.5 Gy between tomotherapy (left) and 3DCRT (right) treatment plans for a patient with Hodgkin lymphoma invading anterior mediastinal lymph nodes treated up to a dose of 36 Gy. This qualitative dosimetric comparison demonstrates an increase of the volumes exposed to a dose of 4 Gy with tomotherapy compared to 3DCRT.

performed. PTV_{tomo} 30 Gy and PTV 36 Gy were contoured separately (Figure 1-4). PTV_{tomo} 30 Gy in tomotherapy therefore corresponded to PTV 30 Gy in 3DCRT minus PTV 36 Gy with a 5 mm margin between PTV_{tomo} 30 Gy and PTV 36 Gy. With the SIB technique, treatments of PTV_{tomo} 30 Gy and PTV 36 Gy were combined in a single treatment plan. An alternative schedule to the sequential schedule was therefore defined: by using the linear quadratic model of cell survival, we calculated the total dose and the dose per fraction for PTV_{tomo} 30 Gy and PTV 36 Gy to ensure that they were biologically equivalent to the total dose delivered to PTV 30 Gy and PTV 36 Gy by 2 Gy fractions in the sequential schedule. A α/β ratio of 10 Gy was chosen for tumour response and a α/β ratio of 3 Gy was chosen for late response of normal tissues. A dose of 30.5 Gy in

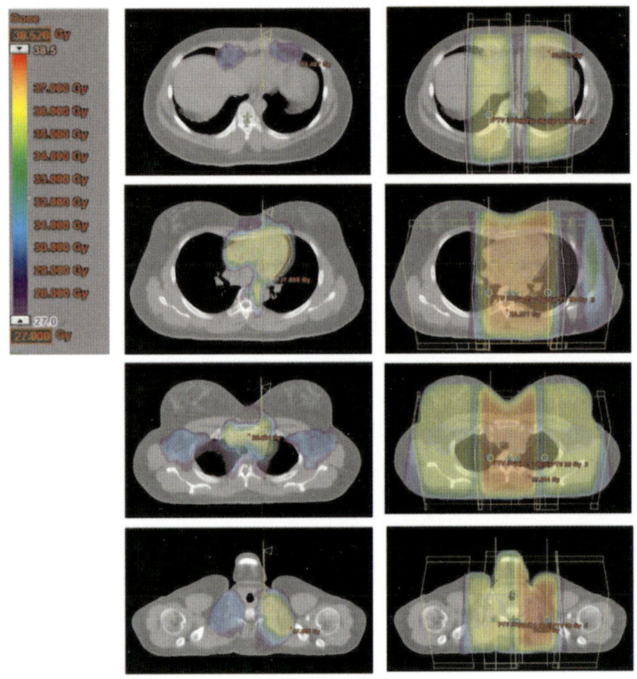

Figure 3: Comparison of isodoses from 27 Gy (90% of the dose to PTV 30 Gy) to 38.5 Gy (107% of the dose to PTV 36 Gy) between tomotherapy (left) and 3DCRT (right) treatment plans for a patient with Hodgkin lymphoma invading anterior mediastinal lymph nodes treated up to a dose of 36 Gy. This qualitative dosimetric comparison demonstrates an improvement of the conformation and homogeneity of the dose with tomotherapy compared to 3DCRT.

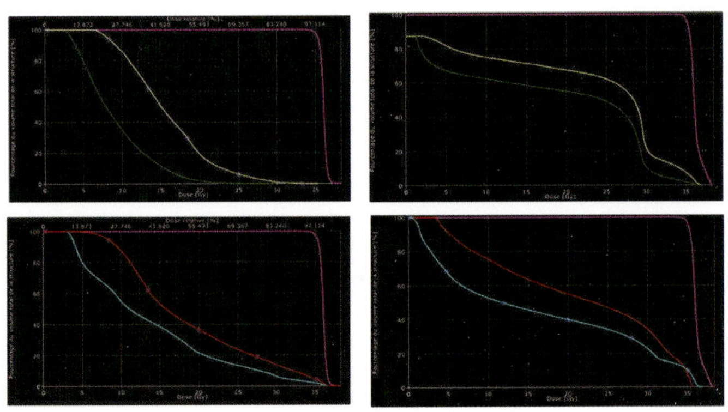

Figure 4: Comparison of dose-volume histograms of the tomotherapy (left) and 3DCRT (right) treatment plans for the same patient with Hodgkin lymphoma invading anterior mediastinal lymph nodes treated up to a dose of 36 Gy. Tomotherapy allowed a reduction of the volumes of heart (red) and lungs (blue), right breast (green) and left breast (yellow) exposed to high doses with a corresponding increase of the volumes exposed to low doses.

Paramètres	3D-CRT	Tomotherapy	P
PTV 30 Gy			
- Mean Dose	30.1 (± 0.4)	30.3 (± 0.9)	NS*
- V_{90} (%)	98.1 (± 2.3)	99.9 (± 0.1)	0.03
- V_{95} (%)	94.7 (± 4.4)	98,7 (± 0.8)	0.03
- V_{100} (%)	63 (± 16.5)	52.2 (± 5)	NS
- V_{107} (%)	1.2 (± 1.7)	0	NS
- Conformity index	2.9 (± 0.8)	1.4 (± 0.2)	0.01
- Homogeneity index	2.9 (± 4.2)	0.5 (± 0.07)	0.03

*NS: non-significant

Table 3: Comparison of doses to the target volume.

Parameters	3D-CRT				P
	Mean	Median	Mean	Median	
Right breast					
- Mean dose (Gy)	2.3	1.6	3.6	3.6	NS*
- Maximum dose (Gy)	26.4	29.5	18.4	20.4	0.03
- $V_{4\ Gy}$ (%)	8.1	6.9	35.4	30.6	0.01
- $V_{10\ Gy}$ (%)	7.3	5.3	10.5	6.1	NS
- $V_{15\ Gy}$ (%)	5	3.9	2.1	0.6	0.03
- $V_{20\ Gy}$ (%)	3.9	2.6	0.1	0.1	0.03
- $V_{30\ Gy}$ (%)	0.5	1.3	0	0	NS
Left breast					
- Mean dose (Gy)	5	1.9	5.6	4.5	NS
- Maximum dose (Gy)	27.6	30.9	25	28.4	NS
- $V_{4\ Gy}$ (%)	22.3	8.2	41.2	35	0.01
- $V_{10\ Gy}$ (%)	18	5.7	22.8	15.8	NS
- $V_{15\ Gy}$ (%)	14.9	3.2	10.9	6.4	NS
- $V_{20\ Gy}$ (%)	13.1	2.6	5.5	1.6	NS
- $V_{30\ Gy}$ (%)	1.1	0.5	0.3	0	NS

*NS: non-significant

Table 4: Comparison of mean and median dosimetric parameters for the breasts.

17 fractions (1.8 Gy per fraction) was therefore prescribed to PTV_{tomo} 30 Gy and a dose of 35.7 Gy in 17 fractions (2.1 Gy per fraction) was prescribed to PTV 36 Gy.

Dosimetries were calculated by inverse planning with Tomotherapy software. For each patient, tomotherapy treatment plans were optimized in order to be able to deliver irradiation under real conditions.

Evaluation

Three dosimetric studies were performed:

- Comparison of 3DCRT and tomotherapy treatment plans for 7 patients with no residual tumour treated at the dose of 30 Gy
- Comparison of 3DCRT and tomotherapy treatment plans for 7 patients with residual tumour treated at the dose of 30 Gy with a 6 Gy boost to the residual tumour.
- Comparison of 3DCRT and tomotherapy treatment plans for all patients (N=14)

Summation of 3DCRT treatment plans comprising PTV 30 Gy and PTV 36 Gy was performed to allow dosimetric comparison with SIB tomotherapy plans.

3DCRT and tomotherapy plans were compared quantitatively by analysis of physical doses on dose-volume histograms and qualitatively by visualization of isodose curves. The parameters analysed for PTV included mean dose, $V_{90\%}$, $V_{95\%}$, $V_{100\%}$, $V_{107\%}$ of the prescribed dose, Conformity Index (CI) and Homogeneity Index (HI).

The RTOG (Radiation Therapy Oncology Group) conformity index (CI) was defined by the following formula [15]:

$$Conformity\ index_{RTOG} = \frac{V_{RI}}{TV}$$

(TV: Target volume; V_{RI}: prescription isodose volume)

The RTOG homogeneity index (HI) was defined by the following formula:

$$Homogeneity\ index_{RTOG} = \frac{Imax}{RI}$$

(*Imax:* Maximum isodose in the target volume; *RI:* Reference Isodose)

Parameters analysed for organs at risk included: mean dose, maximum dose, V_{4Gy}, V_{10Gy}, V_{20Gy}, V_{30Gy} and V_{36Gy} for the right breast, left breast, lungs, heart, origin of the right coronary artery, origin of the left coronary artery, oesophagus and healthy tissues. The following parameters were analysed for the thyroid: mean dose, median dose, V_{18Gy}, V_{26Gy} and the parameters analysed for the spinal canal and trachea were maximum dose and mean dose, respectively.

Statistical analysis

Median values for each dosimetric parameter derived from dose-volume histograms of 3DCRT and tomotherapy treatment plans were compared by a nonparametric test for paired series (Wilcoxon test) using GraphPad Prism 5 software (Graph Pad Software, San Diego, CA, USA). Differences were considered to be significant for $p<0.05$.

Results

Evaluation of tomotherapy and 3DCRT treatment plans at the dose of 30 Gy

Doses to target volumes: The mean doses delivered to the PTV 30 Gy were equivalent with 3DCRT and tomotherapy with significantly improved V_{90} and V_{95}. The Conformity Index (CI) was better with tomotherapy (1.4) than with 3DCRT (2.9) ($p=0.01$). The homogeneity index was also better on tomotherapy plans ($p=0.03$) (Table 3).

Doses to organs at risk

- Right and left breasts

No significant difference in terms of the mean dose to the right breast and the left breast was observed between 3DCRT and tomotherapy, but, as expected, the V_4 was higher with tomotherapy than with 3DCRT. Tomotherapy allowed a reduction of the maximum dose and a reduction of V_{15Gy} and V_{20Gy} for the right breast only ($p=0.03$) (Table 4).

- Lungs

Tomotherapy did not allow any reduction of the mean dose to the lungs. Volumes exposed to low doses were increased with tomotherapy and volumes exposed to doses greater than or equal to 20 Gy were increased with 3DCRT. The median V_{20Gy} with tomotherapy and 3DCRT was therefore 16.2% and 23.9%, respectively ($p=0.01$) (Table 5).

- Heart and origins of the coronary arteries

A reduction of the mean doses to the heart and V_{15Gy} and V_{20Gy} was

Parameters	3D-CRT		Tomotherapy		P
	Mean	Median	Mean	Median	
Lungs					
- Mean dose (Gy)	9.6	8.7	9.5	11.1	NS*
- Maximum dose (Gy)	31.6	31.4	32.5	32.3	NS
- $V_{4\ Gy}$ (%)	42.4	35.55	62	63.8	0,03
- $V_{10\ Gy}$ (%)	31.7	28.9	38.2	46.3	0,04
- $V_{15\ Gy}$ (%)	28.2	26.1	24.8	27.7	NS
- $V_{20\ Gy}$ (%)	25.6	23.9	16.2	16.1	0,01
- $V_{30\ Gy}$ (%)	9.8	6.8	2.3	1.4	0,04

* non sigificant

Table 5: Comparison of mean and median dosimetric parameters for the lungs.

Parameters	3D-CRT		Tomotherapy		P
	Mean	Median	Mean	Median	
Heart					
- Mean dose (Gy)	11.7	8.4	9	7	0.03
- Maximum dose (Gy)	30.3	30.6	30	31	NS*
- $V_{4\ Gy}$ (%)	45	35.2	51.2	43.7	NS
- $V_{10\ Gy}$ (%)	39.6	29.9	33.7	26.2	NS
- $V_{15\ Gy}$ (%)	36.4	26.5	24.7	13.1	0.03
- $V_{20\ Gy}$ (%)	34.1	23.1	18.6	6.6	0.01
- $V_{30\ Gy}$ (%)	16.6	0.3	3.4	0.2	NS
Origin of right coronary artery					
- Mean dose (Gy)	24.4	29.6	21.4	25.8	NS
- Maximum dose (Gy)	25.4	29.8	22.9	27	NS
- $V_{4\ Gy}$ (%)	85.7	100	85.7	100	NS
- $V_{10\ Gy}$ (%)	85.7	100	77.9	100	NS
- $V_{15\ Gy}$ (%)	84.2	100	71.4	100	NS
- $V_{20\ Gy}$ (%)	81.2	100	71.4	100	NS
- $V_{30\ Gy}$ (%)	37.6	31.8	25	0	NS
Origin of left coronary artery					
- Mean dose (Gy)	24.6	26.7	22.9	24.1	NS
- Maximum dose (Gy)	26.4	30	25.6	27.4	NS
- $V_{4\ Gy}$ (%)	85.7	100	96.8	100	NS
- $V_{10\ Gy}$ (%)	84.2	100	85.5	100	NS
- $V_{15\ Gy}$ (%)	82.1	100	84.2	100	NS
- $V_{20\ Gy}$ (%)	79.7	100	77	100	NS
- $V_{30\ Gy}$ (%)	34.1	19.9	30	0	NS

* non-significant

Table 6: Comparison of mean and median dosimetric parameters for the heart and the origins of the coronary arteries.

observed with tomotherapy compared to 3DCRT (p=0.03, p=0.03 and p=0.01, respectively). No significant difference was observed between tomotherapy and 3DCRT in terms of dosimetric parameters of the origins of the coronary arteries (Table 6).

- Oesophagus

No significant difference in terms of dosimetric parameters of the oesophagus was observed between tomotherapy and 3DCRT (Table 7).

- Spinal canal, trachea and thyroid

The maximum dose to the spinal canal was lower with tomotherapy than with 3DCRT (21.3 Gy vs 31.2 Gy; p=0.01). No significant difference in terms of the mean dose to the trachea was demonstrated, while the mean dose to the thyroid was lower with tomotherapy (26.1 Gy vs 28 Gy; p=0.03) (Table 8).

Healthy tissues

A significant increase in the volumes exposed to a dose of 4 Gy was observed with tomotherapy compared to 3DCRT (62.4% vs 35.1%; p=0.03). On the other hand, larger volumes were exposed to doses greater than or equal to 15 Gy with 3DCRT compared to tomotherapy (p=0.01) (Table 9).

Evaluation of tomotherapy and 3DCRT treatment plans at the dose of 30 Gy with a 6 Gy boost to the residual tumour

Doses to target volumes

Dosimetric parameters of the PTV 30 Gy were equivalent with 3DCRT and tomotherapy. For PTV 36 Gy, the conformity index (CI) was better with tomotherapy than with 3DCRT (1.2 vs 5; p=0.01), with no difference in terms of the homogeneity index (Table 10).

Doses to organs at risk

- Right and left breasts

No significant difference in terms of mean dose to the right breast and the left breast was observed between 3DCRT and tomotherapy. Maximum doses were significantly lower with tomotherapy (p=0.01). V_{4Gy} and V_{10Gy} were significantly increased with tomotherapy compared to 3DCRT (p=0.01), while V_{20Gy} and V_{30Gy} were significantly decreased (Table 11).

- Lungs

Tomotherapy did not decrease the mean dose delivered to the

ParametersAR	3D-CRT		Tomotherapy		P
	Mean	Median	Mean	Median	
Esophagus					
- Mean dose (Gy)	22.8	24	21.1	22	NS*
- Maximum dose (Gy)	31.4	31.5	31.9	31.8	NS
- $V_{4\ Gy}$ (%)	80.3	84.1	81.3	85.4	NS
- $V_{10\ Gy}$ (%)	76.9	80.8	73.2	74.5	NS
- $V_{15\ Gy}$ (%)	75.7	79.3	70	71.9	NS
- $V_{20\ Gy}$ (%)	73.4	77.9	65.8	67.6	NS
- $V_{30\ Gy}$ (%)	37.1	20.6	32.7	31.6	NS

* Non-significant

Table 7: Comparison of mean and median dosimetric parameters for the esophagus.

Parameters	3D-CRT		Tomotherapy		P
	Mean	Median	Mean	Median	
Spinal canal					
- Maximum dose (Gy)	31.6	31.2	22.6	21.3	0.01
Trachea - Mean dose (Gy)	31.4	28.7	31.5	28	NS*
Thyroid					
- Mean dose (Gy)	26	28	24	26.1	0.03
- $V_{18\ Gy}$ (%)	85.9	97.6	76	84.9	NS
- $V_{25\ Gy}$ (%)	75	80.3	66.7	68.5	NS

* Non-significant

Table 8: Comparison of mean and median dosimetric parameters for the spinal canal, trachea and thyroid.

Parameters	3D-CRT		Tomotherapy		P
	Mean	Median	Mean	Median	
Healthy tissue					
- Mean dose (Gy)	8.2	7	7.9	8.1	NS*
- Maximum dose (Gy)	32.5	32.1	33.4	33.4	NS
- $V_{4\ Gy}$ (%)	35.8	35.1	54.2	62.4	0,03
- $V_{10\ Gy}$ (%)	28	23.8	29.8	29.1	NS
- $V_{15\ Gy}$ (%)	24.6	21	18.7	16.5	0,01
- $V_{20\ Gy}$ (%)	21.7	18.4	11.7	9.6	0,01
- $V_{30\ Gy}$ (%)	7	4.7	1.1	1	0,01

* Non-significant

Table 9: Comparison of mean and median dosimetric parameters for healthy tissues.

Parameters	3D-CRT	Tomotherapy	P
PTV 30 Gy			
- V_{90} (%)	99.9 (± 0.3)	99.8 (± 0.3)	NS*
- V_{95} (%)	98.8 (± 1.5)	99 (± 0.9)	NS
- V_{100} (%)	86.7 (± 13.2)	79.9 (± 8.1)	NS
PTV 36 Gy			
- Mean dose	36.5 (± 0.2)	36 (± 0,1)	0.01
- V_{90} (%)	99.6 (± 0.5)	100	NS
- V_{95} (%)	98.6 (± 2.1)	99 (± 1.5)	NS
- V_{100} (%)	80 (± 12.6)	54.9 (± 3.9)	0.03
- V_{107} (%)	0	0	NS
- Conformity index	5 (± 1.2)	1.2 (± 0.2)	0.01
- Homogeneity index	0.7 (± 0.2)	0.5 (± 0.1)	NS

* Non-significant

Table 10: Comparison of doses to target volumes.

Parameters	3D-CRT		Tomotherapy		P
	Mean	Median	Mean	Median	
Right breast					
- Mean dose (Gy)	52.1	1.9	4.3	3	NS*
- Maximum dose (Gy)	32.29	32.4	21.8	21.8	0.01
- $V_{4\,Gy}$ (%)	19.5	8	39.8	24.1	0.01
- $V_{10\,Gy}$ (%)	15.8	6	11.6	4.7	NS
- $V_{15\,Gy}$ (%)	13.8	3.9	4.3	1.9	NS
- $V_{20\,Gy}$ (%)	12.5	3.2	1.2	0	0.01
- $V_{30\,Gy}$ (%)	3.2	0.9	0	0	0.03
- $V_{36\,Gy}$ (%)	0	0	0	0	–
Left breast					
- Mean dose (Gy)	6,5	2	5.9	2.6	NS
- Maximum dose (Gy)	34.3	34.8	26.6	16,2	0.01
- $V_{4\,Gy}$ (%)	23.8	8.3	41.5	25.7	0.01
- $V_{10\,Gy}$ (%)	19.3	6.2	22.5	0.4	NS
- $V_{15\,Gy}$ (%)	17.4	5.1	13.6	0	NS
- $V_{20\,Gy}$ (%)	16	4.1	6.2	0	0.04
- $V_{30\,Gy}$ (%)	6.7	4.5	0.4	0	0.03
- $V_{36\,Gy}$ (%)	1.6	0	0.1	0	NS

* Non-significant

Table 11: Comparison of mean and median dosimetric parameters for the breasts.

lungs. Volumes exposed to low doses were significantly increased with tomotherapy (V_{4Gy} and V_{10Gy}) and volumes exposed to doses greater than or equal to 20 Gy were significantly increased with 3DCRT (Table 12).

- Heart and origins of the coronary arteries

A reduction of V_{20Gy} for the heart was only observed with tomotherapy compared to 3DCRT (23.6% vs 35.9%; p=0.01). No significant difference in terms of dosimetric parameters of the origins of the coronary arteries was observed between tomotherapy and 3DCRT (Table 13).

- Oesophagus

Tomotherapy allowed a slight reduction of the mean dose delivered to the oesophagus compared to 3DCRT (21.7 Gy vs 26 Gy; p=0.01). No significant difference was observed between tomotherapy and 3DCRT for the other dosimetric parameters of the oesophagus (Table 14).

- Spinal canal, trachea and thyroid

A significant reduction of the maximum dose to the spinal canal was observed with tomotherapy compared to 3DCRT (24.2 Gy vs 36.9 Gy; p=0.01) and a reduction of the mean dose to the trachea was observed with tomotherapy compared to 3DCRT (27.1 Gy vs 31.5 Gy; p=0.01). The mean dose to the thyroid was significantly increased with tomotherapy (23.6 Gy vs 15.4 Gy; p=0.03) (Table 15).

- Healthy tissues

A significant increase of volumes exposed to a dose of 4 Gy was observed with tomotherapy compared to 3DCRT (58.9% vs 31.2%; p=0.01), while significantly larger volumes were exposed to doses greater than or equal to 15 Gy with 3DCRT compared to tomotherapy (Table 16).

Evaluation of tomotherapy and 3DCRT treatment plans for the 14 patients

Right and left breasts: No significant difference in terms of the mean dose to the right breast and left breast was observed between

Parameters	3D-CRT		Tomotherapy		P
	Mean	Median	Mean	Median	
Lungs					
- Mean dose (Gy)	9.7	8.6	10.3	10.3	NS*
- Dmax (Gy)	36.8	37.4	37.3	37.5	NS
- $V_{4\,Gy}$ (%)	40.9	36.6	66.3	60.9	0.01
- $V_{10\,Gy}$ (%)	31.6	29.6	44.4	42.8	0.01
- $V_{15\,Gy}$ (%)	28.1	27.2	24.5	27.7	NS
- $V_{20\,Gy}$ (%)	25.2	25.6	16	16.6	0.01
- $V_{30\,Gy}$ (%)	13.4	12.4	3.6	3.3	0.01
- $V_{36\,Gy}$ (%)	1.4	1.1	0.2	0.1	0.03

* Non-significant

Table 12: Comparison of mean and median dosimetric parameters for the lungs.

Parameters	3D-CRT		Tomotherapy		P
	Mean	Median	Mean	Median	
Heart					
- Mean dose (Gy)	11.4	12.2	10.5	10.7	NS*
- Maximum dose (Gy)	34.2	35.3	34.4	34.2	NS
- $V_{4\,Gy}$ (%)	45.5	45	54.2	44.7	NS
- $V_{10\,Gy}$ (%)	39.4	40.6	41.6	37.6	NS
- $V_{15\,Gy}$ (%)	34.8	38.4	30.9	31.1	NS
- $V_{20\,Gy}$ (%)	31.8	35.9	23.2	23.6	0,01
- $V_{30\,Gy}$ (%)	14.7	10.1	8.3	7.2	NS
- $V_{36\,Gy}$ (%)	1.3	0	0.4	0	NS
Origin of right coronary artery					
- Mean dose (Gy)	28.8	32.2	29.3 (± 10.7)	32,3	NS
- Maximum dose (Gy)	29,5 (± 11.9)	34	30.9 (± 9.8)	34	NS
- $V_{4\,Gy}$ (%)	85.7 (± 37.8)	100	97.7 (± 6.1)	100	NS
- $V_{10\,Gy}$ (%)	85.7 (± 37.8)	100	85.7 (± 37.8)	100	–
- $V_{15\,Gy}$ (%)	85.7 (± 37.8)	100	85.7 (± 37.8)	100	–
- $V_{20\,Gy}$ (%)	85.7 (± 37.8)	100	85.7 (± 37.8)	100	–
- $V_{30\,Gy}$ (%)	71.4 (± 38.8)	100	74.8 (± 43.5)	100	NS
- $V_{36\,Gy}$ (%)	16.8 (± 37.2)	0	18.8 (± 23.7)	0	NS
Origin of left coronary artery					
- Mean dose (Gy)	26.8	29.5	26.9	28.3	NS
- Maximum dose (Gy)	29.9	30	28.2	29.7	NS
- $V_{4\,Gy}$ (%)	98.5	100	100	100	NS
- $V_{10\,Gy}$ (%)	93.2	100	100	100	NS
- $V_{15\,Gy}$ (%)	86.1	100	100	100	NS
- $V_{20\,Gy}$ (%)	77.1	100	86	100	NS
- $V_{30\,Gy}$ (%)	42.9	0.8	40.5	0	NS
- $V_{36\,Gy}$ (%)	0	0	10.2	0	NS

* Non-significant

Table 13: Comparison of mean and median dosimetric parameters for the heart and the origins of the coronary arteries.

Parameters	3D-CRT		Tomotherapy		P
Esophagus	Mean	Median	Mean	Median	
- Mean dose (Gy)	25.5	26	22,1	21.7	0.01
- Maximum dose (Gy)	36.6	36.7	36	36.9	NS*
- $V_{4\ Gy}$ (%)	84	90	85,2	85.5	NS
- $V_{10\ Gy}$ (%)	79,4	80.3	77,1	74.3	NS
- $V_{15\ Gy}$ (%)	76.9	78.6	70,7	66.8	NS
- $V_{20\ Gy}$ (%)	74.5	76.6	64,5	63.8	NS
- $V_{30\ Gy}$ (%)	54.9	52.6	36,7	35.1	NS
- $V_{36\ Gy}$ (%)	12.7	9,8	3.7	3.4	NS

* Non-significant

Table 14: Comparison of mean and median dosimetric parameters for the esophagus.

Parameters	3D-CRT		Tomotherapy		P
	Mean	Median	Mean	Median	
Spinal canal - Maximum dose (Gy)	36.1	36.9	23.6	24.2	0.01
Trachea - Mean dose (Gy)	30.4	31.5	27	27.1	0.01
Thyroid - Mean dose (Gy) - $V_{18\ Gy}$ (%) - $V_{25\ Gy}$ (%)	20.4 59.5 58.1	15.4 45.8 43.1	20.1 58.4 47.8	23.6 59.5 37.3	0,03 NS* NS

* Non-significant

Table 15: Comparison of mean and median dosimetric parameters for the spinal canal, trachea and thyroid.

Parameters	3D-CRT		Tomotherapy		P
	Mean	Median	Mean	Median	
Healthy tissue					
- Mean dose (Gy)	8.5	8.3	8.5	8.3	NS*
- Maximum dose (Gy)	38	37.9	37.4	38.1	NS
- $V_{4\ Gy}$ (%)	32.4	31.2	58.4	58.9	0.01
- $V_{10\ Gy}$ (%)	27.2	27.3	33.7	33.6	NS
- $V_{15\ Gy}$ (%)	24.2	24.6	18.7	16.4	0.01
- $V_{20\ Gy}$ (%)	21.7	22.7	14.6	12.3	0.04
- $V_{30\ Gy}$ (%)	11.2	12.2	2.7	1.3	0.02
- $V_{36\ Gy}$ (%)	1.5	0.6	0.2	0.1	0.01

* Non-significant

Table 16: Comparison of mean and median dosimetric parameters for healthy tissues.

tomotherapy and 3DCRT, but a significant increase of V_{4Gy} (p=0.0001) and a significant reduction of V_{20Gy} and V_{30Gy} were observed with tomotherapy compared to 3DCRT (Table 17).

Lungs: Tomotherapy did not allow any reduction of the mean dose to the lungs. Volumes exposed to low doses (V_{4Gy} and V_{10Gy}) were significantly increased with tomotherapy and volumes exposed to doses greater than or equal to 20 Gy were significantly increased with 3DCRT (Table 18).

Heart

Tomotherapy allowed a reduction of the mean dose to the heart compared to 3DCRT (7.4 Gy vs 9.6 Gy; p=0.02). V_{4Gy} was significantly increased with tomotherapy and volumes exposed to doses greater than or equal to 20 Gy were significantly increased with 3DCRT (Table 19).

Oesophagus

Tomotherapy allowed a slight reduction of the mean dose delivered to the oesophagus compared to 3DCRT (21.9 Gy vs 24.7 Gy; p=0.005) together with a reduction of V_{20Gy} (65.6% vs 76.5%; p=0.02) (Table 20).

Spinal canal, trachea and thyroid

A significant reduction of the maximum dose to the spinal canal was observed with tomotherapy compared to 3DCRT (23.7 Gy vs 33.4 Gy; p=0.0001). A significant reduction of the mean dose to the trachea was observed with tomotherapy compared to 3DCRT (28.1 Gy vs 30.1 Gy; p=0.02). The thyroid volume receiving a dose of 25 Gy (V_{25Gy}) was significantly decreased with tomotherapy (53.9% vs 80.3%; p=0.005) (Table 21).

Healthy tissues

No significant difference in mean doses to healthy tissues was observed between tomotherapy and 3DCRT treatment plans. A significant increase of V_{4Gy} and V_{10Gy} was observed with tomotherapy compared to 3DCRT. Significantly larger volumes were exposed to doses greater than or equal to 15 Gy with 3DCRT compared to tomotherapy (Table 22).

Discussion

Compared to 3DCRT, tomotherapy delivered low doses of 4 Gy to

Parameters	3D-CRT		Tomotherapy		P
	Mean	Median	Mean	Median	
Right breast					
- Mean dose (Gy)	3.7	1.9	4	3.3	NS*
- Maximum dose (Gy)	29.7	30.8	20.1	20.8	0.0002
- $V_{4\ Gy}$ (%)	15.2	8.6	37.2	24.9	0.0001
- $V_{10\ Gy}$ (%)	11.6	6.3	11.1	5.4	NS
- $V_{15\ Gy}$ (%)	9.4	4.2	3.2	1.3	0.004
- $V_{20\ Gy}$ (%)	8.2	3.4	0.7	0	0.0002
- $V_{30\ Gy}$ (%)	1.9	0	0	0	0.01
Left breast					
- Mean dose (Gy)	5.7	2.5	5.7	4.6	NS
- Maximum dose (Gy)	31	31.5	25.8	27	0.0009
- $V_{4\ Gy}$ (%)	23	10.8	41.9	33.5	0.0001
- $V_{10\ Gy}$ (%)	18.7	7.8	22.7	13.8	NS
- $V_{15\ Gy}$ (%)	16.2	5	12.2	4.7	NS
- $V_{20\ Gy}$ (%)	14.5	4	5.8	1.5	0.0024
- $V_{30\ Gy}$ (%)	3.9	1	0.4	0	0.01

* Non-significant

Table 17: Comparison of mean and median dosimetric parameters for the breasts.

Parameters	3D-CRT		Tomotherapy		P
Lungs	Mean	Median	Mean	Median	
- Mean dose (Gy)	9.6	9.5	9.9	10.5	NS*
- Maximum dose (Gy)	34.2	32.8	34.9	35.6	NS
- $V_{4\ Gy}$ (%)	41.6	38.3	64.1	62.3	0.0002
- $V_{10\ Gy}$ (%)	31.7	32	41.3	42.9	0.0004
- $V_{15\ Gy}$ (%)	28.1	28.9	26.7	27.7	NS
- $V_{20\ Gy}$ (%)	25.4	26.3	16.1	16.3	0.0001
- $V_{30\ Gy}$ (%)	11.6	12.1	2.9	2.8	0.0006

* Non-significant

Table 18: Mean comparison and dosimetric parameter medians for the lungs.

Parameters	3D-CRT		Tomotherapy		P
	Mean	Median	Mean	Median	
Heart					
- Mean dose (Gy)	11.5	9.6	9.7	7.4	0,02
- Maximum dose (Gy)	32.3	31.6	32.2	31.9	NS*
- V4 Gy (%)	45.2	42.4	54.7	44.2	0.002
- $V_{10\ Gy}$ (%)	39	33.6	37.6	27.9	NS
- $V_{15\ Gy}$ (%)	35.6	31.1	27.8	21.1	0.02
- $V_{20\ Gy}$ (%)	33	28.5	20.9	16	0.0001
- $V_{30\ Gy}$ (%)	15.6	5.2	5.8	2.7	0.04

* Non-significant

Table 19: Comparison of mean and median dosimetric parameters for the heart.

Parameters	3D-CRT		Tomotherapy		P
Esophagus	Mean	Median	Mean	Median	
- Mean dose (Gy)	24.1	24.7	21.6	21.9	0.005
- Maximum dose (Gy)	34	33.9	34	33.4	NS*
- $V_{4\ Gy}$ (%)	82.1	84.2	83.2	85.5	NS
- $V_{10\ Gy}$ (%)	78.1	79.8	75.2	74.4	NS
- $V_{15\ Gy}$ (%)	76.3	78.2	70.3	69.5	NS
- $V_{20\ Gy}$ (%)	74	76.5	65.1	65.6	0.02
- $V_{30\ Gy}$ (%)	46	50.8	34.7	33.5	NS

* Non-significant

Table 20: Comparison of mean and median dosimetric parameters for the esophagus.

Parameters	3D-CRT		Tomotherapy		P
	Mean	Median	Mean	Median	
Spinal canal - Maximum dose (Gy)	33.9	33.4	23.1	23.7	0.0001
Trachea - Mean dose (Gy)	29.6	30.1	27.5	28.1	0.02
Thyroid - Mean dose (Gy) - $V_{18\ Gy}$ (%) - $V_{25\ Gy}$ (%)	23.2 72.7 66.6	28 97 80.3	22.4 67.2 57.3	24.1 75 53.9	NS* NS 0.005

* Non-significant

Table 21: Comparison of mean and median dosimetric parameters for the spinal canal, trachea and thyroid.

Parameters	3D-CRT		Tomotherapy		p
	Mean	Median	Mean	Median	
Healthy tissue					
- Mean dose (Gy)	8.3	7.8	8.1	8.2	NS*
- Maximum dose (Gy)	35.2	35.8	35.4	34.5	NS
- $V_{4\ Gy}$ (%)	34.1	31.7	56.3	60.3	0.0002
- $V_{10\ Gy}$ (%)	27.6	26.1	31.8	29.7	0.02
- $V_{15\ Gy}$ (%)	24.4	23.5	19.7	16.4	0.005
- $V_{20\ Gy}$ (%)	21.7	21.3	13.1	9.8	0.0004
- $V_{30\ Gy}$ (%)	9.1	9.4	1.9	1.3	0.001

* Non-significant

Table 22: Comparison of mean and median dosimetric parameters for healthy tissues.

larger volumes of the breast, lungs and healthy tissues, while decreasing the volumes exposed to intermediate-to-high doses. No correlation was observed between breast volumes and the dose received by the breasts in this study.

The heart was also more effectively spared by tomotherapy, as the mean dose to the heart was comparable to that delivered by 3DCRT, but with a 27% reduction of V_{20Gy} (23.2% vs 31.8%; p=0.01). Although tomotherapy allowed better protection of the heart and therefore a lower risk of cardiac complications, it failed to lower the risk of coronary artery disease.

The relative reduction of the maximum dose received by the spinal canal was 32% (23.1 Gy vs 33.9 Gy; p=0.0001); this dose reduction was related to dose constraints determined before inverse planning. Reduction of the dose delivered to the spinal cord can be useful when subsequent irradiation is necessary.

Quantitative comparisons with dosimetric studies performed according to the "involved-field" concept comparing IMRT and 3DCRT techniques are difficult due to the small number of patients included, the variable total radiation doses and the use of different dosimetric parameters in these studies

Better heart sparing, especially in the presence of anterior mediastinal invasion, has been reported by other dosimetric studies evaluating IMRT. In the study by Goodman et al., IMRT allowed a reduction of the mean dose to the heart and lungs [10]. According to Girinsky et al., the mean V_{30Gy} to the heart was 14% with IMRT and 19.7% with 3DCRT, which corresponds to a 29% relative reduction [11]. Nieder et al. reported that IMRT failed to improve coverage of target volumes compared to 3DCRT, but allowed a reduction of the median dose to the heart, a reduction of the breast volumes exposed to high doses and an increase of breast volumes exposed to low doses [16]. De Sanctis et al. also reported an increase of the breast volumes exposed to low-dose irradiation (V_{5Gy} and V_{10Gy}) [12].

This reduction of the doses delivered to the heart with tomotherapy was achieved at the cost of an increased volume of organs at risk exposed to low doses, especially the breasts and lungs. Although a reduction of the volumes exposed to intermediate-to-high doses with 3DCRT may be associated with a decreased risk of second cancer, the effect of an increased volume of healthy tissues exposed to low doses of radiotherapy remains unknown at the present time [17-19]. Consequently, in the absence of data concerning the risk of second cancer, the benefit-risk balance of "involved-field" tomotherapy appears to be favourable when the heart is included in irradiation fields in order to decrease long-term cardiac toxicities, but with no associated reduction of the risk of coronary artery disease and myocardial infarction [20,21]. More generally, age at the time of diagnosis, the presence of cardiac or pulmonary comorbidity, the patient's anatomy and staging of Hodgkin lymphoma must be taken into account in the choice of radiotherapy technique in order to achieve an optimal benefit-risk balance.

In order to lower the risk of subsequent breast cancer, it may be recommended to contour the mammary gland and store the dose-volume histogram in the patient's file, especially in the case of young women under the age of 30 due to the increased radio sensitivity of the breast at this age.

The choice of radiotherapy technique to treat supradiaphragmatic Hodgkin lymphoma must be based on individual criteria such as anatomy, age at the time of diagnosis and the presence of cardiac or pulmonary comorbidity. Approaches comprising the use of IMRT techniques and reduction of irradiation volumes by "involved-node" radiotherapy are currently under evaluation in order to further reduce late toxicities of irradiation for patients with Hodgkin lymphoma [22].

Conclusion

This is the first study to evaluate the impact of "involved-field" tomotherapy on coverage of target volumes and sparing of organs at risk. This study demonstrated improvement of the conformity index and homogeneity index for PTV 30 Gy and improvement of the conformity index for PTV 36 Gy. The dosimetric study also demonstrated dosimetric advantages of tomotherapy in terms of cardiac protection, particularly in patients with anterior mediastinal lymph node invasion. Tomotherapy allowed better sparing of breast, lung and healthy tissue volumes exposed to high doses.

References

1. Hasenclever D, Diehl V (1998) A prognostic score for advanced Hodgkin's disease. International Prognostic Factors Project on Advanced Hodgkin's Disease. N Engl J Med 339: 1506-1514.
2. Ng AK (2011) Review of the cardiac long-term effects of therapy for Hodgkin lymphoma. Br J Haematol 154: 23-31.
3. Hancock SL, Donaldson SS, Hoppe RT (1993) Cardiac disease following treatment of Hodgkin's disease in children and adolescents. J Clin Oncol 11: 1208-1215.
4. Avilés A, Neri N, Nambo JM, Huerta-Guzman J, Talavera A, et al. (2005) Late cardiac toxicity secondary to treatment in Hodgkin's disease. A study comparing doxorubicin, epirubicin and mitoxantrone in combined therapy. Leuk Lymphoma 46: 1023-1028.
5. Myrehaug S, Pintilie M, Yun L, Crump M, Tsang RW, et al.(2010) A population-based study of cardiac morbidity among Hodgkin lymphoma patients with pre-existing heart disease. Blood. 116: 2237-2240.
6. Hodgson DC, Gilbert ES, Dores GM, Schonfeld SJ, Lynch CF, et al. (2007) Long-term solid cancer risk among 5-year survivors of Hodgkin's lymphoma. J Clin Oncol 25: 1489-1497.
7. Travis LB, Hill DA, Dores GM, Gospodarowicz M, van Leeuwen FE, et al. (2003) Breast cancer following radiotherapy and chemotherapy among young women with Hodgkin disease. JAMA 290: 465-475.
8. Paumier A, Khodari W, Beaudre A, Ghalibafian M, Blanchard P, Al Hamokles H, et al. (2011) Optimisation de l'« involved-node radiotherapy » par l'utilisation de la modulation d'intensité dans le lymphome hodgkinien localisé : expérience de l'institut Gustave-Roussy. Cancer/Radiothérapie. 15: 709-715.
9. Fermé C, Eghbali H, Meerwaldt JH, Rieux C, Bosq J, et al. (2007) Chemotherapy plus involved-field radiation in early-stage Hodgkin's disease. N Engl J Med 357: 1916-1927.
10. Goodman KA, Toner S, Hunt M, Wu EJ, Yahalom J (2005) Intensity-modulated radiotherapy for lymphoma involving the mediastinum. Int J Radiat Oncol Biol Phys 62: 198-206.
11. Girinsky T, Pichenot C, Beaudre A, Ghalibafian M, Lefkopoulos D (2006) Is intensity-modulated radiotherapy better than conventional radiation treatment and three-dimensional conformal radiotherapy for mediastinal masses in patients with Hodgkin's disease, and is there a role for beam orientation optimization and dose constraints assigned to virtual volumes? Int J Radiat Oncol Biol Phys. 64: 218-226.
12. De Sanctis V, Bolzan C, D'Arienzo M, Bracci S, Fanelli A, et al. (2012) Intensity modulated radiotherapy in early stage Hodgkin lymphoma patients: is it better than three dimensional conformal radiotherapy? Radiat Oncol Lond Engl. 7:129.
13. Antoni D, Natarajan-Ame S, Meyer P, Niederst C, Bourahla K, et al. (2013) Contribution of three-dimensional conformal intensity-modulated radiation therapy for women affected by bulky stage II supradiaphragmatic Hodgkin disease. Radiat Oncol Lond Engl. 8: 112.
14. Yahalom J, Mauch P (2002) The involved field is back: issues in delineating the radiation field in Hodgkin's disease. Ann Oncol 13 Suppl 1: 79-83.
15. Feuvret L, Noël G, Mazeron JJ, Bey P (2006) Conformity index: a review. Int J Radiat Oncol Biol Phys 64: 333-342.
16. Nieder C, Schill S, Kneschaurek P, Molls M (2007) Comparison of three different mediastinal radiotherapy techniques in female patients: Impact on heart sparing and dose to the breasts. Radiother Oncol J Eur Soc Ther Radiol Oncol. 82: 301-307.
17. Hall EJ, Wuu CS (2003) Radiation-induced second cancers: the impact of 3D-CRT and IMRT. Int J Radiat Oncol Biol Phys 56: 83-88.
18. Hall EJ (2006) Intensity-modulated radiation therapy, protons, and the risk of second cancers. Int J Radiat Oncol Biol Phys. 65: 1-7.
19. Kry SF, Salehpour M, Followill DS, Stovall M, Kuban DA, et al. (2005) The calculated risk of fatal secondary malignancies from intensity-modulated radiation therapy. Int J Radiat Oncol Biol Phys 62: 1195-1203.
20. Gagliardi G, Constine LS, Moiseenko V, Correa C, Pierce LJ, et al. (2010) Radiation dose-volume effects in the heart. Int J Radiat Oncol Biol Phys 76: S77-85.
21. Mulrooney DA, Yeazel MW, Kawashima T, Mertens AC, Mitby P, et al. (2009) Cardiac outcomes in a cohort of adult survivors of childhood and adolescent cancer: retrospective analysis of the Childhood Cancer Survivor Study cohort. BMJ 339: b4606.
22. Girinsky T, van der Maazen R, Specht L, Aleman B, Poortmans P, et al. (2006) Involved-node radiotherapy (INRT) in patients with early Hodgkin lymphoma: concepts and guidelines. Radiother Oncol 79: 270-277.

Adoptive Immunotherapy for Acute Myeloid Leukemia: From Allogeneic Hematopoietic Cell Transplantation to CAR T Cells

Merav Bar[1,2*]

[1]Division of Clinical Research, Fred Hutchinson Cancer Research Center, USA
[2]Department of Medicine, University of Washington, Seattle, WA, USA

Abstract

Allogeneic Hematopoietic Cell Transplantation (allo-HCT) has improved outcome of patients with high risk Acute Myeloid Leukemia (AML), but it harbors a risk of morbidity and mortality due to damage to normal cells and tissues by the high intensity conditioning or due to Graft Versus Host Disease (GVHD). As a major component of the curative potential of allo-HCT is derived from the response of the donor immunity against the malignant cells through the so called Graft Versus Leukemia effect (GVL), novel adoptive immunotherapy strategies have been developed to generate immune response against the leukemic cells, while sparing GVHD.

Keywords: Graft Versus Host Disease (GVHD); Hematopoiesis; Leukemic cells

Allogeneic Hematopoietic Cell Transplantation

The principle of anti-leukemic adoptive immunotherapy, as coined by Georges Mathé in 1965, is an activity of allogeneic immunologically competent cells against the host's leukemic cells [1]. The best known model and the most commonly used method of anti-leukemic adoptive immunotherapy is allogeneic Hematopoietic Cell Transplantation (allo-HCT). The initial goal of allo-HCT was to eradicate leukemic cells by high doses of chemo or radiation therapy, which also destroys normal hematopoiesis, and then rescue the patient with a healthy hematopoietic progenitor cells from an allogeneic donor. However, it is now clear that the potential curative effect of allogeneic HCT is derived not only from the intense cytotoxic therapy, but also from the response of the donor's immune cells against the leukemic cells, through a so called graft versus leukemia (GVL) effect.

The evidence to support GVL effect of allo-HCT are: (i) lower relapse rate among recipients of HLA-identical sibling transplants than recipients of syngeneic transplants [2-5]; (ii) decrease relapse rate among patients who develop Graft Versus Host Disease (GVHD) after allo-HCT [2,6]; (iii) decreased GVHD, but increased relapse rate after T cell depleted allo-HCT [7,8]; (iv) anti-leukemic effect and curative potential of Donor Lymphocyte Infusion (DLI) in patients with relapse leukemia after transplant [9,10]; and (v) effectiveness of nonmyeloablative HCT [11].

GVL is mediated through the immunologic activity of donor T cells and Natural Killer (NK) cells recognizing Leukemia-Associated Antigens (LAA), minor histocompetability antigens (mHag), and in case of mismatch or haploidentical transplants also major histocompetability antigens that are expressed by the malignant cells [12,13].

Donor immunity may contribute to the cure of the leukemia by allo-HCT, but is also the cause of GVHD, mediated by donor T cell recognizing antigens expressing by normal cells. GVHD is a major cause of morbidity and mortality after transplant, and it was recently demonstrated that the beneficial effect of GVL may be outweighed by the morbidity and mortality caused by GVHD [11]. Thus, therapies that provide potent GVL while sparing GVHD are needed.

NK cell-mediated anti-leukemic adoptive immunotherapy

Clinical observations have shown that donor NK cells may contribute to GVL activity in HLA-mismatched allogeneic HCT. NK cells display a number of activating and inhibitory receptors that interact with a wide variety of ligands on target cells, and the function of the NK cell depends on the net effect of the activating and inhibitory receptors [14]. Among the NK cells inhibitory receptors are Killer Immunoglobulin Receptors (KIRs) that recognize certain groups of HLA class I molecules on the target cell. It has been demonstrated that donor NK cells expressing KIRs that are mismatched with the recipient HLA class I and therefore are not inhibited by the HLA molecules of the recipient, so called alloreactive NK cells, are associated with decreased relapse and decreased GVHD rates after T cell-depleted HLA-mismatched or HLA-matched HCT in patients with Acute Myeloid Leukemia (AML) [15-18]. A number of early stage clinical trials have demonstrated that NK cells can be safely infused in AML patients following immunosuppressive chemotherapy and, in some cases, clinical responses without GVHD have been observed [19-21]. The results of these clinical trials demonstrate that NK cell-based therapy, which may provide anti-leukemic effect without GVHD, is a potential strategy to consolidate leukemia remission in high-risk AML, without the need of allo-HCT.

T Cell Mediated Anti-Leukemic Adoptive Immunotherapy

A potential approach to generate GVL is by identifying and expending donor T cells that recognize LAA or mHags expressing on the malignant cells. Cytotoxic T lymphocyte (CTL) clones specific for hematopoietic restricted mHags have been shown to have anti-

***Corresponding author:** Merav Bar, Fred Hutchinson Cancer Research Centre, PO Box 19024 Seattle, WA 98109-1024, USA, E-mail: mbar@u.washington.edu leukemic activity when used to treat patients with relapse leukemia after allo-HCT [22]. T cell clones specific for LAA as WT1, CD45, and PR1 have been generated to target leukemic cells [23-25], and recently Greenberg and colleagues reported results from a clinical trial using *ex vivo* expanded HLA-A*0201-restricted WT1-specific donor-derived CD8 CTL clones for treatment of relapsed or high-risk leukemia after allo-HCT [26]. This clinical trial demonstrated long term persistence and potential anti-leukemic activity of donor CTL clones specific for WT1. However, isolation and *ex vivo* expansion of high avidity mHag or LAA-specific T cell clones is challenging process, as it relies on the individual donor T cell repertoire and may result in products with variable quality and wide range of avidity, persistence, and function *in vivo*.

A potential way to circumvent the challenge of isolation and expansion of antigen-specific high avidity T cells is by using gene transfer technologies to genetically engineer T cell to express a unique high-affinity T cell receptor (TCR). The first successful TCR gene transfer to human peripheral blood lymphocytes conferring anti-tumor reactivity was reported by Clay and colleagues in 1999, using a TCR specific for an HLA-A2-restricted epitope of the MART-1 antigen, which is highly expressed by malignant melanomas [27]. Since then, several studies have demonstrated that transfer of a tumor antigen-specific TCR into T cells has successfully led to generation of an antigen-specific T cell population [28-41]. However there are a number of limitations to this approach:

1. The TCR recognizes a peptide fragment of its target antigen only when the peptide is presented by an HLA Class I molecule on the surface of the target cell. Therefore, antigen specific T cells are restricted to specific HLA allele, requires generation of patient-specific product. To date, most TCR gene transfer studies have focused on TCRs restricted to HLA-A2, as it is the most common HLA class I, present in ~50% of Caucasians [42,43].

2. Mispairing of the transduced and the endogenous TCR α and β chains that may lead to generation of non-specific TCR. A potential way to overcome this difficulty is insertion of point mutations into the constant regions of the transduced TCR α and β chains to create complementary cystein residues that form an inter-chain disulfide bond, which promotes preferential pairing between the transduced TCR chains and significantly reduces mispairing [44,45].

3. Downregulation of HLA class I expression by some leukemic cells have been reported [46], which may prevent recognition of the antigenic target by the TCR, and thus inhibits the antileukemic function of the T cell.

4. Chimeric Antigen Receptor (CAR) is another approach to T cell gene therapy. CAR is a genetically engineered molecule composed of an antigen-specific extracellular binding domain, fused to a transmembrane domain and intracellular T cell-specific signalling domain. The CARs are transduced into T cells, which become "CAR T cells" with specific target based on the CAR binding domain. Upon CAR binding to an antigen on the cell surface of a target cell, the CAR T cell induces apoptosis of the target cell using the same mechanisms of ordinary T cell. In contrast to a TCR, which recognizes a peptide fragment of an antigen only when the peptide is presented by an HLA Class I molecule on the surface of target cells, a CAR molecule recognizes an intact cell surface antigen, and it is HLA independent. Thus, the same CAR molecule may be used in a broad range of patients with different HLA types. CARs can target any cell surface antigen including carbohydrate and lipid moieties, which increases the repertoire of potential targets for CAR-base therapy. However CARs target only cell surface antigens, therefore, CAR T cells cannot target intracellular mutated or over expressed proteins.

Since the CAR concept was first introduced by Eshhar and colleagues in 1989 [47], CAR T cells have been generated to target several antigens on malignant cells [48-64], and a number of clinical trials are currently evaluating the use of CAR T cells, originated from allogeneic donors or patients, for treatment of different malignancies. In haematological malignancies there have been promising reports of using CAR-modified anti-CD19 T cells for treatment of B-cell malignancies [65-70]. CAR T cell targeting AML antigens as CD33 and CD123 have been reported [71,72], and recently early phase small clinical trial has demonstrated persistence and potential anti-leukemic effect of CAR T cell against the LeY antigen in AML [73].

Conclusions

Adoptive immunotherapy has the potential to provide long-term survival and even cure in patients with leukemia. The well-established allogeneic hematopoietic cell transplantation has improved outcome of patient with high risk AML, however it harbors the risk of morbidity and mortality due to damage to normal cells and tissues by the high intensity conditioning or due to graft versus host disease. Novel approaches using NK cells and T cells have been developed to provide more direct anti-leukemic therapy while sparing the risk of toxicity to normal tissues. However several obstacles need to be overcome in order to improve *in vivo* survival and antileukemic function of the transferred cells. Additionally, reliable large scale manufacturing of the therapeutic cells is essential to allow large clinical trials to evaluate the efficacy of various novel strategies before these therapies can be adopted for routine use to treat AML patients.

References

1. Mathé G, Amiel JL, Schwarzenberg L, Cattan A, Schneider M (1965) Adoptive immunotherapy of acute leukemia: experimental and clinical results. Cancer Res 25: 1525-1531.
2. Weiden PL, Sullivan KM, Flournoy N, Storb R, Thomas ED (1981) Antileukemic effect of chronic graft-versus-host disease: contribution to improved survival after allogeneic marrow transplantation. N Engl J Med 304: 1529-1533.
3. Gale RP, Horowitz MM, Ash RC, Champlin RE, Goldman JM, et al. (1994) Identical-twin bone marrow transplants for leukemia. Ann Intern Med 120: 646-652.
4. Horowitz MM, Gale RP, Sondel PM, Goldman JM, Kersey J, et al. (1990) Graft-versus-leukemia reactions after bone marrow transplantation. Blood 75: 555-562.
5. Sullivan KM, Fefer A, Witherspoon R, Storb R, Buckner CD, et al. (1987) Graft-versus-leukemia in man: relationship of acute and chronic graft-versus-host disease to relapse of acute leukemia following allogeneic bone marrow transplantation. Prog Clin Biol Res 244: 391-399.
6. Sullivan KM, Weiden PL, Storb R, Witherspoon RP, Fefer A, et al. (1989) Influence of acute and chronic graft-versus-host disease on relapse and survival after bone marrow transplantation from HLA-identical siblings as treatment of acute and chronic leukemia. Blood 73: 1720-1728.
7. Weiden PL, Flournoy N, Thomas ED, Prentice R, Fefer A, et al. (1979) Antileukemic effect of graft-versus-host disease in human recipients of allogeneic-marrow grafts. N Engl J Med 300: 1068-1073.
8. Martin PJ, Hansen JA, Buckner CD, Sanders JE, Deeg HJ, et al. (1985) Effects of in vitro depletion of T cells in HLA-identical allogeneic marrow grafts. Blood 66: 664-672.

9. Marmont AM, Horowitz MM, Gale RP, Sobocinski K, Ash RC, et al. (1991) T-cell depletion of HLA-identical transplants in leukemia. Blood 78: 2120-2130.

10. Kolb HJ1, Mittermüller J, Clemm C, Holler E, Ledderose G, et al. (1990) Donor leukocyte transfusions for treatment of recurrent chronic myelogenous leukemia in marrow transplant patients. Blood 76: 2462-2465.

11. Bar M, Sandmaier BM, Inamoto Y, Bruno B, Hari P, et al. (2013) Donor lymphocyte infusion for relapsed hematological malignancies after allogeneic hematopoietic cell transplantation: prognostic relevance of the initial CD3+ T cell dose. Biol Blood Marrow Transplant 19: 949-957.

12. Storb R, Gyurkocza B, Storer BE, Sorror ML, Blume K, et al. (2013) Graft-versus-host disease and graft-versus-tumor effects after allogeneic hematopoietic cell transplantation. J Clin Oncol 31: 1530-1538.

13. Kolb HJ (2008) Graft-versus-leukemia effects of transplantation and donor lymphocytes. Blood 112: 4371-4383.

14. Velardi A (2012) Natural killer cell alloreactivity 10 years later. Curr Opin Hematol 19: 421-426.

15. Lanier LL (1998) NK cell receptors. Annu Rev Immunol 16: 359-393.

16. Farag SS, Fehniger TA, Ruggeri L, Velardi A, Caligiuri MA (2002) Natural killer cell receptors: new biology and insights into the graft-versus-leukemia effect. Blood 100: 1935-1947.

17. Ruggeri L, Capanni M, Urbani E, Perruccio K, Shlomchik WD, et al. (2002) Effectiveness of donor natural killer cell alloreactivity in mismatched hematopoietic transplants. Science 295: 2097-2100.

18. Moroi K, Sato T (1975) Comparison between procaine and isocarboxazid metabolism in vitro by a liver microsomal amidase-esterase. Biochem Pharmacol 24: 1517-1521.

19. Ruggeri L, Mancusi A, Capanni M, Urbani E, Carotti A, et al. (2007) Donor natural killer cell allorecognition of missing self in haploidentical hematopoietic transplantation for acute myeloid leukemia: challenging its predictive value. Blood 110: 433-440.

20. Kalos M, Levine BL, Porter DL, Katz S, Grupp SA, et al. (2011) T cells with chimeric antigen receptors have potent antitumor effects and can establish memory in patients with advanced leukemia. Sci Transl Med 3: 95ra73.

21. Hsu KC, Keever-Taylor CA, Wilton A, Pinto C, Heller G, et al. (2005) Improved outcome in HLA-identical sibling hematopoietic stem-cell transplantation for acute myelogenous leukemia predicted by KIR and HLA genotypes. Blood 105: 4878-4884.

22. Miller JS, Soignier Y, Panoskaltsis-Mortari A, McNearney SA, Yun GH, et al. (2005) Successful adoptive transfer and in vivo expansion of human haploidentical NK cells in patients with cancer. Blood 105: 3051-3057.

23. Rubnitz JE1, Inaba H, Ribeiro RC, Pounds S, Rooney B, et al. (2010) NKAML: a pilot study to determine the safety and feasibility of haploidentical natural killer cell transplantation in childhood acute myeloid leukemia. J Clin Oncol 28: 955-959.

24. Curti A, Ruggeri L, D'Addio A, Bontadini A, Dan E, et al. (2011) Successful transfer of alloreactive haploidentical KIR ligand-mismatched natural killer cells after infusion in elderly high risk acute myeloid leukemia patients. Blood 118: 3273-3279.

25. Warren EH, Fujii N, Akatsuka Y, Chaney CN, Mito JK, et al. (2010) Therapy of relapsed leukemia after allogeneic hematopoietic cell transplantation with T cells specific for minor histocompatibility antigens. Blood 115: 3869-3878.

26. Guo Y, Niiya H, Azuma T, Uchida N, Yakushijin Y, et al. (2005) Direct recognition and lysis of leukemia cells by WT1-specific CD4+ T lymphocytes in an HLA class II-restricted manner. Blood 106: 1415-1418.

27. Amrolia PJ, Reid SD, Gao L, Schultheis B, Dotti G, et al. (2003) Allorestricted cytotoxic T cells specific for human CD45 show potent antileukemic activity. Blood 101: 1007-1014.

28. Ma Q, Wang C, Jones D, Quintanilla KE, Li D, et al. (2010) Adoptive transfer of PR1 cytotoxic T lymphocytes associated with reduced leukemia burden in a mouse acute myeloid leukemia xenograft model. Cytotherapy 12: 1056-1062.

29. Chapuis AG, Ragnarsson GB, Nguyen HN, Chaney CN, Pufnock JS, et al. (2013) Transferred WT1-reactive CD8+ T cells can mediate antileukemic activity and persist in post-transplant patients. Sci Transl Med 5: 174ra27.

30. Clay TM, Custer MC, Sachs J, Hwu P, Rosenberg SA, et al. (1999) Efficient transfer of a tumor antigen-reactive TCR to human peripheral blood lymphocytes confers anti-tumor reactivity. J Immunol 163: 507-513.

31. Stanislawski T, Voss RH, Lotz C, Sadovnikova E, Willemsen RA, et al. (2001) Circumventing tolerance to a human MDM2-derived tumor antigen by TCR gene transfer. Nat Immunol 2: 962-970.

32. Morgan RA, Dudley ME, Yu YY, Zheng Z, Robbins PF, et al. (2003) High efficiency TCR gene transfer into primary human lymphocytes affords avid recognition of melanoma tumor antigen glycoprotein 100 and does not alter the recognition of autologous melanoma antigens. J Immunol 171: 3287-3295.

33. Jolly RD, Thompson KG, Winchester BG (1975) Bovine mannosidosis--a model lysosomal storage disease. Birth Defects Orig Artic Ser 11: 273-278.

34. Schaft N, Willemsen RA, de Vries J, Lankiewicz B, Essers BW, et al. (2003) Peptide fine specificity of anti-glycoprotein 100 CTL is preserved following transfer of engineered TCR alpha beta genes into primary human T lymphocytes. J Immunol 170: 2186-2194.

35. Marniemi J, Parkki MG (1975) Radiochemical assay of glutathione S-epoxide transferase and its enhancement by phenobarbital in rat liver in vivo. Biochem Pharmacol 24: 1569-1572.

36. Zhao Y, Zheng Z, Robbins PF, Khong HT, Rosenberg SA, et al. (2005) Primary human lymphocytes transduced with NY-ESO-1 antigen-specific TCR genes recognize and kill diverse human tumor cell lines. J Immunol 174: 4415-4423.

37. Cohen CJ, Zheng Z, Bray R, Zhao Y, Sherman LA, et al. (2005) Recognition of fresh human tumor by human peripheral blood lymphocytes transduced with a bicistronic retroviral vector encoding a murine anti-p53 TCR. J Immunol 175: 5799-5808.

38. Parkhurst MR, Joo J, Riley JP, Yu Z, Li Y, et al. (2009) Characterization of genetically modified T-cell receptors that recognize the CEA:691-699 peptide in the context of HLA-A2.1 on human colorectal cancer cells. Clin Cancer Res 15: 169-180.

39. Frankel TL, Burns WR, Peng PD, Yu Z, Chinnasamy D, et al. (2010) Both CD4 and CD8 T cells mediate equally effective in vivo tumor treatment when engineered with a highly avid TCR targeting tyrosinase. J Immunol 184: 5988-5998.

40. Chinnasamy N, Wargo JA, Yu Z, Rao M, Frankel TL, et al. (2011) A TCR targeting the HLA-A*0201-restricted epitope of MAGE-A3 recognizes multiple epitopes of the MAGE-A antigen superfamily in several types of cancer. J Immunol 186: 685-696.

41. Straetemans T, van Brakel M, van Steenbergen S, Broertjes M, Drexhage J, et al. (2012) TCR gene transfer: MAGE-C2/HLA-A2 and MAGE-A3/HLA-DP4 epitopes as melanoma-specific immune targets. Clin Dev Immunol 2012: 586314.

42. Hillerdal V, Nilsson B, Carlsson B, Eriksson F, Essand M (2012) T cells engineered with a T cell receptor against the prostate antigen TARP specifically kill HLA-A2+ prostate and breast cancer cells. Proc Natl Acad Sci U S A 109: 15877-15881.

43. Tsuji T, Yasukawa M, Matsuzaki J, Ohkuri T, Chamoto K, et al. (2005) Generation of tumor-specific, HLA class I-restricted human Th1 and Tc1 cells by cell engineering with tumor peptide-specific T-cell receptor genes. Blood 106: 470-476.

44. Heemskerk MH, Hoogeboom M, Hagedoorn R, Kester MG, Willemze R, et al. (2004) Reprogramming of virus-specific T cells into leukemia-reactive T cells using T cell receptor gene transfer. J Exp Med 199: 885-894.

45. Xue SA, Gao L, Hart D, Gillmore R, Qasim W, et al. (2005) Elimination of human leukemia cells in NOD/SCID mice by WT1-TCR gene-transduced human T cells. Blood 106: 3062-3067.

46. Krausa P, Brywka M 3rd, Savage D, Hui KM, Bunce M, et al. (1995) Genetic polymorphism within HLA-A-02: significant allelic variation revealed in different populations. Tissue Antigens 45: 223-231.

47. Cohen CJ, Li YF, El-Gamil M, Robbins PF, Rosenberg SA, et al. (2007) Enhanced antitumor activity of T cells engineered to express T-cell receptors with a second disulfide bond. Cancer Res 67: 3898-3903.

48. Schmoldt A, Benthe HF, Haberland G (1975) Digitoxin metabolism by rat liver microsomes. Biochem Pharmacol 24: 1639-1641.

49. Kuball J, Dossett ML, Wolfl M, Ho WY, Voss RH, et al. (2007) Facilitating matched pairing and expression of TCR chains introduced into human T cells. Blood 109: 2331-2338.

50. Demanet C, Mulder A, Deneys V, Worsham MJ, Maes P, et al. (2004) Down-regulation of HLA-A and HLA-Bw6, but not HLA-Bw4, allospecificities in leukemic cells: an escape mechanism from CTL and NK attack? Blood 103: 3122-3130.

51. Gross G, Waks T, Eshhar Z (1989) Expression of immunoglobulin-T-cell receptor chimeric molecules as functional receptors with antibody-type specificity. Proc Natl Acad Sci U S A 86: 10024-10028.

52. Finney HM, Lawson AD, Bebbington CR, Weir AN (1998) Chimeric receptors providing both primary and costimulatory signaling in T cells from a single gene product. J Immunol 161: 2791-2797.

53. Brentjens RJ, Latouche JB, Santos E, Marti F, Gong MC, et al. (2003) Eradication of systemic B-cell tumors by genetically targeted human T lymphocytes co-stimulated by CD80 and interleukin-15. Nat Med 9: 279-286.

54. Imai C, Mihara K, Andreansky M, Nicholson IC, Pui CH, et al. (2004) Chimeric receptors with 4-1BB signaling capacity provoke potent cytotoxicity against acute lymphoblastic leukemia. Leukemia 18: 676-684.

55. Lamers CH, Sleijfer S, Vulto AG, Kruit WH, Kliffen M, et al. (2006) Treatment of metastatic renal cell carcinoma with autologous T-lymphocytes genetically retargeted against carbonic anhydrase IX: first clinical experience. J Clin Oncol 24: e20-22.

56. Till BG, Jensen MC, Wang J, Chen EY, Wood BL, et al. (2008) Adoptive immunotherapy for indolent non-Hodgkin lymphoma and mantle cell lymphoma using genetically modified autologous CD20-specific T cells. Blood 112: 2261-2271.

57. Zhao Y, Wang QJ, Yang S, Kochenderfer JN, Zheng Z, et al. (2009) A herceptin-based chimeric antigen receptor with modified signaling domains leads to enhanced survival of transduced T lymphocytes and antitumor activity. J Immunol 183: 5563-5574.

58. Morgan RA, Yang JC, Kitano M, Dudley ME, Laurencot CM, et al. (2010) Case report of a serious adverse event following the administration of T cells transduced with a chimeric antigen receptor recognizing ERBB2. Mol Ther 18: 843-851.

59. Krause A, Guo HF, Latouche JB, Tan C, Cheung NK, et al. (1998) Antigen-dependent CD28 signaling selectively enhances survival and proliferation in genetically modified activated human primary T lymphocytes. J Exp Med 188: 619-626.

60. Pule MA, Savoldo B, Myers GD, Rossig C, Russell HV, et al. (2008) Virus-specific T cells engineered to coexpress tumor-specific receptors: persistence and antitumor activity in individuals with neuroblastoma. Nat Med 14: 1264-1270.

61. Maher J, Brentjens RJ, Gunset G, Rivière I, Sadelain M (2002) Human T-lymphocyte cytotoxicity and proliferation directed by a single chimeric TCRzeta /CD28 receptor. Nat Biotechnol 20: 70-75.

62. Katari UL, Keirnan JM, Worth AC, Hodges SE, Leen AM, et al. (2011) Engineered T cells for pancreatic cancer treatment. HPB (Oxford) 13: 643-650.

63. Carpenito C, Milone MC, Hassan R, Simonet JC, Lakhal M, et al. (2009) Control of large, established tumor xenografts with genetically retargeted human T cells containing CD28 and CD137 domains. Proc Natl Acad Sci U S A 106: 3360-3365.

64. Lefkowitz RJ (1975) Identification of adenylate cyclase-coupled beta-adrenergic receptors with radiolabeled beta-adrenergic antagonists. Biochem Pharmacol 24: 1651-1658.

65. Park JR, Digiusto DL, Slovak M, Wright C, Naranjo A, et al. (2007) Adoptive transfer of chimeric antigen receptor re-directed cytolytic T lymphocyte clones in patients with neuroblastoma. Mol Ther 15: 825-833.

66. Chinnasamy D, Yu Z, Theoret MR, Zhao Y, Shrimali RK, et al. (2010) Gene therapy using genetically modified lymphocytes targeting VEGFR-2 inhibits the growth of vascularized syngenic tumors in mice. J Clin Invest 120: 3953-3968.

67. Chekmasova AA, Rao TD, Nikhamin Y, Park KJ, Levine DA, et al. (2010) Successful eradication of established peritoneal ovarian tumors in SCID-Beige mice following adoptive transfer of T cells genetically targeted to the MUC16 antigen. Clin Cancer Res 16: 3594-3606.

68. Kershaw MH, Westwood JA, Parker LL, Wang G, Eshhar Z, et al. (2006) A phase I study on adoptive immunotherapy using gene-modified T cells for ovarian cancer. Clin Cancer Res 12: 6106-6115.

69. Song DG, Ye Q, Carpenito C, Poussin M, Wang LP, et al. (2011) In vivo persistence, tumor localization, and antitumor activity of CAR-engineered T cells is enhanced by costimulatory signaling through CD137 (4-1BB). Cancer Res 71: 4617-4627.

70. Porter DL, Levine BL, Kalos M, Bagg A, June CH (2011) Chimeric antigen receptor-modified T cells in chronic lymphoid leukemia. N Engl J Med 365: 725-733.

71. Brentjens RJ, Rivière I, Park JH, Davila ML, Wang X, et al. (2011) Safety and persistence of adoptively transferred autologous CD19-targeted T cells in patients with relapsed or chemotherapy refractory B-cell leukemias. Blood 118: 4817-4828.

72. Grupp SA, Kalos M, Barrett D, Aplenc R, Porter DL, et al. (2013) Chimeric antigen receptor-modified T cells for acute lymphoid leukemia. N Engl J Med 368: 1509-1518.

73. Mardiros A, Dos Santos C, McDonald T, Brown CE, Wang X, et al. (2013) T cells expressing CD123-specific chimeric antigen receptors exhibit specific cytolytic effector functions and antitumor effects against human acute myeloid leukemia. Blood 122: 3138-3148.

12

Dysregulation of the antigen-induced NF-κB signaling pathway in the development of human B-cells lymphomas

Nassima Messali[#], Pierre Génin[#] and Robert Weil*

Institut Pasteur, Unité de Signalisation Moléculaire et Activation Cellulaire, CNRS URA 2582, 75724 Paris Cedex 15, France
[#]Authors Contributed Equally to this Work

Abstract

The adaptive immune response is initiated when microbial or tumor-specific molecules are recognized by antigen receptors present at lymphocyte cell surface. Engagement of these immunoreceptors induces signaling cascades that ultimately activate the transcription factors NF-κB (Nuclear Factor-κB) and NFAT (nuclear factor of activated T-cells) responsible for the establishment of gene expression programs controlling the stimulation, proliferation and survival of activated lymphocytes. Cloning the products of three distinct translocation events found in lymphoma of mucosa-associated lymphoid tissue (MALT lymphoma) led to the identification and characterization of a novel NF-κB-activating complex following antigenic stimulation composed by the CARMA1, BCL10, and MALT1 proteins and called the CBM complex. Since the identification of this complex, other regulatory components were discovered which greatly improve our understanding of this signaling pathways.

Interestingly, CBM complex activity is not only altered in MALT lymphomas but also in a subtype of activated B cell-like (ABC) of diffuse large B-cell (DLBCL) lymphoma. In this review, we described the key players involved in antigen-induced NF-κB activation and covered the recent advances in the molecular mechanisms that are responsible for the regulation of the components of the CBM complex. Understanding these mechanisms is critical for the elucidation of the role of this NF-κB signaling network in both normal and pathologic conditions and we described how dysregulation of this network leads to the uncontrolled activation of NF-κB and development of two particular subtypes of human B cell lymphomas: the MALT and the DLBCL lymphomas.

Keywords: NF-κB; CARMA1; BCL10; MALT1; DLBCL; MALT Lymphoma

Introduction

The immune system can be roughly divided in two groups, the innate and the adaptive immunity. Innate immunity constitutes the first line of defense against invading organisms and refers to nonspecific defense mechanisms that are rapidly triggered upon infection. The adaptive immune response is initiated upon recognition of microbial or tumor-specific molecules by antigen receptors present at the lymphocyte cell surface. Antigen-receptor engagement leads to signaling events that trigger gene expression programs controlling activation of the stimulated lymphocytes and their clonal proliferation and survival. The nuclear factor (NF)-κB transcription factor participates in both innate and adaptive immunity as a critical regulator of the expression of target genes including those encoding anti-apoptotic molecules, cell cycle regulators, cytokines and surface receptors. In resting cells, NF-κB proteins are sequestered in the cytoplasm due to their interaction with the IκB inhibitors. Antigenic stimulation of B- or T-lymphocytes or recognition of bacterial and viral products by Toll-like receptors present on the surface or in the endosomes of immune cells leads to the activation of a cytoplasmic kinase complex composed of two catalytic subunits, the kinases IKKα and IKKβ and a regulatory subunit called NEMO, that induces phosphorylation, followed by ubiquitination and, consequently, proteasome-mediated degradation of IκB proteins. Free NF-κB dimers subsequently translocate to the nucleus and activate their target genes.

Nuclear factor-κB (NF-κB) is activated upon triggering of a wide variety of antigen-dependent receptors, including T-cell receptor (TCR), B-cell receptor (BCR), Fc receptors (FcRs), NK cell receptors, and various immunoglobulin (Ig)- or C-type lectin- family receptors specifically expressed on myeloid cells that associate with cytoplamic ITAMs (Immunoreceptor Tyrosine-based activation motifs)-containing signaling chains (such as: CD3s, Igα and Igβ, FcRγ and DAP12) [1]. Engagement of these receptors initiate a signal-activation cascade that includes phosphorylation of two specific tyrosine residues located in the ITAM by the Src family kinases [1]. Tyrosine kinase Syk or ZAP-70 (zeta-chain-associated protein 70 kD) are then recruited to the phosphorylated ITAM through their tandem Src homology 2 (SH2) regions, initiating downstream signaling cascades that lead to the stimulation of mitogen-activated protein kinase (MAPK) activities and ultimately to the activation of the transcription factors NF-κB and NF-AT (nuclear factor of activated T-cells).

An outstanding issue of lymphocyte activation was the identification of a complex of proteins comprising CARMA1, BCL10 and MALT1 (also called the CBM complex) as critical regulators of the immunoreceptor signaling pathways. In this review, we will focus on the recent advances concerning the role of the CBM function in antigen-induced NF-κB signaling and detail how this pathway may selectively become dysregulated in lymphoma.

The key players of antigen-mediated NF-κB activation

Antigen receptor activation initiates a phosphorylation cascade that promotes assembly of the CBM signalosome complex composed of CARMA1, BCL10, and MALT1 that ultimately activates the NEMO/IKK complex to promote NF-κB transcription (Figure 1). In this

***Corresponding author:** Robert Weil, Unité de Signalisation Moléculaire et Activation Cellulaire, CNRS URA 2582, Institut Pasteur, 75724 Paris Cedex 15, France; E-mail: rweil@pasteur.fr paragraph, we provide a description of the CBM components and detail the molecular mechanisms of their regulation.

CARMA1

CARMA1 (CARD 11/Bimp3) belongs to a family of proteins including CARMA2 (also called CARD14 or Bimp2) and CARMA3/CARD10/Bimp1 that were initially identified based on bioinformatics analyzes of their CARD domain homology [2,3]. Among this family, only CARMA1 is specifically expressed in hematopoietic cells. CARMA1 contains multiple protein-protein association domains that individually contribute to the formation of protein complexes required for transduction of these signaling pathways. Indeed, CARMA1 contains N-terminal caspase-recruitment (CARD) and coiled-coil (CC) domains and a C-terminal membrane-associated kinase (MAGUK) domain [2,3]. Because of this last domain, CARMA1 belongs to the MAGUK family, characterized by their C-terminal PDZ-SH3-GUK tripartite modular domains. CARMA1 resides in lymphocytes in a closed, latent state by an auto-inhibitory mechanism involving an inhibitory domain (ID), positioned between the coiled-coil and PDZ domains and requiring intra-molecular interactions with the CARD and coiled-coil domains. Using mice deficient for CARMA1 or expressing mutated forms of this protein, studies demonstrated an important role of this protein *in vivo* after TCR/BCR signaling (Table 1). These mice exhibit immunodeficiency, defective B lymphocyte development and lymphocyte proliferation probably as a consequence of the impairment of NF-κB and JNK activation [4-7]. Other studies have shown that phosphorylation of CARMA1 (mediated by PKCβ or PKCθ and CaMKII) activates the NF-κB pathway by promoting the formation and stabilization of the CBM complex [8-10]. As a consequence of BCR or TCR engagement, PKC-mediated phosphorylation of the ID allows a conformational change leading to binding of the CARD motif of CARMA1 to BCL10 and to recruitment of several signaling molecules including the paracaspase MALT1, the E3 ligase TRAF6, the kinases TAK1 and IKKα/β and the protease caspase-8 [11]. Accordingly, mutations of the coiled-coil, CARD, or LATCH (a short 19 amino acids region between the CARD and the coiled-coil) domain disrupt the ID binding and constitute dominant-active forms of CARMA1 that result (when overexpressed) in increased association and co-localization with BCL10 and IKK and constitutive NF-κB activation [12]. As a post-inductional repression mechanism, the CBM/IKK/NF-κB signal pathway can be negatively regulated by the phosphatase PP2A regulatory subunit PPP2R1A by binding to CARMA1 and removal of the PKCθ-dependent phosphorylation of CARMA1 [13].

CARD9, another CARD protein, is structurally similar to the CARMA family members [14]. As for the CARMA family of proteins, CARD9 contains N-terminal CARD and coiled-coil domains, but lacks the C-terminal MAGUK domain. In contrast, CARD9 is mostly expressed in myeloid cells including dendritic cells and macrophages. CARD9 is a critical mediator of the innate immune response to fungal infections, but is dispensable for antigen receptor-induced signaling pathway that involves BCL10 and MALT1. In contrast, recent studies

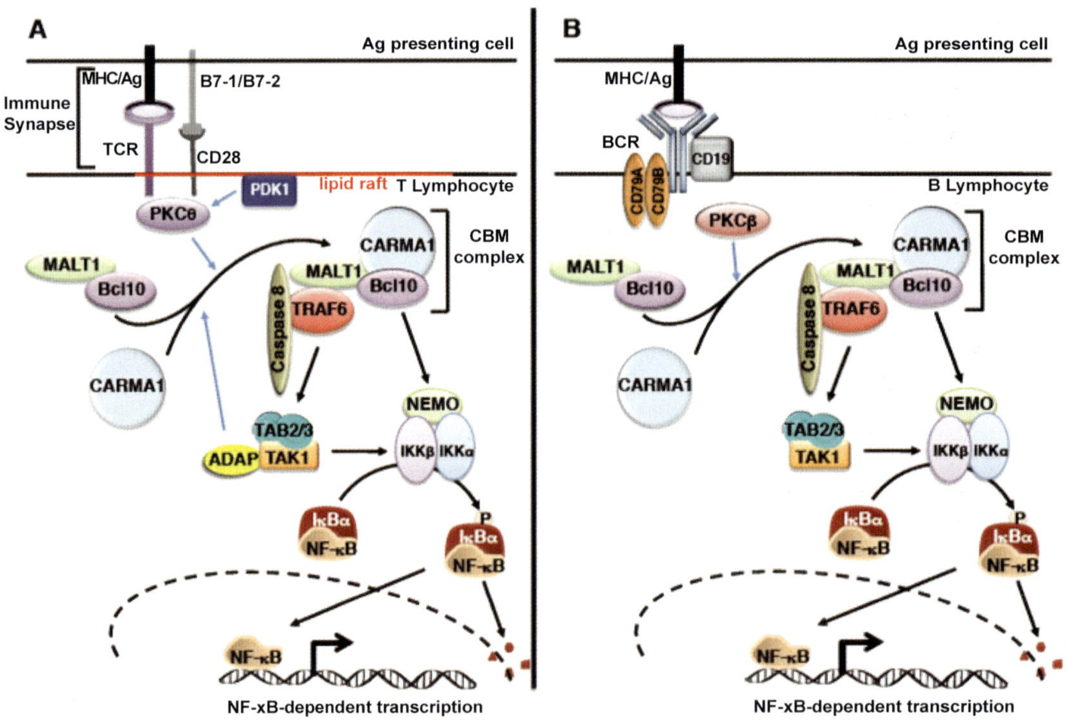

Figure1: Immunoreceptor-mediated activation of the NF-κB pathway in T cells (A) and B cells (B).Activation of the CBM/NF-κB signalling pathway occurred following engagement of the TCR by the antigen-MHC complex and CD28-B7 interaction in T cells and after recognition of the antigen-MHC complex by the BCR in B cells. These early events lead to the formation of the CBM complex (CARMA1, BCL10 and MALT1) through the PKC-θ- or PKC-β-mediated phosphorylation of CARMA1, in T and B cells, respectively. In T cells, assembly of this complex also involves the activation of PKC-θ by the kinase PDK1 and the association of the adaptor ADAP with both CARMA1 and the NF-κB activating kinase TAK1. In B and T cells, CBM complex formation triggers the ubiquitination of NEMO through TRAF6/Caspase-8 complex and the phosphorylation of IKKβ by TAK1. Once activated, the NEMO/IKKs complex promotes the phosphorylation and degradation of the inhibitor proteins IκBs and the release and nuclear translocation of the transcription factor NF-κB that can activate expression of the target genes.

KO mice	Phenotype	Signaling pathways affected	References
CARMA1	- Defective TCR-mediated lymphocyte proliferation - Reduced number of mature B cells and complete absence of B1 cells - Defective BCR-mediated proliferation	- Impaired TCR / BCR-mediated NF-κB and JNK activation - Deficient IL-2 production	[4-7]
BCL10	- Defective TCR-mediated lymphocyte proliferation - Reduced number of B1 cells. - Impaired B cell development and activation - Impaired neuronal-tube closure	- Impaired TCR/BCR-mediated NF-κB activation - Deficient IL-2 production	[17,18]
MALT1	- Defective TCR-mediated lymphocyte proliferation - Reduced number of B1 cells - Defective BCR-mediated proliferation	- Deficient IL-2 production - Impaired TCR/BCR-mediated NF-κB activation. - Effect on in JNK activation remains controversial	[18,27]
PKCθ	- Normal development of naïve CD4 and CD8 cells in thymus - Normal CD8⁺ proliferation and defective CD4⁺ proliferation following TCR-mediated activation - Resistance to bacteria and virus pathogens	- Impaired NF-κB, NF-AT and AP1 activation - Deficient IL-2 production	[44,47-52]
PKCβ	- Reduced number of mature B cells and B1 cells	- Impaired NF-κB activation	[53]
Caspase-8	- Defective hematopoietic development in bone marrow - T cell-specific age-dependant lethal lympho-proliferative and lympho-infiltrative immune disorder - Resting T cell proliferation - Defective antigen-induced T cell proliferation	- Impaired antigen-receptor-induced NF-κB activation - Reduced IL-2 responses	[68,69-71]
PDK1	- Impaired T cell differentiation in thymus		[59]

Table 1: Mouse knockout and gene expression phenotypes for genes involved in antigen-mediated NF-κB activity.

suggest that CARD9 forms a complex with MALT1 and BCL10 that was found to be involved in the C-type lectin receptor (CLR)-induced signaling pathways after fungal stimulation and to activate the IKK complex, leading to activation of NF-κB [15,16].

BCL10

B cell lymphoma 10 (BCL10) is an adaptor protein containing a N-terminal caspase recruitment domain and a C-terminal Ser/Thr-rich region. BCL10, identified as a novel member of a family of proteins containing a CARD domain, was initially suggested to act as a regulator of the proapoptotic signaling pathways, as many proteins containing a CARD motif were originally involved in the control of apoptosis. Analyzes of the BCL10 deficient mice did not substantiate these hypotheses, but rather revealed unexpected roles of this protein in innate and adaptive immune responses, in antigen-induced proliferation of T and B cells and in NF-κB activation. In addition, BCL10 is critical not only for the function, but also for the maturation of B cells, since knockout of its expression leads to reduced number of follicular and marginal cells of the B cell zone (Table 1) [17]. Furthermore, BCL10-deficient mice show defects in neural tube closure [18]. In concert with activation of NF-κB by TCR, proteolysis of BCL10 occurs and this degradation is a specialized function of differentiated T cells, since it was not observed in naïve T cells. Although these studies suggested that BCL10 degradation might constitute a regulatory mechanism to reduce NF-κB activation by TCR, the molecular mechanism responsible for BCL10 degradation remains highly controversial since several groups published data supporting different BCL10 proteolysis mechanisms [19-23]. Thus, BCL10 was shown to be phosphorylated at several Ser and Thr residues and then degraded through the ubiquitin-dependent proteasome machinery [20]. However, BCL10 degradation is only partially altered by proteasome inhibitors and may involved ubiquitin conjugation and subsequent lysosomes trafficking, since BCL10 degradation is preceded by its localization in vesicular compartments identified as late endosomes or lysosomes [21]. A recent study indicated that TCR stimulation induces autophagy and that inhibition of autophagy enhances TCR-mediated NF-κB activation [24]. Interestingly, BCL10 can be degraded via selective autophagy, thus limiting the NF-κB-dependent responses through reduction of TCR-mediated activation of NF-κB. Actually, upon TCR stimulation, BCL10 undergoes K63-linked polyubiquitination of its CARD domain, an event required for NF-κB activation. Selective autophagy of K63-modified BCL10 requires the autophagy adaptor protein p62 and inhibition of p62 expression not only altered BCL10 degradation, but also impaired NF-κB activation [24]. The attachment of K63-linked ubiquitin chains on BCL10 can also be recognized by NEMO (a subunit in the IKK complex) leading to the increased interaction efficiency between components of the IKK complex and the CBM complex [22]. Using genetically deficient B cell lines, it has been recently shown that CARMA1 and TAK1, but not IKKβ are necessary for antigen receptor- (or phorbol esters)- mediated BCL10 degradation, further suggesting that TAK1 functions as an adaptor for the E3 ligases ITCH and NEDD4 (involved in K63-ubiquitination of BCL10) and plays a feedback role for BCR-mediated NF-κB activation [25].

MALT1

The human paracaspase MALT1 has also been recently identified as a caspase-like protein involved in NF-κB activation [26-29]. Like BCL10, MALT1 was originally found as interactant of CARMA1 and inducer of the NF-κB signaling pathway following the characterization of the *IGH-BCL10, IGH-MALT1* and *API2-MALT1* translocations [30,31]. MALT1 contains a N-terminal death domain (DD), two immunoglobulin (Ig)-like domains and a C-terminal caspase-like domain. The interaction between BCL10 and MALT1 that requires the central Ig-like domains of MALT1 and a region C-terminal to the CARD domain of BCL10 induces the oligomerization of MALT1. Because of its caspase-like domain, MALT1 was further identified as a member of the paracaspase family. For long times, MALT1 was thought to act solely as a scaffolding protein, but many groups have recently shown that the caspase-like domain of MALT1 exhibits important proteolytic activities. This protease cleaves specific substrates following arginine residues unlike conventional caspases that cleave after aspartate residues, and promotes T cell activation [32]. Thus, MALT1 cleaves and inactivates negative regulators of the canonical NF-κB pathway, such as RelB, A20 (TNFAIP3) and CYLD [33]. MALT1 also targets BCL10 for proteolysis, potentiating the NF-κB signaling pathway [34]. In addition, this specific cleavage was shown to play an important role in T-cell antigen receptor-induced integrin adhesion.

Structure of the human MALT1 caspase-like domain in complex with a peptide inhibitor showed that the paracaspase domain adopts a fold similar to that of classical caspases. The crystal structure of the MALT1 caspase-like domain further provided clues about the mechanism of MALT1 activation: in the absence of stimulation, MALT1 is not active by itself, since the caspase-like domain is autoinhibited by its interaction with the Ig3 domain. Its activation requires a first dimerization step and a second step in which caspase substrate binding causes substantial structural reorganization, allowing the release of the caspases like domain of MALT1 from the Ig3 inhibitory domain [35]. Using mice lacking MALT1, two different studies reported impaired TCR-mediated NF-κB activation, defective lymphocyte proliferation and decreased IL-2 production (Table 1). However, they present conflicting results regarding the role of MALT1 in BCR-mediated NF-κB and JNK activation [18,27].

Regulation of the CBM complex

Role of Ubiquitination in the CBM function

Ubiquitination plays a crucial role in the NF-κB activation pathway. The presence of isopeptide linkages at each of the seven lysine residues of ubiquitin has been reported and the type of conjugated polyubiquitin seems to determine the mode of regulation of conjugated proteins. In particular, the role of lysine 63-linked chains in NF-κB activation has been extensively studied. CBM assembly promotes polymerization of lysine 63-linked ubiquitin chains and subsequent activation of TAK1 to stimulate NF-κB-mediated transcription [36]. It is also clear that formation of the CBM complex is required for the inducible lysine 63 ubiquitination of NEMO. Like NEMO, TRAF6, MALT1, and BCL10 constitute targets for Lys-63 polyubiquitination. Their primary ubiquitination sites have been mapped and were shown to be critical for NF-κB activation [37]. Ubiquitination of BCL10 has also been first suggested to facilitate TCR activation, and thereafter to limit NF-κB activation, this discrepancy remaining to be clarified (see above). The lysine 63 polyubiquitination of BCL10 is required for NEMO recruitment via its ubiquitin-binding domain (UBD) and for the subsequent activation of the IKK kinase complex. In response to T cell activation, TRAF6 associates with MALT1 and therefore co-purifies with the CBM complex in TCR-activated cells. In addition, TRAF6 can function *in vitro* and *in vivo* as an E3 ligase for MALT1, catalyzing its lysine 63-linked ubiquitination [38]. Recently, linear polyubiquitin chains, in which the C-terminal glycine of one ubiquitin is conjugated to the amino group of the N-terminal methionine of another ubiquitin, were reported to be involved in NF-κB activation. A unique ligase complex named LUBAC generates linear polyubiquitin chains. It is composed of three subunits: HOIL-1, HOIP and Sharpin. LUBAC has been shown to bind to NEMO in the IKK complex and to conjugate linear chains to NEMO, this process being critical for TNF-α-mediated NF-κB activation. Interestingly, a recent study indicates that HOIL-1-deficient patients present clinical features of autoinflammation and immunodeficiency, which correlates with a defect in the activation of NF-κB in B cells (and also in fibroblasts), whereas monocytes from these patients present an abnormal sensitivity to stimulation by IL1-β [39]. An interesting future issue will be therefore to determine the role played by linear polyubiquitin chains in antigen-mediated NF-κB signaling.

Ubiquitination is a covalent modification that can be reversed by deubiquitinating enzymes (DUBs). Not surprisingly, DUBs were shown to be critical for repressing NF-κB activation. Among those, the cylindromatosis tumour suppressor protein CYLD was found to interfere with IKK activation by cleaving K63-linked polyubiquitin chains on several proteins, including TRAF2, TRAF6 and NEMO [40]. Several other reports have established that another DUB called A20 acts as an inhibitor of NF-κB activity by forming a complex with three partners, TAX1BP1 and the E3 ligases Itch and RNF11 [41]. Interestingly, A20 is constitutively expressed in lymphoid cells, in contrast to other cell types in which A20 is induced by NF-κB providing a negative-feedback mechanism to prevent sustained NF-κB signaling. MALT1-induced A20 cleavage was thereafter proposed as a mechanism responsible for A20 inactivation and thereby upregulation of antigen-mediated NF-κB activation.

Role of other regulatory components

Besides post-translational modifications that could affect components of the CBM complex, other proteins were shown to play a regulatory role.

PKCθ and PKCβ: PKCθ and PKCβ are members of two different subfamilies of protein kinase C family [42]. The role of PKCθ has been well established by studies on knock-out mice showing its major role in the development and function of both effector T cells and regulatory T cells (Table 1) through the regulation of NF-κB, AP-1 and NF-AT activation [43-53]. In order to be fully activated, PKCθ requires the engagement of both TCR and CD28 receptors. Thus, binding of PKCθ to the DAG that is released upon TCR simulation is sufficient to promote its localization to the plasma membrane and CD28 engagement leads to the formation of a tripartite CD28-LCK-PKCθ complex allowing the recruitment of PKCθ to the immune synapse [54-56]. Roles of PKCθ and PKCβ in NF-κB activation have been reported in different studies. For example, it has been shown that PKCθ and PKCβ phosphorylate the serine 645 and 552 of the linker domain of human CARMA1, triggering its activation and subsequent interaction with BCL10-MALT1 [8,9].

PDK1: PDK1 possesses a pleckstrin homology (PH) domain that binds to the second messenger PtdIns(3,4,5)P_3. Recent studies have established that PDK1 is critical for efficient activation of PKCθ in T cells and PKCβ in B cells by the PI3K pathway. PDK1 is also required for the subsequent assembly of the CBM complex to activate NF-κB during coordinated stimulation of the TCR and co-stimulatory receptor CD28 or during activation of the BCR [57-59]. PDK1 phosphorylates PKCθ and has a dual role in TCR-mediating NF-κB activation by recruiting PKCθ and CARMA1 into lipid rafts [60]. Using B-cell specific conditional PDK1 knock-out mice (Table 1) and chemical inhibitor approaches, it was demonstrated that PDK1 plays a critical role in B-cells by promoting transduction of the BCR signalings that are essential for the activation of both NF-κB and Foxo transcription factors. PDK1 is required for the survival of resting and activated B cells through the activation of Foxo and NF-κB respectively [57].

ADAP: ADAP (adhesion- and degranulation-promoting adaptor protein) was identified as an adapter protein that becomes tyrosine phosphorylated upon association with the TCR complex, creating docking sites for the SH2 domains of the Fyn kinase and SLP-76 protein [61,62]. ADAP contains two regions exhibiting similarities with the SH3 domains and mediating interaction with a proline-independent motif of SKAP55 [63]. Through this interaction, ADAP has been shown to play an important role in T-cell receptor mediated integrin activation. As PDK1, ADAP plays a role in TCR-induced NF-κB activation, although ADAP is not involved in the activation of PKCθ [64]. ADAP participates to the assembly of the CARMA1–BCL10–MALT1 complex by interacting with the C-terminal region of

CARMA1 through its N-terminal helical SH3 domain and E/K-rich region. Interestingly, a site in the C-terminal end of ADAP is critical for recruitment of TAK1 [65]. This TAK1 binding sites is required for IKKα/β phosphorylation, whereas ADAP-binding sites of CBM components regulate NEMO ubiquitination. Finally, using resting naive T cells from ADAP$^{-/-}$ mice reconstituted with ADAP mutant constructs, it was demonstrated that formation of the ADAP/SKAP55 complex required for integrin activation is dispensable for CBM complex assembly, suggesting differential control of integrin and NF-κB-dependent pathways by ADAP [66].

Caspase-8: Caspase-8 was first characterized by its critical role in death receptor-mediated apoptosis. Activation of caspase-8 leads to stimulation of effector caspase activities and ultimately to cell death. Besides its apoptotic function, caspase-8 is also involved in antigen receptor-induced NF-κB activation, as caspase-8 is essential for lymphocyte proliferation in response to antigen stimulation [67-71]. TCR-mediated activation of NF-κB is impaired in T cells from caspase-8 deficient patients or mice as well as in caspase-8 deficient Jurkat cells [68]. Caspase-8 deficient patients show clear defects in T and B lymphocytes and NK cells activations that were accompanied by recurrent sinopulmonary herpes simplex virus infections and poor responses to immunization [72]. Not only NF-κB signaling is impaired in caspase-8 deficient T cells, but also in their human B and NK cells, as shown by the inability of B and NK cells from these patients to translocate p65 to the nucleus upon BCR engagement [68]. These effects appeared to be selective for antigen signaling pathway, since caspase-8 inhibitor or knockdown caspase-8 expression did not affect TNF-α-induced NF-κB activation. The same study identified active caspase-8 as a critical link between the CBM and IKK complexes leading to NF-κB activation in both lymphoid cell lines and isolated human lymphocytes. Actually, TCR stimulation induces caspase-8 interaction with the BCL10- MALT1 complex followed by recruitment of IKK. Subsequently, the E3 ubiquitin ligase TRAF6 was shown to interact and activate caspase-8, unraveling a novel role of TRAF6 in induction of apoptosis [73], but also to interact with CARMA1 in association with caspase-8 following TCR stimulation, an event that facilitates the movement of caspase-8 into lipid rafts [74]. Interactions of caspase-8 and TRAF6 with CARMA1 were enhanced when the inhibitory domain (ID) of CARMA1 was deleted. Strikingly, TRAF6, caspase-8, NEMO and TAK1 may associate with CARMA1 in a BCL10-independent manner, as suggested by the mapping of the domains required for the association of these proteins with the activated form of CARMA1. The caspase-8 function in TCR-induced NF-κB signaling seems to involved the caspase-8 dependent cleavage of cFLIPL into a p43^{FLIP} isoform that exhibits a greater capacity to recruit RIP1 and TRAF2 compared to its uncleaved counterpart, resulting in enhanced NF-κB activation and IL-2 production [75,76]. Altogether, these studies demonstrate that caspase-8 and TRAF6 are both required for programmed cell death and antigen-mediated NF-κB activation.

CaMKII: CaMKII could also be involved in TCR-mediated NF-κB activation since treatment with CaM or CaMKII inhibitors blocks this signaling pathway. Upon cross-linking of the TCR, CaMKII is recruited to the immunological synapse where it interacts with and phosphorylates both BCL10 and the CARD domain of CARMA1. These phosphorylations facilitate the interaction between CARMA1 and BCL10 and enhance NF-κB activation [10,77]. Interestingly, CARMA1 interacted constitutively with BCL10 when CaMKII was over-expressed.

Casein kinase 1α (CK1α): CK1α was identified using a mass spectrometry screen of CARMA1 protein interactants [78]. Silencing CK1α reduces TCR-induced IL-2 production while it had no effect on TNF-α signaling, underscoring the selective involvement of this kinase in the TCR-NF-κB pathway. Moreover, CK1α associates with CARMA1 independently of PKCθ and BCL10 and has also a negative regulatory role on TCR-mediated NF-κB activation, since it promotes the phosphorylation and inactivation of CARMA1.

Three dimensional requirement for TCR-mediated NF-κB activation

The area formed at the contact site between T cells and antigen-presenting cells (APC) has been termed the 'immunological synapse' (IS), formation of this synapse being correlated with a dramatic induction of cell polarity. Over the past few years, several groups have shown that the signaling components of TCR-mediated NF-κB activation are localized in the IS. Indeed, the immunological synapse appears essential for the organization of the CBM complex and subsequent NF-κB activation. The molecular mechanisms responsible for the recruitment and activation of the CBM complex to the immunological synapse are not fully understood. Over the last several years, new approaches using various cell imaging techniques have been used to address the spatial and dynamic characteristics of these events [79]. They clearly demonstrated that intracellular signaling molecules, adaptors and cytoskeletal proteins associated with highly spatially and temporally organized structures called supra-molecular activation clusters (SMACs).

Importance of IS for the positive regulation of antigen-mediated NF-κB activation

CARMA1 is a member of the membrane-associated guanylate kinase (MAGUK) family of proteins, characterized by their association with membrane proteins. CARMA1 is localized in specialized parts of the membrane called lipid rafts, where NF-κB signaling pathways are initiated. Following TCR stimulation, CARMA1 is recruited to the IS (and therefore enriched in the lipid rafts), where it colocalizes with BCL10 [80,81]. Analyses of mutants of the transmembrane and cytoplasmic domains of the TCR-β chain reveal that the integrity of the TCR-β chain is critical for recruitment of CARMA1 and BCL10, and consequently NF-κB activation [82]. Besides its involvement in BCL10 recruitment to the IS, CARMA1 may also be important for the IS localization of PKCθ following TCR stimulation [83,84]. However, this conclusion is in contradiction with data showing that PKCθ recruitment to central and peripheral IS normally occurs in CARMA1 deficient T cells [85]. Two other components of the IS, SAP and the receptor SLAM, would also be involved in PKCθ recruitment to the IS [86].

Finally, the NEMO/IKK complex is also recruited to the IS and associates with the TCR following stimulation [87]. Accordingly, artificial targeting of NEMO to the IS is sufficient to activate NF-κB following TCR stimulation. Recruitment of NEMO/IKK complex to the IS is also supported by the finding that CARMA1 is important for recruitment of IKK into cSMAC and for its activation [81,85].

Importance of IS for the negative regulation of antigen-mediated NF-κB activation

It is now generally admitted that the IS constitutes a specialized domain of the membrane where sustained engagement and signaling of TCR take place. Increasing evidences indicate that the IS is not only the area where TCR signaling pathways are initiated, but also the place where TCR-induced protein ubiquitination and degradation of key activation molecules occur [88,89]. Whether components of the TCR-activated NF-κB signaling pathway are also degraded in the IS remains to be investigated.

Although, it remains unclear how CARMA1 is recruited to the IS, an expression-cloning screen for regulators of CARMA1 identified GAKIN as a protein that can remove CARMA1 from the central IS. Interestingly, GAKIN interacts with CARMA1 in an inducible manner following TCR activation, competes with BCL10 for the association with CARMA1 and ultimately downregulates NF-κB activation [90]. Altogether these data indicate that GAKIN dynamically localizes to the IS and regulates the duration of CARMA1 occupancy to the IS at the benefit of the peripheral IS.

Localization and function of PKC-θ in the IS

Although the relationship between the IS and lipid rafts remains to be determined, several studies have pointed that PKCθ colocalizes with rafts at the central region of the IS [91,92]. In naive CD4⁺ T cells, TCR-mediated signals are sufficient to induce the capping of PKCθ to the area of the TCR, although CD28-mediated signals seem also to be required for the localization of PKCθ to the SMAC of the synapse [92].

Studies of PKCθ-deficient T cells on lipid bilayers containing pMHC and ICAM1 demonstrated that there is a clear relationship between TCR signaling, IS assembly and motility [93]. Those studies were the first to document T cells migrating, while engaging agonist pMHC complexes on bilayers, and to show that cells lacking PKCθ were less mobile. This observation suggests that autonomous signals within the T cell enhanced motility and that a stable synapse can be observed upon inhibition of PKCθ. More recently, it was demonstrated that motility arrest is not required for TCR signaling to take place [94,95].

Microclusters in the IS

The structure of the IS is highly ordered and dynamic. Imaging microscopy techniques have shown that TCR and its signaling molecules aggregate onto dynamic microclusters, formed at the periphery of the IS (at the peripheral SMAC or pSMAC) and migrating toward its center (at the centralized SMAC or cSMAC) [96-98]. Although the TCR microclusters can also include molecules like CD2, CD4, CD8, and CD28, they exclude the tyrosine phosphatase CD45 [55,99]. The dynamics of cluster coalescence may involve multiple mechanisms. Although a centralized cluster (cSMAC) is typically always formed, different events may coordinately act to give the final aggregated structure. While membrane movement may constrain aggregation cluster within a given domain, the contact between individual membrane may also be required to reorganize contacts in the IS [100]. The activity of microclusters progressively decreases as they are centralized toward the cSMAC, where they are ultimately internalized [99].

Formation of the IS also requires stabilization of the interaction between the T cell and the APC [101]. Such stabilization can be achieved by the binding of the adhesion molecule LFA-1 (lymphocyte function associated antigen 1) located on T cells with its ligand ICAM-1 (intercellular adhesion molecule 1) present on the APC, the binding affinity between these molecules being greatly enhanced by the structural change induced following antigen recognition and signaling by the TCR.

Molecular requirements for the polarization of the IS

A hallmark of T-cell activation is the reorientation of the microtubule organizing center (MTOC) to a position beneath the IS [102] and therefore the MTOC constitutes a marker of changes in T-cell polarization in response to antigen stimulation. In fact, TCR stimulation induces actin polymerization at the immune synapse and MTOC reorientation [103]. In addition, direct contact of the MTOC with the IS plays a critical role by allowing directed secretion of cytotoxic granules by killer lymphocytes [104]. The formation of microclusters and SMACs depends on the actin cytoskeleton [99,105]. Recently, it was shown that clathrin, a protein involved in endocytic processes, in intracellular compartments and vesicle formation, as well as in the formation of late endosomes termed multivesicular bodies (MVBs), is recruited to and regulates actin accumulation at the IS suggesting that some interactions might occur between MVBs and the IS [106]. Actin polymerization occurs and is enhanced at the edge of the synapse, as the cell spreads to achieve synapse formation [94]. Actin polymerization then appeared to be a key factor in the migration of microclusters. Interestingly, the adaptor ADAP is linked to the actin cytoskeleton and, upon antigenic stimulation, is recruited to the actin-rich periphery of the immune synapse, where it associates with the microtubule motor dynein [107]. Furthermore, ADAP was shown to play a role in the relocation of the MTOC to the IS through its interaction with dynein.

Molecular requirements for the spatio-temporal organization of the IS

The time-dependent molecular composition and the functional role of the SMAC and the IS are under intense investigation. For example, following complete or partial activation, the kinetics of intracellular protein recruitment to the T-cell-APC contact site may be correlated with specific functions of a signaling molecule. In addition, the spatial segregation of intracellular proteins in distinct areas of the cSMAC and pSMAC correlates with their importance in the activation pathway. Thus, TCR-mediated tyrosine kinase activities primarily occurs at the periphery of the synapse and is terminated before mature IS is formed.

NF-κB and lymphoma

NF-κB transcription factors can be uncoupled from their normal regulation and promote tumorigenesis in different ways. For example, mutations of the key components of the antigen-mediated signaling pathways are associated with constitutive CBM-mediated signaling, and with the development of particular subtypes of human B-cell lymphomas, including MALT and DLBCL lymphomas [108].

MALT lymphoma

B-cell lymphomas of mucosa-associated lymphoid tissue, which represent the most common extranodal lymphomas (8% of all non-Hodgkin's lymphomas), occur in different anatomic sites including stomach, ocular adnexa (conjunctiva and orbit), lung and thyroid [108]. Several molecular events involved in the lymphomagenesis of MALT lymphomas, where chronic antigenic stimulation plays a pivotal role, have been described. This chronic inflammation is induced by microbial infection, i.e. *Helicobacter pylori* (*Hp*) for gastric lymphomas and *Chlamydia psittaci* (*Cp*) for ocular adnexa lymphoma, or autoimmune disorders. Because the majority of cases arise in the stomach, most of our understanding comes from studies on gastric MALT lymphoma. In chronic inflammation and early stages of lymphoma development, an antigen-driven expansion of polyclonal B-cell and specific T cells is induced, promoting an interaction between normal BCL10 and MALT1 proteins that leads to NF-κB activation [109]. A subclone with molecular genetic abnormalities may eventually emerge, eliminating the need for persistent infection and/or chronic inflammation. Moreover, at early stage, eradicating the source of infection can successfully treat gastric lymphomas. However, recurrent cytogenetic alterations can promote disease progression. The most common alteration in gastric lymphoma and first-described chromosomal abnormality found in MALT lymphoma is t(11;18)(q21;q21), which fused the gene encoding the *inhibitor of apoptosis 2* (API2; also known as *cIAP2)* with *MALT1.12-14*. Another translocation t(1;14)(p22;q32) places the *BCL10* gene under the control of the immunoglobulin (Ig) heavy-chain enhancer promoter element (*IGH-BCL10*) leading to its overexpression [110,111]. The most common in ocular adnexa lymphoma is t(14;18)(q32;q21) which was originally found in MALT lymphoma of the liver and skin and involves the placement of the *MALT1* gene under the control of the Ig heavy chain enhancer (*IGH-MALT1*) [112]. Others have been reported including trisomy 3 or 18 occurring most frequently in intestinal and salivary gland MALT lymphoma [113] and, more recently, t(3;14)(p14.1;q32), involving the *IGH* and *forkhead box protein P1* (*FOXP1*), that was also reported in DLBCL [114]. Forkhead box P1 contains a N-terminal glutamine-rich region, a zinc finger, a leucine zipper, a forkhead and an acid-rich domain. By its involvement in the regulation of Rag1 and Rag2 expression, FoxP1 is essential for B cell development [115]. Given that MALT lymphoma and some types of DLBCL are characterized by constitutive NF-κB activation, it has been speculated that Foxp1 may be a regulator of NF-κB activation. Accordingly, various Foxp1 isoforms are capable of activating the NF-κB reporter in both B and T cell lines [109]. Recently, the deubiquitinase A20 was also implicated in the arising of MALT lymphomas. Importantly, A20 was found inactivated by somatic deletion, mutation or promoter methylation in around 30% of translocation-negative ocular adnexal MALT lymphoma [109,116]. These A20 alterations were also significantly associated with increased expression of NF-κB target genes CCR2, TLR6 and BCL2 [116]. Interestingly, it has been shown that ocula MALT lymphoma have preferential loss of the *TNFAIP3/A20* region.

BCL10 relocalisation from the cytosol to the nucleus is strongly observed in the nuclei from lymphomas carrying t(1;14)(p22;q32)/*BCL10-IGH* and moderately in gastric and pulmonary MALT lymphomas with t(11;18)(q21;q21)/*API2-MALT1* fusion and is highly predictive of *Helicobacter pylori*-independent status in high-grade gastric MALT lymphoma [117-120]. BCL10 does not contain any identified nuclear localization signal and the mechanisms responsible for BCL10 nuclear localization are not fully understood, although several factors regulating BCL10 stability or nucleus-to-cytoplasm shuttling have been identified. For example, MALT1 contains nuclear export signals and can export BCL10 from the nucleus to the cytoplasm, and the subcellular localization of BCL10 depends upon the relative ratio of BCL10 and MALT1 expression [121]. API2 is an E3 ubiquitin ligase of BCL10 that targets it for degradation. In the t(11;18)(q21;q21)/*API2-MALT1* translocation, the API2-mediated BCL10 degradation is likely compromised resulting in its nuclear localization. Interestingly, BCL10 degradation can be also affected by mutation of IKK-dependent phosphorylation sites leading to BCL10 nuclear accumulation and to increased IL-2 production after T cell antigen-receptor activation [20]. Although nuclear function of BCL10 remains to be determined, BCL10 could be involved in the regulation of NF-κB transcriptional activities through its association with BCL3, a coactivator of NF-κB.

There is growing evidence indicating that chromosome translocations alone, including those identified in MALT lymphomas, do not account for full malignant transformation. Indeed, lymphoma was not observed in mice in which API2-MALT1 or BCL10 were expressed in B lymphocytes, suggesting that NF-κB activation may not be sufficient to promote malignant transformation [122,123]. Additional factors, such as surface receptor activation, should act in cooperation with these chromosome translocations to induce MALT lymphoma development. Lack of cellular models of human-like MALT lymphoma has hindered a better understanding of the disease pathogenesis and the development of MALT-specific therapies. However, a recent study has shown that mice in which MALT1 is specifically expressed in the hematopoietic stem/progenitor cells can constitute models of human lymphoma pathogenesis and tools for developing and testing MALT1 inhibitors [124]. This work also indicates that MALT1 signaling is required for the survival of murine lymphoma cells.

DLBCL

Gene expression profiling revealed three main molecular subtypes of DLBCL reflecting the signature of this lymphoma from B-cells at different stages of differentiation [125]: the ABC-DLBCL and the germinal-center B-cell-like (GCB) subtypes, as well as primary mediastinal B-cell lymphoma (PMBL) [126-129]. These subtypes are characterized by their gene expression, response to chemotherapy and clinical progression and are associated with distinct genetic lesions, indicating the involvement of different oncogenic pathways [125]. The ABC subtype of DLBCL is characterized by chronic active B-cell receptor signaling and constitutive activation of the NF-κB pathway and, for this reason, we therefore focus only on this subtype of lymphoma. ABC-DLBLCL is associated with poor overall survival, since patients have a five years survival rate of only 30% [130]. While MALT1 and BCL10 have been described as key factors in the pathogenesis of MALT lymphoma subtypes with *MALT1* or *BCL10* chromosomal translocations (see above), the role of the CBM/NF-κB signaling pathway in other B-cell lymphoma development was largely unknown until recently. Indeed, it was recently shown that a hallmark of ABC-DLBCL is the constitutive signaling of the NF-κB pathway, linked to mutations in various genes regulating NF-κB, such as activating mutations of CARMA1, CD79A, CD79B, MyD88, and inactivating mutations of TNFAIP3/A20 [131]. Remarkably, most of the genes affecting by these mutations are critical for the survival of ABC-DLBCL through their involvement in NF-κB signaling. Additional translocation/inactivation, including BCL6 translocations and inactivation of the acetyltransferase genes CREBBP and EP300, are shared by ABC-DLBCL and GCB-DLBCL [132]. The B-cell receptor is composed of the antigen-binding IgH and IgL chains and the two signaling subunits, CD79A and CD79B. Over 20% of ABC lymphomas have mutations in *CD79A* or *CD79B* leading to chronic active B-cell receptor signaling. Interestingly, the PKCβ activator PDK1 was shown to be essential for NF-κB activation and survival of a DLBCL cell line carrying a mutation in the BCR signaling subunit CD79B [133]. Downstream of CD79A/B, PKCβ propagates BCR signaling to the CBM complex. Using a loss-of function screen to identify genes that are required for proliferation and survival of DLBCL cells, Ngo and coworkers elegantly demonstrated that shRNAs targeting the NF-κB pathway were critical for the survival of ABC-DLBCL, but not for that of GCB-DLBCL [134]. This screen uncovered a previously unsuspected role for CARMA1 in the pathogenesis of ABC-DLBCL and identified also BCL10 and CARMA1 as critical components for ABC-DLBCL survival. Indeed, approximately 10% of ABC-DLBCLs harbors activating missense mutations within the coiled-coil domain of CARMA1 and expression of these mutants leads to constitutive and enhanced antigen receptor-dependent activation of NF-κB [12,135,136]. It was further showed that these mutations alter the intra- and inter-molecular interactions that depend on the auto-inhibitory domain of CARMA1, thereby promoting constitutive NF- κB activity (see above). Furthermore, CARMA1 expression levels are consistently elevated in primary tumor biopsies of ABC-DLBCL lymphomas.

Whole-exome sequencing (WES) and genome-wide high-density single nucleotide polymorphism (SNP) array were also used to discover new non-silent mutations implicated in DLBCL pathogenesis [137]. The genes identified by these approaches include most of the known genes implicated in the pathogenesis of DLBCL, in addition to a few genes that have never been implicated in cancers. It was found that MALT1 is not mutated or translocated in ABC-DLBCL, while ABC-DLBCL cell lines are dependent on MALT1 catalytic activity [134,138,139]. Consequently, A20 and BCL10 are constitutively processed in these last lymphoma subtypes. Interestingly, MALT1 protease inhibitor, by preventing A20 and BCL10 cleavage, reduces NF-κB activity resulting in cell death and growth retardation. This study further suggests that MALT1 protease activity is a potential target for pharmacological treatment of ABC-DLBCL. Using MALT1 activity assay, diverse MALT1 inhibitors were found and tested on ABC-DLBCL [140]. Notably, one of these inhibitors (MI-2) displayed a selective activity against ABC-DLBCL. As mentioned above, constitutive activity of PI3K and PDK1, its downstream kinase, is required for survival of a subset of ABC-DLBCL cell lines that carry mutations in the gene encoding the BCR signaling adaptor CD79B. By a pharmacological inhibitory approach, it was further demonstrated that PI3K/PDK1 activity was also required for constitutive MALT1 protease activity and subsequently for NF-κB activity in a subgroup of ABC-DLBCL [133]. Interestingly, additional screening uncovered that CK1α is selectively lethal for ABC-DLBCL cell lines [78], however, no mutations of its gene has been reported so far. Although, inactivation of the deubiquitinase A20 results in increased NF-κB activity in ABC-DLBL cells, supression of A20 alone is not sufficient for tumor development, suggesting that tumors bearing A20 inactivation rely on additional mechanisms to activate NF-κB signaling, such as chronic active B-cell receptor signaling or CARMA1 gene mutations.

Ngo and colleagues discovered that a leucine (CTG) to proline (CCG) exchange at position 265 (L265P) of the myeloid differentiation primary response gene 88 (MYD88) occurred in 29% of ABC-DLBCL biopsies [134]. MYD88 has not been implicated in antigen-mediated NF-κB activation, but is an adaptor protein that transduces signals from most of the Toll-like receptors and receptors for interleukin (IL)-1and IL-18 [141]. Recently, whole-exome sequencing studies have revealed that MYD88 is a recurrently mutated gene in DLBCL cases [142,143]. However, the incidence of MYD88 L265P mutation in Korean patients with DLBCL did not give the same incidence (6.5%) [144]. Finally, several FoxP1 isoforms and especially its smaller isoforms, are expressed at much higher levels in the ABC-DLBCL compared to the GCB-DLBCL lymphomas [145].

Concluding Remarks

For the last 10 years, our understanding of the signaling pathways that control normal physiologic processes and can lead to tumor and cancer development when perturbed, have considerably progressed, especially due to the characterization of well-established models of cancer such as MALT and DLBCL lymphomas. Indeed, identification of the alterations involved in development of these lymphoma subtypes led to the discovery of a novel complex of proteins, the CBM complex and highlighted the role of the CBM/NF-κB axis in both normal and pathological responses. Future works will certainly aim at designing therapeutic molecules or approaches that specifically target the CBM/NF-κB pathways to prevent the constitutive activation of NF-κB signaling as a treatment of lymphomas that are dependent on NF-κB hyperactivation. Therapies targeting the anti-apoptotic aspect of the NF-κB pathway would be particularly of great interest, given the growing number of studies involving this pathway in lymphoma development.

Acknowledgments

We thank all the members of the laboratory for helpful discussions. RW, PG were supported by CNRS and NM by the Ministère de la Recherche. Work in the RW's team is supported by Institut National du cancer (INCa).

References

1. Weiss A, Littman DR (1994) Signal transduction by lymphocyte antigen receptors. Cell 76: 263-274.
2. Gaide O, Martinon F, Micheau O, Bonnet D, Thome M, et al. (2001) Carma1, a CARD-containing binding partner of Bcl10, induces Bcl10 phosphorylation and NF-kappaB activation. FEBS Lett 496: 121-127.
3. Bertin J, Wang L, Guo Y, Jacobson MD, Poyet JL, et al. (2001) CARD11 and CARD14 are novel caspase recruitment domain (CARD)/membrane-associated guanylate kinase (MAGUK) family members that interact with BCL10 and activate NF-kappa B. J Biol Chem 276: 11877-11882.
4. Jun JE, Wilson LE, Vinuesa CG, Lesage S, Blery M, et al. (2003) Identifying the MAGUK protein Carma-1 as a central regulator of humoral immune responses and atopy by genome-wide mouse mutagenesis. Immunity 18: 751-762.
5. Egawa T, Albrecht B, Favier B, Sunshine MJ, Mirchandani K, et al. (2003) Requirement for CARMA1 in antigen receptor-induced NF-kappa B activation and lymphocyte proliferation. Curr Biol 13: 1252-1258.
6. Newton K, Dixit VM (2003) Mice lacking the CARD of CARMA1 exhibit defective B lymphocyte development and impaired proliferation of their B and T lymphocytes. Curr Biol 13: 1247-1251.
7. Hara H, Wada T, Bakal C, Kozieradzki I, Suzuki S, et al. (2003) The MAGUK family protein CARD11 is essential for lymphocyte activation. Immunity 18: 763-775.
8. Sommer K, Guo B, Pomerantz JL, Bandaranayake AD, Moreno-García ME, et al. (2005) Phosphorylation of the CARMA1 linker controls NF-kappaB activation. Immunity 23: 561-574.
9. Matsumoto R, Wang D, Blonska M, Li H, Kobayashi M, et al. (2005) Phosphorylation of CARMA1 plays a critical role in T Cell receptor-mediated NF-kappaB activation. Immunity 23: 575-585.
10. Ishiguro K, Green T, Rapley J, Wachtel H, Giallourakis C, et al. (2006) Ca2+/calmodulin-dependent protein kinase II is a modulator of CARMA1-mediated NF-kappaB activation. Mol Cell Biol 26: 5497-5508.
11. Thome M, Weil R (2007) Post-translational modifications regulate distinct functions of CARMA1 and BCL10. Trends Immunol 28: 281-288.
12. Chan W, Schaffer TB, Pomerantz JL (2013) A quantitative signaling screen identifies CARD11 mutations in the CARD and LATCH domains that induce Bcl10 ubiquitination and human lymphoma cell survival. Mol Cell Biol 33: 429-443.
13. Eitelhuber AC, Warth S, Schimmack G, Düwel M, Hadian K, et al. (2011) Dephosphorylation of Carma1 by PP2A negatively regulates T-cell activation. EMBO J 30: 594-605.
14. Hara H, Saito T (2009) CARD9 versus CARMA1 in innate and adaptive immunity. Trends Immunol 30: 234-242.
15. Gross O, Gewies A, Finger K, Schäfer M, Sparwasser T, et al. (2006) Card9 controls a non-TLR signalling pathway for innate anti-fungal immunity. Nature 442: 651-656.
16. Saijo S, Fujikado N, Furuta T, Chung SH, Kotaki H, et al. (2007) Dectin-1 is required for host defense against Pneumocystis carinii but not against Candida albicans. Nat Immunol 8: 39-46.
17. Xue L, Morris SW, Orihuela C, Tuomanen E, Cui X, et al. (2003) Defective development and function of Bcl10-deficient follicular, marginal zone and B1 B cells. Nat Immunol 4: 857-865.
18. Ruland J, Duncan GS, Elia A, del Barco Barrantes I, Nguyen L, et al. (2001) Bcl10 is a positive regulator of antigen receptor-induced activation of NF-kappaB and neural tube closure. Cell 104: 33-42.

19. Hu S, Du MQ, Park SM, Alcivar A, Qu L, et al. (2006) cIAP2 is a ubiquitin protein ligase for BCL10 and is dysregulated in mucosa-associated lymphoid tissue lymphomas. J Clin Invest 116: 174-181.

20. Lobry C, Lopez T, Israël A, Weil R (2007) Negative feedback loop in T cell activation through IkappaB kinase-induced phosphorylation and degradation of Bcl10. Proc Natl Acad Sci U S A 104: 908-913.

21. Scharschmidt E, Wegener E, Heissmeyer V, Rao A, Krappmann D (2004) Degradation of Bcl10 induced by T-cell activation negatively regulates NF-kappa B signaling. Mol Cell Biol 24: 3860-3873.

22. Wu CJ, Ashwell JD (2008) NEMO recognition of ubiquitinated Bcl10 is required for T cell receptor-mediated NF-kappaB activation. Proc Natl Acad Sci U S A 105: 3023-3028.

23. Zeng H, Di L, Fu G, Chen Y, Gao X, et al. (2007) Phosphorylation of Bcl10 negatively regulates T-cell receptor-mediated NF-kappaB activation. Mol Cell Biol 27: 5235-5245.

24. Paul S, Kashyap AK, Jia W, He YW, Schaefer BC (2012) Selective autophagy of the adaptor protein Bcl10 modulates T cell receptor activation of NF-κB. Immunity 36: 947-958.

25. Moreno-García ME, Sommer K, Rincon-Arano H, Brault M, Ninomiya-Tsuji J, et al. (2013) Kinase-independent feedback of the TAK1/TAB1 complex on BCL10 turnover and NF-κB activation. Mol Cell Biol 33: 1149-1163.

26. Dufner A, Schamel WW (2011) B cell antigen receptor-induced activation of an IRAK4-dependent signaling pathway revealed by a MALT1-IRAK4 double knockout mouse model. Cell Commun Signal 9: 6.

27. Ruefli-Brasse AA, French DM, Dixit VM (2003) Regulation of NF-kappaB-dependent lymphocyte activation and development by paracaspase. Science 302: 1581-1584.

28. Ruland J, Duncan GS, Wakeham A, Mak TW (2003) Differential requirement for Malt1 in T and B cell antigen receptor signaling. Immunity 19: 749-758.

29. Tusche MW, Ward LA, Vu F, McCarthy D, Quintela-Fandino M, et al. (2009) Differential requirement of MALT1 for BAFF-induced outcomes in B cell subsets. J Exp Med 206: 2671-2683.

30. Lucas PC, Yonezumi M, Inohara N, McAllister-Lucas LM, Abazeed ME, et al. (2001) Bcl10 and MALT1, independent targets of chromosomal translocation in malt lymphoma, cooperate in a novel NF-kappa B signaling pathway. J Biol Chem 276: 19012-19019.

31. Uren AG, O'Rourke K, Aravind LA, Pisabarro MT, Seshagiri S, et al. (2000) Identification of paracaspases and metacaspases: two ancient families of caspase-like proteins, one of which plays a key role in MALT lymphoma. Mol Cell 6: 961-967.

32. Kirchhofer D, Vucic D (2012) Protease activity of MALT1: a mystery unravelled. Biochem J 444: e3-5.

33. Hailfinger S, Nogai H, Pelzer C, Jaworski M, Cabalzar K, et al. (2011) Malt1-dependent RelB cleavage promotes canonical NF-kappaB activation in lymphocytes and lymphoma cell lines. Proc Natl Acad Sci U S A 108: 14596-14601.

34. Rebeaud F, Hailfinger S, Posevitz-Fejfar A, Tapernoux M, Moser R, et al. (2008) The proteolytic activity of the paracaspase MALT1 is key in T cell activation. Nat Immunol 9: 272-281.

35. Wiesmann C, Leder L, Blank J, Bernardi A, Melkko S, et al. (2012) Structural determinants of MALT1 protease activity. J Mol Biol 419: 4-21.

36. Bhoj VG, Chen ZJ (2009) Ubiquitylation in innate and adaptive immunity. Nature 458: 430-437.

37. Wertz IE, Dixit VM (2010) Signaling to NF-kappaB: regulation by ubiquitination. Cold Spring Harb Perspect Biol 2: a003350.

38. Oeckinghaus A, Wegener E, Welteke V, Ferch U, Arslan SC, et al. (2007) Malt1 ubiquitination triggers NF-kappaB signaling upon T-cell activation. EMBO J 26: 4634-4645.

39. Boisson B, Laplantine E, Prando C, Giliani S, Israelsson E, et al. (2012) Immunodeficiency, autoinflammation and amylopectinosis in humans with inherited HOIL-1 and LUBAC deficiency. Nat Immunol 13: 1178-1186.

40. Sun SC (2010) CYLD: a tumor suppressor deubiquitinase regulating NF-kappaB activation and diverse biological processes. Cell Death Differ 17: 25-34.

41. Shembade N, Harhaj EW (2012) Regulation of NF-κB signaling by the A20 deubiquitinase. Cell Mol Immunol 9: 123-130.

42. Baier G (2003) The PKC gene module: molecular biosystematics to resolve its T cell functions. Immunol Rev 192: 64-79.

43. Coudronniere N, Villalba M, Englund N, Altman A (2000) NF-kappa B activation induced by T cell receptor/CD28 costimulation is mediated by protein kinase C-theta. Proc Natl Acad Sci U S A 97: 3394-3399.

44. Pfeifhofer C, Kofler K, Gruber T, Tabrizi NG, Lutz C, et al. (2003) Protein kinase C theta affects Ca2+ mobilization and NFAT cell activation in primary mouse T cells. J Exp Med 197: 1525-1535.

45. Baier-Bitterlich G, Uberall F, Bauer B, Fresser F, Wachter H, et al. (1996) Protein kinase C-theta isoenzyme selective stimulation of the transcription factor complex AP-1 in T lymphocytes. Mol Cell Biol 16: 1842-1850.

46. Sakaguchi S, Yamaguchi T, Nomura T, Ono M (2008) Regulatory T cells and immune tolerance. Cell 133: 775-787.

47. Kong KF, Yokosuka T, Canonigo-Balancio AJ, Isakov N, Saito T, et al. (2011) A motif in the V3 domain of the kinase PKCθ determines its localization in the immunological synapse and functions in T cells via association with CD28. Nat Immunol 12: 1105-1112.

48. Yokosuka T, Kobayashi W, Sakata-Sogawa K, Takamatsu M, Hashimoto-Tane A, et al. (2008) Spatiotemporal regulation of T cell costimulation by TCR-CD28 microclusters and protein kinase C theta translocation. Immunity 29: 589-601.

49. Isakov N, Altman A (2012) PKC-theta-mediated signal delivery from the TCR/CD28 surface receptors. Front Immunol 3: 273.

50. Park SG, Long M, Kang JA, Kim WS, Lee CR, et al. (2013) The kinase PDK1 is essential for B-cell receptor mediated survival signaling. PLoS One 8: e55378.

51. Park SG, Schulze-Luehrman J, Hayden MS, Hashimoto N, Ogawa W, et al. (2009) The kinase PDK1 integrates T cell antigen receptor and CD28 coreceptor signaling to induce NF-kappaB and activate T cells. Nat Immunol 10: 158-166.

52. Lee KY, D'Acquisto F, Hayden MS, Shim JH, Ghosh S (2005) PDK1 nucleates T cell receptor-induced signaling complex for NF-kappaB activation. Science 308: 114-118.

53. da Silva AJ, Li Z, de Vera C, Canto E, Findell P, et al. (1997) Cloning of a novel T-cell protein FYB that binds FYN and SH2-domain-containing leukocyte protein 76 and modulates interleukin 2 production. Proc Natl Acad Sci U S A 94: 7493-7498.

54. Musci MA, Hendricks-Taylor LR, Motto DG, Paskind M, Kamens J, et al. (1997) Molecular cloning of SLAP-130, an SLP-76-associated substrate of the T cell antigen receptor-stimulated protein tyrosine kinases. J Biol Chem 272: 11674-11677.

55. Wang H, Rudd CE (2008) SKAP-55, SKAP-55-related and ADAP adaptors modulate integrin-mediated immune-cell adhesion. Trends Cell Biol 18: 486-493.

56. Medeiros RB, Burbach BJ, Mueller KL, Srivastava R, Moon JJ, et al. (2007) Regulation of NF-kappaB activation in T cells via association of the adapter proteins ADAP and CARMA1. Science 316: 754-758.

57. Srivastava R, Burbach BJ, Mitchell JS, Pagán AJ, Shimizu Y (2012) ADAP regulates cell cycle progression of T cells via control of cyclin E and Cdk2 expression through two distinct CARMA1-dependent signaling pathways. Mol Cell Biol 32: 1908-1917.

58. Burbach BJ, Srivastava R, Medeiros RB, O'Gorman WE, Peterson EJ, et al. (2008) Distinct regulation of integrin-dependent T cell conjugate formation and NF-kappa B activation by the adapter protein ADAP. J Immunol 181: 4840-4851.

59. Maelfait J, Beyaert R (2008) Non-apoptotic functions of caspase-8. Biochem Pharmacol 76: 1365-1373.

60. Su H, Bidère N, Zheng L, Cubre A, Sakai K, et al. (2005) Requirement for caspase-8 in NF-kappaB activation by antigen receptor. Science 307: 1465-1468.

61. Chun HJ, Zheng L, Ahmad M, Wang J, Speirs CK, et al. (2002) Pleiotropic defects in lymphocyte activation caused by caspase-8 mutations lead to human immunodeficiency. Nature 419: 395-399.

62. He L, Wu X, Siegel R, Lipsky PE (2006) TRAF6 regulates cell fate decisions by

inducing caspase 8-dependent apoptosis and the activation of NF-kappaB. J Biol Chem 281: 11235-11249.

63. McCully RR, Pomerantz JL (2008) The protein kinase C-responsive inhibitory domain of CARD11 functions in NF-kappaB activation to regulate the association of multiple signaling cofactors that differentially depend on Bcl10 and MALT1 for association. Mol Cell Biol 28: 5668-5686.

64. Lens SM, Kataoka T, Fortner KA, Tinel A, Ferrero I, et al. (2002) The caspase 8 inhibitor c-FLIP(L) modulates T-cell receptor-induced proliferation but not activation-induced cell death of lymphocytes. Mol Cell Biol 22: 5419-5433.

65. Safa AR, Pollok KE (2011) Targeting the Anti-Apoptotic Protein c-FLIP for Cancer Therapy. Cancers (Basel) 3: 1639-1671.

66. Oruganti SR, Edin S, Grundström C, Grundström T (2011) CaMKII targets Bcl10 in T-cell receptor induced activation of NF-κB. Mol Immunol 48: 1448-1460.

67. Bidère N, Ngo VN, Lee J, Collins C, Zheng L, et al. (2009) Casein kinase 1alpha governs antigen-receptor-induced NF-kappaB activation and human lymphoma cell survival. Nature 458: 92-96.

68. Kupfer A, Kupfer H (2003) Imaging immune cell interactions and functions: SMACs and the Immunological Synapse. Semin Immunol 15: 295-300.

69. Gaide O, Favier B, Legler DF, Bonnet D, Brissoni B, et al. (2002) CARMA1 is a critical lipid raft-associated regulator of TCR-induced NF-kappa B activation. Nat Immunol 3: 836-843.

70. Wang D, Matsumoto R, You Y, Che T, Lin XY, et al. (2004) CD3/CD28 costimulation-induced NF-kappaB activation is mediated by recruitment of protein kinase C-theta, Bcl10, and IkappaB kinase beta to the immunological synapse through CARMA1. Mol Cell Biol 24: 164-171.

71. Teixeiro E, Daniels MA, Hausmann B, Schrum AG, Naeher D, et al. (2004) T cell division and death are segregated by mutation of TCRbeta chain constant domains. Immunity 21: 515-526.

72. Hayashi K, Altman A (2007) Protein kinase C theta (PKCtheta): a key player in T cell life and death. Pharmacol Res 55: 537-544.

73. Weil R, Israël A (2006) Deciphering the pathway from the TCR to NF-kappaB. Cell Death Differ 13: 826-833.

74. Hara H, Bakal C, Wada T, Bouchard D, Rottapel R, et al. (2004) The molecular adapter Carma1 controls entry of IkappaB kinase into the central immune synapse. J Exp Med 200: 1167-1177.

75. Cannons JL, Yu LJ, Hill B, Mijares LA, Dombroski D, et al. (2004) SAP regulates T(H)2 differentiation and PKC-theta-mediated activation of NF-kappaB1. Immunity 21: 693-706.

76. Weil R, Schwamborn K, Alcover A, Bessia C, Di Bartolo V, et al. (2003) Induction of the NF-kappaB cascade by recruitment of the scaffold molecule NEMO to the T cell receptor. Immunity 18: 13-26.

77. Lee KH, Dinner AR, Tu C, Campi G, Raychaudhuri S, et al. (2003) The immunological synapse balances T cell receptor signaling and degradation. Science 302: 1218-1222.

78. Wiedemann A, Müller S, Favier B, Penna D, Guiraud M, et al. (2005) T-cell activation is accompanied by an ubiquitination process occurring at the immunological synapse. Immunol Lett 98: 57-61.

79. Lamason RL, Kupfer A, Pomerantz JL (2010) The dynamic distribution of CARD11 at the immunological synapse is regulated by the inhibitory kinesin GAKIN. Mol Cell 40: 798-809.

80. Bi K, Tanaka Y, Coudronniere N, Sugie K, Hong S, et al. (2001) Antigen-induced translocation of PKC-theta to membrane rafts is required for T cell activation. Nat Immunol 2: 556-563.

81. Huang J, Lo PF, Zal T, Gascoigne NR, Smith BA, et al. (2002) CD28 plays a critical role in the segregation of PKC theta within the immunologic synapse. Proc Natl Acad Sci U S A 99: 9369-9373.

82. Sims TN, Soos TJ, Xenias HS, Dubin-Thaler B, Hofman JM, et al. (2007) Opposing effects of PKCtheta and WASp on symmetry breaking and relocation of the immunological synapse. Cell 129: 773-785.

83. Beemiller P, Jacobelli J, Krummel MF (2012) Integration of the movement of signaling microclusters with cellular motility in immunological synapses. Nat Immunol 13: 787-795.

84. Friedman RS, Beemiller P, Sorensen CM, Jacobelli J, Krummel MF (2010) Real-time analysis of T cell receptors in naive cells in vitro and in vivo reveals flexibility in synapse and signaling dynamics. J Exp Med 207: 2733-2749.

85. Campi G, Varma R, Dustin ML (2005) Actin and agonist MHC-peptide complex-dependent T cell receptor microclusters as scaffolds for signaling. J Exp Med 202: 1031-1036.

86. Hashimoto-Tane A, Yokosuka T, Sakata-Sogawa K, Sakuma M, Ishihara C, et al. (2011) Dynein-driven transport of T cell receptor microclusters regulates immune synapse formation and T cell activation. Immunity 34: 919-931.

87. Yokosuka T, Sakata-Sogawa K, Kobayashi W, Hiroshima M, Hashimoto-Tane A, et al. (2005) Newly generated T cell receptor microclusters initiate and sustain T cell activation by recruitment of Zap70 and SLP-76. Nat Immunol 6: 1253-1262.

88. Varma R, Campi G, Yokosuka T, Saito T, Dustin ML (2006) T cell receptor-proximal signals are sustained in peripheral microclusters and terminated in the central supramolecular activation cluster. Immunity 25: 117-127.

89. Gérard A, Beemiller P, Friedman RS, Jacobelli J, Krummel MF (2013) Evolving immune circuits are generated by flexible, motile, and sequential immunological synapses. Immunol Rev 251: 80-96.

90. Dustin ML, Springer TA (1989) T-cell receptor cross-linking transiently stimulates adhesiveness through LFA-1. Nature 341: 619-624.

91. Kupfer A, Dennert G (1984) Reorientation of the microtubule-organizing center and the Golgi apparatus in cloned cytotoxic lymphocytes triggered by binding to lysable target cells. J Immunol 133: 2762-2766.

92. Bunnell SC, Kapoor V, Trible RP, Zhang W, Samelson LE (2001) Dynamic actin polymerization drives T cell receptor-induced spreading: a role for the signal transduction adaptor LAT. Immunity 14: 315-329.

93. Stinchcombe JC, Majorovits E, Bossi G, Fuller S, Griffiths GM (2006) Centrosome polarization delivers secretory granules to the immunological synapse. Nature 443: 462-465.

94. Kaizuka Y, Douglass AD, Varma R, Dustin ML, Vale RD (2007) Mechanisms for segregating T cell receptor and adhesion molecules during immunological synapse formation in Jurkat T cells. Proc Natl Acad Sci U S A 104: 20296-20301.

95. Calabia-Linares C, Robles-Valero J, de la Fuente H, Perez-Martinez M, Martín-Cofreces N, et al. (2011) Endosomal clathrin drives actin accumulation at the immunological synapse. J Cell Sci 124: 820-830.

96. Combs J, Kim SJ, Tan S, Ligon LA, Holzbaur EL, et al. (2006) Recruitment of dynein to the Jurkat immunological synapse. Proc Natl Acad Sci U S A 103: 14883-14888.

97. Rosebeck S, Rehman AO, Lucas PC, McAllister-Lucas LM (2011) From MALT lymphoma to the CBM signalosome: three decades of discovery. Cell Cycle 10: 2485-2496.

98. Du MQ (2011) MALT lymphoma: many roads lead to nuclear factor-Î°b activation. Histopathology 58: 26-38.

99. Willis TG, Jadayel DM, Du MQ, Peng H, Perry AR, et al. (1999) Bcl10 is involved in t(1;14)(p22;q32) of MALT B cell lymphoma and mutated in multiple tumor types. Cell 96: 35-45.

100. Zhang Q, Siebert R, Yan M, Hinzmann B, Cui X, et al. (1999) Inactivating mutations and overexpression of BCL10, a caspase recruitment domain-containing gene, in MALT lymphoma with t(1;14)(p22;q32). Nat Genet 22: 63-68.

101. Streubel B, Lamprecht A, Dierlamm J, Cerroni L, Stolte M, et al. (2003) T(14;18)(q32;q21) involving IGH and MALT1 is a frequent chromosomal aberration in MALT lymphoma. Blood 101: 2335-2339.

102. Streubel B, Simonitsch-Klupp I, Müllauer L, Lamprecht A, Huber D, et al. (2004) Variable frequencies of MALT lymphoma-associated genetic aberrations in MALT lymphomas of different sites. Leukemia 18: 1722-1726.

103. Streubel B, Vinatzer U, Lamprecht A, Raderer M, Chott A (2005) T(3;14)(p14.1;q32) involving IGH and FOXP1 is a novel recurrent chromosomal aberration in MALT lymphoma. Leukemia 19: 652-658.

104. Hu H, Wang B, Borde M, Nardone J, Maika S, et al. (2006) Foxp1 is an essential transcriptional regulator of B cell development. Nat Immunol 7: 819-826.

105. Bi Y, Zeng N, Chanudet E, Huang Y, Hamoudi RA, et al. (2012) A20 inactivation in ocular adnexal MALT lymphoma. Haematologica 97: 926-930.

106. Liu H, Ye H, Dogan A, Ranaldi R, Hamoudi RA, et al. (2001) T(11;18)(q21;q21) is associated with advanced mucosa-associated lymphoid tissue lymphoma that expresses nuclear BCL10. Blood 98: 1182-1187.

107. Maes B, Demunter A, Peeters B, De Wolf-Peeters C (2002) BCL10 mutation does not represent an important pathogenic mechanism in gastric MALT-type lymphoma, and the presence of the API2-MLT fusion is associated with aberrant nuclear BCL10 expression. Blood 99: 1398-1404.

108. Ye H, Dogan A, Karran L, Willis TG, Chen L, et al. (2000) BCL10 expression in normal and neoplastic lymphoid tissue. Nuclear localization in MALT lymphoma. Am J Pathol 157: 1147-1154.

109. Ye H, Liu H, Attygalle A, Wotherspoon AC, Nicholson AG, et al. (2003) Variable frequencies of t(11;18)(q21;q21) in MALT lymphomas of different sites: significant association with CagA strains of H pylori in gastric MALT lymphoma. Blood 102: 1012-1018.

110. Nakagawa M, Hosokawa Y, Yonezumi M, Izumiyama K, Suzuki R, et al. (2005) MALT1 contains nuclear export signals and regulates cytoplasmic localization of BCL10. Blood 106: 4210-4216.

111. Baens M, Fevery S, Sagaert X, Noels H, Hagens S, et al. (2006) Selective expansion of marginal zone B cells in Emicro-API2-MALT1 mice is linked to enhanced IkappaB kinase gamma polyubiquitination. Cancer Res 66: 5270-5277.

112. Li Z, Wang H, Xue L, Shin DM, Roopenian D, et al. (2009) Emu-BCL10 mice exhibit constitutive activation of both canonical and noncanonical NF-kappaB pathways generating marginal zone (MZ) B-cell expansion as a precursor to splenic MZ lymphoma. Blood 114: 4158-4168.

113. Vicente-Dueñas C, Fontán L, Gonzalez-Herrero I, Romero-Camarero I, Segura V, et al. (2012) Expression of MALT1 oncogene in hematopoietic stem/progenitor cells recapitulates the pathogenesis of human lymphoma in mice. Proc Natl Acad Sci U S A 109: 10534-10539.

114. Lenz G, Staudt LM (2010) Aggressive lymphomas. N Engl J Med 362: 1417-1429.

115. Alizadeh AA, Eisen MB, Davis RE, Ma C, Lossos IS, et al. (2000) Distinct types of diffuse large B-cell lymphoma identified by gene expression profiling. Nature 403: 503-511.

116. Rosenwald A, Wright G, Chan WC, Connors JM, Campo E, et al. (2002) The use of molecular profiling to predict survival after chemotherapy for diffuse large-B-cell lymphoma. N Engl J Med 346: 1937-1947.

117. Savage KJ, Monti S, Kutok JL, Cattoretti G, Neuberg D, et al. (2003) The molecular signature of mediastinal large B-cell lymphoma differs from that of other diffuse large B-cell lymphomas and shares features with classical Hodgkin lymphoma. Blood 102: 3871-3879.

118. Wright G, Tan B, Rosenwald A, Hurt EH, Wiestner A, et al. (2003) A gene expression-based method to diagnose clinically distinct subgroups of diffuse large B cell lymphoma. Proc Natl Acad Sci U S A 100: 9991-9996.

119. Lossos IS, Czerwinski DK, Alizadeh AA, Wechser MA, Tibshirani R, et al. (2004) Prediction of survival in diffuse large-B-cell lymphoma based on the expression of six genes. N Engl J Med 350: 1828-1837.

120. Novak U, Rinaldi A, Kwee I, Nandula SV, Rancoita PM, et al. (2009) The NF-{kappa}B negative regulator TNFAIP3 (A20) is inactivated by somatic mutations and genomic deletions in marginal zone lymphomas. Blood 113: 4918-4921.

121. Pasqualucci L, Dominguez-Sola D, Chiarenza A, Fabbri G, Grunn A, et al. (2011) Inactivating mutations of acetyltransferase genes in B-cell lymphoma. Nature 471: 189-195.

122. Kloo B, Nagel D, Pfeifer M, Grau M, Düwel M, et al. (2011) Critical role of PI3K signaling for NF-kappaB-dependent survival in a subset of activated B-cell-like diffuse large B-cell lymphoma cells. Proc Natl Acad Sci U S A 108: 272-277.

123. Ngo VN, Davis RE, Lamy L, Yu X, Zhao H, et al. (2006) A loss-of-function RNA interference screen for molecular targets in cancer. Nature 441: 106-110.

124. Compagno M, Lim WK, Grunn A, Nandula SV, Brahmachary M, et al. (2009) Mutations of multiple genes cause deregulation of NF-kappaB in diffuse large B-cell lymphoma. Nature 459: 717-721.

125. Lenz G, Davis RE, Ngo VN, Lam L, George TC, et al. (2008) Oncogenic CARD11 mutations in human diffuse large B cell lymphoma. Science 319: 1676-1679.

126. Pasqualucci L, Trifonov V, Fabbri G, Ma J, Rossi D, et al. (2011) Analysis of the coding genome of diffuse large B-cell lymphoma. Nat Genet 43: 830-837.

127. Ferch U, Kloo B, Gewies A, Pfänder V, Düwel M, et al. (2009) Inhibition of MALT1 protease activity is selectively toxic for activated B cell-like diffuse large B cell lymphoma cells. J Exp Med 206: 2313-2320.

128. Hailfinger S, Lenz G, Ngo V, Posvitz-Fejfar A, Rebeaud F, et al. (2009) Essential role of MALT1 protease activity in activated B cell-like diffuse large B-cell lymphoma. Proc Natl Acad Sci U S A 106: 19946-19951.

129. Fontan L, Yang C, Kabaleeswaran V, Volpon L, Osborne MJ, et al. (2012) MALT1 small molecule inhibitors specifically suppress ABC-DLBCL in vitro and in vivo. Cancer Cell 22: 812-824.

130. Kawai T, Akira S (2010) The role of pattern-recognition receptors in innate immunity: update on Toll-like receptors. Nat Immunol 11: 373-384.

131. Lohr JG, Stojanov P, Lawrence MS, Auclair D, Chapuy B, et al. (2012) Discovery and prioritization of somatic mutations in diffuse large B-cell lymphoma (DLBCL) by whole-exome sequencing. Proc Natl Acad Sci U S A 109: 3879-3884.

132. Morin RD, Mendez-Lago M, Mungall AJ, Goya R, Mungall KL, et al. (2011) Frequent mutation of histone-modifying genes in non-Hodgkin lymphoma. Nature 476: 298-303.

133. Choi JW, Kim Y, Lee JH, Kim YS (2013) MYD88 expression and L265P mutation in diffuse large B-cell lymphoma. Hum Pathol .

134. Wlodarska I, Veyt E, De Paepe P, Vandenberghe P, Nooijen P, et al. (2005) FOXP1, a gene highly expressed in a subset of diffuse large B-cell lymphoma, is recurrently targeted by genomic aberrations. Leukemia 19: 1299-1305.

135. Sun Z, Arendt CW, Ellmeier W, Schaeffer EM, Sunshine MJ, et al. (2000) PKC-theta is required for TCR-induced NF-kappaB activation in mature but not immature T lymphocytes. Nature 404: 402-407.

136. Berg-Brown NN, Gronski MA, Jones RG, Elford AR, Deenick EK, et al. (2004) PKCtheta signals activation versus tolerance in vivo. J Exp Med 199: 743-752.

137. Giannoni F, Lyon AB, Wareing MD, Dias PB, Sarawar SR (2005) Protein kinase C theta is not essential for T-cell-mediated clearance of murine gammaherpesvirus 68. J Virol 79: 6808-6813.

138. Marsland BJ, Nembrini C, Schmitz N, Abel B, Krautwald S, et al. (2005) Innate signals compensate for the absence of PKC-{theta} during in vivo CD8(+) T cell effector and memory responses. Proc Natl Acad Sci U S A 102: 14374-14379.

139. Valenzuela JO, Iclozan C, Hossain MS, Prlic M, Hopewell E, et al. (2009) PKCtheta is required for alloreactivity and GVHD but not for immune responses toward leukemia and infection in mice. J Clin Invest 119: 3774-3786.

140. Kingeter LM, Schaefer BC (2008) Loss of protein kinase C theta, Bcl10, or Malt1 selectively impairs proliferation and NF-kappa B activation in the CD4+ T cell subset. J Immunol 181: 6244-6254.

141. Su TT, Guo B, Kawakami Y, Sommer K, Chae K, et al. (2002) PKC-beta controls I kappa B kinase lipid raft recruitment and activation in response to BCR signaling. Nat Immunol 3: 780-786.

142. Kang TB, Ben-Moshe T, Varfolomeev EE, Pewzner-Jung Y, Yogev N, et al. (2004) Caspase-8 serves both apoptotic and nonapoptotic roles. J Immunol 173: 2976-2984.

143. Salmena L, Hakem R (2005) Caspase-8 deficiency in T cells leads to a lethal lymphoinfiltrative immune disorder. J Exp Med 202: 727-732.

144. Salmena L, Lemmers B, Hakem A, Matysiak-Zablocki E, Murakami K, et al. (2003) Essential role for caspase 8 in T-cell homeostasis and T-cell-mediated immunity. Genes Dev 17: 883-895.

145. Hinton HJ, Alessi DR, Cantrell DA (2004) The serine kinase phosphoinositide-dependent kinase 1 (PDK1) regulates T cell development. Nat Immunol 5: 539-545.

Methylated SFRP1,2 and CD25 Expression in Acute Myeloid Leukemia Play an Important Role in the Pathogenesis of the Disease and in Turn in its Treatment

Mohamed Z Abd Elrahman, Dalia Ahmad Nigm* and Azza Abo Elfadle

Department of Clinical Pathology, Assiut University, Egypt

Abstract

Objectives: Recently, hyperactivation of the Wnt signaling pathway has been implicated in leukomogenesis, so we studied the epigenetic dysfunction of SFRP1,2 and expression of interleukin2 receptor α chain (IL2Rα, also known as CD25) and its prognostic impact in acute myeloblastic leukemia (AML).

Methods: We studied the methylation profile of SFRP1,2 in AML cells by methylation-specific polymerase chain reaction (MSP) and the hyper expression of IL2Rα (CD25) by flowcytometry.

Results: We analyzed the methylation profile of SFRP1,2 in 40 de novo AML patients. The percentage of hypermethylation in the patient samples were 37.5% for SFRP1, 12.5% for SFRP2. CD25 was positive in 12(30%) of 40 patients AML. We found that in patients whom 60 years and younger with intermediate risk cytogenetics in de novo AML, hypermethylation of SFRP1 and CD25 were accompanied with relapse (P=0.024).

Conclusion: Our data indicates that in a subgroup of AML patients, hypermethylation of SFRP1 and high expression of CD25 predict relapse.

Introduction

Acute myeloid leukemia is a clonal hematopoietic disease associated by aberrant renewal of hematopoietic stem cells, differentiation arrest at blast cells, peripheral blood infiltration of blasts. It is found that pathogenesis of AML is accompanied by chromosomal translocations and genetic disorders [1]. Recently, epigenetic disorders, like promoter hypermethylation has been integrated in the pathogenesis of leukemia [2]. Wnt signaling pathway is important in the development of different organ systems [3,4] and also a very important factor in cell self renewal, cell proliferation, maturation and hematopoietic stem cell survival [4,5]. Prolonged activation of the Wnt pathway has been detected in AML [6]. SFRP is a tumor suppressor protein that regulates the Wnt signaling pathway. SFRP binds to Wnt protein and in turn inhibits its binding to Wnt-frizzled receptor and in order result in inhibition of Wnt signaling pathway. Thereafter there may be an association between methylation of Wnt signaling antagonist genes (SFRPs) and the activation of this pathway in leukemia [7]. Wnt signaling composed of the canonical pathway with b-catenin as a central factor and the non-canonical pathways including planar cell polarity and calcium ions [8]. If Wnt ligands absent, b-catenin is phosphorylated by glycogen synthase kinase-3b (GSK3b) which leads to its ubiquitination and degradation [9]. Attachment of Wnt to the Frizzled receptor leads to an inhibition of the GSK3b by the protein Dishevelled activation. This leads to b-catenin stabilization and its translocation into the nucleus where it binds to a number of transcription factors, like T-cell factor (TCF) and lymphoid enhancing factor-1 (LEF1) [10]. Elevated b-catenin has been found to block myeloid, lymphoid and erythroid cell maturation associated by an increase of blast cells [11]. In a case of hypermethylation of SFRP genes, its inhibitory effect on wnt singnaling pathway was lost which leads to elevation of cytoplasmic and nuclear levels of β- cathenin and in turn β-cathenin as a transcription factor increases expression of cyclin D and Myc genes that are included in cell cycle regulation [12]. Abnormal Wnt signaling has been detected in AML patients with normal karyotype and in patients with fms-like tyrosine kinase -3(Flt3) mutations [13] CD25 (α chain of interleukin 2 receptor) expression on AML cells has a role in the differentiation and proliferation of myeloid stem cells, cell-to-cell interactions, and the chemoresistant condition of the malignant cells [14]. We aimed to study the prognostic impact of hypermethylated SFRP1,2 and overexpression of CD25 in AML patients.

Patients and Methods

Patients

Twenty five healthy persons as a negative control group and 40 patients with de novo AML were involved in this study. These patients were admitted to Hematology unit, clinical pathology department and south Egypt cancer institute, Assiut University, Egypt, and were grouped depending on morphology and immune phenotyping (FAB classification).

The clinical data consisted of age and sex, laboratory data consisted of hemoglobin level, white blood cell count, platelets count and the recovery after induction chemotherapy were taken from patients' medical records.

Flowcytometric analysis

A panel of monoclonal antibodies was designed against myeloid lineage specific antigens including CD13, CD33, MPO, Cyto MPO,

***Corresponding author:** Dalia Ahmad Nigm, Faculty of medicine, Clinical Pathlogy Department, Assiut University, Egypt; E-mail: dodonigma@yahoo com

CD15, CD14, CD41 and and non-specific antigens including CD45, CD34, CD 11C, CD 117 and HLA-DR. In addition to, CD25 (IL-2Rα) were analyzed on 4 color BD FACSCALIBUR.

Cytogenetic study

Depending on the recommendations of the International System for Human Cytogenetic, cytogenetic analysis was done using short term cultures [15]. At least 20 metaphases were examined. Cytogenetic risk groups were categorized as follows: high risk, −7/ del(7q), −5/ del(5q), abn 3q, complex aberrations (X3 independent aberrations), t(6;9) and t(9;22); low risk, inv(16) and t(8;21); inter- mediate risk, normal karyotype or all other karyotypic abnormalities.

DNA extraction and bisulfite treatment

Genomic DNA was extracted from peripheral blood samples at diagnosis using an Invitrogen PureLink™ Genomic DNA Mini Kit, USA. Then, bisulfite conversion was done with the Invitrogen MethylCode™ Bisulfite Conversion Kit, USA using manufacurer's protocol. By this, methylated cytosine stayed as it where unmethylated cytosine converted to uracil.

Molecular analysis

In FLT3-internal tandem duplication (flt3/ITD) mutation analysis, we added 200 ng of DNA, 50 mM KCL, 10 mM Tris-HCL, pH 8.3, 1.5 mM $MgCL_2$, 200 μM dNTPs, 0.4 μM of forward primer 5'GCAATTTAGGTATGAAAGCCAGC-3'and 0.4 μM reverse primer 5'CTTTCAGCATTTTGACGGCAACC-3', and 1U of polymerase, in a volume of 50 μl [16]. The PCR consisted of an initial incubation step at 95°C for 10 minutes followed by 35 cycles at 94°C for 30 seconds, 57°C for 60 seconds, and 72°C for 90 seconds. The final extension step was at 72°C for 10 minutes. PCR products were analyzed on standard 3% agarose gels. Normal amplification produced a 330 bp product; whereas, FLT3 ITD mutations showed longer PCR products.

MSP methylation analysis

We used MSP (Methylation specific PCR) method to analyze the methylation profile of SFRP1 and SFRP2 genes. MSP is a PCR type used to analyze the CpG islands methylation state. In this technique, we used 2 pairs of primers specific for the methylated or unmethylated residue. Table 1 showed these primers sequences accompanied with product values [17].

In methylation testing, we added 2 μl of bisulfite-treated DNA, 4.5 μl of dH_2O, 12.5 μl of Master mix , 0.5 μl of forward primer(0.91 μM for SFRP1,0.88 μM for SFRP2) and 0.5 μl of reverse primer(0.95 μM for SFRP1,0.87 μM for SFRP2), and in unmethylation testing we added 2 μl of DNA, 8.5 μl of dH_2O, 12.5 μl of master mix , 0.5 μl of forward primer(0.91 μM for SFRP1,0.88 μM for SFRP2), 0.5 μl of reverse primer(0.95 μM for SFRP1,0.87 μM for SFRP2), and 1 μl of $MgCl_2$. In the first step of unmethylated status testing, we put reaction components in pre-thermal condition including 98°C for 1 minute and 96°C for 3 minutes then 40 cycles including 99°C for 10 seconds, 97°C for 20 seconds, 54°C for 30 seconds, while for methylated status testing, we did as previous steps except for the last step (64°C for 30 seconds), then 72°C for 7 minutes (extension). ddH_2O was used as the negative control. Finally, electrophoresis using a 2.5% agarose gel was done for MSP product identification.

We studied the prognostic impact of hypermethylated SFRP1,2 and overexpression of CD25 on the outcome in AML patients (complete remission(CR) which was defined as presence of <5% of blast cells in the bone marrow, Relapse was defined as bone marrow blast ≥ 5%, reappearance of blasts in peripheral blood and/or extramedullary disease and death) [18].

Results

Of the 40 patients, 29 (72.5%) were males and 11 (27.5%) were females (Table 2). Mean age was 35.5 years old (18-60 years). SFRP1 gene was completely unmethylated in 18 patients (45%), hemi-methylated in 7 patients (17.5%), while completely methylated in 15 patients (37.5%), however, SFRP2 gene was completely unmethylated in 29 patients (72.5%), hemi- methylated in 6 patients (15%), and completely methylated in 5 patients (12.5%) (Figure 1). All the control group showed negative methylation in SFRP1 and SFRP2 genes.

In our study, hypermethylation percentage of SFRP1 and SFRP2 genes was 37.5% (15 out of 40 patients) and 12.5% (5 out of 40 patients), respectively (Figure 2). Hypermethylation of SFRP1,2 was found in all FAB classifications of AML, except for M6. Hypermethylation of SFRP1 (P=0.021) gene was found significantly in subtype M0 (Table 3). No significant relationship was found between hypermethylation of SFRP1,2 and clinical data of patients including age, sex, laboratory data including Hb level , white blood cells and platelets count (Table 3). In addition, there was no effect of the SFRP metylation patterns on CR, relapse or death.

Among the 15 patients with hypermethylated SFRP1 there were 5 patients with favorable risk cytogenetics, 8 patients with intermediate risk cytogenetics (5 of 8 patients with normal karyotype P=0.01 and 3 of 8 patients had flt3/ITD mutation P=0.44) (P=0.025), and 2 patients with adverse risk cytogenetics. However, there was no significant relationship between hypermethylated SFRP2 and risk cytogenetics (Table 3). However, we found that there was a significant relationship between methylated SFRP1 and flt3/ITD mutation in AML patients

Primer	Sequence	Annealing temperature	Product size (bp)
SFRP-1 MF	TGTAGTTTTCGGAGTTAGT GTCGCGC	65	126
SFRP-1 MR	CCTACGATCGAAAACGACG CGAACG		
SFRP-1 UF	GTTTTGTAGTTTTTGGAGT TAGTGTTGTGT	54	135
SFRP-1 UR	CTCAACCTACAATCAAAAA CAACACAAACA		
SFRP-2 MF	GGGTCGGAGTTTTTCGGAG TTGCGC	62	138
SFRP-2 MR	CCGCTCTCTTCGCTAAATA CGACTCG		
SFRP-2 UF	TTTTGGGTTGGAGTTTTTT GGAGTTGTGT	64	145
SFRP-2 UR	AACCCACTCTCTTCACTAA ATACAACTCA		

MF: Methylated Forward, MR: Methylated Reverse, UF: Unmethylated Forward, UR: Unmethylated Reverse

Table 1: SFRP-1 and SFRP-2 gene primers sequences, annealing temperature and product size for MSP Assays.

Parameters	AML patients	Control group	P
Number of patients (%)	40	25	
Age(years),(Mean ± SD)	35.3 ± 11.55	36.1 ± 11.3	0.643
Sex (%)			
Male	29 (72.5%)	17 (68%)	
Female	17(68%)	8 (32%)	0.589
Rural/Urban (%)	16(40)/24(60)	9(36)/16(64)	0.732

Table 2: Demographic characteristics of AML patients and control group.

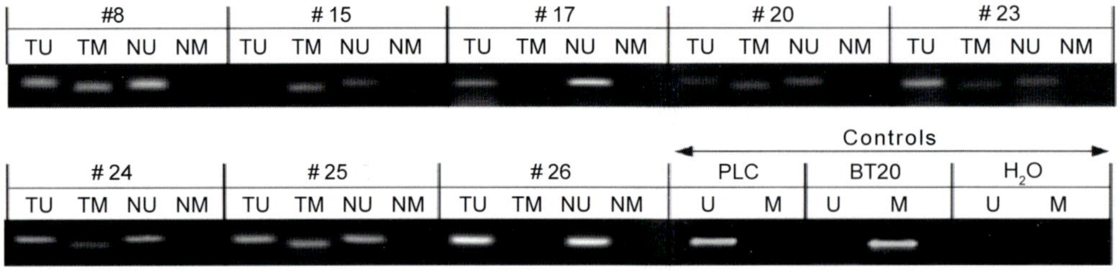

Figure 1: Methylation analysis of SFRP1 AML patients. SFRP1 Methylation-specific PCR (MSP) was performed on bisulphite-treated DNA from AML (T) and matching normal subjects (N). MSP results from eight representative patients are shown. DNA bands in lanes labelled with U indicate PCR products amplified with primers recognising the unmethylated promoter sequence. DNA bands in lanes labelled with M represent amplified products with methylation-specific primers. Human placenta (PL) and *in vitro* methylated DNA (IVD) served as positive controls for the U and M reaction, respectively. Water was used as template in the negative control (NTC). Patient number 15: methylated SFRP1, Patients number 8,20,23,24,25: hemimethylated SFRP1, Patients number 17,26: unmethylated SFRP1.

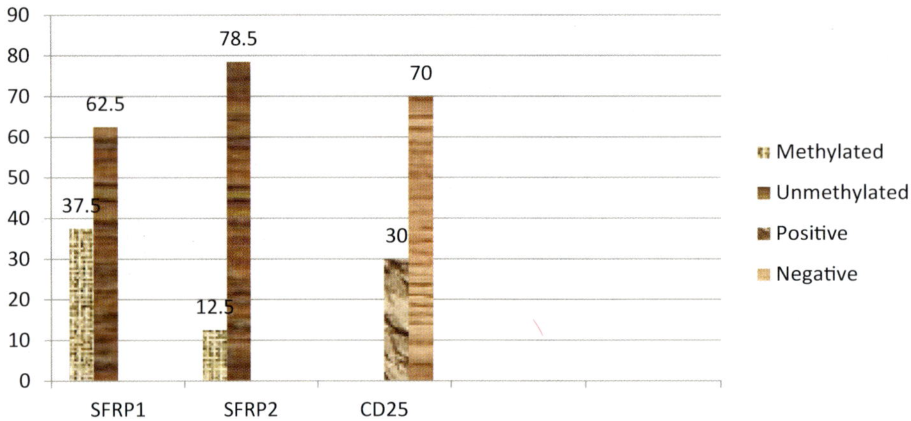

Figure 2: Frequency of promoter methylation of SFRPs and CD25 expression in 40 patients with AML.

Parameters	SFRP1			SFRP2		
	M	U	P	M	U	P
Number of patients (%)	15(37.5)	25(62.5)		5(12.5)	35(87.5)	
Age(years), (Mean ± SD)	34.5 ± 11.8	36 ± 11.3	0.411	33.8 ± 13	35 ± 11.9	0.565
Sex (%)						
Male	12(30)	17(42.5)	0.532	10(25)	19(47.5)	0.443
Female	2(5)	9(22.5)	0.435	1(2.5)	10(25)	0.307
WBCs (Mean ± SD)10^3/µl	145.3 ± 113.3	136.9 ±109	0.526	143 ± 110	150 ± 114	0.639
Hb level (Mean ± SD) g/dl	7.1 ± 1.4	8 ± 1.6	0.732	8.3 ± 1.1	8.7 ± 1.6	0.892
Platelet (Mean ± SD) 10^3/µl	45.8 ± 15.6	47.3 ± 14.6	0.699	46.7 ± 13	48.2 ± 14	0.807
FAB, n (%)						
M0	3(20.0)	0	0.021	0	1(2.8)	0.438
M1	2(13.3)	5(20)	0.657	1(20)	8(22.8)	0.876
M2	4(26.6)	6(24)	0.854	1(20)	7(20)	0.984
M3	1(6.6)	2(8)	0.865	0	6(17.1)	0.054
M4	3(20)	5(20)	0.986	1(20)	8(22.8)	0.876
M5	2(13.3)	4(16)	0.812	1(20)	3(8.6)	0.564
M6	0	2(8)	0.557	0	1(2.8)	0.438
M7	0	1(5.5)	0.732	1(20)	0	0.021
Flt3/ITD, n(%)	3(20)	1(4)	0.042	2(40)	7(22)	0.233
Karyotype, n						
Favourable	5(33.3)	14(56)	0.343	2(40)	17(48.6)	0.877
Intermediate, (normal karyotype)	8(53.3), 5(33.3)	4(16), 1(4)	0.025, 0.01	1(20), 1(20)	11(31.4), 5(14.2)	0.673
Adverse	2(13.3)	7(28)	0.310	2(40)	7(20.0)	0.562
Outcome, n (%)						
CR	4(26.7)	11(44)	0.531	1(20)	14(40)	0.356
Death	7(46.7)	8(32)	0.642	2(40)	12(34.3	0.761
Death	4(26.7)	6(24)	0.858	2(40)	9(25.7)	0.603

Table 3: Clinical and laboratory characteristics in AML patients in relation to methylation profile of sFRP.

(20% of methylated SFRP1 patients had flt3/ITD compared to 4% of unmethylated SFRP1 patients) (Figure 3).

The patients 60 years and younger with intermediate risk cytogenetics, Multivariate analysis indicated that the methylation status was independent adverse prognostic factor for relapse (P=0.024).

Monoclonal antibodies against CD25(IL2Rα) was positive (cutoff of positivity is >20%) in 12 patients (30%). 9(60%) of hypermethylated SFPR1 patients were positive for CD25 and only one Hypermethylated SFPR2 was positive for CD25. There was significant relationship between high expression of CD25 and hypermethylation of SFRP1 (P=0.023). There was significant relationship between Hypermethylated SFPR1 gene and increased expression of Cyto MPO (P=0.046) and CD117 (P=0.044) (Table 4). With regards to CD25, we analyzed the relationships between the level of CD25 expression and clinical (age, gender), laboratory (WBCs, Hb and platelets at diagnosis), FAB classification, cytogenetic risk groups, flt3/ITD and the outcome in patients with de novo AML. Regarding the clinical data there was no significant relationship with high expression CD25, there was 6 patients with overexpressed CD25 had flt3/ITD mutation. With regards to FAB classification and cytogenetic risk groups, there was significant relationship between high expression CD25 and M1 AML patients (P=0.043) and intermediate risk cytogenetics (P=0.026). Furthermore, significant relationship (P=0.022) was found between Relapse and high expression of CD25 (Table 5).

In multivariate analysis hypermethylated SFRP1 with intermediate risk cytogenetics were predictors for relapse in patients showed high expression of CD25 and flt3/ITD mutation (Table 6), the results given as odds ratio {95% Confidence interval}: 2.53{1.38-5.89}P=0.031, 3.1{1.81-6.1}P=0.028 respectively. Furthermore, hypermethylated SFRP1 with intermediate risk cytogenetics were predictors for relapse in patients with increased WBCs (leukocytosis>20 $10^3/\mu l$) 2.1{0.89-4.9} P=0.041.

Discussion

Hypermethylation of tumor suppressor genes is a common epigenetic event in cancers [19]. In our study, we analyzed the methylation profile of SFRP 1 ,2 genes promoters in 40 de novo AML patients and its correlation with karyotying, immunophenotypic features of blast cells, complete remission and relapse in addition to CD25 (IL2αR) expression. As over expression of CD25 was listed before as a standard poor prognostic factor in AML, so we studied the correlation between it and hypermethylated SFRP1,2 in AML patients. In this study we stated that hypermethylation of SFRP1,2 genes occurs with a percentage of 37.5% (15 out of 40 patients) and 12.5% (five out of 40 patients) in de novo AML patients, respectively. While none of the control samples showed hypermethylation. Veeck et al. stated that hypermethylation of SFRP-1 associated with poor prognosis in breast cancer patients [20,21]. SFRP gene promoter hypermethylation has been demonstrated in different hematopoietic malignancies like acute lymphoblastic leukemia (ALL) and Multiple myeloma (MM). Cooper et al. demonstrated that recombinant SFRP1 may be a

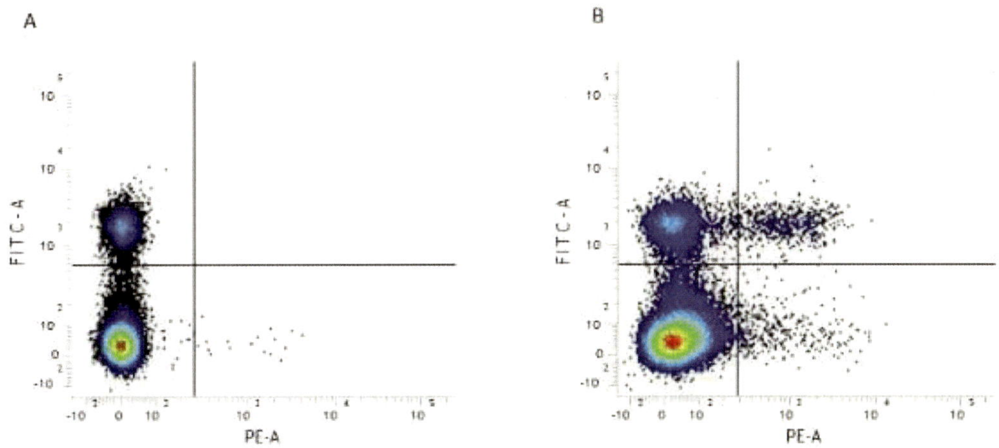

Figure 3: Double immunostaining of leukemia cells using anti-IL-2Rα and anti-CD33 antibodies in a representative patient with AML. The horizontal axis indicates the logarithmic scale of PE- conjugated anti-CD33 binding, and the vertical axis FITC-conjugated anti- IL-2Rα (CD25)binding. A- negative case. B- positive case (cut off of positivity is >20%).

Parameters	SFRP1				SFRP2	
	M	U	P	M	U	P
Number of patients,%	15(37.5)	25(62.5)	5(12.5)		35(87.5)	35(87.5)
Antigens						
HLA DR	11(73.3)	20(80)	0.945	4(80)	32(91.4)	0.872
CD13	12(80)	23(92)	0.864	4(80)	35(100)	0.648
CD33	15(100)	24(96)	0.921	5(100)	31(88.5)	0.611
CD14	5(33.3)	6(24)	0.873	1(20)	5(14.2)	0.754
CD41	1(6.6)	1(4)	0.932	1(20)	2(5.7)	0.081
Cyto MPO	10(66.6)	7(28)	0.046	2(40)	15(42.8)	0.952
CD117	8(53.3)	6(24)	0.44	3(60)	13(37.1)	0.76
CD11c	4(26.6)	8(32)	0.84	2(40)	11(31.4)	0.625

Table 4: Immunophenotyping characteristics of AML patients in relation to methylation profile of sFRP.

Parameters	Positive CD25	Negative CD25	P
Number of patients (%)	12(30)	28(70)	
Age(years), (Mean ± SD)	32.1 ± 12	34.6 ± 12.1	0.839
Sex, %			
Male	8(66.6)	18(64.3)	0.974
Female	5(33.3)	10(35.7)	0.878
WBCs (Mean ± SD) 103/µl	143.5 ± 115.2	144.8 ± 113	0.745
Hb level (Mean ± SD)g/dl	8.3 ± 1.5	8.4 ± 1.4	0.834
Platelet (Mean ± SD) 103/µl	46.3 ± 14.7	48.2 ± 13.8	0.73
FAB, n (%)			
M0	2(16.6)	1(3.6)	0.671
M1	5(41.6)	2(7.1)	0.043
M2	1(8.3)	6(21.4)	0.783
M3	1(8.3)	8(28.5)	0.531
M4	1(8.3)	8(28.5)	0.531
M5	1(8.3)	2(7.1)	0.911
M6	1(8.3)	1(3.6)	0.832
M7	0(0)	0(0)	0.993
Methylated SFRP1	9(60%)	6(30%)	0.023
Karyotype, n			
Favorable	4(33.3)	15(53.6)	0.064
Intermediate (normal karyotype)	6(50) , 4(33.3)	6(21.4) , 2(7.1)	0.026 , 0.01
Adverse	2(16.7)	7(25)	0.837
Flt3/ITD	6(50)	9(36)	0.083
Outcome, n(%)			
CR	4(33.3)	15(53.6)	0.068
Relapse	6(50)	6(21.4)	0.022
Death	2(16.6)	7(25)	0.713

Table 5: Clinical and laboratory characteristics in AML patients in relation to CD25 expression.

Parameters	Relapse			Death		
	*Selected patient					
	Odds Ratio	95% CI	P	Odds Ratio	95%CI	P
Age	0.84	0.35-1.9	0.748	0.34	0.04-1.56	0.332
Positive CD25	2.53	1.38-5.8	0.031	1.06	0.46-2.48	0.713
WBCs	2.1	0.89-4.9	0.041	0.97	0.44-2.13	0.933
Flt3/ITD	3.1	1.81-6.1	0.028	0.83	0.38-1.9	0.811

Table 6: Multivariate analysis for relapse and death in patients with hypermethylated SFRP1 and intermediate cytogenetics risk.

therapeutic policy for patients with suppressed SFRP1 expression [22]. Follow up of hypermethylation status of SFRP genes may help in risk stratification and relapse prediction [23] and as epigenetic changes are pharmacologically reversible, so the demethylating factors may help in reactivation of SFRP1,2 function in patients with hypermethylation induced inhibition of those genes. And so SFRPs could used as biomarkers in monitoring the *in vivo* effects of demethylating factors [24,25].

Because of the 40 patients studied, 7 patients (17.5%) for SFRP1 gene and 6 patients (15%) for SFRP2 gene had one methylated allele, hemi-methylated patients may develop with time and it is an important poor prognostic factor. Hypermethylation of SFRP genes has been found in hematologic malignancies, as Pehlivan et al. stated that hypermethylated SFRP1 can lead to drug resistance in chronic myeloid leukemia(CML) patients treated with imatinib mesylate by inhibition of imatinib mesylate effect on BCR-ABL signaling pathway [26]. Wang found that hypermethylation of SPRP genes in myelodysblastic syndrome (MDS) patients is accompanied with bad prognosis and low survival rate [8]. In this study, we did not found any significant association between hypermethylation of SFRP genes and other prognostic parameters in AML, like WBC count and age. Also no significant relationship was found between hypermethylation of these genes and other parameters like hemoglobin, platelets count and sex. Our results showed that hypermethylation of SFRP genes occurs in all FAB subgroups involving M0, M1,M2, M3, M4 and M5, except M6 and M7. While the highest percentage of hypermethylation of SFRP-1 (P=0.021) was shown in M0 subgroup. Hou et al. observed that FAB M0 subtype patients had the highest percentage of hypermethylation of SFRPs genes, whereas patients with M4, M5 subtype had the lowest percentage [27]. Recently, it has been demonstrated that in AML patients with flt3/ITD mutation are associated with aberrations in Wnt signaling pathway and so we found that there was a significant relationship between patients with hypermethylated SFRP1 and flt3/ITD mutation (P=0.042). In the present study, the high percentage of hypermethylated SFRP1 gene (P=0.025) was found in patients with intermediate risk karyotyping. However, no significant association was found between hypermethylation of SFRPs and complete remission or death after induction therapy.

We also observed that hypermethylation of SFRPs has a poor prognostic factor in 60 years and younger patients with intermediate risk karyotyping. AML is a heterogeneous disease with divergent clinical characteristics, of which karyotyping is the most important prognostic factor. Unfortunately, the intermediate risk group includes a different group of patients either of normal karyotypes or with a variety of other mutations whose prognostic impact is uncertain. Therefore, better discovery of other prognostic factors in this group has been of specific interest in the recent years.

CD25+ CD34+ leukemic cells have been found to be chemotherapy resistant and initiate AML in xenograft models, suggesting a leukemic stem cells (LSC) biology [28]. IL2 increases survival, proliferation and chemotherapy resistance in CD25+ chronic lymphocytic leukemia (CLL) *in vitro* [29]. Regarding the results of CD25 expression in our results, twelve (30%) AML patients were CD25 positive. When comparing CD25+ and CD25- patients, there was a significant relationship between positive CD25 AML patients and intermediate risk karyotype(P=0.026). Moreover, expression of CD25 at diagnosis was a predictor of relapse 6 (50%) CD25+ patients have relapse compared with 6(21.4%) CD25- patients (P=0.022). Jan Cerny, 2013 stated that over expression of CD25 was a strong predictor of induction failure and relapse. Terwijn l 2009 reported that over CD25 expression (>10%) in young AML patients (<60 years) in retrospective study associated with a significant shorter survival and relapse free survival [30].

Our results found that the methylation status of SFRP1 together with CD25+ is a poor prognostic impact in the subgroup of 60 years and younger patients with intermediate risk karyotyping (also only normal karyotyping). And the combination of both markers (hypermethylated SFRP1 and CD25 over expression) together in the same patient may play a stronger role in the poor prognosis for relapse (P=0.031).

References

1. Dohner H, Weisdorf DJ, Bloomfield CD (2015) Acute Myeloid Leukemia. NEJM 373: 1136-1152.

2. Galm O, Herman JG, Baylin SB (2006) The fundamental role of epigenetics in hematopoietic malignancies. Blood Reviews 20: 1-13.

3. Klaus A, Birchmeier W (2008) Wnt signalling and its impact on development and cancer. Nat Rev Cancer 8: 387-398.

4. Huang J, Zhang YL, Teng XM (2007) Down-regulation of SFRP1 as a putative tumor suppressor gene can contribute to human hepato- cellular carcinoma. BMC Cancer 7: 126.

5. Kirstetter P, Anderson K, Porse BT (2006). Activation of the canonical Wnt pathway leads to loss of hematopoietic stem cell repopulation and multilineage differentia- tion block. Nature Immunology 7: 1048-1056.

6. Clevers H (2004) Wnt breakers in colon cancer. Cancer Cell 5: 5-6.

7. Wang H, Fan R, Wang XQ (2013) Methylation of Wnt antagonist genes: a useful prognostic marker for myelodysplastic syndrome. Ann Hematol 92: 199-209.

8. Malbon CC, Frizzleds (2004) new members of the superfamily of G-protein-coupled receptors. Frontiers in Bioscience 9: 1048-1058.

9. Nelson WJ, Nusse R (2004) Convergence of Wnt, beta-catenin, and cadherin pathways. Science 303: 1483-1487.

10. Veeck J, Bektas N, Hartmann A, Kristiansen G, Heindrichs U, et al. (2008) Wnt signalling in human breast cancer: expression of the putative Wnt inhibitor Dickkopf-3 (DKK3) is frequently suppressed by promoter hypermethylation in mammary tumours. Breast Cancer Res 10: R82.

11. Reya T, Duncan AW, Ailles L (2003) A role for Wnt signalling in self-renewal of haematopoietic stem cells. Nature 423: 409-414.

12. Bovolenta P, Esteve P, Ruiz JM (2008) Beyond Wnt inhibition: new functions of secreted Frizzled-related proteins in development and disease. Journal of cell science 121: 737-46.

13. Simon M, Grandage VL, Linch DC, Khwaja A (2005) Constitutive activation of the Wnt/beta-catenin signaling pathway in acute myeloid leukaemia. Oncogene 24: 2410-2420.

14. Jan C, Hongbo Y, Muthalagu R (2013) Expressionof CD25 independently predicts early treatment failure of acute myeloid leukemia (AML) BJH 160: 255-272.

15. Shaffer LG, Tommerup N (2005) ISCN Guidelines for Cancer Cytogenetics. Supplement to: An International System for Human Cytogenetic Nomenclature Karger: Basel.

16. Rombouts WJ, Blokland I, Lowenberg B, Ploemacher RE (2000) Biological characteristics and prognosis of adult acute myeloid leukemia with internal tandem duplications in the Flt3gene. Leukemia 14: 675-683.

17. Wang H, Fan R, Wang XQ (2013) Methylation of Wnt antagonist genes: a useful prognostic marker for myelodysplastic syndrome. Ann Hematol 92: 199-209.

18. Dohner H, Estey EH, Amadori S, Appelbaum FR, Buchner T, et al. (2010) Diagnosis andmanagement of acute myeloid leukemia in adults: recommenda- tions from an international expert panel, on behalf of the European Leukemia Net. Blood 115: 453-474.

19. Nakamoto D, Yamamoto N, Takagi R (2008) Detection of microsatellite al- terations in plasma DNA of malignant mucosal melano- ma using whole genome amplification. Bull Tokyo Dent Coll 49: 77-87.

20. Veeck J, Bektas N, Hartmann A (2008) Wnt signalling in human breast cancer: expression of the putative Wnt inhibitor Dickkopf-3 (DKK3) is frequently suppressed by pro- moter hypermethylation in mammary tumours. Breast Cancer Res 10: R82.

21. Veeck J, Geisler C, Noetzel E (2008) Epigenetic inactivation of the secreted frizzled-related protein-5 (SFRP5) gene in human breast cancer is associated with unfavorable prognosis. Carcinogenesis 29: 991-998.

22. Cooper SJ, Von Roemeling CA, Kang KH (2012) Reexpression of tumor suppressor, sFRP1, leads to antitumor syn- ergy of combined HDAC and methyltransferase in- hibitors in chemoresistant cancers. Mol Cancer Ther 11: 2105-2115.

23. Agrawal S, Unterberg M, Koschmieder S (2007) DNA methylation of tumor suppressor genes in clinical remission predicts the relapse risk in acute myeloid leuke- mia. Cancer Research 67: 1370-1377.

24. Gore SD, Baylin S, Sugar E (2006) Combined DNA methyltransferase and histone deacetylase inhibition in the treatment of myeloid neoplasms. Cancer Research 66: 6361-6369.

25. Yang AS, Doshi KD, Choi SW (2006) DNA methyl- ation changes after 5-aza-2¢-deoxycytidine therapy in patients with leukemia. Cancer Research 66: 5495-5503.

26. Pehlivan M, Sercan Z, Sercan HO (2009) sFRP1 promoter methylation is associated with persistent Philadelphia chromosome in chronic myeloid leukemia. Leuk Res 33: 1062-1067.

27. Hou HA, Kuo YY, Liu CY (2011) Distinct association between ab- errant methylation of Wnt inhibitors and genetic al- terations in acute myeloid leukaemia. Br J Cancer 105: 1927-1933.

28. Saito Y, Kitamura H, Hijikata A (2010) Identification of therapeu- tic targets for quiescent, chemotherapy-resistant human leukemia stem cells. Science translational medicine 2: 17ra9.

29. Decker T, Bogner C, Oelsner M (2010) Antiapoptotic effect of interleukin-2 (IL-2) in B-CLL cells with low and high affinity IL-2 receptors. Annals of hematology 89: 1125-1132.

30. Terwijn M, Feller N, Van Rhenen A (2009) Interleukin-2 receptor alpha-chain (CD25) expression on leukaemic blasts is predictive for outcome and level of residual disease in AML. European Journal of Cancer 45: 1692-1699.

A Rare Presentation of Cutaneous Pseudolymphoma as a Preleukaemic State

Muthu Sivaramakrishnan[1]*, Ronald Kerr[2], Alan Evans[3] and Andrew Affleck[1]
[1]*Department of Dermatology, Ninewells Hospital and Medical School, Dundee, UK*
[2]*Department of Haematology, Ninewells Hospital and Medical School, Dundee, UK*
[3]*Department of Histopathology, Ninewells Hospital and Medical School, Dundee, UK*

Abstract

A patient presented with progressive and unresponsive erythematous rash affecting his trunk and limbs over a period of 5 years. His systemic examination and extensive relevant investigations were normal throughout this period. Skin biopsies at different times showed features of annular erythema, cutaneous pseudolymphoma and sub-acute dermatitis. Five years after the initial presentation, he developed erythroderma, leonine facies, lymphadenopathy and peripheral lymphocytosis. CT chest and abdomen revealed generalised lymphadenopathy. Skin biopsy and immunophenotyping was suggestive of Sezary syndrome. However, peripheral blood smear examination was highly suggestive of T-cell prolymphocytic leukaemia (TPLL). Subsequent molecular genetic analysis was consistent with TPLL. To the best of our knowledge, there are no reports of cutaneous pseudolymphoma transforming to TPLL in the literature. The long indolent course of apparently benign skin disease before transforming into TPLL appears to be unique in our case. An analogy can be made with cutaneous T-Cell lymphoma both in terms of the difficulty in proving the diagnosis-needing multiple skin biopsies, and in the possible link between cutaneous and systemic disease. TPLL should be considered as a rare cause of erythroderma, which may clinically and histologically mimic Sezary syndrome.

Keywords: Erythroderma; Cutaneous; Lymphocytosis

Introduction

Erythroderma is defined as erythema and scaling affecting more than 90% of the body surface. The commonest cause of erythroderma was due to pre-existing inflammatory skin disease with an incidence between 27-68% in various case series [1]. Malignancies were the least common cause of erythroderma in these series, with cutaneous T-cell lymphoma (CTCL) as the most frequent malignant cause of erythroderma with a median incidence of 3% (range, 0-18%) [1]. Such patients with a malignant cause of erythroderma may have non-specific histological features for many years before the actual diagnosis can be established. Cutaneous pseudo-lymphomas are considered as a heterogenous group of benign T-cell or B-cell lympho proliferative process and have many potential causes [2]. There are reports that suggest pseudo lymphomas can progress into overt lymphoma in some patients [3,4]. However it is unclear if these patients were misdiagnosed at the initial stage or developed lymphoma due to persistent antigenic stimulation [5].

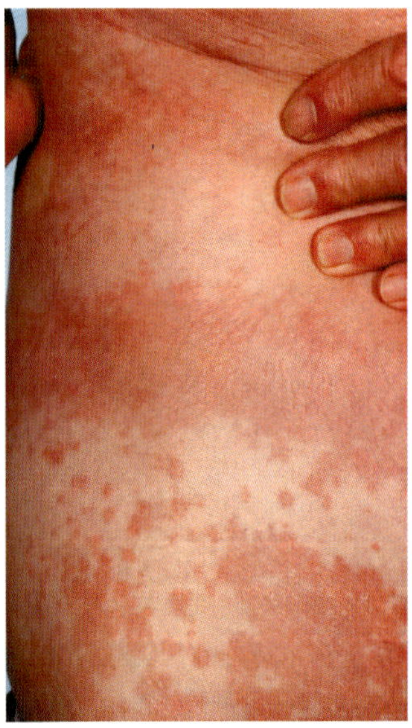

Figure 1: Initial presentation of erythematous patches on the trunk.

Case Report

A 75-year-old male presented with a one year history of a persistent erythematous eruption affecting his trunk and limbs (Figure 1). Systemic examination was normal. An initial diagnosis of a drug eruption to quinine was made; stopping this drug and using super potent topical steroid produced moderate improvement. Over the next 4 years, he developed scaly erythematous papules and plaques affecting his trunk and limbs (Figures 2a and 2b). His disease was gradually progressive becoming more extensive in distribution and persistent despite treatment. Systemic examination, full blood count, peripheral blood film examination, renal and liver functions were normal throughout this period.

Two skin biopsies performed at various stages of presentation during this time showed features of annular erythema and sub-acute

***Corresponding author:** Muthu Sivaramakrishnan, Specialist Registrar, Department of Dermatology, Ninewells Hospital and Medical School, Dundee, DD19SY, UK, E-mail: muthusivaramakrishnan@nhs.net

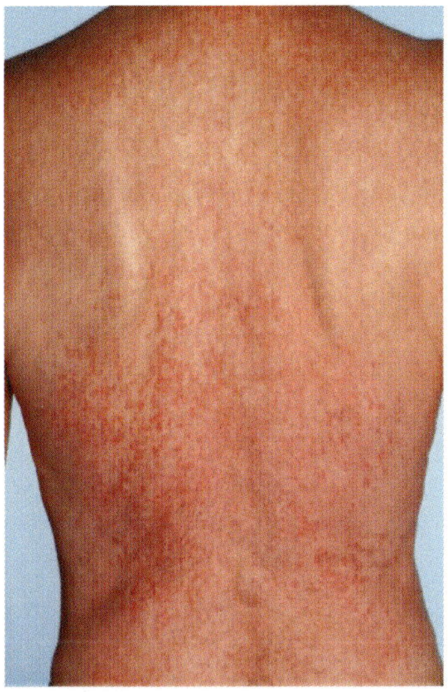

Figure 2a: Progressive skin disease -erythematous papules on the trunk.

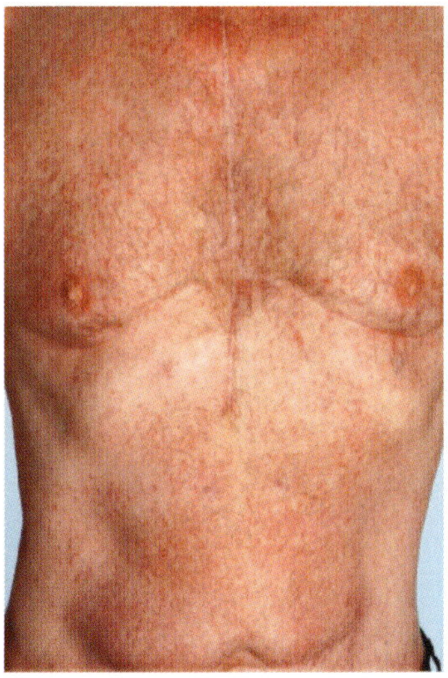

Figure 2b: Progressive skin disease -erythematous papules on the trunk.

dermatitis. A third biopsy showed patchy upper dermal infiltrate composed of lymphoid cells. Most of the lymphocytes were small although showed some degree of nuclear irregularity. In addition, there were a significant number of cells with a blast morphology showing considerable nuclear atypia. Only a small number of lymphocytes extended into the overlying epidermis with some spongiotic reaction noted. Abroad range of immunohistochemical stains showed that the bulk of cells are of T-lineage but a modest population of cells marking as B-cell lineage. The blast cell population were a mixture of T and B cell lineage. Molecular genetic analysis failed to show clonal re-arrangement of T-cell receptor gene. The immunoglobulin gene re-arrangement tests failed. Hence the conclusion at that stage was a reactive pseudo lymphomatous process. He partially improved with narrow band UVB and oral PUVA phototherapy.

Five years after the initial presentation, he developed leonine-like facial swelling and erythroderma (Figures 3a and 3b). Systemic examination showed palpable axillary and inguinal lymphadenopathy. Full blood count demonstrated a marked peripheral lymphocytosis. CT scan showed hepato splenomegaly and generalised lymphadenopathy.

Skin biopsy showed atypical lymphocytes with many cerebriform nuclei in a band like infiltrate in the upper and mid dermis (Figures 4a and 4b), epidermotropism (Figure 4c) and with an immunophenotype pattern of strong staining to CD3 and CD4 but down regulation of other T-cell markers. The clinical picture, laboratory imaging and dermatopathological findings raised a possible diagnosis of Sezary syndrome (SS).

However, peripheral blood smear examination showed large atypical lymphocytes with plentiful cytoplasm and expressing CD2, CD3, CD4, CD5 and CD7 markers, typical of T-cell prolymphocytic leukaemia (TPLL). Subsequent cytogenetic analysis demonstrated a complex karyotype including inversion of the long arm of chromosome 14, consistent with TPLL. Management with dexamethasone produced only moderate and short term response. Subsequent management with

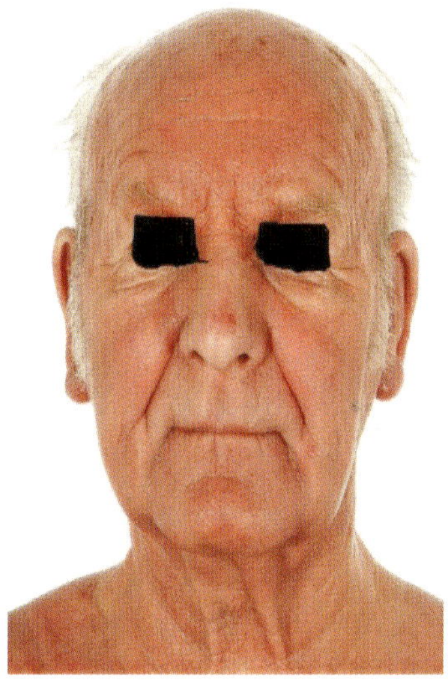

Figure 3a: Leonine facial appearance and erythroderma.

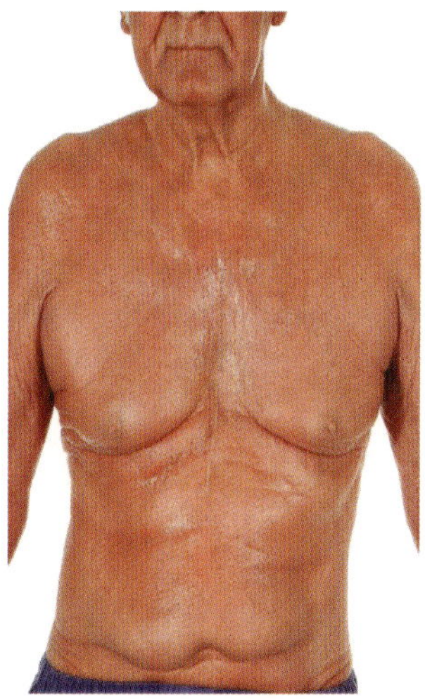

Figure 3b: Leonine facial appearance and erythroderma.

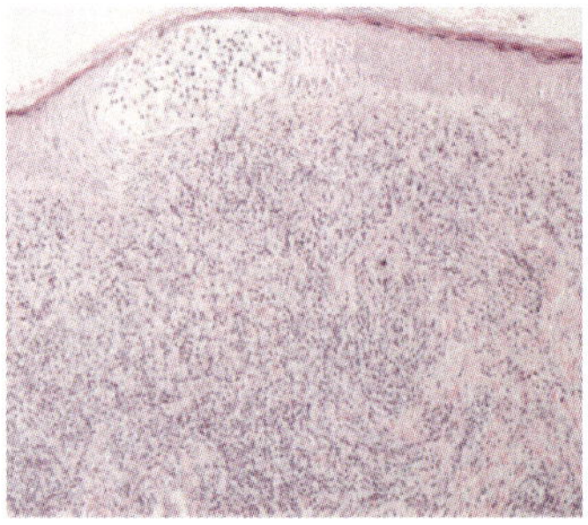

Figure 4a: H&E X40 Band like lymphoid infiltrate in the upper and mid dermis.

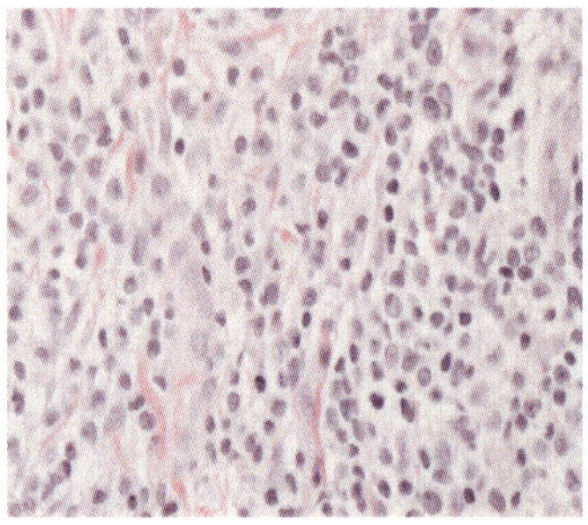

Figure 4b: H&E X40 Band like lymphoid infiltrate in the upper and mid dermis.

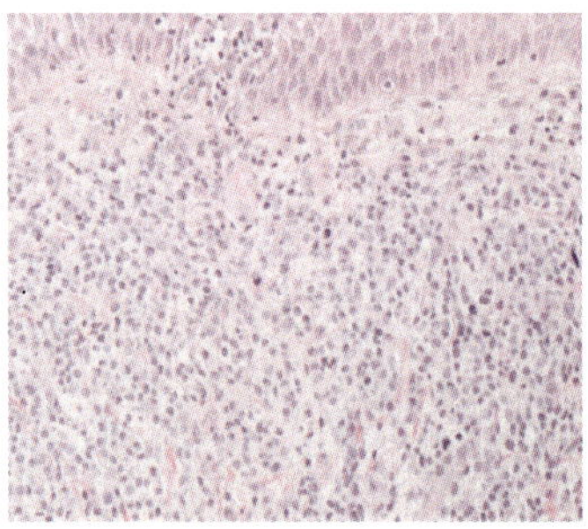

Figure 4c: H&E X100 Epidermotropism.

CAMPATH (alemtuzumab-CD52 monoclonal antibody) produced excellent response initially but the treatment course was not completed due to severe pancytopenia. The disease relapsed and was progressive from that stage leading to death.

Discussion

TPLL is a rare aggressive mature T-cell leukaemia. It accounted for 37.5% of cases in a series of 175 adult patients with mature T-cell malignancies [6]. The characteristic clinical features of TPLL include splenomegaly, lymphadenopathy, skin disease and a high leukocyte count. The cutaneous features occurred in 25-28% of cases of TPLL in various case series [7,8]. Skin disease has been reported at the time of initial diagnosis or later, heralding aggressive clinical course in such cases. The various cutaneous manifestations include facial swelling with erythema, alopecia, symmetrical petechial rash in the periorbital area, nodules and erythroderma [7,9]. Cutaneous histological features include grenz zone, dermal peri-vascular and peri-appendegeal infiltrate composed of medium-sized lymphoid cells with prominent nucleoli, similar to peripheral blood smear examination. Peripheral blood smear examination shows characteristic tumour cells with a prominent nucleolus and deep basophilic cytoplasm but the nuclear contours and prevalence of distinctive central nucleoli are quite variable [10]. The immunophenotype profile is usually positive for CD3, CD2, CD4, CD5, CD7, CD45, and CD45RO. Other markers of immaturity such as CD34, CD1a and terminal deoxynucleotiyl transferase are absent. Expression of T-cell leukaemia (TCL)-1 oncoprotein can be reasonably specific for TPLL [10]. The most distinctive cytogenetic abnormality in TPLL is inversion of the long arm of chromosome 14 [10].

To the best of our knowledge, there are no previous reports of cutaneous pseudolymphoma transforming to TPLL. The long indolent course of apparently benign skin disease before the final diagnosis of TPLL appears to be unique in our case. However, the disease was rapidly progressive from that stage of transformation. In our case, the cutaneous histology was not diagnostic and was suggestive of SS. Peripheral blood smear examination and immune phenotyping was the key in making the diagnosis in our case.

It is impossible to completely prove a link between his pre-existing long term skin condition which we have classified as pseudo-lymphoma and his subsequent development of TPLL. This could only be proved if we had a clonal marker in the initial skin biopsy that was demonstrated to evolve when he developed TPLL. Despite looking for this we could not detect an initial clonal marker in the initial biopsy and if we had, we would not have classified it as pseudo-lymphoma. The characteristics of his skin rash and T-cell phenotype suggest it is likely that the two conditions are linked.

TPLL is an aggressive disease with a median survival of 7 months with conventional treatment [11]. The advent of monoclonal antibodies has improved treatment options in this condition. Alemtuzumab is a humanised IgG1 antibody that targets the CD52 antigen highly expressed on normal, malignant T- and B-lymphocytes and on monocytes but not on haematopoietic stem cells [12]. The mechanism of action is not fully understood but it can cause antibody-dependent cellular cytotoxicity, complement activation and direct apoptosis [12]. A study of 39 patients treated with intravenous alemtuzumab 30 mg 3 times weekly until a maximum response showed complete remission (CR) in 60% of patients, partial remission (PR) in 16% of patients and a median disease free interval of 7 months after the treatment [11]. Further follow-up of this series of patients showed that the median survival was 2 years for patients achieving a CR and 9 months for those in PR [11].

Patients with asymptomatic lymphocytosis who are relatively stable or slowly progressive can be monitored. The first line treatment for rapidly progressive disease is intravenous alemtuzumab which is also effective for the skin disease. Pentostatin (purine analogues) can be considered along with alemtuzumab for patients showing slow response to alemtuzumab on its own. In spite of satisfactory response with alemtuzumab, patients tend to relapse with T-PLL. Autologous and allogenic hematopoietic stem cell transplantation has been found to be useful in such patients [11].

The differential diagnoses of erythroderma due to TPLL include SS, erythrodermic mycosis fungoides (MF) and adult T-cell leukemia-lymphoma (ATLL).SS is characterised by erythroderma, peripheral lymphadenopathy and atypical circulating lymphocytes called as Sezary cells or Lutzner cells [13]. Sezary cells exhibit distinctive cerebriorm nuclear outlines best detected on high magnification [10]. SS can present primarily as erythroderma without pre-existing skin disease or can develop secondarily in patients with mycosis fungoides. The diagnostic criteria for this syndrome are that the circulating monoclonal lymphocyte population should be identified by molecular or cytogenetic methods and there should be an identity between the circulating T-lymphocyte clone and the clone present in the skin, in addition to one of the following: atleast 1,000 Sezary cells per mm3 of peripheral blood, an increased population of CD4+/CD7- in peripheral blood with remarkable predominance of CD4 cells in relation to CD8 cells (CD4/CD8 ratio>10), Sezary cells with a diameter >14 μm representing >20% of the circulating lymphocytes and, aberrant expression of pan T-cell antigens [13]. Patients with MF can sometimes progress to erythroderma without blood findings of SS called as erythrodermic MF [13].

ATLL can present as solitary or widespread papules, nodules, tumours or erythroderma. The clinical features in an acute form of ATLL include marked leucocytosis, lymphadenopathy, hepatoslpenomegaly, skin involvement and hypercalcemia [14]. Skin histology usually shows epidermotropic infiltrate of medium to large cells which have pleomorphic nuclear morphology [14]. The tumour cells in the peripheral blood have characteristic polylobulated nuclei called flower cells [10]. The immunophenotypic profile includes expression of CD2, CD3, CD4 and CD5. Weak expression or absence of CD7, absent CD8 and positive CD25 are features of ATLL [10]. Serologic confirmation of HTLV-1 infection will be present and monoclonal integration of HTLV-1 proviral genome can be demonstrated. No specific cytogenetic abnormalities are noted but most cases exhibit an abnormal karyotype [10].

Our case can be considered analogousto cutaneous T-cell lymphoma both in terms of the difficulty in proving the diagnosis - needing multiple skin biopsies, and possible link between cutaneous and systemic disease that occurred after a latent period. TPLL should be considered as a rare cause of erythroderma, which may clinically and histologically mimic Sezary syndrome.

References

1. Vonderheid EC (2006) On the diagnosis of erythrodermic cutaneous T-cell lymphoma. J Cutan Pathol 33 Suppl 1: 27-42.
2. Ploysangam T, Breneman DL, Mutasim DF (1998) Cutaneous pseudolymphomas. J Am Acad Dermatol 38: 877-895.
3. Nihal M, Mikkola D, Horvath N, Gilliam AC, Stevens SR, et al. (2003) Cutaneous lymphoid hyperplasia: a lymphoproliferative continuum with lymphomatous potential. Hum Pathol 34: 617-622.
4. Sangueza OP, Yadav S, White CR Jr, Braziel RM (1992) Evolution of B-cell lymphoma from pseudolymphoma. A multidisciplinary approach using histology, immunohistochemistry, and Southern blot analysis. Am J Dermatopathol 14: 408-413.
5. Bergman R (2010) Pseudolymphoma and cutaneous lymphoma: facts and controversies. Clin Dermatol 28: 568-574.
6. Matutes E, Catovsky D (1991) Mature T-cell leukemias and leukemia/lymphoma syndrome. Review of our experience in 175 cases. Leukemia Lymphoma 4: 81-91.
7. Mallett RB, Matutes E, Catovsky D, Maclennan K, Mortimer PS, et al. (1995) Cutaneous infiltration in T-cell prolymphocytic leukaemia. Br J Dermatol 132: 263-266.
8. Garand R, Goasguen J, Brizard A, Buisine J, Charpentier A, et al. (1998) Indolent course as a relatively frequent presentation in T-prolymphocytic leukaemia. Groupe Français d'Hématologie Cellulaire. Br J Haematol 103: 488-494.
9. Magro CM, Morrison CD, Heerema N, Porcu P, Sroa N, et al. (2006) T-cell prolymphocytic leukemia: an aggressive T cell malignancy with frequent cutaneous tropism. J Am Acad Dermatol 55: 467-477.
10. Foucar K (2007) Mature T-cell leukemias including T-prolymphocytic leukemia, adult T-cell leukemia/lymphoma, and Sézary syndrome. Am J Clin Pathol 127: 496-510.
11. Dearden C (2012) How I treat prolymphocytic leukemia. Blood 120: 538-551.
12. Gilleece MH, Dexter TM (1993) Effect of Campath-1H antibody on human hematopoietic progenitors in vitro. Blood 82: 807-812.
13. Yamashita T, Abbade LP, Marques ME, Marques SA (2012) Mycosis fungoides and Sézary syndrome: clinical, histopathological and immunohistochemical review and update. An Bras Dermatol 87: 817-828.
14. Burns T, Breathnach S, Cox N, Griffiths C (2010) Rook's Textbook of Dermatology: Wiley-Blackwell, Cutaneous Lymphomas and Lymphocytic Infiltrates.

Chronic Myeloid Leukemia Presenting with Priapism

Farhan S[1], Anjum F[1], Al-Qahtani FS[2] and Al-Anazi KA[3]*

[1]Senior Medical Residents, Section of Hematology, Department of Medicine, College of Medicine and King Khalid University Hospital, King Saud University, Riyadh, Saudi Arabia
[2]Assistant Professor and Consultant Hematopathologist, Division of Hematopathology, Department of Pathology, King Khalid University Hospital, King Saud University, Riyadh, Kingdom of Saudi Arabia
[3]Consultant Hemato-Oncologist, Section of Adult Hematology and Oncology, Department of Medicine, College of Medicine and King Khalid University Hospital, King Saud University, Riyadh, Saudi Arabia

Abstract

Chronic myeloid leukemia is a chronic myeloproliferative neoplasm that usually presents with an elevated white blood cell count and an enlarged spleen. Presentation with priapism is rather exceptional and is usually caused by leukostasis due to hyperleukocytosis. Priapism in chronic myeloid leukemia is a medical emergency that requires local therapies, symptomatic treatment as well as specific measures aimed at rapid control of the leukemia in the form of cytoreductive therapy, early initiation of targeted therapy with tyrosine kinase inhibitors in addition to leukapheresis in order to decrease the elevated leukocytic count as quickly as possible. A young patient with chronic myeloid leukemia who presented with priapism to King Khalid University Hospital in Riyadh is presented. The diagnostic work up and the lines of management are discussed.

Keywords: Chronic myeloid leukemia; Priapism; Hyperleukocytosis; Leukapheresis; Tyrosine kinase inhibitors.

Introduction

Priapism is a medical and surgical emergency that is characterized by prolonged and painful erection of the penis unassociated with any sexual arousal or desire. Approximately 50% of patients having priapism are at risk of impotence, despite appropriate therapy. If untreated, priapism may lead to penile necrosis and permanent erectile dysfunction [1-7]. Priapism can occur at any age. It has bimodal peak incidence with the first peak mainly occurring in children with Sickle Cell Disease (SCD) between 5 and 10 years of age and the second peak developing in sexually active adult males belonging to the age group 20 to 50 years. The incidence of priapism is 1.5 per 100,000 people. Priapism can either be idiopathic or secondary to several medical conditions (Table 1) [1-5,7]. Idiopathic priapism accounts for 64% of all cases of priapism. About 20% of cases of priapism are caused by hematological disorders [2,4,5]. In children, SCD accounts for 67% of cases while leukemia accounts for 15% of cases of priapism. The incidence of priapism in adult leukemia ranges between 1 and 5% [3-6]. In patients with leukemia, 50% of cases of priapism are due to Chronic Myeloid Leukemia (CML) and priapism is less common in patients with acute leukemia than in patients with chronic leukemia. Priapism can be classified into low flow type and high flow priapism (Table 2) [1,2,4,6].

Case Presentation

On 11/06/2013, a previously healthy 38 years Saudi male was referred from a local hospital to King Khalid University Hospital (KKUH) for treatment of painful erection of his penis that had lasted for 30 hours. There was no history of trauma, intake of new medications, exposure to radiation, fever or chills but the patient gave history of weight loss of 20 kg over 6 months in addition to dragging sensation in the abdomen and malaise. There was no history of bleeding from any site, dyspnea, headache, blurring of vision, convulsions or loss of consciousness. On arrival to the emergency room, his vital signs revealed pulse: 109/min, blood pressure: 136/72 mmHg, respiratory rate: 20/minute and temperature: 36.7°C. The physical examination revealed conjunctival pallor, but no: external palpable lymphadenopathy, jaundice, ecchymoses, skin rashes or leg edema. Abdominal examination showed no tenderness, impalpable liver and splenomegaly of 18 cm below the left costal margin. Examination of cardiovascular, respiratory and central nervous systems did not reveal any abnormality. The penis was erect, firm and tender with superficial venous engorgement. The testicles were bilaterally descended. Digital rectal examination revealed no enlargement or tenderness of the prostate. Complete Blood Count (CBC) showed white blood cell (WBC) count: 378×10^9/l, hemoglobin: 105 g/l, platelets: 155×10^9/l. Differential cell count revealed: 57% neutrophils, 15% metamyelocytes, 20% myelocytes, 2% promyelocytes and there were no blast cells on peripheral blood smear. Renal, hepatic and coagulation profiles were all normal. Uric acid was 429 μmol/l, lactic dehydrogenase was 688 u/l.

As the patient presented with priapism and before obtaining the results of CBC, he was initially seen by urologists. Because of the prolonged duration of priapism, treatment was initiated by performing cavernosal aspiration and irrigation. Unfortunately, there was incomplete relief of the erection by the procedure. Then the patient was admitted to KKUH initially under care of urologists. Later on-call hematologists were consulted to see the patient. After reviewing his clinical findings, laboratory investigations and making sure that CML was the most likely cause of his priapism, he was commenced on intravenous fluids, allopurinol and cytoreductive therapy with hydroxyurea 4 g/day. Also, leukapheresis was initiated and the patient received a total of three sessions of leukapheresis. Bone marrow biopsy was performed and it confirmed the diagnosis of CML (Figures 1-4).

***Corresponding author:** Dr. Khalid Ahmed Al-Anazi, Consultant Hemato-Oncologist, Section of Adult Hematology and Oncology, Department of Medicine, College of Medicine, King Khalid University Hospital, King Saud University, P.O. Box: 2925, Riyadh 11461, Saudi Arabia, E-mail: kaa_alanazi@yahoo.com

Idiopathic: no cause is found			
Secondary:			
	a- Trauma to perineum or genitalia		
	b- Infection or inflammation:		Prosatitis
			Mumps orchitis
	c- Malignancy:		Infiltration of penis by cancer
	c- Central nervous system mediated		
	d- Drug induced:		Alcohol ingestion
			Phenothiazines
			Intravenous fat for parenteral nutrition
			Heparin
	e- Thromboembolic diseases:		Systemic lupus erythromatosis
			Protein C deficiency
	f- Hemoglobinopathies:		Sickle cell disease
			Sickle cell trait
	g- Hyperleukocytosis:	* Acute leukemia:	acute lymphoblastic leukemia
			acute myeloid leukemia
		* Chronic leukemia:	chronic myeloid leukemia
			chronic lymphocytic leukemia
	h- Hyperviscosity states:		Polycythemia rubra vera
			Multiple myeloma
			Waldenström's macroglobulinemia
	i- Miscellaneous causes:		Hemodialysis
			Amyloidosis

Table 1: Shows causes of priapism.

Type of priapism	Low flow (ischemic, venous) priapism	High flow (non-ischemic, arterial) priapism
Etiology and associations	- Idiopathic - Drug induced - Neurologically mediated - Tumor infiltration - Hyperviscosity states: thrombophilia, hemoglobinopathies and hyperleukocytosis	- Trauma to perineum or genitalia
Clinical manifestations	- Painful and rigid erection. - Irreversible erectile dysfunction if condition persists longer than 24-48 hours.	- Painless erection at clinical presentation - Irreversible cellular damage and fibrosis are rare
Pathogenesis and course	- Intracavernosal blood sampling: acidosis and low oxygen tension. - Blockade of venous drainage from emissary venules causes intra-cavernosal blood stasis leading to accumulation of deoxygenated blood within the cavernous tissue thus causing trabecular interstitial edema and ultrastructural changes in trabecular smooth muscle. Functional transformation of these cells to fibroblast like cells ultimately causes cellular damage and fibrosis.	- Intracavernosal blood sampling: bright red oxygenated blood. -* Increased blood how in arteries causes an increase in blood flow into cavernosal sinusoids thus overwhelming the venous outflow.
Management	- Local penile or systemic anesthesia: spinal anesthesia, circumferential penile block or subcutaneous local penile shaft block. - Intracavernosal instillation of a sympathomimetic agent e.g. phenlyephedrine to induce detumescence. - Surgical shunt designed to divert blood away from corpus cavernosum is indicated in case of failure of the above measures. - Immediate aspiration and irrigation of the corpora cavernosa. - Anticoagulants and antifibrinolytic agents may be indicated. **- More common; actual medical and surgical emergency.**	- Perineal trauma causes injury to internal pudendal artery and this establishes a fistula between cavernosal artery and corpus cavernesum thus ultimately leading to unregulated blood flow. - Treatment can be given on an elective basis. **- Less Common; not a medical emergency.**

Table 2: Types of priapism, their etiology, pathogenesis and management.

Cytogenetic analysis revealed the presence of philadelphia chromosome and molecular studies confirmed the presence of BCR-ABL transcript, so the patient was commenced on imatinib 400 mg/day. Five days after admission, priapism resolved and his leukocyte count dropped to 53×10^9/l. Later on, the patient became asymptomatic, he remained stable clinically and his WBC count continued to drop which allowed discontinuation of hydroxyurea and allopurinol.

On 11/11/2013, the patient was discharged on imatinib 400 mg/day and he was given regular follow up appointments at the hematology outpatient clinic. Six months after starting imatinib therapy, the patient achieved major molecular response (MMR) of his CML. The patient was last seen on 11/23/2014. He was asymptomatic, his clinical examination showed impalpable spleen and his CBC was normal and his BCR-ABL taken 2 weeks earlier was negative. He was continued on imatinib, given new follow up appointment and was planned for a new molecular evaluation of his disease in 3 months.

Discussion

CML is a chronic myeloproliferative neoplasm, characterized by philadelphia chromosome and results from clonal expansion of pluripotent hematopoietic stem cells containing the active BCR-

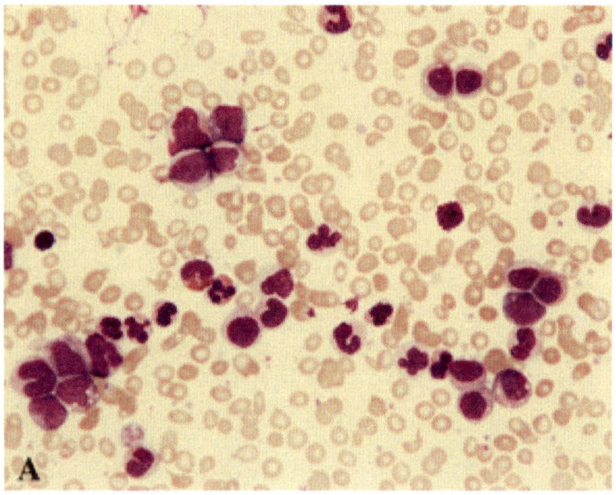

Figure 1: Peripheral blood smear showing: leukocytosis, neutrophils at different stages of maturation and prominent basophilia without evidence of dysplasia.

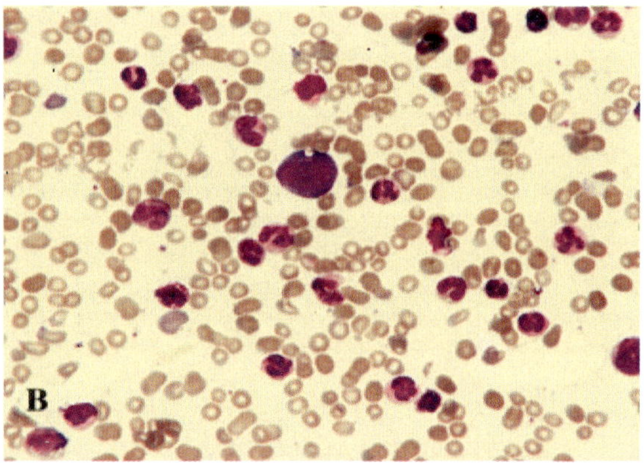

Figure 2: Bone marrow aspirate showing marked granulocytic proliferation with maturation pattern similar to that in the peripheral blood.

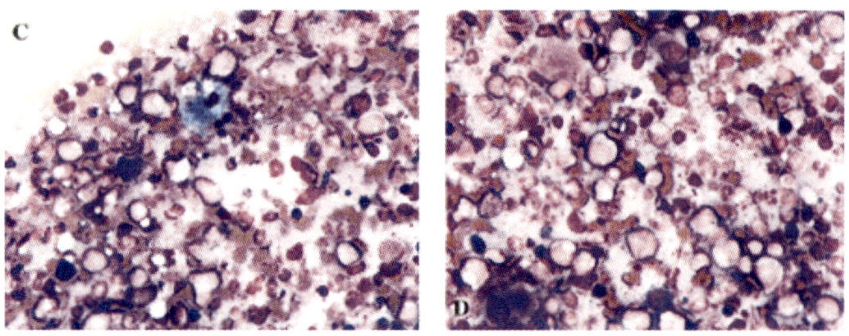

Figure 3: Sea-blue histiocytes are observed in the bone marrow aspirate. These histiocytes are secondary to increased cell turnover and they are derived from the neoplastic clone.

ABL fusion gene which is produced by a reciprocal chromosomal translocation between the ABL oncogene on chromosome 9 and the BCR gene on chromosome 22 [8-12]. The disease is often discovered accidentally when the patient presents with an elevated WBC count and/or an enlarged spleen. The most common clinical manifestations of CML are: anorexia, malaise, weight loss, sweating, bleeding episodes due to platelet dysfunction, abdominal fullness and pain or dragging sensation in the abdomen due to progressive enlargement of the spleen. Involvement of extramedullary tissues or sites such as liver, lymph nodes and skin is generally limited to patients having progressive disease [10]. At times, patients may present with leukostatic complications of hyperleukocytosis such as thromboembolic phenomena, hearing loss or priapism [4,13-15].

Introduction of imatinib and other Tyrosine Kinase Inhibitors (TKIs) has radically improved the outcome of patients with CML and some other diseases with BCR-ABL expression [8]. Imatinib was the first TKI to be licensed for use in treating patients with CML in Chronic-Phase (CP) and its introduction was associated with substantial improvements in response and survival compared with previous therapies [11]. Imatinib was approved by the food and drug authority in the United States of America as first-line treatment for newly diagnosed CML in December 2002, following an International Randomized Study (IRIS) initiated in June 2000 comparing imatinib as a single daily dose of 400 mg to interferon plus cytarabine in newly diagnosed patients with CML in CP [16]. The IRIS study showed the outstanding effectiveness of imatinib and its superiority with respect to the rates of Complete Hematological Response (CHR), Major Cytogenetic Response (McyR) and Complete Cytogenetic Response (CcyR). However, imatinib at dose of 400mg per day is still the gold standard first-line treatment for CML [17]. If the patient has a suboptimal response whilst on imatinib therapy, shifting to a second generation TKI such as dasatinib or nilotinib is justified in order to have a more optimal response as these agents have shown higher efficacy in clinical trials in imatinib-resistant or intolerant CML patients compared to imatinib treatment [10,18]. Other therapeutic options in case of suboptimal response to imatinib include: (1) escalation of the dose of imatinib, (2) allogeneic hematopoietic stem cell transplantation (HSCT), and (3) the use of agents that are being evaluated in clinical trials.

Approximately 20-30% of patients with CML fail imatinib therapy and develop resistance to the drug. These patients require alternative therapies. Therefore, it is vital to identify high risk patients at presentation of CML and start them on appropriate alternative therapies as early as possible [10,19]. Patients with CML harboring specific mutations such as T315 I remain resistant not only to first line but also to second line TKIs and require additional third generation inhibitors such as ponatinib to overcome resistance induced by these point mutations [8,18]. In patients with CML having accelerated phase or blast cell crisis, therapeutic options are limited and survival

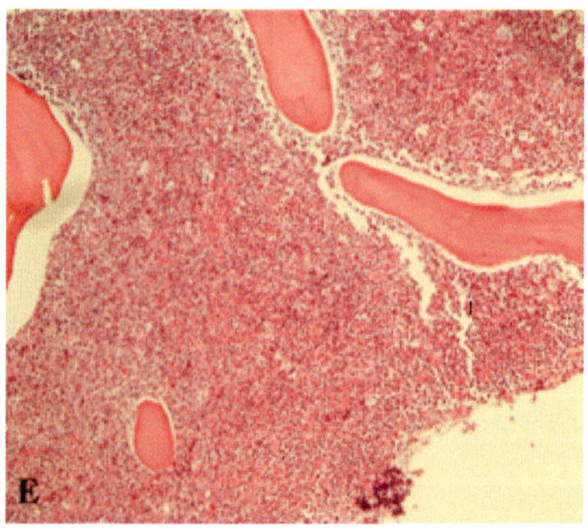

Figure 4: Bone marrow trephine biopsy showing 100% cellularity, increased megakaryopoiesis and granulopoiesis, prominent eosinophils without increase in blast cells.

is significantly shorter than that of patients with CP-CML even in the presence of powerful targeted therapies [20]. Allogeneic HSCT is still the only potentially curative therapy for CML and is the most valid therapeutic option that can be offered before the disease reaches the blastic phase [17].

In a comparative study, the rates of CcyR, MMR and Complete Molecular Response (CMR) in adolescents and young adults with CML treated upfront with TKIs were found to be lower than those in older patients but the overall survival was similar between the two groups. So, additional research in adolescents and young adults is needed to optimize CML treatment in this age group [21]. The aim of TKI therapy in patients with CML is to obtain ideal hematological, cytogenetic and molecular responses at certain and critical time points. Molecular monitoring of BCR-ABL transcripts by performing real time, quantitative, polymerase chain reaction has proven to be the most sensitive available method and has shown prognostic impact with regard to progression-free survival. The depth of response obtained with TKI therapy and the time to achieve this response are important in predicting the prognosis in patients with CML [17,20,22]. Careful and regular monitoring of CML patients on TKI treatment according to the European Leukemia Net CML guidelines and recommendations is of vital importance as timely and accurate monitoring is the key to optimizing patient management [18,20]. Excessive monitoring may have an economic cost, whilst failure to optimize TKI therapy may result in CML disease progression and death. Additionally, achievement of optimal responses and minimizing healthcare costs require full adherence of patients with CML to TKI therapy [23]. The patient presented achieved MMR 6 months after diagnosis and he achieved CMR 12 months after starting imatinib therapy.

Hyperleukocytosis is usually defined as having circulating blast cell count or WBC count exceeding 50 to 100 x 109/l. Hyperleukocytosis is usually encountered at the presentation of acute myeloid leukemia, acute lymphoblastic leukemia, CML or chronic lymphocytic leukemia [14,24,25]. Hyperleukocytosis leads to leukostasis that may be complicated by: hearing loss, papilledema, cerebellar dysfunction, impairment of memory function, intracranial hemorrhage, respiratory depression or failure, acute renal failure and priapism [14,15,24,26-28]. Treatment of hyperleukocytosis and leukostasis includes: cytoreductive therapy with hydroxyurea, cyclophosphamide or cytosine arabinoside, and therapeutic leukapheresis.

Although priapism is a rare and a rather exceptional presentation in male patients with CML, physicians should be aware of this disorder in order to ensure timely management [1,2,6,13]. At times, CML presents with an unexpected emergency such as priapism and the diagnosis of CML can only be made retrospectively after obtaining results of laboratory investigations. Hyperleukocytosis in CML causes formation of leukocyte aggregates or leukostatis which leads to the formation of thrombi in small blood vessels that ultimately causes vascular obstruction [4,13]. In our patient, hyperleokocytosis caused leukostasis and possibly microthrombi in the cavernosal circulation which precipitated priapism. The following five pathophysislogical mechanisms of priapism in CML have been postulated: (1) venous congestion of the corpora cavernosa resulting from mechanical pressure exerted by the enlarged spleen on the abdominal veins, (2) sludging of leukemia cells in the corpora cavernosa and the dorsal veins of the penis, (3) local infiltration of sacral nerves by leukemia cells, (4) central nervous system infiltration by leukemia, and (5) hyperleukocytosis causing elevation of whole-blood viscosity and this ultimately causing complication due to vascular obstruction [2,4].

In a patient presenting with priapism, the following are essential to make diagnosis of the cause of presentation: detailed history, through physical examination, appropriate laboratory investigations including CBC, differential cell count and peripheral blood film, cavernosal blood gas analysis and color duplex ultrasonography [6]. However, early intervention allows the best chance for full recovery. Currently, there are no standard protocols for management of priapism in CML patients and optimal management is still controversial. Old therapies reported in literature included: local radiotherapy, with or without open surgical shunting. New therapies include: (1) cytoreductive therapies with chemotherapeutic agents such as hydroxyurea, (2) leukapheresis in case of hyperleukocytosis, (3) allopurinol, hydration and symptomatic treatment, and (4) early initiation of TKI therapy with agents such as imatinib [3,7]. The patient presented was initially tried on local measures then he received: cytoreductive therapy in the form of high dose hydroxyurea, leukapheresis and TKI therapy in the form of imatinib, which allowed rapid reduction of the disease burden and rapid reversal of his priapism.

Conclusion

Priapism is a rare presentation of CML. Once it is encountered, the diagnostic procedures should be performed urgently and the patient should be commenced on: cytoreductive therapy, TKI therapy and leukapheresis in case of hyperleukocytosis as soon as possible not only to control priapism, but also to prevent further complications.

Acknowledgements

We are grateful to all medical, nursing and technical staff at KKUH who participated in the management of the patient presented.

References

1. Jana K, Aggarwal R, Gawande A, Lal M (2013) Priapism: a chronic myeloid leukemia harbinger in exigency. Ann Trop Med Public Health 6 (5): 583-585.
2. Chang MW, Tang CC, Chang SS (2003) Priapism--a rare presentation in chronic myeloid leukemia: case report and review of the literature. Chang Gung Med J 26: 288-292.
3. Tazi I (2009) Priapism as the first manifestation of chronic myeloid leukemia. Ann Saudi Med 29: 412.
4. Jameel T, Mehmood K (2009) Priapism - an usual presentation in chronic myeloid leukemia: case report and review of the literature. Biomedica 25: 197-199.
5. Yu KP, Hwang WS, Lee WC, Lin JS, Twu BH (1985) Priapism in patients with chronic myeloid leukemia: report of two cases. J Med Sci 6 (1): 87-92.
6. Hazra SP, Priyadarshi V, Gogoi D, Sharma PK, Pal DK, et al. (2013) Pediatric priapism: a rare first manifestation of leukemia. APSP J Case Rep 4: 39.
7. Tsai CH, Tsan YT, Hu SY, Lin TC, Hu WH, et al. (2008) Priapism as an initial manifestation of chronic myeloid leukemia: a case report. J Taiwan Emerg Med 10 (3): 100-104.
8. Trela E, Glowacki S (2014) Therapy of chronic myeloid leukemia: twilight of the imatinib era? ISRN Oncol 2014: 596483.
9. Fausel C (2007) Targeted chronic myeloid leukemia therapy: seeking a cure. J Manag Care Pharm 13: 8-12.
10. Baran Y, Saydam G (2012) Cumulative clinical experience from a decade of use: imatinib as first-line treatment of chronic myeloid leukemia. J Blood Med 3: 139-150.
11. Ferdinand R, Mitchell SA, Batson S, Tumur I (2012) Treatments for chronic myeloid leukemia: a qualitative systematic review. J Blood Med 3: 51-76.
12. Hu B, Savani BN (2014) Impact of risk score calculations in choosing front-line tyrosine kinase inhibitors for patients with newly diagnosed chronic myeloid leukemia in the chronic phase. Eur J Haematol 93: 179-186.
13. Ocheni S, Ibegbulam OG, Olusina DB, Oyekunle AA, Durosinmi MA (2010)

Chronic myeloid leukemia presenting as priapism: a report of 2 cases and review of literature. J Coll Med 15 (2).

14. Rowe JM, Lichtman MA (1984) Hyperleukocytosis and leukostasis: common features of childhood chronic myelogenous leukemia. Blood 63: 1230-1234.

15. Tsai CC, Huang CB, Sheen JM, Wei HH, Hsiao CC (2004) Sudden hearing loss as the initial manifestation of chronic myeloid leukemia in a child. Chang Gung Med J 27: 629-633.

16. Sacha T (2014) Imatinib in chronic myeloid leukemia: an overview. Mediterr J Hematol Infect Dis 6: e2014007.

17. Baccarani M, Pileri S, Steegmann JL, Muller M, Soverini S, et al. (2012) Chronic myeloid leukemia: ESMO Clinical Practice Guidelines for diagnosis, treatment and follow-up. Ann Oncol 23 Suppl 7: vii72-77.

18. Menon H (2013) Issues in current management of chronic myeloid leukemia: Importance of molecular monitoring on long term outcome. South Asian J Cancer 2: 38-43.

19. Deininger MW (2008) Milestones and monitoring in patients with CML treated with imatinib. Hematology Am Soc Hematol Educ Program .

20. Haznedaroglu IC (2014) Monitoring the Response to Tyrosine Kinase Inhibitor (TKI) Treatment in Chronic Myeloid Leukemia (CML). Mediterr J Hematol Infect Dis 6: e2014009.

21. Pemmaraju N, Kantarjian H, Shan J, Jabbour E, Quintas-Cardama A, et al. (2012) Analysis of outcomes in adolescents and young adults with chronic myelogenous leukemia treated with upfront tyrosine kinase inhibitor therapy. Haematologica 97 (7): 1029-1035.

22. Agarwal MB (2014) Importance of early and deeper responses to long-term survival in CML patients: Implications of BCR-ABL testing in management of CML in Indian setting. Indian J Med Paediatr Oncol 35: 10-16.

23. de Almeida MH, Fogliatto L, Couto D (2014) Importance of adherence to BCR-ABL tyrosine-kinase inhibitors in the treatment of chronic myeloid leukemia. Rev Bras Hematol Hemoter 36: 54-59.

24. Blum W, Porcu P (2007) Therapeutic apheresis in hyperleukocytosis and hyperviscosity syndrome. Semin Thromb Hemost 33: 350-354.

25. Galbraith PR, Valberg LS, Gruner PH, Brown GM (1965) The mechanism of the leukocytosis in chronic myeloid leukemia. Ann Inter Med 62 (5): 1085.

26. Resende LS, Coradazzi AL, Rocha-Júnior C, Zanini JM, Niéro-Melo L (2000) Sudden bilateral deafness from hyperleukocytosis in chronic myeloid leukemia. Acta Haematol 104: 46-49.

27. Kapur S, Wax M, Miles L, Hussain A (2013) Permanent sensorineural deafness in a patient with chronic myelogenous leukemia secondary to intracranial hemorrhage. Case Rep Hematol 2013: 894141.

28. Naithani R, Chandra J, Mathur NN, Narayan S, Singh V (2005) Hearing loss in chronic myeloid leukemia. Pediatr Blood Cancer 45: 54-56.

B-cell Chronic Lymphocytic Leukemia/Small Lymphocytic Lymphoma, without the Development of Richter's Syndrome, with Neoplastic Cells Lacking CD20 Antigen Expression after Rituximab Treatment

Shingo Yanagiya[1], Kazuya Sato[2], Nodoka Tsukada[2], Junki Inamura[2], Satoshi Ito[3], Motohiro Shindo[3], Keisuke Sato[4], Koji Sakurai[4], Eisuke Shiozawa[5], Toshiko Yamochi[5], Hidekazu Ota[5] and Takaaki Hosoki[2]

[1]*Junior resident of Asahikawa Kosei Hospital, 1-24, Asahikawa, 078-8211, Japan*
[2]*Department of Hematology/Oncology, Asahikawa Kosei Hospital, Japan*
[3]*Division of Gastroenterology and Hematology/Oncology, Department of Medicine, Asahikawa Medical University, Japan*
[4]*Department of Pathology, Asahikawa Kosei Hospital, 1-24, Asahikawa, 078-8211, Japan*
[5]*Department of Pathology and Laboratory Medicine, Showa University School of Medicine, Japan*

Abstract

A 40-year-old man was admitted to our hospital with systemic swelling of the lymphnodes (LNs). The histopathological findings of the neck LNs revealed a diffuse proliferation of neoplastic small lymphocytes. LN and bone marrow (BM) cells were subjected to immunostaining and flow cytometric analysis of the cell surface, showing CD5, CD19, CD20, and CD23 positivity and CD3, CD10, and cyclin D1 negativity. The patient was diagnosed with B-cell chronic lymphocytic leukemia/small lymphocytic lymphoma (B-CLL/SLL). He received a cycle of CHOP (cyclophosphamide, doxorubicin, vincristine, and prednisolone) and 6 cycles of RFC (rituximab, fludarabine, and cyclophosphamide), after which complete remission was obtained. Fifteen months after the diagnosis, the lymphoma relapsed and massive systemic LN swelling and BM infiltration were observed, characterized by a lack of CD20 antigen expression in the neoplastic cells. Two salvage chemotherapy regimens proved ineffective and the lymphoma progressed. The patient died two months after the relapse. The pathological findings at autopsy revealed the multiple organ infiltration of CLL/SLL cells which lacked CD20 expression. There were no evidence of Richter's syndrome. Patients with relapsed B-CLL/SLL who are undergoing rituximab-containing therapy should be monitored for the loss of CD20 antigen expression in the neoplastic cells.

Keywords: B-cell chronic lymphocytic leukemia/small lymphocytic lymphoma; CD20 antigen loss; rituximab

Introduction

B-cell chronic lymphocytic leukemia/small lymphocytic lymphoma (B-CLL/SLL) is a mature B-cell lymphoid neoplasm characterized by the proliferation of monoclonal mature B-cell in the peripheral blood, bone marrow, and lymph nodes (LNs) [1-3]. SLL is typically characterized by the proliferation of neoplastic cells, mainly in the LNs, which is not accompanied by cytopenia due to bone marrow infiltration. In many ways, SLL is similar to CLL. The similarities include the characteristics of the neolpastic cells [1]. The B-CLL/SLL neoplastic cells strongly express CD5 and CD23 and weakly express cell-surface IgM/IgD, CD11c, CD19, CD20, CD22, and CD79a [4]. Approximately 3-15% of all B-CLL/SLL cases experience the transformation into diffuse large B-cell lymphoma (DLBCL), which is also known as Richter's syndrome (RS) in the narrow sense of the term [5]. Mauro et al. [6] reported the development of 22 RS patients, including 18 cases of DLBCL and 4 of Hodgkin's Lymphoma (HL), in their analysis of 1,011 B-CLL/SLL patients. It has been previously demonstrated that B-CLL/SLL transforms into DLBCL, HL, and hairy cell leukemia [1,6,7] and into high-grade lymphoma, which is also known as RS in the wider sense of the term [1]. The prognosis of patients who develop RS is very poor, with survival rate of 7 to 8-month, even in the patient treated with R-CHOP (rituximab, cyclophosphamide, doxorubicin, vincristine, and prednisolone), hyper-CVAD (cyclophosphamide, vincristine, doxorubicin, and dexamethasone) or a purine analogue regimen [1]. Aggressive cases of B-CLL/SLL, which develop into RS with cells that lack CD20 antigen expression have also been reported [8-10]. However, the cases of B-CLL/SLL with cells that lack CD20 antigen expression without RS development, are not fully understood.

We herein report a relapsed case of B-CLL/SLL, in which RS did not develop, which presented an aggressive clinical course due to presence of neoplastic cells that lacked CD20 antigen expression after the treatment with a rituximab-containing regimen.

Case report

A 40-year-old man was referred to our hospital for lymphadenopathy. A physical examination revealed systemic lymphadenopathy including neck and axillary LN swelling. A computed tomography (CT) scan (Figure 1) showed multiple lymphadenopathy of the neck (A), axilla (B), mediastinum and the abdomen (C). The results of a blood test performed on admission (Table 1) were as follows: white blood cells (WBC) 3300/μl (neutrophils 38.1%, lymphocytes 58.6%); red blood cells (RBC) 347 × 10^4/μl; hemoglobin (Hb) 12.4 g/dl; platelet (Plt) 21.3 × 10^4/μl; total protein (TP) 5.7 g/dl; albumin (ALB) 3.9 g/dl; LDH 221 IU/l; creatinine (CRE) 0.48 mg/dl; CRP 0.78 mg/dl; and soluble interleukin-2 receptor (sIL-2R) 2880 IU/l. The pathological findings of a cervical LN biopsy specimen (Figure 2) revealed the destruction of the basic structure of the LN and the diffuse proliferation of atypical

***Corresponding author:** Kazuya Sato, MD, PhD, Department of Hematology/Oncology, Asahikawa Kosei Hospital1jodoori 24 chome 111-3, Asahikawa, Hokkaido, 078-8210, Japan; E-mail: satofam@wine.plala.or.jp

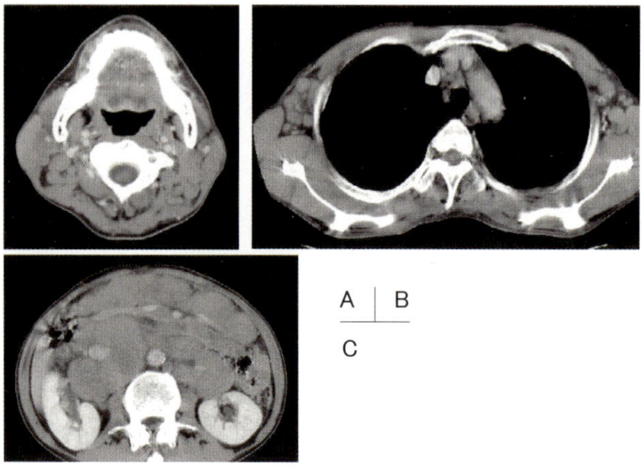

Figure 1: CT showed swelling of the cervical (A), axillary (B), and mesenteric lymph nodes.

WBC	3300/µl	TP	5.7g/dl	APTT	28sec
Neu	38.1%	Alb	3.9g/dl	PT	13.2 sec
Lym	58.6	T-bil	0.7mg/dl	PT-%	0.877
Mono	2	D-bil	0.1mg/dl	PT-INR	1.06
Baso	0.7	AST	21IU/l	FDP	2.5 mg/dl
Eos	0.6	ALT	11IU/l	D-dimer	0.6 mg/dl
RBC	347×10^4/C	LDH	221IU/l		
Hb	12.3g/dl	BUN	11.4mg/dl	FBS	108 mg/dl
Ht	36%	Cre	0.48mg/dl	HbA1c(NGSP)	4.8
MCV	103.7fl	Na	142mEq/l		
MCH	35.5pg	K	4mEq/l	RPR	(-)
MCHC	34.2%	Cl	104mEq/l	HBsAg	(-)
Plt	21.3×10^4/µl	CRP	0.78mg/dl	HCVAb	(-)
				HTLV-1Ab	(-)
				EBVVCA IgG	×80
				sIL-2R	2880 IU/l

Table 1: Laboratory data at diagnosis.

lymphocytes via hematoxylin and eosin (HE) staining (Figures 2A and 2B). The immunostaining of these atypical cells revealed that they were positive for CD5, CD20, CD23, and CD79a (Figures 2C-F), but negative for CD3, CD10, and cyclin D1. A flow cytometric analysis using Peripheral Blood (PB) was not performed at the time of the initial diagnosis because there were no atypical lymphocytes in the PB. Bone marrow mononuclear cells (BMCs) were found to be positive for CD5, CD19 (Figure 3A), CD20 (Figure 3B), CD23, CD25, and the λ-chain of the immunoglobulin light chain and negative for CD3 and CD10 by a cell surface marker analysis using flow cytometry. We were unable to make a definitive diagnosis at that point, however, DLBCL was initially doubted based on the histopathologic findings. Because the patient's LNs became further enlarged, CHOP therapy was administered as an initial treatment, and thereafter the LNs decreased in size. We obtained a second opinion consultation of his tissue samples from the Department of Pathology and Laboratory Medicine, Showa University School of Medicine. A definitive diagnosis of B-CLL/SLL was made according to the findings of diffuse proliferation of small and medium-sized atypical lymphocytes with a B-cell phenotype, of which 20% were found to be positive for Ki67 immunostaining. Furthermore, the long-arm deletion of chromosome 11 [del (11q)] was detected in 15 of 20 BMCs by the G-banding method. His clinical staging was determined to be intermediate risk II by the modified Rai classification [11], and B by the Binet classification [12]. We modified the treatment strategy to the RFC regimen (rituximab, fludarabine, and cyclophosphamide) after the definitive diagnosis. He achieved complete remission after

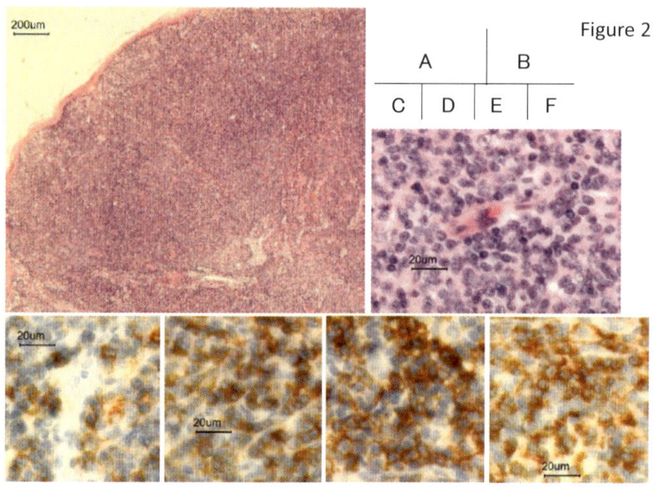

Figure 2: The pathological findings of the cervical lymph nodes at diagnosis. HE staining (2×) (A), (B) (20×) and immunostainings (20×) demonstrate positivity for CD20 (C), CD5 (D), CD23 (E) and CD79a (F).

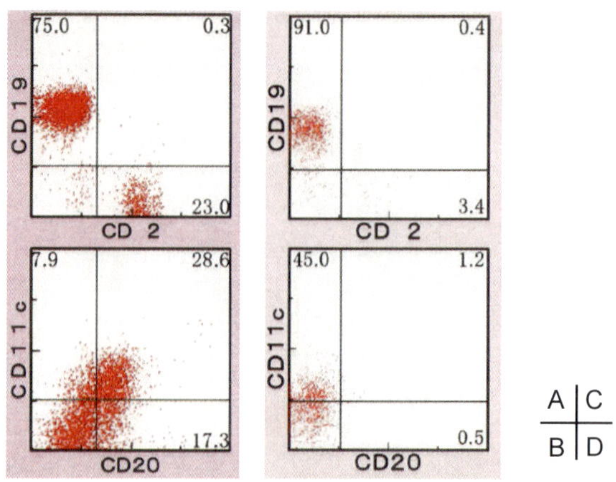

Figure 3: The immunophenotyping by flowcytometry of the bone marrow cells at diagnosis and at relapse after rituximab-including treatment. Before rituximab treatment, the neoplastic cells expressed CD19 (A) and CD20 (B). At relapse after treatment with the rituximab regimen, the tumor cells were positive for CD19 (C), but exhibited the loss of CD20 expression (D). These analyses were performed by SRL Inc., Tokyo, Japan.

6 cycles of RFC. Fourteen months after the first admission, he felt an abdominal distension and CT revealed the presence of multiple enlarged abdominal LNs, and he was thus readmitted to our hospital. On this occasion, the blood test results were as follows: WBC 2100/μl (neutrophils 73.0%, lymphocytes 24.0%, monocytes 1.0%, eosinophiles 1.0%, and atypical lymphocytes 1.0%); RBC 289 × 10^4/μl; Hb 9.5 g/dl; Plt 4.2 × 10^4/μl; LDH 307 IU/l; CRP 3.2 mg/dl; and sIL-2R 1420 U/ml. The bone marrow examination showed that 90.6% of the total BMCs were atypical mature lymphocytes. Furthermore, the bone marrow neoplastic cells were positive for CD5, CD19 (Figure 3C), CD23, CD25, and λ-chain of immunoglobulin light chain and negative for not only CD3 and CD10, but also for CD20 (Figure 3D), which was found to be positive at the initial diagnosis (Figure 3B) by the cell surface marker analysis using flow cytometry. Complicated chromosomal abnormalities including abnormalities in chromosomes 3, 6, 7, 8, 9, 13, 15, 16, 17, and 19, were detected in 15 of 20 analyzed BMCs by the G-banding method. The abnormalities in chromosome 11, which were detected at the initial diagnosis, were not included. We ultimately determined that the patient had relapsed due to B-CLL without RS and with the loss of CD20 antigen expression.

Figure 4 shows the clinical course of the patient after the initial admission. He received one cycle of bendamustine monotherapy as the initial treatment of the salvage therapy, however, the number of bone marrow neoplastic cells increased. Afterwards, he received a cycle of hyper-CVAD; however, he presented life-threatening pneumonitis during the period of prolonged bone marrow suppression. Although the patient received several antibiotics and antifungal drugs with the support of mechanical ventilation, he died from a pulmonary hemorrhage associated with the pneumonitis 16 months after the initial admission. The pathological findings by HE staining at autopsy Figure 5 revealed the massive infiltration of neoplastic cells in the mesenteric LN (A), bone marrow (B), kidney (C), and Glisson's capsule of the liver (D). Both lungs showed diffuse hemorrhages and fluid retention. The weights of the right and left lungs were 1.7 kg and 1.3 kg, respectively. Lung parenchyma and intra vessels demonstrated the dissemination of Candida and focal pneumonitis. The stomach, colon and kidney

Figure 4

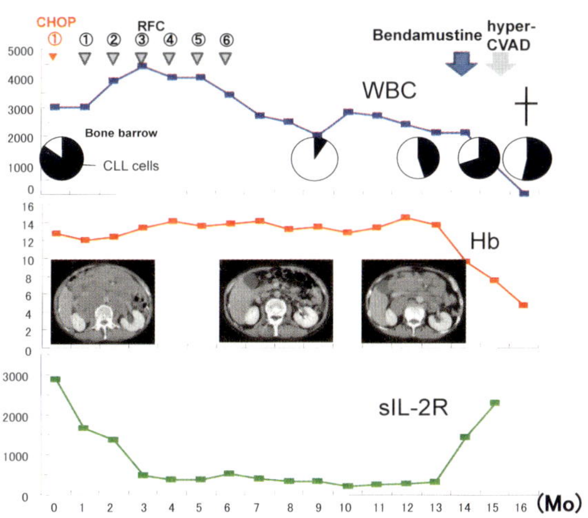

Figure 4: The clinical course. CHOP: cyclophosphamide, doxorubicin, vincristine, and prednisolone; RFC: rituximab, fludarabine, and cyclophosphamide; hyper-CVAD: cyclophosphamide, vincristine, doxorubicin, and dexamethasone; CLL: chronic lymphocytic leukemia; Mo: months.

Figure 5

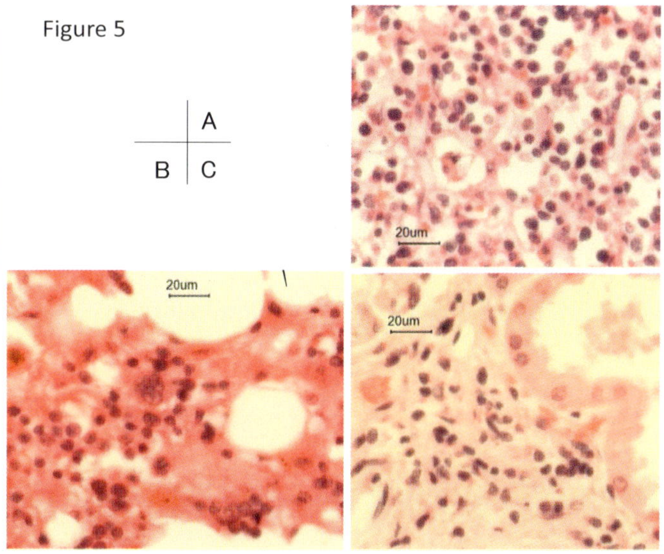

Figure 5: The pathological findings via HE staining (20X) at autopsy. Massive neoplastic cell infiltration was observed in the mesenteric lymph node (A), bone marrow (B), kidney (C).

Figure 5D

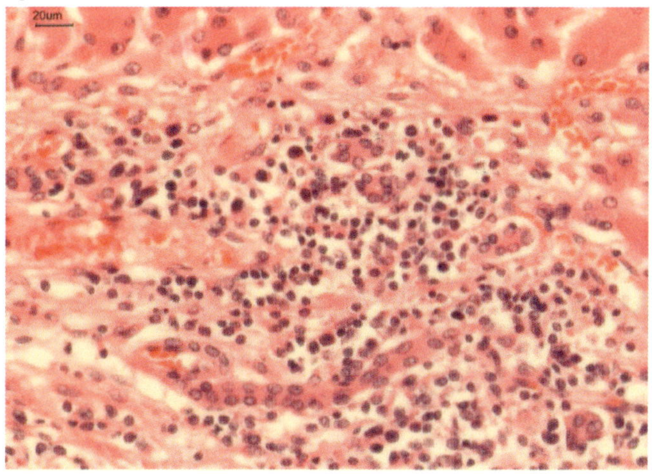

Figure 5D: Glisson's capsules of the liver

were also hemorrhagic. The cause of death was determined to be respiratory failure due to lung bleeding and pneumonia. Figure 6 shows the pathological findings of the mesenteric LN at autopsy. The atypical lymphocytes show negativity for CD20 (A) and positivity for CD5 (B), CD23 (C) and CD79a (D) by immunostaining, which was consistent with the characteristic B-CLL/SLL findings, without evidence of RS (including DLBCL). We ultimately concluded that the neoplastic B-CLL/SLL cells lost the expression of the CD20 antigen after the rituximab treatment.

Discussion

A recent search of the MEDLINE database revealed a limited number of cases of B-CLL/SLL demonstrating the loss of CD20 antigen expression after rituximab treatment. Including the present case, only

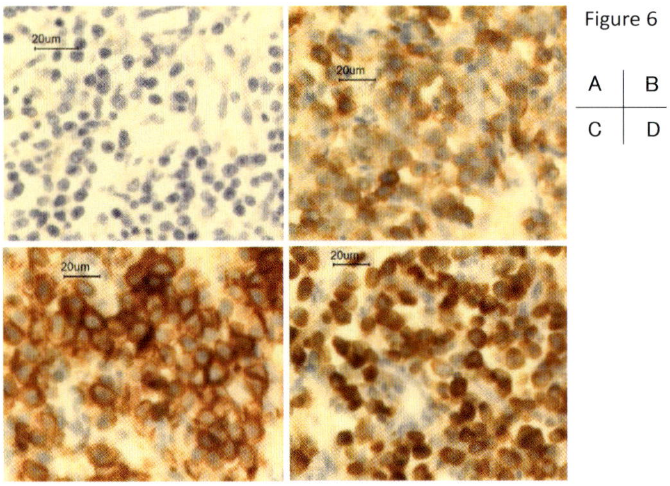

Figure 6: The pathological findings of the mesenteric lymph node at autopsy (20X). The immunostainings demonstrate negativity for CD20 expression (A) and positivity for the expression of CD5 (B), CD23 (C) and CD79a (D).

a small number of cases have been reported thus far [9,12-15]. The characteristics of 11 patients (including 6 males) whose details were described are listed in Table 2. Treatment regimens that included rituximab, such as R-CHOP or fludarabine-based regimens, were chosen for patients with B-CLL/SLL before the loss of CD20 expression was demonstrated. The expression of B-cell markers other than CD20, such as CD19, CD22 or CD23, were observed in the neoplastic cells after CD20 loss. Most cases received salvage chemotherapies according to the aggressive lymphomas after CD20 loss. Three of the eight confirmed cases developed into RS. In the five cases where survival was described, 3 cases (including 2 which developed into RS), died within 1-4 months after the loss of CD20 expression. Moreover, 1 of the 3 cases (the present case) which did not develop into RS showed chemoresistance and died within a short period of time. Although a further accumulation of cases is needed to clarify the prognosis of B-CLL/SLL that does not develop into RS, but demonstrates the loss of CD20 expression after rituximab treatment, the existence of such patients must be recognized.

It is not well understood how frequently CD20 antigen loss in tumor cells occurs in B-CLL/SLL patients after rituximab therapy. D'Auria et al. [9] reported that 4 of 8 (50%) tested CLL/SLL patients demonstrated CD20 antigen loss, half of whom later developed RS. Goteri et al. [13]

Case No. [references]	Age/ Sex	Status at Rituximab (R) therapy	R-regimen (cycles)	Response to R-regimen	Cell surface antigens after CD20 loss	Further clinical course after CD20 loss (final status)	Development of RS	Final outcome	Survival after CD20 loss (Mo)
1 [9]	67/M	Rel2 after CB and Flu	R-CHOP-like (6)	PR	CD5+,19+, 23+, 52+, Lambda+	Al, Ben → CD20+(PR)	no	A	26+
2 [9]	68/M	Rel1 after FC	R (6) + CB	PR	CD5+,19+, 23+, 52+, Lambda+	Al → CD20+→ R-Ben (PR)	no	A	25+
3 [9]	74/F	Rel1 after CB	R-FC (5)	NR	CD5+,19+, 23+, 52+, Lambda+	Evolution into CD20+ high grade lymphoma (RS) →R-CHOP (PD)	yes	D	1
4 [9]	61/M	Rel2 as CD20+ RS after FC and R-Ben	R-CHOP (4)	PR	CD5+,19+, 23+, 52+, Kappa+	CD20- high grade lymphoma (RS) → 4 regimens including ASCT	yes	D	4
5 [12]	64/F	Rel1 as RS after multiple CT	R-CHOP (6)	PR→PD	CD45+	Evolution into CD20- DLBCL (PD)	yes	N/A	NA
6 [14]	53/F	NA	NA	NA	CD5+, 19+, 22+	NA	NA	A	NA
7 [14]	42/M	NA	NA	NA	CD79a+	NA	NA	A	NA
8 [14]	77/F	NA	NA	NA	CD5+, 19+, 22+	NA	NA	A	NA
9 [15]	54/M	Initial treatment	R (2)	NA	NA	C-MOPP (PR)	no	N/A	NA
10 [15]	52/F	Treatment after CHOP and COP	R-CEPP (7)	NA	NA	R-ESHAP, CHASE, R-ESHAP + ASCT, R → (PR)	no	N/A	NA
11 [our case]	40/M	Initial treatment	CHOP (1) + R-FC (6)	CR	CD5+,19+, 23+, 11c+, 25+ Lambda+	Ben, Hyper-CVAD (PD)	no	D	2

Table 2: Cases with B-cell chronic lymphocytic leukemia/small lymphocytic lymphoma showing the loss of CD20 antigen expression after rituximab treatment. No: Number; M: male; F: female; R: rituximab; RS: Richter's syndrome; CB: chlorambucil; Flu: fludarabine; CHOP: cyclophosphamide, vincristine, doxorubicin, prednisone; Al: alemtuzumab; PR: partial response; FC: fludarabine, cyclophosphamide; Ben: bendamustine; NR: no response; Hyper-CVAD: cyclophosphamide (high dose), vincristine, doxorubicin, dexamethasone; ASCT: autologous stem cell transplantation; CVP: cyclophosphamide, vincristine, prednisone; CR: complete remission; SD: stable disease; PD: progressive disease; R-B: rituximab, bendamustine; NA: not available; C-MOPP: cyclophosphamide, vincristine, prednisone, procarbazine; COP: cyclophosphamide, vincristine, prednisone; CEPP: cyclophosphamide, etoposide, prednisone, procarbazine; ESHAP: etoposide, methylprednisolone, high-dose cytarabine, cisplatin; CHASE: cyclophosphamide, high-dose cytarabine, dexamethasone, etoposide; CT: chemotherapy; Rel1: first relapse; A: alive; D: died.

indicated that 4 of 5 patients (80%) with CLL/SLL showed the loss of CD20 antigen expression after rituximab treatment in their investigation of 26 low-grade, non-Hodgkin's lymphoma (NHL) patients. Seliem et al. retrospectively analyzed the immunophenotypic changes in patients with B-cell NHL after rituximab therapy and showed a reduction or significant decrease in the CD20 expression of 5 patients, including 3 patients with B-CLL/SLL. Taken together, it appears that a certain percentage of B-CLL/SLL patients develop the loss (or reduction of the level) of CD20 antigen expression on the neoplastic cells after rituximab treatment.

Several mechanisms for the loss of CD20 antigen expression

on the neoplastic cells have been demonstrated in patients with B-CLL/SLL receiving rituximab therapy. Jilani et al. [16] tested the presence of rituximab on the surface of CLL lymphocytes using anti-mouse immunoglobulin antibodies to detect rituximab and found its presence in 3 of 65 B-CLL patients, despite the fact that most of them had no detectable CD20 expression. They speculated that the disappearance of CD20 expression may not only be due to a masking effect by rituximab, but also due to the down-modulation of CD20 expression or its internalization. Conversely, Hiraga et al. [17] proposed the epigenetic modulation of the CD20 antigen as an alternative explanation of the phenomenon. Moreover, Takei, et al. [18] demonstrated clonal selection and the expansion of CD20-negative cells in CLL/SLL patients after rituximab treatment. The fact that the neoplastic cells with chromosomal types that differed from the initial diagnosis developed after rituximab treatment in the present case may support this hypothesis. Although we cannot definitively determine which mechanism or mechanisms are associated with the loss of CD20 antigen on the neoplastic cells in the present case of B-CLL/SLL patients after rituximab treatment, the mechanism(s) should be further clarified in future investigations.

We chose bendamustine monotherapy as the salvage chemotherapy in the present case due to the loss of CD20 expression on the neoplastic cells. However, it was not effective for the present case. One of the other potential therapies may include the use of the humanized anti-CD52 monoclonal antibody alemtuzumab, which has been reported to be an active agent for CLL patients with high-risk genetic markers including del (17p) [3]. Moreover, D'Auria et al. [9] reported two cases of B-CLL in whom alemtuzumab was effective survived for more than 2 years after the loss of CD20 antigen expression following rituximab treatment (Case Nos. 1 and 2 in Table 2). However, it is not easy to administer alemtuzumab because it is not currently approved in Japan. Another potential therapy would be use of ofatumumab, a fully humanized antibody targeting a unique epitope on the CD20 molecule, which results in an increased binding affinity to CD20 and increased (in comparison to rituximab) cellular killing due to a greater CDC activity and similar ADCC activity [3]. It has been previously demonstrated that ofatumumab is effective for B-CLL/SLL cells expressing even low levels of CD20 [3]. The last choice may have been to perform an allogeneic stem cell transplantation (allo-SCT) before the present patient's relapse. In fact, we had considered performing allo-SCT at his first CR due to his age and risk factors, including del (11q), and we had searched for an HLA-identical sibling donor. There was no appropriate sibling donor, and we had to wait until the patient agreed to search for unrelated donors. Although the optimal therapeutic strategy for this case is unknown, further investigations are required to identify the risk factors for the loss of CD20 expression on the neoplastic cells in B-CLL/SLL patients after rituximab treatment.

References

1. Müller-Hermelink HK, Montserrat E, Catovsky D, Martinez A (2008) Chronic lymphocytic leukaemia/small lymphocytic lymphoma.WHO Classification of Tumours of Haematopoietic and Lymphoid Tissues. Lyon, France: IARC Press. 180–182.
2. Tandra P, Krishnamurthy J, Bhatt VR, Newman K, Armitage JO, et al. (2013) Autoimmune cytopenias in chronic lymphocytic leukemia, facts and myths. Mediterr J Hematol Infect Dis 5: e2013068.
3. Hallek M (2013) Chronic lymphocytic leukemia: 2013 update on diagnosis, risk stratification and treatment. Am J Hematol 88: 803-816.
4. Rossi M, Fuligni F, Ciccone M, Agostinelli C, Righi S, et al. (2013) Hsa-miR-15a and Hsa-miR-16-1 expression is not related to proliferation centers abundance and other prognostic factors in chronic lymphocytic leukemia. Biomed Res Int 2013: 715391.
5. Parikh SA, Habermann TM, Chaffee KG, Call TG, Ding W, et al. (2015) Hodgkin transformation of chronic lymphocytic leukemia: Incidence, outcomes, and comparison to de novo Hodgkin lymphoma. Am J Hematol 90: 334-338.
6. Mauro FR, Foa R, Giannarelli D, Cordone I, Crescenzi S, et al. (1999) Clinical characteristics and outcome of young chronic lymphocytic leukemia patients: a single institution study of 204 cases. Blood 94: 448-454.
7. Gribben JG, O'Brien S (2011) Update on therapy of chronic lymphocytic leukemia. J Clin Oncol 29: 544-550.
8. Mankai A, Bordron A, Renaudineau Y, Martins-Carvalho C, Takahashi S, et al. (2008) Purine-Rich Box-1-Mediated Reduced Expression of CD20 Alters Rituximab-Induced Lysis of Chronic lymphocytic Leukemia B cells. Cancer Res 68:7512-7519.
9. D'Auria F, Guariglia R, Villani O, Mansueto G, Grieco V, et al. (2010) Modulation of CD20 antigen expression after rituximab treatment: a retrospective study in patients with chronic lymphocytic leukemia. Clin Ther 32: 1911-1916.
10. Rai KR. (1987) A critical analysis of staging in CLL. In: Gale RP, Rai KR, eds. Chronic Lymphocytic Leukemia: Recent Progress and Future Directions. New York, NY: Liss :253-264.
11. Binet JL, Auquier A, Dighiero G, Chastang C, Piguet H, et al. (1981) A new prognostic classification of chronic lymphocytic leukemia derived from a multivariate survival analysis. Cancer 48: 198-206.
12. Haidar JH, Shamseddine A, Salem Z, Mrad YA, Nasr MR, et al. (2003) Loss of CD20 expression in relapsed lymphomas after rituximab therapy. Eur J Haematol 70: 330-332.
13. Goteri G, Olivieri A, Ranaldi R, Lucesole M, Filosa A, et al. (2006) Bone marrow histopathological and molecular changes of small B-cell lymphomas after rituximab therapy: Comparison with clinical response and patients outcome. Int J Immunopathol Pharmacol 19:421–431.
14. Seliem RM, Freeman JK, Steingart RH, Hasserjian RP (2006) Immunophenotypic changes and clinical outcome in B-cell lymphomas treated with rituximab. Appl Immunohistochem Mol Morphol 14: 18-23.
15. Maeshima AM, Taniguchi H, Nomoto J, Maruyama D, Kim SW, et al. (2009) Histological and immunophenotypic changes in 59 cases of B-cell non-Hodgkin's lymphoma after rituximab therapy. Cancer Sci 100: 54-61.
16. Jilani I, O'Brien S, Manshuri T, Thomas DA, Thomazy VA, et al. (2003) Transient down-modulation of CD20 by rituximab in patients with chronic lymphocytic leukemia. Blood 102: 3514-3520.
17. Hiraga J, Tomita A, Sugimoto T, Shimada K, Ito M, et al. (2009) Down-regulation of CD20 expression in B-cell lymphoma cells after treatment with rituximab-containing combination chemotherapies: Its prevalence and clinical significance. Blood 113: 4885–4893.
18. Takei K, Yamazaki T, Sawada U, Ishizuka H, Aizawa S (2006) Analysis of changes in CD20, CD55, and CD59 expression on established rituximab-resistant B-lymphoma cell lines. Leuk Res 30: 625-631.

Detection of a High Frequency of e1a3/BCR-ABL in Chronic Myeloid Leukemia Patients of Sulaimania Province by RT-PCR

Gaza F Salih*

Department of Biology, University of Sulaimania, Sulamania, KRG, Iraq

Abstract

Introduction: In order to detect the mutation variants of BCR-ABL fusion genes that lead to leukemia in human, 30 blood samples from chronic myeloid leukemia patients and 10 blood samples from apparently healthy people (as control) were collected and tested hematologically, morphologically and by amplification of the fusion mRNA by RT-PCR. The e1a3 variant was detected by amplification of 309 bp from the fusion of exons 1 of bcr and exon 3 of abl gene.

Materials and method: Application of RT-PCR assay to detect the prevalence and frequency of ela3 and ela2 variants in CML patients and in routine diagnosis of the most common leukemia translocations.

Results: The RT-PCR showed that out of 30 patients, 23 (76.6%) were with e1a3 mutation variant and 7 (23.3%) were negative for e1a2 and e1a3 variants. All the 10 control samples showed no mutations related to these variants.

Conclusion: The e1a3 variant was detected by amplification of 309 bp from the fusion of exons 1 of bcr and exon 3 of abl gene and the RT-PCR showed that out of 30 patients, 23 (76.6%) were with e1a3 mutation variant and 7 (23.3%) were negative for e1a2 and e1a3 variants, while the 10 control samples showed no mutations related to these variants.

Keywords: Chronic myeloid leukemia (CML); ela2; ela3; RT-PCR

Introduction

Chronic Myeloid Leukemia (CML) is a myeloproliferative disorder of hematopoietic stem cells [1]. It has been observed following exposure to high doses of ionizing radiation [2]. It is also believed that Abelson murine leukemia virus (A-MuLV) which is originated from recombination between Moloney murine leukemia virus (M-MuLV) and the cellular proto-oncogene c-abl [3] is usually defective in replication, but can transform host cells following re-infection [4] CML is generally associated with Philadelphia (Ph') chromosome that is resulted from translocation between chromosomes 9q34.1 and 22q11.21[g]. On Ph' chromosome the bcr-abl fusion gene encodes a constitutively active tyrosine kinase [5], which causes malignant transformation of leukocytes [6]. Duplication of Ph' chromosome, an isochromosome 17 [7], as well as MYC gene over-expression as a consequence of trisomy 8 or gene amplification are also found [2].

Clinical symptoms are usually nonspecific, and include fatigue, weight loss, anorexia, headache [1], fever, bone pain and splenomegaly [7]. Up to 50% of patients may be asymptomatic [1]. Complete blood count (CBC) shows an increased number of white blood cells, low number of red blood cells or blood platelets [8]. Blood films show pathologic left shift with the appearance of a large number of granulocytes at all stages of differentiation including promyelocytes and myeloblasts [9]. Bone marrow shows marked hyper-cellularity due to myeloid hyperplasia [9].

The chimeric protein encoded by bcr-abl fusion gene varies depending on the breakpoint in the bcr gene. Three breakpoint cluster regions have been characterized to date; major (M-*bcr*), minor (m-*bcr*) and micro (mu-*bcr*) [10]. The majority of CML patients have p210 BCR-ABL (M-bcr), whose mRNA transcripts have b2a2 and/or b3a2 junction [11], which is associated with granulocytic leukemia. A small group has p190 BCR-ABL (m-bcr), whose mRNA transcripts have e1a2 and/or e1a3 variants [10], which is principally associated with monocytic leukemia [10]. CML resulting from a p230 BCR-ABL (mu-bcr) is also rare, and has been associated with the CNL and/or with marked thrombocytosis [10].

Since the introduction of imatinib (Gleevec), the outlook of patients with CML has improved dramatically. Many patients can remain in remission for many years while on this drug [11]. Imatinib is a selective inhibitor not only for ABL kinase but also for PDGFR kinases and c-kit tyrosine kinases [12,13] and it exerts significant anti-leukemic activity in the majority of CML patients.

Reverse transcription polymerase chain reaction (RT-PCR) assay is important to evaluate benefits of bone marrow transplantation and minimal residual disease (MRD) monitoring [14]. RT-PCR assay is rapid and accurate affording the ability to make crucial therapeutic decisions [14] the requirement for dividing cells is not needed and providing a sensitive marker for subsequent MRD testing [15]. In this case there is no need to wait for cytogenetic studies that require a longer time and has a lower sensitivity [14].

The bcr-abl fusion gene counts for the major molecular marker for leukemia in molecular pathology laboratories [14]. Recent WHO classification announced that genetic analysis of leukemia has prognostic and therapeutic implications, which require accurate genetic diagnosis that can be rapidly obtained by molecular approaches

***Corresponding author:** Gaza F Salih, Faculty of Science, Department of Biology, University of Sulaimania, Sulamania, KRG, Iraq; E-mail: gazasalih@home.se

[15]. RT-PCR assays are designed to detect specific fusions, and it would be extremely labor intensive to evaluate leukemia via a panel of individual monoplex assays. This can be circumvented by the use of multiplex RT-PCR assays [16].

This study aimed at detecting the prevalence of e1a3 and e1a2 variants in CML patients of Sulaimani province and the frequency of each variant through using RNA amplification technique by reverse transcription polymerase chain reaction (RT-PCR) and to apply RT-PCR assay in routine diagnosis of the most common leukemia translocation.

Method

The genomic RNA was efficiently extracted by filter-based method. This method was used in RNA extraction of blood, which is rapid, safe and inexpensive [17]. Then all RNA samples (30 CML patients and 10 controls) were reversely transcribed to cDNA according to Bioneer RT PreMix protocol. Eight µl of genomic RNA, 2.5 µl of R-ABL (N6) [TGTTGACTGGCGTGATGTAGTTGC] primer, 1.5 µl of R-actβ [GCATACCCCTCGTAGATGGG] as internal control and 3 µl of nuclease free D.W. were mixed in a 0.2 ml PCR tube and then the mixture was put in thermal cycler. RT1 reaction includes denaturation of genomic RNA at 65°C for 5 min. and then the reaction was hold at 4°C. The RT PreMix was dissolved with 5 µl of D.W. and then RT1 mixture was added to this mixture in a final volume 20 µl of RT2. RT2 reaction includes cDNA synthesis at 42°C for 1h, heat inactivation at 95°C for 5 min (according to Bioneer RT PreMix protocol), then the reaction was hold at 4°C.

The cDNA region from bcr-abl fusion gene was amplified by PCR using specific oligonucleotide primers. All 30 patient samples and 10 control samples were tested for the fusion using 1 µl 10 µM of F-BCR (N2) [ACCGCATGTTCCGGGACAAAAG] (0.5 µM), 1 µl 10 µM of R-ABL (N6) (0.5 µM), 0.5 µl 10 µM of F-actβ [TATGTGGGCGACGAGGCCCA] (0.25 µM), 0.5 µl 10 µM of R-actβ (0.25 µM) and 4 µl of cDNA sample were used in a final volume of 20 µl. Amplification includes initial denaturation for 4 min. at 94°C, then 35 cycles: each cycle consists of 94°C for 44 sec., 63°C for 30 sec. (according to primer manufacturer), and 72°C for 40 sec., final extension 72°C for 5 min. and then the reaction was hold at 4°C. The amplification products were analyzed on 2% of agarose gel stained with ethidium bromide and run at 90 V, 100 mA, 9 W for 90 min.

Results

Ten local healthy subjects were tested for hemoglobin (Hb), white blood cells (WBC), and platelet count and bcr-abl fusion gene. They included 6 males and 4 females; their age ranged 18-62 years. All showed normal ranges of Hb, WBC and platelet count [18] and they were negative for e1a2 and e1a3 fusion variants (Table 1). Results for 30 subjects diagnosed clinically as CML patients showed different Hb, WBC and platelet count (Table 2).

From the specific primer typing, the prevalence of the two studied fusion variants (e1a2 and e1a3) and their distribution among CML patients of Sulaimani province is shown in Table 3. The only variant detected with a primer set F-BCR (N2) and R-ABL (N6) was e1a3 variant 76.6% while e1a2 appeared in 0% of total patients.

Blood film of patients on diagnosis showed leukocytosis and a pathologic left shift [7] with the appearance of immature granulocytopoietic cells at all stages of differentiation including promyelocytes and myeloblasts [7]. Basophilia and eosinophilia were present in the peripheral blood and confirmed the diagnosis (Figures 1A and 1B) [9]. In addition, individual granulocytes showed qualitative changes such as anisocytosis [7].

No.	A	S	Hb* g/dL	WBC**×10³/µl	Plt.***×10³/µl	bcr-abl: e1a2, e1a3
1	21	M	14.8	5.0	166	-ve
2	34	M	14.3	6.2	265	-ve
3	56	M	15	7.2	304	-ve
4	18	M	16.4	7.0	293	-ve
5	46	F	13.6	6.2	224	-ve
6	62	F	12	5.2	228	-ve
7	33	F	12.3	6.6	234	-ve
8	26	M	14.1	8.5	448	-ve
9	12	M	12.5	7.3	294	-ve
10	19	F	13	5.8	374	-ve
M			13.8	6.5	283	

*: Normal range of Hb for female (12.0-16.0 g/dL)
*: Normal range of Hb for male (14.0-18.0 g/dL)
**: Normal range of WBC (4.3-10.0×10³ cells/ µl)
***: Normal range of platelet (140-440×10³ cells/ µl)
m: male; f: female; M: Mean; -ve: Negative

Table 1: Hb, WBC, platelet and bcr-abl fusion gene of control samples, those with normal CBC.

No.	A	S	Hb* g/dL	WBC**×103/ µl	Plt.***×103/ µl	bcr-abl: e1a3	Therapy
1	35	M	12.9	4.7	164	+ve	Glivec
2	46	F	10.4	6.2	477	+ve	Glivec
3	68	F	13.2	5.7	152	+ve	Glivec
4	54	M	13.8	6.5	148	+ve	Glivec
5	64	M	7.8	189	95	+ve	-
6	45	M	14	6.5	202	+ve	Glivec
7	53	F	13.3	4.5	175	-ve ★	Glivec
8	62	M	6.6	1.7	63	-ve ★	Glivec
9	42	F	8.9	122	126	+ve	-
10	35	M	15	7.0	242	+ve	Glivec
11	33	F	13.8	5.5	182	-ve ★	Glivec
12	52	M	11.4	5.8	140	-ve ★	Glivec
13	65	F	11.6	3.7	133	+ve	Glivec
14	57	F	12	5.6	149	+ve	Glivec
15	47	M	12.2	4.8	153	+ve	Glivec
16	54	F	11.3	9.7	284	+ve	Glivec
17	60	M	12.1	11.6	504	+ve	Glivec
18	45	F	10.3	8.3	500	+ve	Glivec
19	41	F	10.1	5.1	129	+ve	Glivec
20	65	M	12.8	7.4	255	+ve	Glivec
21	45	F	10.1	8.5	218	+ve	Glivec
22	58	F	10.9	7.7	128	+ve	Glivec
23	50	M	12.6	5.5	119	+ve	Glivec
24	52	F	12.5	6.5	21	+ve	Glivec
25	36	M	13.4	5.6	187	-ve ★	Glivec
26	51	M	11.2	6.3	145	-ve ★	Glivec
27	65	F	13	5.5	147	+ve	Glivec
28	47	M	14.2	6.5	212	+ve	Glivec
29	65	F	7.2	1.8	72	-ve ★	Glivec
30	50	F	11	5.8	143	+ve	Glivec

Table 2: Hb, WBC, platelet and bcr-abl fusion gene of those diagnosed clinically as CML patients.

Subjects	Number of Subjects	Ela 3 variant No. (%)	Ela 2 variant No. (%)	Negative Samples*
Males	14	10 (33.3)	0	4 (13.3)
Females	16	13 (43.3)	0	3 (10)
Total	30	(76,6)	0	7 (23.3)

*: No of Mutations For the two variants ela3 and ela2 was detected

Table 3: Distribution of bcr-abl fusion variants among 30 CML patients of Sulaimani province.

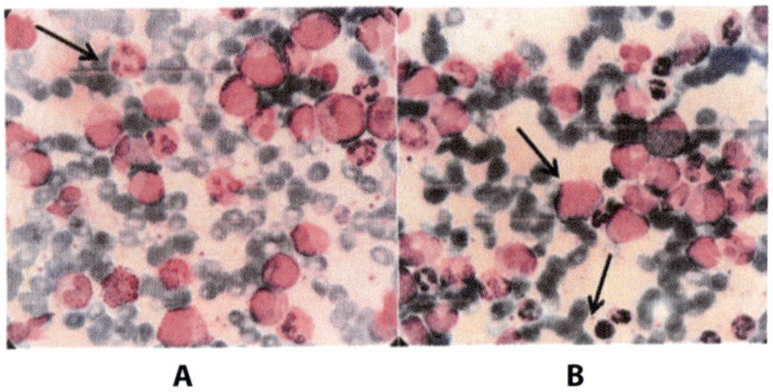

Figure 1: Agarose gel electrophoresis of BCR- ABL fusion gene in controls with IC .kb M: DNA ladder (2 kb); Lanes 1-6 PCR products of controls. 353 bp fragments are actβ (IC).

Discussion

Out of 30 patients, 2 were new cases and appeared to have leukocytosis [18], and they were positive for e1a3 fusion because they were newly diagnosed and they did not take CML treatment [2]. In this case, the hemoglobin and platelet of patients were decreased in favor of granulocytopoiesis [7]. The BCR-ABL negative cases that form 23.3% of total patients may have molecular remission or may be of other variants that occur between different exons of both genes and require specific primer set to diagnose. Out of 30 patients, two had leukocytopenia, low Hb, and platelet count and were negative for e1a2 and e1a3 fusion variants because they might take overdose of Glive. The other five negative cases have good prognosis, which means that they have response to Glivec and didn't contain a mutation that affect ATP binding site of ABL kinase [19].

Although the primers used in this research were also used by Rosline et al. [20] but they did not get e1a3 variant with respect to the 309 bp fragments produced (Figures 2 and 3). They rather got e1a2/ 481 bp (as they determined) by using the same primer set; however, the fusion was at different site, e1a2/ BCR exon1-ABL exon2 while e1a3/ BCR exon1-ABL exon3. This means that the reverse primer anneals with exon 3 of ABL gene.

Heterozygous detection is reliable by RT-PCR method; specific primer sets for normal bcr and abl loci are required as well as the used primer set for bcr-abl fusion gene [21]. Gene silencing that caused by alteration of the methylation pattern of DNA on the related chromosome leads to prevent transcription [22] but it does not affect its DNA detection.

Out of 30 clinically diagnosed CML patients, 7 were negative for the two variants. The seven negative subjects have appeared to be negative for the two variants studied and to confirm their negativity another primer set is required. So either they are other variants or they are negative due to imatinib treatment leading to affect their fusion gene detection [23].

CML is one of the most common human cancers, being present in high frequencies especially in countries with high radiation rate [24,25]. It is a common hematologic cancer worldwide especially in the regions after nuclear disaster [11]. More than 50 different point mutations in Abl kinase domain have been described [26]. However, many of these mutations are relatively rare, and the most common, affecting residues Gly250, Tyr253, Glu255, Thr315, Met351 and Phe359, account for 60–70% of all mutations [27]. With regard to the incidence, the frequency of CML by order is white, black, American Indian/ Alaska Native, Hispanic and Asian/ Pacific Islander respectively [28]. In north India the b3a2 BCR-ABL transcripts were most commonly detected (66.82%) followed by b2a2 (28.84%), b3a2+b2a2 (3.36%), b3a2+e19a2 (0.48%) and b2a2+e19a2 (0.48%) (29). In Pakistani patients, 64% expressed b3a2 while 36% expressed b2a2 transcript [29,30]. In Iran the majority of the patients express one of the p210 BCR-ABL transcripts (b3a2, 62% and b2a2, 20%), while the remaining showed one of the transcripts of b3a3, b2a3, e1a2 or co-expression of b3a2 and b2a2. The rate of co-expression of the b3a2 and b2a2 was 5% 29. In Turkey the most frequent type of transcriptions was p210 76%, p190 16.5% and p190 with p210 transcripts 7.5%. The most common type of p210 was b3a2 transcript (54%), p190 was e1a3+e1a2 (36%), p210+p190 was b3a2+e1a3 (40%), and b3a2+e1a3+e1a2 (40%) [31]. The prevalence of e1a3 is common (76.6%) in Sulaimani patients (Table 3). Sulaimani province mostly inhabited by Kurdish people and in general e1a3 is a common variant in Kurdish population of Sulaimani province.

The new cases appeared to have leukocytosis, with anemia and

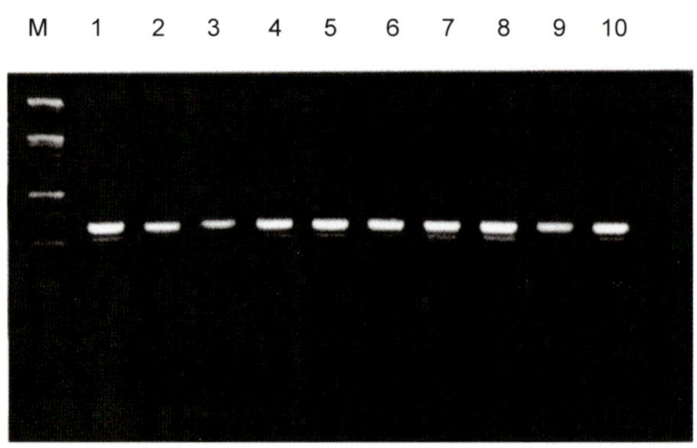

Figure 2: Agarose gel electrophoretic pattern of PCR amplification of BCR-ABL fusion gene in patients with internal control (IC). M: DNA ladder marker (2 kb); Lanes 1-10 amplification products of patients; BCR-ABL fusion gene Ela3 (309 bp) and internal control (353 bp).

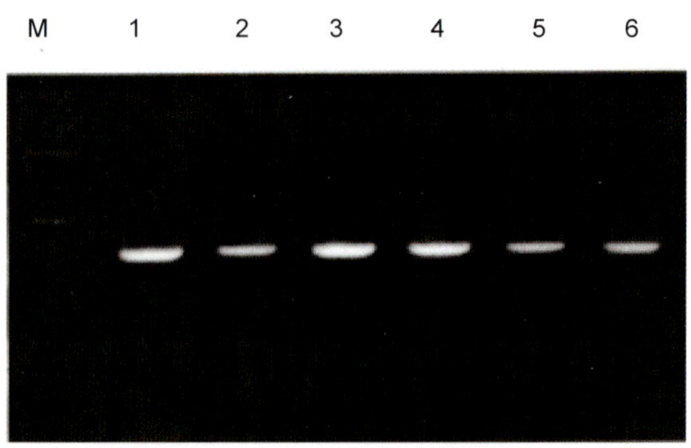

Figure 3: Agarose gel electrophoresis of BCR- ABL fusion gene in controls with IC .kb M: DNA ladder (2 kb); Lanes 1-6 PCR products of controls. 353 bp fragments are actβ (IC).

thrombocytopenia, in favor of granulocytopoiesis that dominated the cell picture [7]. In blastic phase, the blast cells were found in greater frequency, they were in excess of 20% of the circulating leukocytes [9,32]. During this phase, smears showed elevated number of blast cells that resulted from malignant transformation of bone marrow stem cells [5,32]. For those patients that have response to treatment, these cells were little or absent.

References

1. Timothy PH, David MR, Junia VM (2014) Handbook of Chronic Myeloid Leukemia, ISBN: 978-3-319-08350-6.
2. Schulz WA (2007) In Molecular Biology of Human Cancers. Dordrecht, Netherlands pp: 219-242.
3. Patel M, Philip V, Fazel F (2012) Human immunodeficiency virus infection and chronic myeloid leukemia. Leukemia Research 36: 1334-1338.
4. Macdonald F, Ford CH, Casson AG (2004) Molecular Biology of Cancer. Garland Science/ BIOS Scientific Publishers, United Kingdom, London.
5. George PR (2008) In Encyclopedia of Genetics, Genomics, Proteomics, and Informatics. 3rd ed. Springer. Columbia pp: 1097-1098.
6. Voncken JW, Van Schaick H, Kaartinen V (1995) Increased neutrophil respiratory burst in bcr-null mutants. Cell 80: 719-728.
7. Loffler H, Rastetter J, Haferlach T (2005) In Atlas of Clinical Hematology, 6th ed. Springer-Verlag. Berlin, Germany 144-145.
8. Baccarani M, Cortes J, Pane F, Niederwieser D (2009) European LeukemiaNet. Chronic myeloid leukemia: an update of concepts and management recommendations of European LeukemiaNet. J Clin Onco 27: 6041-6051.
9. Kantarjian H, Cortes J (2008) Chronic myeloid leukemia. In: Abeloff MD, Armitage JO, Niederhuber JE, editors. Abeloff's Clinical Oncology, 4th ed. Elsevier Churchill-Livingstone. Philadelphia, PA p: 107.
10. Provan D, Singer RJ, Baglin T, Lilleyman J (2004) Chronic myeloid leukemia. In Oxford Handbook of Clinical Haematology. 2nd ed. Oxford University Press. New York, USA pp: 164-165.
11. Melo JV (1997) BCR-ABL gene variants. In Bailliere's Clinical Hematology 10: 203-222.
12. Kantarjian H, O'Brien S (2011) The chronic leukemias. Chap 190, 24th ed. Saunders Elsevier, Philadelphia pp: 190.
13. Druker BJ, Talpaz M, Resta DJ (2001) Efficacy and safety of a specific inhibitor of the BCR-ABL tyrosine kinase in chronic myeloid leukemia. N Engl J Med 344: 1031-1037.
14. Buchdunger E, Matter A, Druker BJ (2001) Bcr-Abl inhibition as a modality of CML therapeutics. Biochim Biophys Acta 1551: 11-28.
15. Manuel S, Suresh GS, Bernice B (2003) Multiplex RT-PCR for the detection of leukemia-associated translocations: validation and application to routine molecular diagnostic practice 5: 231-236.
16. Bagg A (2001) Commentary: minimal residual disease: how low do we go? Mol Diagn 6: 155-160.
17. Suh SP, Kee SJ, Lim WH (2000) Multiplex in-cell RT-PCR for the simultaneous detection of p210 and p190 BCR-ABL mRNAs in chronic myeloid leukemia and Philadelphia- positive acute lymphoblastic leukemia cell lines. Clin Chem Lab Med 38: 939-944.
18. Bama CM, Aditi B, Sunipa M (2006) Molecular Profiling of Chronic Myeloid Leukemia in Eastern India. American Journal of Hematology 11: 845-849.
19. Theml H, Diem, Haferlach T (2004) Procedures, assays and normal values. Georg Thieme Verlag. Stuttgart, Germany pp: 12-13.
20. Rosline H, Majdan R, Wan ZA (2008) Real Time Polymerase Chain Reaction in Diagnosis of Chronic Myeloid Leukemia. APJMBB 16: 41-44.
21. Wolf-KH, Letetia CJ, Nathan AL (2002) Acute lymphoblastic leukemia resistant to the tyrosine kinase inhibitor STI571 has a unique BCR-ABL gene mutation. Blood 99: 1860-1862.
22. Diamond J, Goldman JM, Melo JV (1995) BCR-ABL, ABL-BCR, BCR, and ABL Genes Are All Expressed in Individual Granulocyte-Macrophage Colony-Forming Unit Colonies Derived From Blood of Patients With Chronic Myeloid Leukemia. Blood 85: 2171-2175.
23. Capdeville R, Buchdunger E, Zimmermann J, Matter AG (2002) Arationally developed, targeted anticancer drug. Nature Rev. Drug Discov 1: 493-502.
24. Sachs RK, Hlatky LR, Trask BJ (2000) Radiation-produced chromosome aberrations: colourful clues. Trends Genet 4: 143-146.
25. Obe G, Natarajan AT (2004) In Chromosome Aberrations. Günter Obe and Adyapalam T. Natarajan, Karger S editor. In Medical and Scientific Publishers. Basel, Switzerland 104: 393-394.
26. Rourmiantsev S, Shah NP, Gorre ME, Nicoll J (2002) Clinical resistance to the kinase inhibitor STI-571 in chronic myeloid leukemia by mutation of Tyr-253 in the ABL kinase domain P-loop. Proc Natl Acad Sci 99: 10700-10705.
27. Ellen W, Paul WM, Sandra WC, Andreas H, James DG (2007) Second generation inhibitors of BCR-ABL for the treatment of imatinib-resistant chronic myeloid leukemia. Nature Reviews 7: 345-356.
28. Howlader N, Noone AM, Krapcho M (2012) SEER Cancer Statistics Review: 1975-2010, National Cancer Institute.
29. Maninder SA, Neelam V, Subhash V, Kamer SR, Pankaj M, et al. (2012) Cytogenetic and molecular analyses in adult chronic myelogenous leukemia patients in north India. Indian J Med Res 135: 42-48.
30. Zafar I, Fatima M, Mudassar I (2011) Frequency of Bcr-Abl Fusion Oncogene Splice Variants Associated with Chronic Myeloid Leukemia. JCT 2: 176-180.
31. Marjan Y, Seyed HG, Ardashir G (2008) Frequency of BCR-ABL Fusion Transcripts in Iranian Patients with Chronic Myeloid Leukemia. Arch Iranian Med 11: 247-251.
32. Torsten H, Ulrike B, Wolfgang KS, Claudia H (2007) Diagnostic pathways in acute leukemias: a proposal for a multimodal approach. Ann Hematol 86: 311-327.

18

Association of Chronic Lymphocytic Leukemia and Acute Myeloid Leukemia in Three Patients: Cases with the Concomitant Presence of Two Different Malignant Clones

Mehmet Yilmaz[1], Salih Sertac Durusoy[2], Alperen Kizikli[3], Mahmut Yeral[4], Ilknur Kozanoglu[4], Salih Subari[3]*, Azer Abiyev[3] and Sibel Cangi[5]

[1]*SANKO University School of Medicine, Department of Hematology Gaziantep, Turkey*
[2]*Gaziantep University Department of Hematology, Gaziantep, Turkey*
[3]*Gaziantep University Department of Internal Medicine, Gaziantep, Turkey*
[4]*Baskent University School of Medicine Department of Hematology Adana, Turkey*
[5]*Gaziantep University Department of Pathology, Gaziantep, Turkey*

Abstract

In this report we present three patients who are 70, 50 and 55 years of ages with complaints of fatigue, pallor, weakness and epistaxis. The Peripheral Blood (PB) smear and bone marrow aspiration (BMA) showed circulating blast cells, lymphocytes, and smudge cells. In first and second cases flow cytometric (FC) analysis demonstrated that blasts were associated with co-expression of Chronic Lymphocytic Leukemia (CLL) and Acute Myeloid Leukemia (AML) immunophenotyping. In the third case Bone Marrow Biopsy (BMB) showed megaloblastic and dysplastic changes in eryhtroid, megakaryocytic and myeloid lineages. The concomitant occurrence of AML and CLL might be a common stem cell defect, a consequence of leukomogenic factors or a genetic predisposition in some patients. CLL development after the diagnosis of Myelodysplastic Syndrome (MDS) or AML was not reported in the literature. From this point of view this is the first case in the literature. Duration of the treatment, intensity and nature of the given agent might explain development AML but not CLL. However, CLL might have developed during the initial leukomogenic process of the disease. The two cases support the idea that AML and CLL might demonstrate two separate disease processes originating from abnormal different clones.

Keywords: Peripheral blood; Leukemia; Stem cell

Introduction

The coexistence of AML and CLL has occasionally been reported [1]. Most of these cases occur as a secondary event in patients receiving chemotherapy or radiotherapy [2]. CLL disease is known to be associated with immunoglobulin deficiencies and increases the risk of secondary malignancies [3]. In addition, CLL patients with co-existent solid tumors have been reported to develop MDS and AML. AML developed after CLL treatment is called therapy-related AML. Some AML patients are diagnosed concomitantly with CLL disease. The development of flow cytometry has increased the diagnosis of coexistence [4-8].

In this study we present 3 cases of CLL&AML and CLL&MDS/AML co-existences without previous exposure to cytotoxic, immunosuppressive drugs or radiation.

Case Presentations

Case 1

A 70-year-old male presented to our clinic with complaints of fatigue, pallor and weakness. On physical examination, 5 cm splenomegaly and 2 cm hepatomegaly were noted. Laboratory studies showed hemoglobin (Hb), 10.8 g/dL; white blood cell (WBC), 49×10^9/L; platelet count, (PLT) 58×10^9/L. The peripheral blood (PB) smear showed 60% circulating blast cells and 30% lymphocytes, with smudge cells. Bone marrow examination and flow cytometric analyses demonstrated that blasts expressed CD117, HLA-DR, CD13, CD33, MPO and lymphocytes showed a typical CLL immunophenotype which was CD5+CD19, CD20, CD22 positive; and CD200, CD10, CD23, CD25, FMC7 negative (Figure 1, Figure 2A and 2B). Polymerase chain reaction (PCR) assay, CLL cytogenetic studies, AML specific genetic abnormalities panel including t(8;21), t(15;17), inv(16), FLT3-

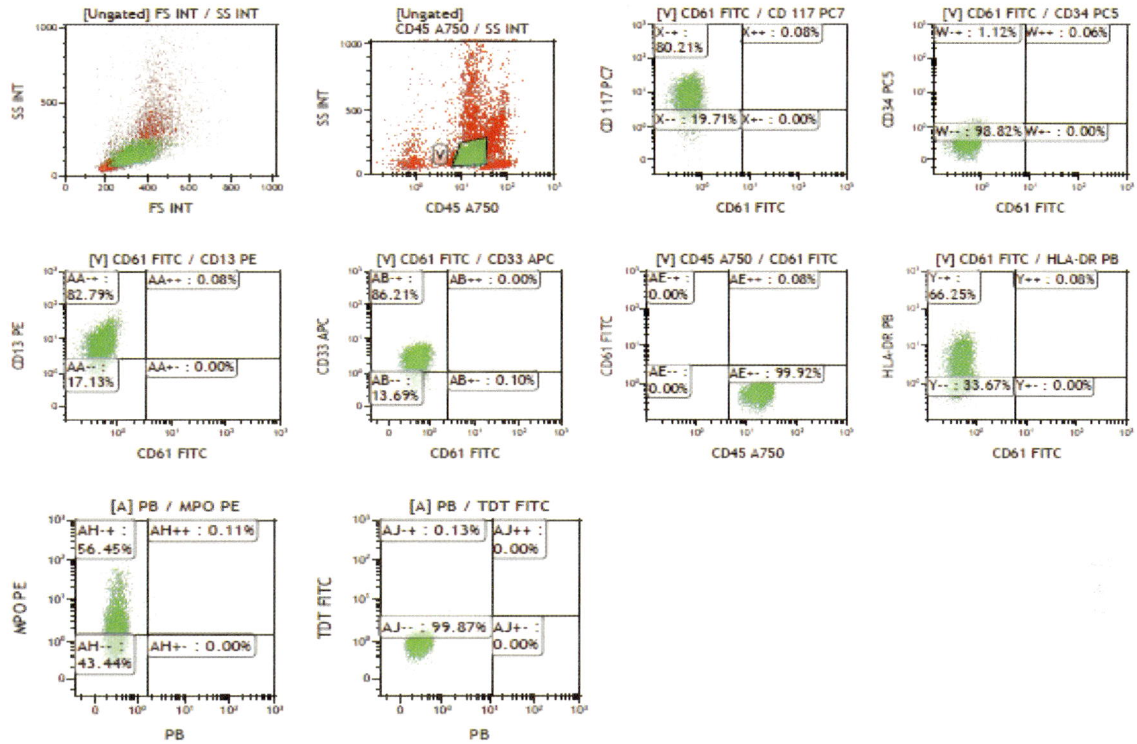

Figure 2A: Flow cytometric analysis of bone marrow demonstrated that blasts were characterized by the expression of CD117, HLA-DR, CD13, CD33, MPO.

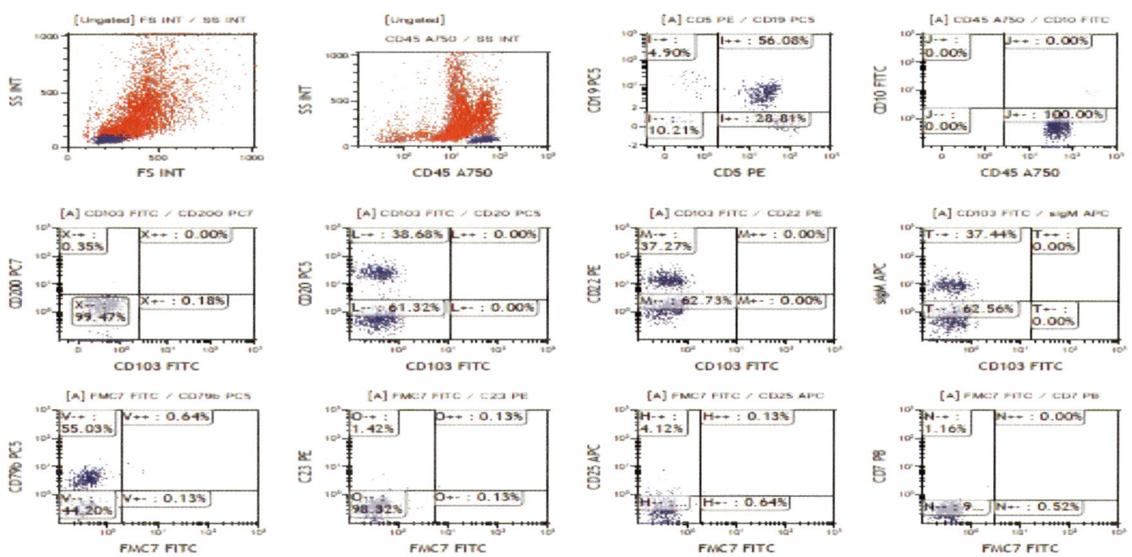

Figure 2B: Flow cytometric analysis of bone marrow lymphocytes were characterized by a typical CLL immunophenotype; CD5+CD19, CD20, CD22 positive; and CD200, CD10, CD23, CD25, FMC7 negative.

final diagnosis. Cytarabine and daunorubucin treatment (5+2) was administered. Remission was obtained after treatment. After that, dose adjusted FLAG (fludarabine + high-dose cytarabine + G-CSF) was given since FLAG is effective both AML and CLL clones. The aim was to consolidate AML and to eradicate CLL clones because of the agressive course of the disease. Examination of bone marrow aspiration, biopsy and peripheral blood smear after the second cycle of chemotherapy showed increased blast counts. A Hypometylating agent with low dose cytarabine treatment was planned. During the follow-up period patient developed pneumonia and heart failure. Treatment targeting heart failure and pneumonia was started. The patient responded the therapy, however refused further hypometylating agents and cytarabine therapy and unfortunately died 5 months after the diagnosis.

Case 2

A-50-year old female presented with weakness and epistaxis.

Laboratory studies showed Hb, 10.8 g/dL; WBC, 3.8 $\times 10^9$/L; PLT, 17 $\times 10^9$/L. The peripheral blood smear showed lymphocytes with smudge cells, normoblasts, and 35% circulating blasts. Bone marrow aspiration showed 32% blastic cells which expressed CD34, CD33, CD13, CD117, CD45, CD16 and 52% lymphocytes with positive CD45, CD5+CD19, CD20, CD23, CD200 and negative CD10 expression (Figure 3A and 3B, Figure 4A and 4B). Cytogenetic studies were negative for CLL and AML panels. PCR assays for AML specific genetic abnormalities such as t(8;21), t(15;17), inv (16), FLT3-ITD, FLT3D835 and NPM1 del(17) (p13.1), del(13)(q14.3), del(11) (q22.3) were negative. Patient classified as intermediate risk group for AML. Cytarabine and Idarubucin (7+3) treatment was administered. After this treatment, bone marrow aspiration and biopsy showed remission status, and Minimal residual disease (MRD) was negative. A fungal infection and retinal hemorrhage developed during the follow up period. After resolving of infection and retinal hemorrhage, allogeneic stem cell transplantation was performed from an HLA-matched sibling. Grade 1 graft versus host disease developed. On the 100th day chimerism was 99% and there was a CLL clone (20%, CD5+CD19, CD200 positivity). Cyclosporine was stopped at 6th month. The patient was in remission at 23th month of allogeneic hematopoietic stem cell transplant without treatment.

Case 3

A-55-year-old man was referred to our hospital with complaint of weakness. The laboratory studies showed Hb, 8.2 g/dL; WBC, 2.8 $\times 10^9$/L; PLT, 17 $\times$ 10^9/L. Serum vitamin B12 and folic acid levels were in normal range. The peripheral blood smear showed neutrophil hypersegmentation and blastic cells. On physical examination 3 cm splenomegaly was found. Bone marrow biopsy showed megaloblastic and dysplastic changes in erythroid, megakaryocytic and myeloid lineages. Besides, neoplastic small lymphocyte cluster in the middle of blastic myeloid area was seen. Percentage of myeloid blasts was 15%. The pathological diagnosis of bone marrow evaluation was a coexistence of AML/KLL diseases (Figure 5A-3C). Flow cytometric analysis revealed HLA-DR, CD13, CD33, GlyA, MPO positivity. Expression rates of CD117 were 15 % and CD34 was 6 %. CD5+CD19, CD20, CD22, CD23 and CD200 were negative (Figure 6A). Diagnosis of MDS with excess blasts was considered. Decitabine treatment was started. After 4 cycles of decitabine, bone marrow aspiration and biopsy were remade. CD34, CD117, MPO were positive and blast cell number was around 30%. Lymphocytic cells activity increased at around 35%. In the concurrent flow cytometry result, the analysis of HLA-DR, CD5+CD19, CD20,

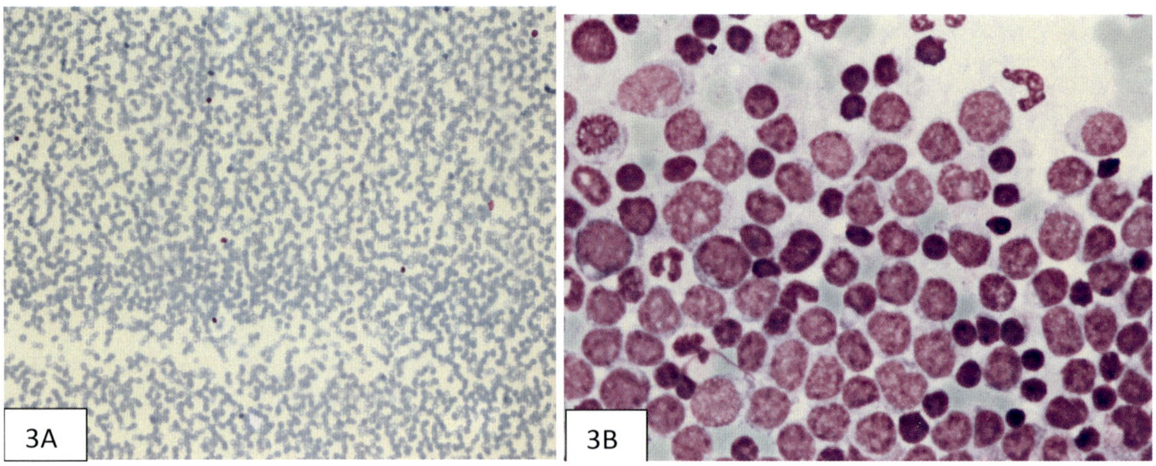

Figure 3: A. Mature apparent lymphocytes, normoblast, and circulating blasts in peripheral blood with Giemsa staining **B.** Blastic cells (32%) which are expressed CD34, CD33, CD13, CD117 CD45, CD16 and lymphocytes (52%) CD45, CD5, CD19, CD20, CD23, CD200 positivity and negative for CD10 in bone marrow.

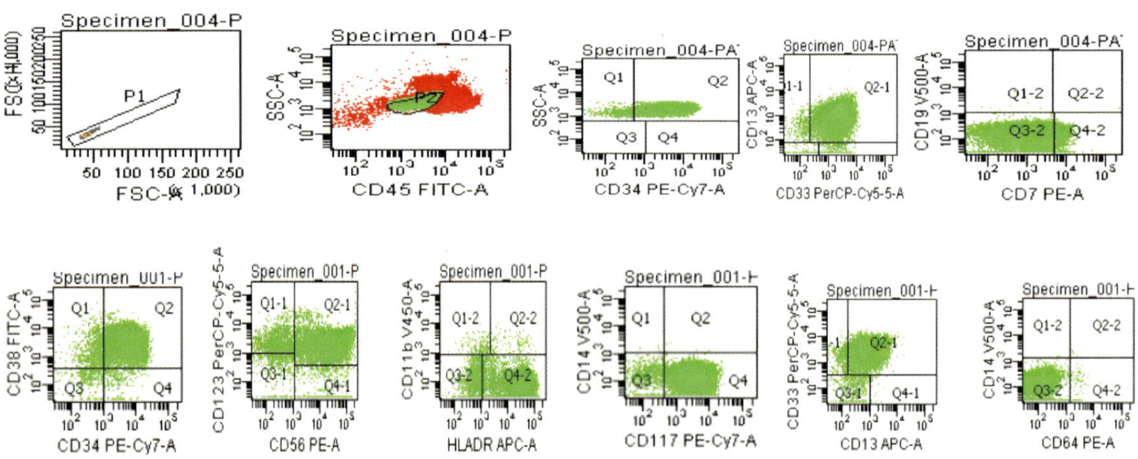

Figure 4A: Flow cytometric analysis of bone marrow aspiration showed blastic cells which are expressed CD34, CD33, CD13, CD117 CD45, CD56.

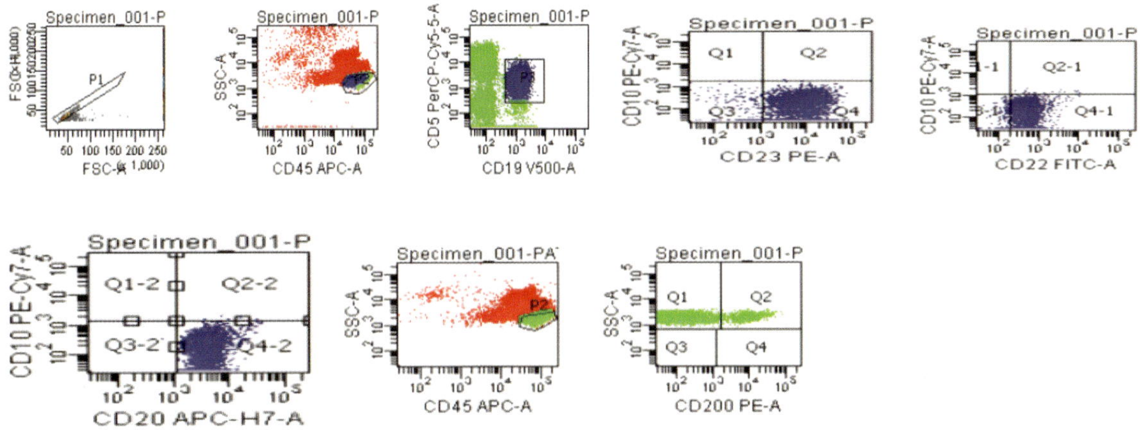

Figure 4B: Flow cytometric analysis of bone marrow aspiration showed lymphocytes which are expressed CD45, CD5+CD19, CD20, CD23, CD200 positivity and negative for CD10.

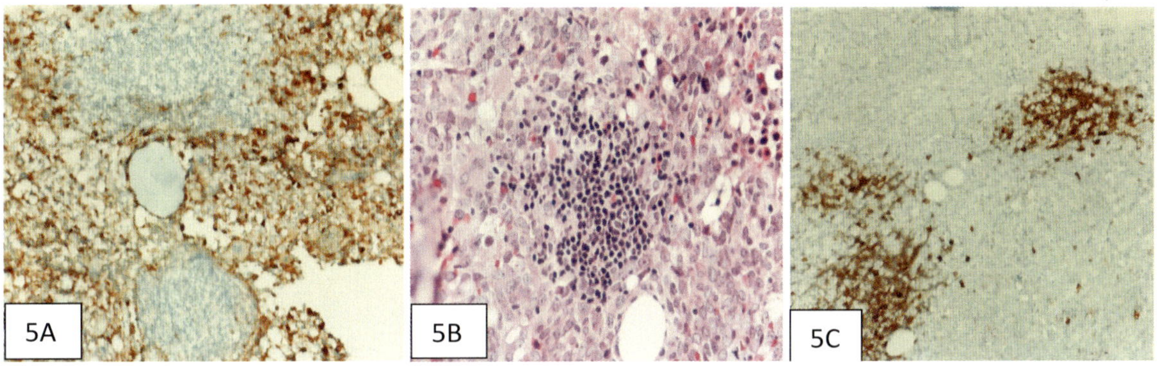

Figure 5: Bone marrow sampling A. Myeloid cells are (+) with MPO immunostaining (x200), B. Neoplastic small lymphocyte cluster in the middle of blastic myeloid area (x400, H-E), C. Lymphoid cells are (+) with CD20 immunostaining (x200).

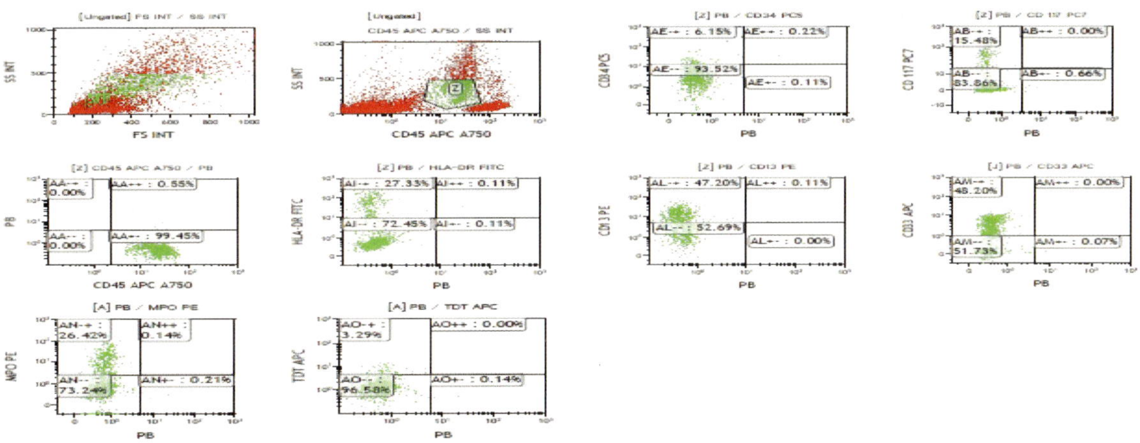

Figure 6A: Flow cytometric analysis of bone marrow aspiration revealed that HLA-DR, CD13, CD33, GlyA, MPO positivity and expression rate of CD117 15 %, CD34 %6. There was no positivity of CD5+19, CD20, CD22, CD23 and CD200.

CD22 were positive (Figure 6B). PCR assays for AML and CLL specific genetic abnormalities which were t(8;21), t(15;17), inv(16), FLT3-ITD, FLT3D835 NPM1, del(17)(p13.1), del(13)(q14.3), del(11)(q22.3), and centromere 12 were negative. Cytarabine and mitoxantrone (7+3) treatment was started. After cytarabine and mitoxantrone regimen control bone marrow aspiration and biopsy showed partial remission with 12% percent of blasts. FLAG regimen was applied to eradicate CLL clone. After the second FLAG regimen neutropenic fever and pneumonia developed and could not be controlled by antibiotics and supportive treatment. The patient died after 14 months of the diagnosis.

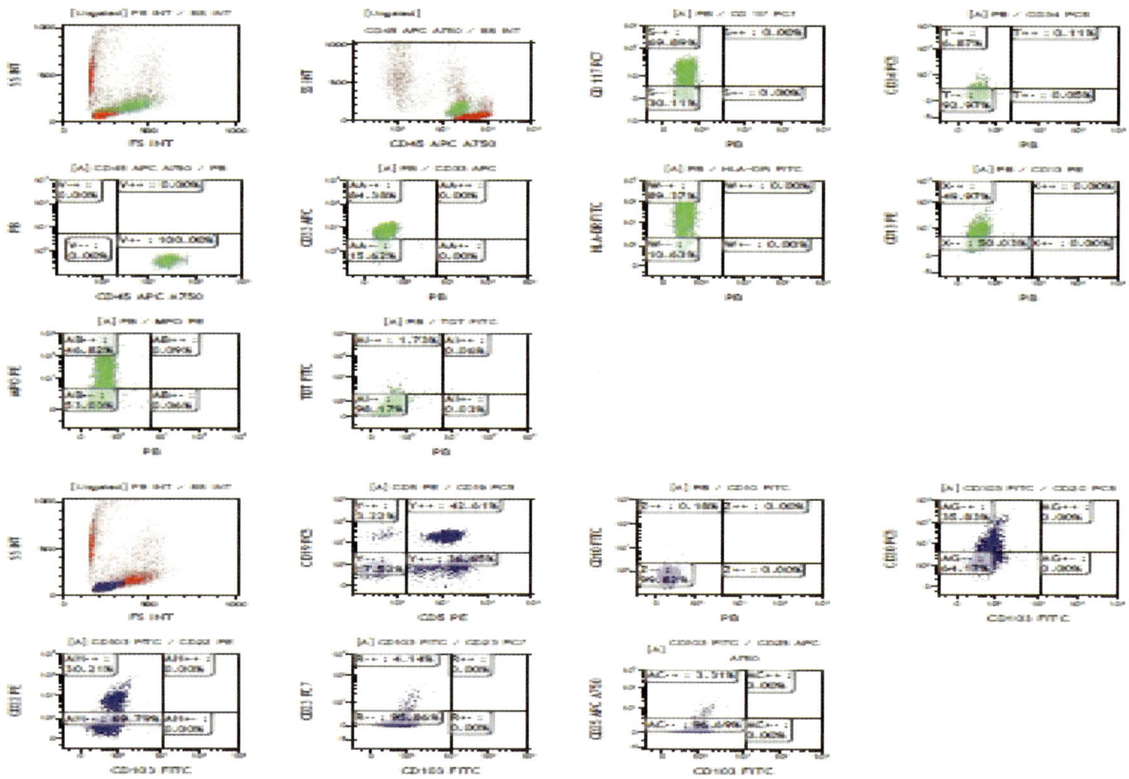

Figure 6B: Flow cytometric analysis of bone marrow aspiration showed, CD117, MPO were positive and Lymphocytic cells activity increased at around %35.In the concurrent flow cytometry result, the analysis of lymphocytes showed HLA-DR, CD5+CD19, CD20, CD22 positivity.

Discussion

The association of AML and CLL has previously been reported. AML is considered to develop as a secondary leukemia after CLL treatment likewise that after having given alkylating agents particularly chlorambucil, melphelan, nitrosureas and radiotherapy [9]. In the present study history of the patients did not reveal any known leukomogenic drug, radiotherapy and CLL treatment exposure before the diagnosis MDS and AML. Acute myeloblastic leukemia and CLL, which are two different and unrelated malignancies, have occasionally been diagnosed simultaneously in treatment-naive patients. AML is about 10 to 50 times more frequent in CLL patients than in the age-matched general population. In one report, eleven patients developed AML during the course of untreated CLL, whereas AML and CLL were diagnosed concomitantly in 16 patients [10]. The concomitant occurrence of AML and CLL might stem from a common stem cell defect, leukomogenic factors or from a genetic predisposition in some patients. We found no cytogenetic abnormalities in our cases; however, Hematopoietic Stem Cells (HSCs) with multiple genetic abnormalities might have caused the development of several myeloid and lymphoid progenitors that consequently turned into leukemic stem cells. Recently it was reported that CLL cells did not originate from differentiated mature lymphocytes but rather from primitive HSC [11]. Aberrant Wnt signaling is observed in both CLL and AML patients and might play a role in transforming pre-leukemic stem cells into the leukemic stem cells [12]. Our cases support the idea that AML and CLL might demonstrate two separate disease processes, which is CLL originates from abnormal CD5+CD19 positive lymphoid clone whereas AML originates from myeloid from CD34, CD117, CD13, CD33, and MPO positive myeloid clone. Lu CM et al. showed that in a patient AML and CLL developed from different clones [13]. We only showed immunophenotypic features of AML and CLL were different. This phenotypic difference does not rule out a possibility that two clones might be related. Kikushige et al. reported that the tendency to generate clonal B cells had already been acquired at the HSC stage in CLL patients [11]. In this setting, HSCs might be considered as the critical cellular target in the oncogenic process. This is an arguable subject that needs to be elucidated.

Most cases have been diagnosed based on morphology and cytochemical evidence. Both methods have questionable limitations. After the development of multi-color flow cytometric analysis elucidation of different malignant clones became evident [8]. Common usage of cytometric analysis might reveal greater incidence than expected especially in elderly patients with a low number of monoclonal lymphocytes. In the patient, we tried to treat the AML clone at the beginning. We observed remission in both AML and CLL clones. However, after the second cycle with dose-adjusted FLAG regimen relapse occurred. This might be explained by advanced age due possibly to developing genetic abnormalities. In the second case allogeneic stem cell transplantation was performed from HLA-matched sibling. At least 27 months after transplantation patient is alive and has complete hematologic cytogenetical remission for AML and CLL. Regarding the allogeneic stem cell transplantation limited number of transplanted patients has been reported and optimal transplant time is unclear [14]. If adverse prognosis is considered allogeneic stem cell transplantation might be the best option in transplant-eligible patient who are under 60 years old. Such patients should be transplanted after remission is obtained. It is questionable to perform allogeneic stem cell transplantation to obtain a remission for both AML and CLL clones. It seems reasonable to achieve remission for AML clone after performing allogeneic transplantation because of the aggressive course of the disease. Prospective studies are needed to prove this hypothesis. The third case showed 15% of blastic cells and was diagnosed as MDS with excess blast type II, however after 4 cycles of decitabine treatment transforming to AML and CLL was noticed. CLL development after the diagnosis of MDS or AML was not found in the literature. This is the first case from this point of view. It might be questionable that AML developed after administration of decitabine. The nature, duration and intensity of the treatment might explain the development AML but not CLL. CLL might have developed during the initial leukomogenic process of the disease.

As a conclusion, we reported 3 cases presented concomitant AML and CLL diseases, which have no exposure to radiation and cytotoxic agents. These cases support the idea that AML and CLL might demonstrate two separate disease processes originating from abnormal different clones. Allogeneic transplant should be an option in transplant eligible patient.

Disclosure

The authors have no relevant conflicts of interest to disclose.

References

1. Gottardi M, Valter G, Degan M, Bomben R, Zucchetto A, et al. (2006) Concomitant chronic lymphocytic leukemia andacute myeloid leukemia: Evidence of simultaneousexpansion of two independent clones. Leuk Lymphoma 5: 885-889.
2. Stern N, Shemesh J, Ramot B (1981) chronic lymphocytic leukemia terminating in acute myeloid leukemia: review of the literature. Cancer 47: 1849-1851.
3. Royle JA, Baade PD, Joske D, Girschik J, Fritschi L (2011) Second cancer incidence and cancer mortality among chronic lymphocytic leukemia patients: a population based study. Br J Cancer 105: 1076-1081.
4. Tambaro FP, Garcia-Manero G, O'Brien SM, Faderl SH, Ferrajoli A, et al. (2016) Outcomes for patients with chronic lymphocytic leukemia and acute leukemia or myelodysplastic syndrome. Leukemia 30: 325-330.
5. Hamilton PJ (1976) Concomitant myeloblastic and lymphocytic leukemia. Lancet 14: 373.
6. Hull MT, Griep JA (1980) Mixed leukemia lymphoid and myelomonocytic. Am J Clin Pathol 74: 473-475.
7. Conlan MG, Mosher DF (1989) Concomitant chronic lymphocytic leukemia, acute myeloid leukemia, and thrombosis with protein C deficiency. Case report and review of the literature. Cancer 63: 1398-1401.
8. Tamul KR Meyers DC, Bentley SA, Folds JD (1994) Two color flow cytometric analysis of concomitant acute myeloid leukemia and chronic lymphocytic leukemia. Cytometry 18: 30-34.
9. Rund D, Ben-Yehuda D (2004) Therapy related leukemia and myelodisplasia: evolving concepts of pathogenesis and treatment. Hematology 9: 179-187.
10. Ito S, Fujiwara SI, Mashima K, Umino K, Minakata D, et al. (2017) Development of acute myeloid leukemia in patients with untreated chronic lymphocytic leukemia. Ann Hematol 96: 719-724.
11. Kikushige Y, Miyamoto T (2014) Hematopoetic stem cell aging and chronic lymphocytic leukemia pathogenesis. Int J Hematol 4; 335-340.
12. Staal FJ, Famili F, Garcia Perez L, Pike-Overzet K (2016) Abberant Wnt Signaling in leukemia. Cancers 8:78.
13. Lu CM, Murata-Collins JL, Wang E, Siddiqi I, Lawrence H (2006) Concurrent acute myeloid leukemia with inv(16)(p13.1q22) and chronic lymphocytic leukemia: molecular evidence of two separate diseases. Am J Hematol 12: 963-968
14. DeFilipp Z, Huynh DV, Fazal, S, Sahovic E (2012) Allogeneic stem cell transplantation for acute myeloid leukemia with del (7q) following untreated chronic lymphocytic leukemia. Hematol Oncol Stem Cell Ther 5: 165-168.

Genetic Heterogeneity and Clonal Evolution of Tumor Cells and their Impact on Precision Cancer Medicine

Hatem E Sabaawy[1-3*]

[1]Department of Medicine, Rutgers-Robert Wood Johnson Medical School, USA

[2]Department of Cellular and Molecular Pharmacology, Rutgers-Robert Wood Johnson Medical School, USA

[3]Rutgers Cancer Institute of New Jersey, New Brunswick, NJ 08903-2681, USA

Abstract

The efficacy of targeted therapies in leukemias and solid tumors depends upon the accurate detection and sustained targeting of initial and evolving driver mutations and/or aberrations in cancer cells. Tumor clonal evolution of the diverse populations of cancer cells during cancer progression contributes to the longitudinal variations of clonal, morphological, anatomical, and molecular heterogeneity of tumors. Moreover, drug-resistant subclones present at initiation of therapy or emerging as a result of targeted therapies represent major challenges for achieving success of personalized therapies in providing meaningful improvement in cancer survival rates. Here, I briefly portray tumor cell clonal evolution at the cellular and molecular levels, and present the multiple types of genetic heterogeneity in tumors, with a focus on their impact on the implementation of personalized or precision cancer medicine.

Keywords: Genetic heterogeneity; Clonal evolution; Precision medicine

Introduction

The lifetime risk of a clinical cancer diagnosis in humans is around one in three, with more than 10 million cases diagnosed each year [1]. The oldest description of cancer dates back to Ancient Egypt around 1600 BC when a number of breast cancer patients were described to be surgically treated by cauterization. Since then, surgical resection and adjuvant therapy can cure well-confined primary tumors, however, metastatic disease is largely incurable because of its systemic nature and resistance to existing therapies. Currently, cancer is a leading cause of death globally, and more than 90% of mortality from cancer is attributable to metastasis, not the primary tumors from which these lesions arise. In the case of leukemias, once leukemic cells are less confined to the bone marrow or the thymus, and are found in the peripheral blood, the disease is already a systemic disease. Despite the significant investment in cancer research and clinical trials over several decades around the world and in the US, especially after enabling the National Cancer Act in 1971, only few targeted therapies in leukemias and some solid tumors deemed therapeutically effective in phase III trials, and most current advanced cancer therapies have marginal improvement in survival. A better understanding of tumor development and better classification of tumor types at the cellular and genetic levels might provide improved strategies to suppress progression of prenoplastic lesion towards the malignant and the metastatic state(s) and offer more specific targets for drug development that would lead to more effective and personalized cancer therapy.

It has been known that a large number of patients treated for cancer don't respond to therapy given to them. This indicates that every drug does not work similarly in every patient, given that every patient has a unique biology and unique tumor architectures. These variations should be reflected in their choice of therapy to improve efficacy and minimize side effects. Several molecular mechanisms have been implicated in the development of neoplastic lesions and therapy resistance, and novel targeted agents to treat these neoplasms after diagnosis and/or relapse have been developed. However, variable efficacy has been observed in late-stage clinical trials, most likely because of the lack of complete understanding of the tumor development process and the biological heterogeneity of these tumors. The key response to the long-term disappointments in the fight against cancer must be revolutionary and lies in implementation of personalized or precision medicine where cancer therapy is tailored to each patient's biology and tumor signatures to achieve the best medicinal outcome for that individual.

Precision cancer medicine traditionally involves determining the biological status of an individual tumor before therapy by assessing genetic signatures, hormone metabolism, and signaling activity, and then directing tailored treatment accordingly. The recent surge in Next Generation Sequencing (NGS) of cancer genomes has supported the expansion of molecular cancer profiling to support precision cancer medicine. However, translation of these genetic and metabolic findings into clinically valuable genetic, epigenetic, proteomic, biochemical, metabolic and imaging biomarkers for diagnosis, prognosis, and response to therapy is an extended intricate process that remains critical for the wide implementation of precision medicine in cancer therapy. The remaining central challenges for this approach include selection of optimal drug targets, evaluation of genetic profiles and genetic interactions, determining proper combinations of therapies, implementing clinical platforms in phase I studies, and resolving the organizational, commercial, regulatory, and societal challenges facing these precision cancer medicine approaches. To name a few, organizational challenges include structure and administration of personalized clinical trials, commercial concepts of personalized therapy such as pay for performance of multiple tailored treatments replacing blockbuster drugs, regulatory evaluation of outcome of personalized medicine, ethical considerations of genetic testing,

***Corresponding author:** Sabaawy HE, M.D., Ph.D. Rutgers Cancer Institute of New Jersey, 195 Little Albany Street, Room 4557, New Brunswick, NJ 08903-2681, USA, E-mail: sabaawhe@cinj.rutgers.edu and level of acceptance of cancer patients to the new paradigm of personalized medicine studies. Ultimately, a better understanding of the tumor and metastatic developmental process, and an optimum design of targeted tailored therapies are instrumental in the success of precision cancer medicine. Two concepts have recently gained a great deal of attention, and remain at the center stage of our understanding of tumor development for designing better-tailored therapies; these are tumor cell clonal evolution and tumor heterogeneity.

Tumor Cell Clonal Evolution

NGS for cancer samples is now widely accessible, increasingly affordable, and provides a transformative influence on cancer care with a particular insight into the complexity of the cancer genome [2]. With it, we came to realize the true meaning of the statement that cancer is a disease of the genome. Neoplasms in general represent abnormal outgrowth of tumor cells that gain selective advantages in cell growth, survival, and metabolism. Their sustained growth kinetics lead to the formation of dominant neoplastic clones that compete with, and override normal and preneoplastic cells for space, energy, and nutrient requirements utilizing their genetic and non-genetic drivers for selective advantage. Sequencing of genomes from tumor cells within these clones revealed that tumors have partially or fully transformed cells that harbor hundreds to thousands of genetic mutations, chromosomal alterations, and epigenetic aberrations. The majority of these mutations represents neutral (passenger) mutations, while the selection and propagation of dominant clones of tumor cells that ultimately lead to malignant transformation are both successively and may be independently sustained by multiple different combinations of driver mutations. The orchestrated and sustained signaling actions of these driver mutations during the process of clonal evolution provide, at each stage, a selection advantage, and allow dominant tumor cell clones to finally control various interactions with microenvirmental clues at the eminent stages of tumor development (Figure 1) [3,4]. Intrinsic changes in Tumor Initiating Cells (TICs) result partially from ineffective DNA repair mechanisms [5] and deregulated stem cell differentiation signals [6]. The repertoire of these intrinsic changes in preneoplastic TICs confers neoplastic features of uncontrolled proliferation, unlimited self-renewal, sustained angiogenesis, abnormal differentiation, and tissue invasion and metastasis making hallmarks of cancer [3]. These mutations act as drivers for transformation of cells primed with genetic and epigenetic changes to form preleukemic clones. The preleukemic clones proceed in evolution with additional mutations and clonal selection causing occult leukemias and solid tumors [7-9]. Sequencing studies revealed about 140 genes that when altered by intragenic mutations can act as driver mutations during tumorigenesis [10]. A typical tumor contains two to eight driver mutations, while the remaining are passenger mutations that do not directly confer selective advantages [10], but might play critical roles in orchestrating the genetic interactions between driver mutations and the microenvironment towards tumor progression. The numbers of driver and passenger mutations that were revealed by sequencing vary among tumor types and even from patient to patient. Genome sequencing studies have also found that pediatric leukemias harbor on average 9.6 mutations per tumor, while melanomas and lung cancer might harbor more than 200 mutations per tumor [10]. The latter might reflect effects of environmental factors such as smoking and UV radiation that play significant roles in the etiology of lung cancer and melanomas, respectively.

It is believed that leukemia and neoplasms in general are abnormal outgrowth from a TIC(s) whose progeny sequentially accumulate nested genetic and epigenetic mutations in cancer genes, over an extended period of time during clonal evolution [11], that generate cellular diversity [12] and clonal expansion [13-15]. TICs are the cellular drivers of clonal expansion that can predict aggressive disease, and the TICs stem cell signature was shown to influence leukemia clinical outcome [16]. TICs (sometimes referred to as Cancer Stem Cells (CSCs), however, the CSCs term may only be used when self-renewal potential is a recognized feature of the described cell type, i.e. some TICs may not be self-renewing stem cells) were initially revealed through transplantation of subfractions of leukemic cells in mice [17]. While the existence of CSCs is human tumors is still contentious, the evidence for a central role of TICs in tumor development and resistance to therapy was recently solidified by lineage tracing studies in mice [18-20]. Longitudinal tracking of single cell-derived tumor cell clonal formation and monitoring of tumor development from TICs are unfeasible at the current level of knowledge. Therefore, there has been no consensus on the frequencies of TICs in the same tumor types and whether they are rare or frequent cells within each tumor. Understandably, the frequencies of TICs are most likely dynamic variables that reflect changes during the different phases of each tumor growth and also in response to changes in the tumor microenvironment [21,22].

In addition to genetic drivers, non-genetic drivers of clonal tumor cell selection during clonal evolution are also recognized, and among them are activation of alternative signaling, cell quiescence and epigenetic drivers. The first of these non-genetic drivers of formation of dominant clones during clonal evolution include the activation of alternative or downstream signaling pathway through signaling plasticity to achieve growth advantage or resistance to targeted therapy, a phenomenon termed oncogenic bypass [23]. Additional mechanisms of selection and drug resistance that are developed by TICs during clonal evolution of therapy resistance clones include cell quiescence of tumor stem cells [24], whereas these cells remain dormant awaiting further activating signals. Cell quiescence or cell dormancy is a mechanism also employed by disseminated tumor cells that shed from primary tumors and may lie dormant in distant tissues for long periods of time while retaining their potential for clonal activation resulting in metastatic growth [25]. Epigenetic changes affecting DNA methylation or chromatin proteins are likely to exert major influences on clonal evolution by mediating abnormal DNA methylation, histone modifications and/or nucleosome remodeling [26]. Cancer epigenome revealed simultaneous global losses and abnormal gains in DNA methylation. The rates of these epigenetic changes are estimated to be significantly higher than gene mutations [27]. However, unlike genetic changes in the DNA, DNA methylation varies between different cell types, developmental stages, and with aging [28]. Moreover, criteria for distinguishing epigenetic changes that would represent driver changes and provide selective advantages during clonal evolution are less established. Additionally, targeting epigenetic drivers with current and future epigenetic cancer therapy depends on adjusting treatment concepts towards dose optimization to avoid widespread toxicities [29]. The progression of clonal evolution of cancer, driven by genetic and non-genetic drivers from frequent preneoplastic lesions, is a highly inefficient process, and is frequently aborted before formation of occult malignancies [30]. When genetic sequences from multiple subclones were compared using single cell sequencing, the branched clonal structures of these cancers were revealed [31]. Furthermore, the evolutionary relationship and clonal architecture of Acute Lymphoblastic Leukemia (ALL) examined in stem cell populations demonstrated repeated independent copy number alteration within the same leukemic tumors [32]. Evidence for clonal evolution from ancestral clones was revealed earlier in non-

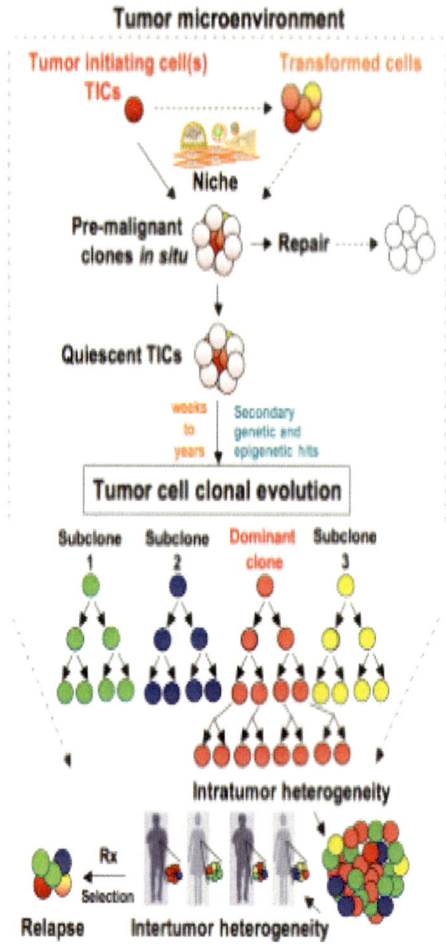

Figure 1: **Tumor intiating cells, tumor cell clonal evolution, and tumor heterogeneity**. A simplified diagram displaying the different tumor evolution processes under review. Within the tumor microenvironment, Tumor intiating cells (TICs) initiate premalignant clones through the interactions with the niche cells. The premalignant clones may generate frequent sublinical lesions such as carcinoma in situ (or preleukemic conditions) that are either in most cases repaired at the cellular levels through cell death mechanisms, and at the genetic levels through DNA repair of driver genetic mutations. The premalignant clones may alternatively remain harboring quiescent TICs that can then undergo tumor cell differentiation and/or plasticity within the competitive clonal evolution process to compete for space, nutrients, and proximity to vascular supply. Acquisition of secondary genetic and epigenetic changes in TICs or supportive tumor cells that favor enhanced self-renewal and clonal growth allows premalignant lesions to become a clinically diagnosed malignancy. This tumor evolution process can take from weeks to several years or even decades depending on the tumor type and the the host genetic and enviromental exposure factors. TICs are the units of clonal evolution and their diversity seed the recently identified tumor heterogeneity within each tumor (intratumor heterogeneity) (represented by a dominant clone in red, and three additional subclones in green, blue and yellow in the model). I proposed one dominat clone and three subclones for simplicity. Indeed, the frequency of subclones can be unlimited and dependes on the sensetivity of the detection assays. Neverthless, only detectable clones are thought to have clinical implications. Genetic and phenotypic variations are also detected between individuals with the same tumor type (Intertumor heterogeneity), and occur due to the diversity of clones generated during tumor cell clonal evolution. Upon treatment (Rx), relapse might occur from the diagnostic dominant clone that acquired more selective and drug resistance features, or from sublones that have acquired or inherited resistance to therapy. Therefore, detecting clonal heterogeneity and mechanisms of development of therapy resistant clones is critical for tailoring combination therapies for personalized cancer medicine. Solid arrows indicate defined pathways while dashed arrows indicate suggested mechanisms.

Hodgkin's lymphoma [33], and more recently in BCR-ABL1 ALL [34], ALL in twins [32], T-cell ALL [35], and during leukemic relapse [36]. Therefore, mapping and targeting tumor clones without driving additional clonal evolution and/or development of resistant clones is an optimum goal for cancer therapy.

Tumor Heterogeneity

Tumor heterogeneity is recently recognized in leukemias and solid tumors [37], and is attributed to multiple levels of heterogeneity at the cellular, molecular, genetic, and therapeutic response levels. Variations between tumors arising at the same site accounts for intertumoral heterogeneity, while variations in clonal growth, functional properties or expression markers delineate intratumoral heterogeneity. Genetic heterogeneity between different tumor clones and even within the same clones is a common feature in many tumor types [38]. Moreover, cells within single genetic clones were deemed to display functional variability in tumor propagation potential when single lentivirus-marked lineages were examined for copy number alterations, sequencing, and lentiviral lineage tracking [39]. This study revealed another layer of functional complexity beyond the genetic heterogeneity that drives the intratumoral heterogeneity, and might define responses to therapy (Figure 1).

The recognition that driver mutations frequently encode protein kinases has led the recent use of EGFR inhibitors [40], ALK inhibitors [41], BRAF inhibitors [42], and PARP inhibitors [43] in cancers that are proven to harbor these mutations, or their signaling pathway such as BRCA gene mutations in the case of PARP inhibitors. Combination therapy utilizing these and other newer drugs that target multiple components of driver signaling pathways should be tailored to fit the genetic interactions [44] within individual genomic repertoire of each patient in personalized or precision medicine approach. Alternative approaches may target the TICs, the microenvironment, or to keep tumors clinically manageable without selection of resistance clones utilizing modified dosing regimen and intermittent therapy. Addressing the key challenges of defining the order of events during tumor progression, the roles of driver and/or passenger mutations in clonal selection and heterogeneity, and mechanisms of development of therapy resistant clones will lead to significant advances in cancer care.

Acknowledgement

The work of the author is supported by the New Jersey Commission on Cancer Research, Department of Defense Congressionally directed Medical Research Program (Synergy award PC111595), and National Institutes of Health (NIH) under grant number P30CA072720 (PI: R. DiPaola) and Department of Defense (DOD), grant number W81XWH-12-1-0249 (PI: H. Sabaawy).

References

1. Siegel R, Naishadham D, Jemal A (2013) Cancer statistics, 2013. CA Cancer J Clin 63: 11-30.
2. Stratton MR (2011) Exploring the genomes of cancer cells: progress and promise. Science 331: 1553-1558.
3. Hanahan D, Weinberg RA (2011) Hallmarks of cancer: the next generation. Cell 144: 646-674.
4. Gatenby RA, Gillies RJ (2008) A microenvironmental model of carcinogenesis. Nat Rev Cancer 8: 56-61.
5. Illingworth CJ, Mustonen V (2011) Distinguishing driver and passenger mutations in an evolutionary history categorized by interference. Genetics 189: 989-1000.
6. Knoblich JA (2008) Mechanisms of asymmetric stem cell division. Cell 132: 583-597.
7. Sabaawy HE, Azuma M, Embree LJ, Tsai HJ, Starost MF, et al. (2006) TEL-AML1 transgenic zebrafish model of precursor B cell acute lymphoblastic leukemia. Proc Natl Acad Sci U S A 103: 15166-15171.

8. Quijano CA, Moore D 2nd, Arthur D, Feusner J, Winter SS, et al. (1997) Cytogenetically aberrant cells are present in the CD34+CD33-38-19- marrow compartment in children with acute lymphoblastic leukemia. Leukemia 11: 1508-1515.

9. Greaves MF (1986) Differentiation-linked leukemogenesis in lymphocytes. Science 234: 697-704.

10. Vogelstein B, Papadopoulos N, Velculescu VE, Zhou S, Diaz LA Jr, et al. (2013) Cancer genome landscapes. Science 339: 1546-1558.

11. Greaves M, Maley CC (2012) Clonal evolution in cancer. Nature 481: 306-313.

12. González-García I, Solé RV, Costa J (2002) Metapopulation dynamics and spatial heterogeneity in cancer. Proc Natl Acad Sci U S A 99: 13085-13089.

13. Nowell PC (1976) The clonal evolution of tumor cell populations. Science 194: 23-28.

14. Sieber OM, Heinimann K, Tomlinson IP (2003) Genomic instability--the engine of tumorigenesis? Nat Rev Cancer 3: 701-708.

15. Rajagopalan H, Lengauer C (2004) CIN-ful cancers. Cancer Chemother Pharmacol 54 Suppl 1: S65-68.

16. Eppert K, Takenaka K, Lechman ER, Waldron L, Nilsson B, et al. (2011) Stem cell gene expression programs influence clinical outcome in human leukemia. Nat Med 17: 1086-1093.

17. Dick JE (2008) Stem cell concepts renew cancer research. Blood 112: 4793-4807.

18. Driessens G, Beck B, Caauwe A, Simons BD, Blanpain C (2012) Defining the mode of tumour growth by clonal analysis. Nature 488: 527-530.

19. Chen J, Li Y, Yu TS, McKay RM, Burns DK, et al. (2012) A restricted cell population propagates glioblastoma growth after chemotherapy. Nature 488: 522-526.

20. Schepers AG, Snippert HJ, Stange DE, van den Born M, van Es JH, et al. (2012) Lineage tracing reveals Lgr5+ stem cell activity in mouse intestinal adenomas. Science 337: 730-735.

21. Bissell MJ, Labarge MA (2005) Context, tissue plasticity, and cancer: are tumor stem cells also regulated by the microenvironment? Cancer Cell 7: 17-23.

22. Rosen JM, Jordan CT (2009) The increasing complexity of the cancer stem cell paradigm. Science 324: 1670-1673.

23. Solit D, Sawyers CL (2010) Drug discovery: How melanomas bypass new therapy. Nature 468: 902-903.

24. Goff D, Jamieson C (2010) Cycling toward elimination of leukemic stem cells. Cell Stem Cell 6: 296-297.

25. Pantel K, Alix-Panabières C, Riethdorf S (2009) Cancer micrometastases. Nat Rev Clin Oncol 6: 339-351.

26. Baylin SB, Jones PA (2011) A decade of exploring the cancer epigenome - biological and translational implications. Nat Rev Cancer 11: 726-734.

27. Siegmund KD, Marjoram P, Woo YJ, Tavaré S, Shibata D (2009) Inferring clonal expansion and cancer stem cell dynamics from DNA methylation patterns in colorectal cancers. Proc Natl Acad Sci U S A 106: 4828-4833.

28. Pelizzola M, Ecker JR (2011) The DNA methylome. FEBS Lett 585: 1994-2000.

29. Azad N, Zahnow CA, Rudin CM, Baylin SB (2013) The future of epigenetic therapy in solid tumours--lessons from the past. Nat Rev Clin Oncol 10: 256-266.

30. Mori H, Colman SM, Xiao Z, Ford AM, Healy LE, et al. (2002) Chromosome translocations and covert leukemic clones are generated during normal fetal development. Proc Natl Acad Sci U S A 99: 8242-8247.

31. Navin N, Kendall J, Troge J, Andrews P, Rodgers L, et al. (2011) Tumour evolution inferred by single-cell sequencing. Nature 472: 90-94.

32. Anderson K, Lutz C, van Delft FW, Bateman CM, Guo Y, et al. (2011) Genetic variegation of clonal architecture and propagating cells in leukaemia. Nature 469: 356-361.

33. Sabaawy HE, Sandoval C, Guo Q, Yin C, Kulangara A, et al. (2007) Lymphoproliferative clonal origin of AIDS-related non-Hodgkin's lymphoma. Leuk Lymphoma 48: 812-815.

34. Notta F, Mullighan CG, Wang JC, Poeppl A, Doulatov S, et al. (2011) Evolution of human BCR-ABL1 lymphoblastic leukaemia-initiating cells. Nature 469: 362-367.

35. Clappier E, Gerby B, Sigaux F, Delord M, Touzri F, et al. (2011) Clonal selection in xenografted human T cell acute lymphoblastic leukemia recapitulates gain of malignancy at relapse. J Exp Med 208: 653-661.

36. Mullighan CG, Phillips LA, Su X, Ma J, Miller CB, et al. (2008) Genomic analysis of the clonal origins of relapsed acute lymphoblastic leukemia. Science 322: 1377-1380.

37. Gerlinger M, Rowan AJ, Horswell S, Larkin J, Endesfelder D, et al. (2012) Intratumor heterogeneity and branched evolution revealed by multiregion sequencing. N Engl J Med 366: 883-892.

38. Marusyk A, Polyak K (2010) Tumor heterogeneity: causes and consequences. Biochim Biophys Acta 1805: 105-117.

39. Kreso A, O'Brien CA, van Galen P, Gan OI, Notta F, et al. (2013) Variable clonal repopulation dynamics influence chemotherapy response in colorectal cancer. Science 339: 543-548.

40. Sharma SV, Bell DW, Settleman J, Haber DA (2007) Epidermal growth factor receptor mutations in lung cancer. Nat Rev Cancer 7: 169-181.

41. Kwak EL, Bang YJ, Camidge DR, Shaw AT, Solomon B, et al. (2010) Anaplastic lymphoma kinase inhibition in non-small-cell lung cancer. N Engl J Med 363: 1693-1703.

42. Chapman PB, Hauschild A, Robert C, Haanen JB, Ascierto P, et al. (2011) Improved survival with vemurafenib in melanoma with BRAF V600E mutation. N Engl J Med 364: 2507-2516.

43. Irshad S, Ashworth A, Tutt A (2011) Therapeutic potential of PARP inhibitors for metastatic breast cancer. Expert Rev Anticancer Ther 11: 1243-1251.

44. Ashworth A, Lord CJ, Reis-Filho JS (2011) Genetic interactions in cancer progression and treatment. Cell 145: 30-38.

Immune Thrombocytopenic Purpura Following Acute Lymphoblastic Leukemia in Remission

Olaniyi John A[1]*, Ogundeji Peter S[1] and Ogbaro Daniel D[2]

[1]*University College Hospital, Ibadan, Nigeria*
[2]*Babcock University, Ilisan-Remo, Ogun State, Nigeria*

Abstract

This is a case report of a 19 year old male undergraduate with a background diagnosis of polycystic kidney and hypertension. Two years thereafter, he was diagnosed to have ALL L1 morphology which responded to induction chemotherapy using Vincristine and Prednisolone (V+P). He later proceeded to India where the same diagnosis was confirmed and molecular study pointed to standard risks ALL. Following successful Induction Remission and Consolidated therapy, he was sent to us to follow up his maintenance therapy. Patient defaulted severally. He represented with severe thrombocytopenia and thrombocytopenic bleeding with blood film and marrow being devoid of blasts but rather marrow showed numerous smooth, non-budding, cytoplasmic basophilic megakaryocytes in keeping with ITP. He responded rapidly to steroid therapy. Patient remains stable as at now after 3 months of steroid therapy. ITP following ALL in remission is an uncommon occurrence, hence this report.

Keywords: ALL; ITP; Chemotherapy; Bleeding

Abbreviations: Immune Thrombocytopenic Purpura (ITP); Acute Lymphoblastic Leukemia (ALL); Chronic Lymphocytic Leukemia (CLL); Systemic Lupus Erythematosus (SLE); Acute Myeloid Leukemia (AML)

Introduction

Immune Thrombocytopenic Purpura (ITP) is known to be associated with an abnormal autoantibody, usually immunoglobulin G (IgG) with specificity for GPIIb/IIIa and GPIb/IX or more platelet membrane glycoproteins; which bind to circulating platelet membrane [1-3] Auto-antibody coated platelets induce Fc receptor mediated phagocytosis by mononuclear macrophages primarily in the spleen [2]. The resultant thrombocytopenia manifests as bleeding tendency, easy bruising (purpura), or extravasations of blood from capillaries into skin and mucous membrane (petechiae). Therefore thrombocytopenia and its sequelae are common to both ITP and acute leukemia in general.

An unexpected relationship between diseases was previously documented. In 1978; Ihara et al. [4] reported a case of AML in a 29 year old female in 10 years course of ITP with episodes of splenectomy and of safe delivery of a baby girl. Also reported was AML that strangely emerged from a diagnosed breast carcinoma patient within one month of diagnosis [5]. Also, an unusual case of AML masquerading as ITP was reported in this center [6]. A detailed literature search did not reveal any link in respect of existing pathogenesis between AML and ITP as well as any direct link between ALL and ITP except for a report of nine cases of ITP in children with ALL; three of them were acute ITP, and rest were chronic ITP [7]. Hence, the need for this case report which hereby suggests a possible link between ALL in remission and ITP by its clinical presentation and laboratory profile.

Case Presentation

The case is that of a 19 years old man, an undergraduate who was seen in the University College Hospital Ibadan in March 2012. He presented with a day history of total haematuria and gum bleed, prolonged bleeding from punctured sites and redness of both eyes. There was no previous history of bleeding diasthesis. There was no family history of cancers.

He was diagnosed with adult polycystic kidney disease in India 2 years previously following severe systemic hypertension and has been on anti-hypertensive – Tabs Valsartan 160 mg daily and Tabs Carvedilol 25 mg bd. His mother had adult polycystic kidney disease post renal transplantation in India. He is the 2nd of three children in a monogamous family setting.

The physical examination at presentation revealed a young man who was well built, fully conscious and alert, not pale, afebrile, anicteric with extensive bilateral sub-conjunctival haemorrhages, petechiae haemorrhages on the lips, gum bleeds, a left lower cervical lymphadenopathy and no pedal edema.

The chest examination revealed no abnormalities. The Cardiovascular system revealed a pulse of 100 beats per minute, blood pressure was 160/120 mmHg with heart sounds I and II only. The abdomen was full and moves with respiration, moderate generalized tenderness and guarding, both kidneys were bimanually palpable but there was no palpably enlarged liver and spleen.

He was admitted and managed by the Haematology and Nephrology teams. Complete blood counts at presentation showed haematocrit of 0.38, white cell of 6.5×10^9/L, platelet count of 6.0×10^9/L, Neutrophils-61%, lymphocytes-29%, monocytes-8%, Eosinophils-1% and Basophils-1%. The peripheral blood film review showed red blood cells with moderate hypochromia and severe microcytosis (Figure 1). The white cells showed primitive intermediate sized lymphoblasts with high nucleo-cytoplasmic ratio and pale blue agranular cytoplasm. Some of these cells have 1-2 prominent nucleoli. These lymphoblasts constitute about 40% of all circulating white cells. There was also

***Corresponding author:** John Ayodele Olaniyi, University of Ibadan University College Hospital, Ibadan, Oyo Nigeria, E-mail: ayodeleolaniyi8@gmail.com

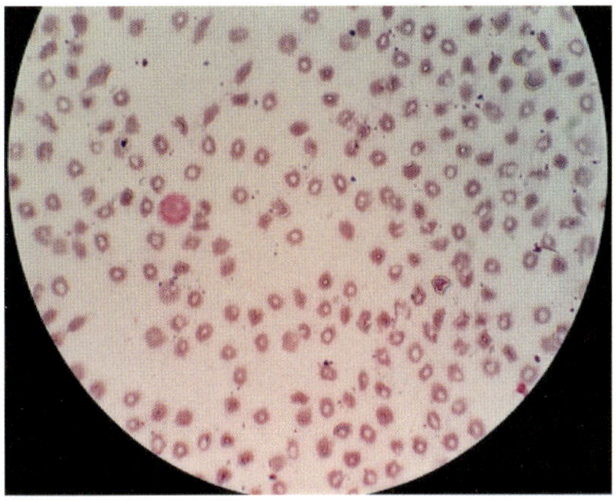

Figure 1: Initial peripheral blood photomicrograph showing severely hypochromic and microcytic red cells and a circulating lymphoblast with prominent nucleolus.

neutrophil left shift and toxic granulations. Platelets estimate was less than 10 × 10^9/L.

The bone marrow aspiration cytology showed intermediate to large sized lymphoblasts with high nucleo-cytoplasdmic ratio (Figure 2). Myelopoiesis showed sequential maturation along the cell lines. Megakaryocytes were not seen. The lymphoblasts constituted 60% of bone marrow nucleated elements. A diagnosis of acute lymphoblastic leukemia (ALL) (L1-FAB) was therefore made. Other results of investigations normal electrolyte and urea but a uric acid 0.43 mmol/L, hyperuricaemia, Calcuim- 2.15 mmol/L, and phosphate- 0.94 mmol/L. Liver function tests showed total bilirubin-41.7 μmol/L, direct bilirubin-8.3 μmol/L, total protein-72 g/L, albumin-44 g/L, AST-37 iu/l, ALT-21uI/L. Retroviral screening was non-reactive and hepatitis B surface antigen was negative. Coagulation profile showed Prothrombin time of 19 seconds, control 14 seconds, INR-1.5, APTT TEST -29 seconds, and control- 30 seconds. Abdominal ultrasound revealed an enlarged liver with a cranio-caudal span of 16.3 cm at MCL. It shows normal parenchymal echogenicity with no intrahepatic mass lesion or ductal dilatation seen. Both kidneys were enlarged with heterogeneous parenchymal echogenicity. They show multiple well defined, non-communicating anechoic oval shaped structure consistent with cyst. Some of the cysts show hyper echoic collections within them suggestive of intra-lesional haematoma. The central sinus is however well preserved. Other available investigations serum iron-32.1 μmol/l (12.0-30.0), serum transferrin-1.7 g/l (1.6-3.2), % saturation 73.8% (20.0-55), serum ferritin 488.3 μg/l (20-300).

The patient was resuscitated with red cell and platelet concentrate infusion and then commenced on pre-induction chemotherapy with intravenous Vincristine weekly and tablet prednisolone 20 mg tds (V+P) for 4 weeks. He had a significant response to the V+P therapy by normalization of platelets counts to 335×10^9/L.

He subsequently went to India where he was further evaluated and the diagnosis of ALL was sustained as evidenced by about 10% and 20% lymphoblasts in the peripheral blood and bone marrow respectively. A molecular study was in keeping with standard risk. He had Hyper CVAD (Cylophosphamide 1200 mg, Doxorubicin 100 mg, Vincistine 2 mg, Dexamethasone 40 mg daily×4 days) and intra-theca (IT) 12.5 mg methotrexate in April 9, 2013. He also had IV Asparaginase 5000 IU in April 17, 2013. In May 2103 he had high dose ARA-C (2G alternate days for 3 days from 02/05/13), followed by high dose methotrexate (6 gm) on 23/5/2013. He was subsequently commenced on maintenance 6 Mercaptopurine and per oral methotrexate. He was then referred back to us for follow up.

At the second presentation in July 2013, his complete blood count showed haematocrit of 0.34 white blood cell count of 2.9×10^9/L (neutrophil-46%, lymphocyte-50%, eosinophils-2% and momocyte-2%) and platelets count of 153×10^9/L. The peripheral blood film review still showed about 30% lymphoblasts in circulation. He was thus assessed not to be in remission. He was thereafter lost to follow up.

He presented for the third time in December 2013 for re-assessment and a repeat bone marrow examination showed a normo-cellular marrow with micro-normoblastic erythropoiesis, sequential maturation of the myeloid series and adequate Megakaryocyte with evidence of platelet budding (Figure 3). Also present were degenerating lymphoid cells constituting about 10% of the marrow elements. The assessment of ALL in partial remission was made. He continued with the maintenance therapy with oral methotrexate and 6 Mercaptopurine but again he was lost to follow up.

He represented in January 2015, while still on his maintenance therapy, on account of a repeat total haematuria and sub-conjunctival haemorrhage. The peripheral blood film review showed marked thrombocytopaenia without evidence of circulating lymphoblast. A bone marrow aspiration cytology at this time revealed normo-cellular marrow with micro-normoblastic erythropoiesis, sequential maturation of the myeloid series. Megakaryocytopoieis was increased

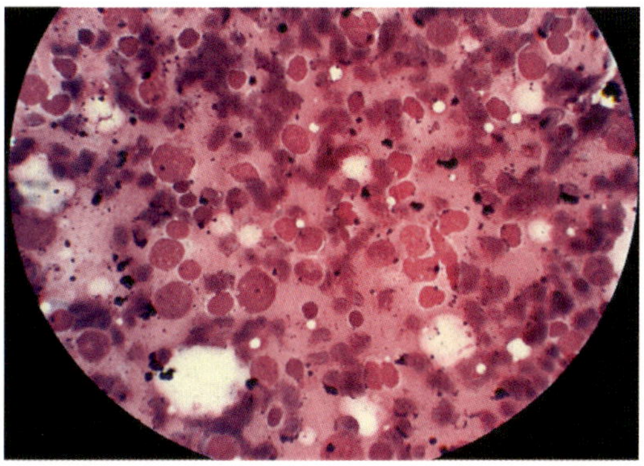

Figure 2: Initial bone marrow film showing numerous lymphoblasts and absence megakaryocytes.

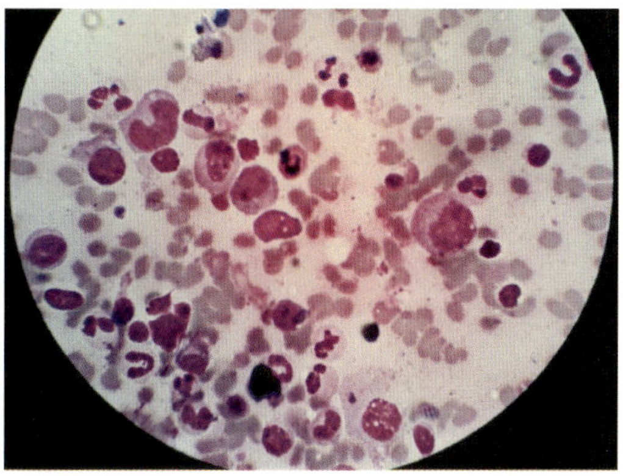

Figure 3: Second repeat bone marrow photomicrograph showing a normal marrow while on maintenance chemotherapy.

with 5-7 megakayocytes seen per × 10 objective and they were of low ploidy, cytoplasmic basophilia and have smooth non-budding nuclei (Figure 5). The assessment of Immune Thrombocytopenic purpura was made. He was commenced on steroid therapy with oral prednisolone 20 mg tds which he responded to with normalization of platelets counts and resolution of bleeding. The patient has remained in remission after being treated with prednisolone for a total period of three months but would require regular follow up to monitor progress.

Discussion

While acute leukemia is known to be an aggressive disease that usually presents with features of bone marrow failure, presence of excess of blasts in the bone marrow, spillage of blasts into the peripheral circulation and evidence of multiple tissue infiltration [8-12]; ALL is a malignant disorder of lymphopoietic stem cells that originates in the lymphoid precursor of marrow, thymus and lymph nodes. Untreated ALL is usually fatal within 6 months, but with the best therapy 70-80% of children and 20- 30% of adults survive beyond 5 years [13]. Acute leukemia in remission followed by ITP was not found in the course of our literature even though, found documented are many ITP associated disorders [14,15] involving lymphocyte abnormalities like large granular lymphocyte syndrome, lymphoproliferative disorders like Chronic Lymphocytic Leukemia (CLL) and lymphomas, others include autoimmune lymphoproliferative disorders, autoimmune haemolytic anaemias, Systemic Lupus Erythematosus (SLE) and antiphospholipid syndrome; direct link of ALL with ITP is yet to be reported in literature. The closest reported was AML masquerading as ITP [6].

The patient, when diagnosed of ALL mainly by the thrombocytopenic bleeding, presence of solitary cervical lymphadenopathy, finding of lymphoblast on blood smears and bone marrow smears, was not acutely ill, not anaemic and there was no neutropaenia.

Immunophenotyping and molecular studies would have helped in characterizing the disease but facilities for such studies were not readily available. However, further evaluation of this patient in India still confirmed ALL for which Induction chemotherapy, followed by consolidated chemotherapy for ALL were instituted. He was back to Nigeria while on Maintenance chemotherapy. All these reinforced the diagnosis of ALL.

This patient remained well and was fit enough to cope with his undergraduate studies over the three years of diagnosis except for the notable two episodes of bleeding. The recent re-presentation with total haematuria, florid petechiae haemorrhage, with a platelet count of 10,000/mm^3, blood and marrow smears being devoid of lymphoblasts created a puzzle. However the finding of numerous, smooth non-budding megakaryocytes of up to six at low power and about two at high power objective suggested ITP (Figure 4).

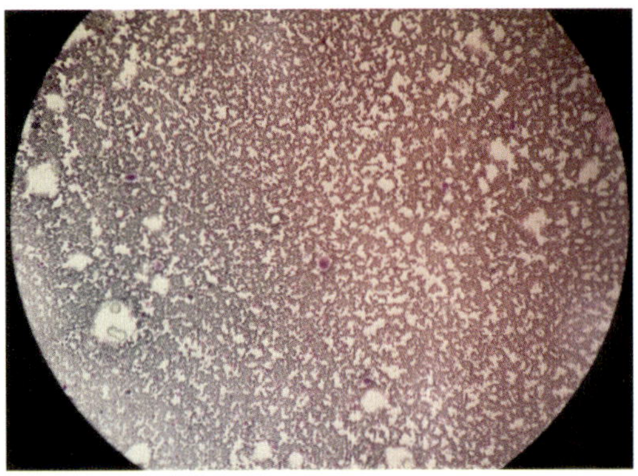

Figure 4: Bone marrow photomicrograph taken in February 2015 showing 6 megakaryocytes. X10 lens objective.

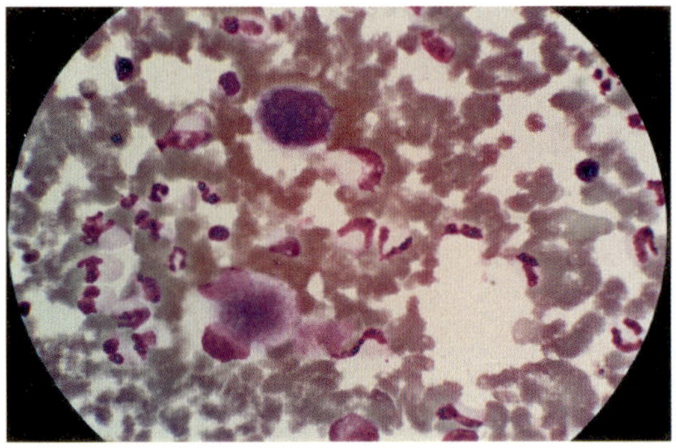

Figure 5: Bone marrow photomicrograph showing Megakaryocytes with low ploidy, cytoplasmic basophilia and smooth non-budding nuclei.

Therefore the substantive question to answer at this point is what is the link between ALL and ITP? A prospective study of ITP in 245 adults, carried out in 2003 [16] showed an overall incidence 1.6/100,000/yr., median age 56, F:M 1.2:1, 12% presented with bleeding, 28% asymptomatic, 18% needed no treatment, only 12% needed splenectomy, 63% in remission (plts>100×10^9/L) at end of follow up period (6-78 months, median 60), 87% had at least partial remission (plts>30×10^9/L) and freedom from symptoms, 1.6% died from complications of disease or its treatment. This study did not report any association between acute leukemia and ITP.

In conclusion this case report strongly suggests that a possible pathogenetic link exists between acute leukemia and ITP which requires detail investigation.

References

1. Stasi R, Evangelista ML, Stipa E, Buccisano F, Venditti A (2008) Idiopathic thrombocytopenic purpura: current concept in pathophysiology and management. Thromb Haemost 1: 4-13.
2. McMillan R (2007) The pathogenesis of chronic immune thrombocytopenic purpura. Semin hematol 44: 3-11.
3. Chan H, Moore JC, Finch CN, Warkintin TE, Kelton JG (2003) The IgG of subclasses of platelet- associated auto-antibodies directed against platelet glycoproteins IIb/IIIa in patients with idiopathic thrombocytopaenic purpura. Br J Haemato 1: 818-824.
4. Ihara A, Shimizu N, Okada K, Kamada N, Kuramoto A, et al. (1978) A case of acute myelogenous leukemia (AML) in 10 years course of thrombocytopenia (ITP) with episodes of splenectomy and of delivery (author's transl). Rinsho Ketsueki 19: 295-303.
5. Mishra PP, Mahapatra M, Choudhry VP, Saxena R, Pati H, et al. (2004) Synchronous occurrence of breast carcinoma and acute myeloid leukemia: case report and review of the literature. Ann Hematol 83: 541-543.
6. Olaniyi JA (2009) An Acute Leukaemia Masquerading as Immune Thrombocytopaenic Purpura (ITP)? A Case Report. Clin Med Case Rep 2: 31-34.
7. Horino S, Rikiishi T, Niizuma H, Abe H, Watanabe Y, et al. (2009) Refractory chronic immune thrombocytopenic purpura in a child with acute lymphoblastic leukemia. Int J Hematol 90: 483-485.
8. AV Hoffbrand and JE Pettit (2000) Acute Leukaemia. in Essential Haematology. (3rdedn), Blackwell Science.
9. Albert S, Child M (1977) Familial cancer in the general population. Cancer 40: 1674-1679.

10. Zuelzer WW, Cox DE (1969) Genetic aspects of leukemia. Semin Hematol 6: 228-249.

11. http://en.wikipedia.org/wiki/Fanconi_anemia

12. Abkowitz JL, Fialkow PJ, Niebrugge DJ, Raskind WH, Adamson JW (1984) Pancytopenia as a clonal disorder of a multipotent hematopoietic stem cell. J Clin Invest 73: 258-261.

13. Hoelzer D (1993) Acute lymphoblastic leukemia--progress in children, less in adults. N Engl J Med 329: 1343-1344.

14. Carey RW, McGinnis A, Jacobson BM, Carvalho A (1976) Idiopathic thrombocytopenic purpura complicating chronic lymphocytic leukemia. Arch Intern Med 136: 62-66.

15. Ertem M, Uysal Z, Yavuz G, Gözdaşoğlu S (2000) Immune thrombocytopenia and hemolytic anemia as a presenting manifestation of Hodgkin disease. Pediatr Hematol Oncol 17: 181-185.

16. Rodeghiero F, Francesco MR (2007) First-line Idiopathic Thrombocytopenic Purpura Therapies- Benefits and Limitations. Brit J Haematol 122: 966-968.

Interferon Gamma/IL10 Ratio Production in Response to Host Antigens may Predict Acute Graft Versus Host Disease after Allogeneic Stem Cell Transplantation from a Sibling

Azza M Kamel[1]*, Nahla M El-Sharkawy[1], Eman K Abd El-Fattah[1], Raafat M Abd El-Fattah[2], Mohammed A Samra[2], Paul K Wallace[3] and Hossam K Mahmoud[2]

[1]*Department of Clinical Pathology, NCI, Cairo University, Egypt*
[2]*Department of Medical oncology, NCI, Cairo University, Egypt*
[3]*Flow Cytometry Lab, Roswell Park Cancer Institute, USA*

Abstract

Background: Graft versus host disease (GVHD) continues to be the main concern of transplanters. Cytokines' contribution to its pathogenesis has been widely addressed in the literature. Previous studies have mainly evaluated the cytokine's level after the actual occurrence of GVHD. In this work, we investigated the possibility of predicting the occurrence of acute GVHD through an experimental setup to mimic the response of the immune cells of the graft to the host antigens expressed by interferon gamma (IFNγ) and interleukin 10 (IL10) production.

Methods: The study included 45 patients receiving allogeneic HSCT from an identical sibling. An aliquot from the graft prior to infusion was used for in vitro culture for 3 days with patients' mitomycin treated mononuclear cells. IFNγ and IL10 were measured in culture supernatant using microbead array technology.

Results: Acute GVHD was encountered in 14 cases. IFNγ was detectable in the culture supernatant of 9/14 (64.3%) cases with GVHD at a level of 6.2 - 19.000 with a median of 159.3 pg/ml versus 3/31 (9.6%) cases without GVHD at a level of 1.1, 8.1 and 80.01 pg/ml ($p<0.001$). IL10 was detectable in the culture supernatant of 7/14 (50%) cases with GVHD at a level of 9.5 – 858.5 with a median of 128 pg/ml versus 6/31 (19.3%) cases without GVHD at a level of 14.0 – 359.0 with a median of 45.39 pg/ml ($p<0.05$). At a cutoff of 1.13, IFNγ/IL10 ratio could predict GVHD with a sensitivity of 85.7%, specificity of 83.3% and a total accuracy of 84.6%.

Conclusion: *In vitro* cytokine production by graft immune cells in response to host antigens is extremely variable. IFNγ production apparently reflects potential development of acute GVHD while IL10 production is apparently protective. When both are produced the IFNγ/IL10 ratio is more informative than either alone.

Keywords: GVHD; HSCT; IFNγ; IL10; Cytokines

Abbreviations: HSCT: Hematopoietic Stem Cell Transplantation; GVHD: Graft Versus Host Disease; IFN γ: Interferon Gamma; IL10: Interleukin 10; BMT: Bone Marrow Transplantation; PBSCT: Peripheral Blood Stem Cell Transplantation; MHC: Major Histocompatibility. IL2: Interleukin 2; TGF β: Transforming Growth Factor β; Th: T Helper

Introduction

Stem cell transplantation is a widely used therapeutic modality [1]. Graft versus host disease (GVHD) continues to be the main concern of transplanters [1-3]. If not, so far, preventable, prediction of its occurrence will help proper management and reducing its severity.

The conditioning regimen with radiation and chemotherapy produces host tissue injury leading to release of chemokines and cytokines and the host dendritic cells in spleen and peripheral target tissues (skin, liver, gut) are activated. This cytokine storm initiates a cascade of immune reactions leading to Th1-polarized immune response [4]. These events are followed by the generation of cytotoxic and inflammatory cytokines, cytotoxic effector cells, large granular lymphocytes, and nitric oxide. Interactions of innate and adaptive immune responses lead to organ damage.

On the other hand, these effector mechanisms are accompanied by endogenous release of IL10 and other Th2 cytokines [5,6]. There is substantial evidence to implicate that different cytokines play a major role in GVHD induction and grade. GVHD was reported to be associated with increased production of IFN γ [7], IL2 [8] and IL10 [9]. IL 10 has been used as a predictor of GVHD [10]. Other reports demonstrated a protective role for IL10 [11]; the increased level may be a physiological response to counteract the effect of Th1 cytokines. A very good positive correlation between the frequency of Th1 and Th2 ($r=0.951$, $p=0.001$) in acute GVHD has been reported [12]. In general cytokines associated with Th1 response are claimed to be contributing to the occurrence and severity of acute GVHD while those associated with Th2 response are claimed to be protective [13]. All reports addressed the roles of cytokine(s) individually and, in most, the evaluation was performed after the actual occurrence of GVHD. We hypothesized that it is the balance between Th1 and Th2 rather than either alone would determine the potential occurrence and severity of GVHD. In the present study, we attempted to develop an experimental setup to mimic the response of the immune cells of the graft to the host antigens expressed by Th1 (IFNγ) and Th2 (IL10) cytokine production

***Corresponding author:** Azza M Kamel, Department of Clinical Pathology, NCI, Cairo University, Egypt, E-mail: azzamkamel@yahoo.com and study the potential impact of the pattern of production of each cytokine separately and the balance between both on the development of acute GVHD. We also aimed to verify if this pattern could possibly predict the occurrence of acute GVHD.

Patients and Methods

Forty five patients who received fully matched allogeneic peripheral blood stem cell transplantation from a sibling donor at Nasser Institute, Cairo, Egypt in the period from November 2008 until May 2010 were enrolled in the study. They included 26 males and 19 females with an age range from 6 to 41 with a mean of 22.5 ± 9.3 and a median of 22 years. Eighteen patients had Acute Myeloid Leukemia, 15 had Chronic Myeloid Leukemia, 4 had Acute Lymphoblastic Leukemia, 4 had aplastic anemia, 3 had Myelodysplastic Syndrome and one patient had Fanconi's anemia. All CML patients were transplanted in chronic phase 1 except one case (case 21) that was transplanted in accelerated phase. Of the 18 AML patients, 9 were transplanted in first and 9 in second remission. Two of the four ALL cases were transplanted in first, one was transplanted in second and one in third remission. All patients and donors were ABO compatible. Conditioning regimen and GVHD prophylaxis were applied as previously reported [14]. The different conditioning regimens according to age and diagnosis are displayed in table 1. GVHD prophylaxis consisted of Cyclosporin-A (CSA) 3 mg/kg IV from day –1 to be changed to oral form (3 mg/kg) once the patient can swallow for 9-12 months post-transplant; as well as a short course of IV methotrexate (15 mg/m^2 day 1 and 10 mg/m^2 days 3 and 6) with leucovorin rescue.

The work was performed according to Helsinki declaration and the protocol was approved by the IRB of the NCI, Cairo University. Under informed consent, a heparinized venous blood sample was obtained from the patient before conditioning, mononuclear cells separated by Ficoll-Hypaque density gradient centrifugation and cryopreserved. On the day of transplant, the cryopreserved cells were thawed, viability test was done and cells were incubated with 200 µl/ml of mitomycin C (MUTAMYCIN (5 mg) Bristol Mayers Squibb) at a concentration of 50 µg/ml at room temperature for one hour then washed in RPMI and readjusted to 5 × 10^6/ml to serve as stimulators while the mononuclear cells of the graft at a concentration of 5 × 10^{6}cells/ ml served as responders in a mixed lymphocyte culture setup. Culture plates were incubated for 3 days at 37°C in a CO_2 incubator; the culture supernatant was collected and stored at -80°C till tested. IFNγ and IL10 were measured by microbead array technology using Luminex 200 and Flourokine MAP kit provided by R&D Company (Human multianalyte profiling base kit A and Human multianalyte profiling base kit B).

Patients were followed up for at least one year; development of acute and chronic GVHD was recorded.

Data was analyzed using SPSSwin statistical package version 16. Numerical data were expressed as mean ± standard deviation, median and range. Qualitative data were expressed as frequency and percentage. Chi square test (Fisher's Exact test) was used to examine the relation between qualitative variables. For quantitative data, comparison between two groups was done using Mann Whitney test (non-parametric t test). ROC curve was used to determine the appropriate cut off levels for the different markers; then sensitivity and specificity were calculated.

Results

Fourteen/45 patients developed acute GVHD, 4 grade I, six grade II and 4 grade III. Seven patients developed chronic GVHD; 3 of them on top of acute GVHD. Patients who developed chronic GVHD showed no statistically significant differences in any of the tested parameters and will not be mentioned any more.

IFN γ and IL10 were measured in the culture supernatant. Both cytokines were significantly higher in the 14 cases that developed as compared to the 31 cases that did not develop GVHD (Table 2). Both cytokines were more frequently detected in the culture supernatant of the cases that developed GVHD and at a significantly higher level as compared to those who did not develop GVHD (Table 3).

In the culture supernatant, cytokines were below the detection limit in 25/31 (80.6%) cases who did not and in 3/14 (16.13%) cases who did develop acute GVHD. The level of cytokines in the other cases varied widely. Of the 11 cases that showed cytokine production, 4 produced IFNγ only and two produced IL10 only. The other 5 cases produced both; IL10 was higher in one case; in the other 4 cases, IFNγ was much higher (Table 4). In the 6/31 cases without GVHD, IL10 only was detected in 3 cases. The other 3 cases produced both; IFNγ was higher in one, in the other two cases IL10 was much higher (Table 5).

All patients were positive for anti CMV IgG except two cases; both had undetectable cytokines in the culture supernatant and both did not

Disease	Age Group	
	≤18 years	>18 years
AML	BU/CY	FLU/BU
ALL	BU/CY	FLU/BU
	TBI/CY	TBI/CY
CML	BU/CY	FLU/BU
MDS	BU/CY	FLU/ALK
SAA	FLU/CY	FLU/CY
FA	FLU/CY/ATG	---

AML: Acute Myeloid Leukemia, ALL: Acute lymphatic leukemia, CML: Chronic myeloid leukemia, MDS: Myelodysplastic syndrome, SAA: Severe aplastic Anemia, FA: Fanconi's Anemia
BU: Busulphan CY Cyclophosphamide, TBI: Total Body Irradiation,
FLU: Fludarabine, ATG: Antithymocyte Globulin, ALK: Alkeran.

Table 1: Conditioning regimens used in allogeneic stem cell transplantation according to diagnosis.

Parameter	GVHD	No GVHD	p value
No	14	31	
IFNγ pg/ml	1652.5 ± 5051.7* 0.0-19000 56.43	2.88 ± 14.4 0-80.1 0	<0.001
IL10 pg/ml	119.6 ± 254.3 0-858.6 2.27	19.7 ± 67.5 0-359.0 0	<0.05

*Mean + SD, Range, Median

Table 2: Level of IFN and IL10 in MLC supernatant in patients with and without GVHD after allogeneic PBSCT from a sibling.

Parameter	GVHD	No GVHD	p value
IFNγ: No (%)	9/14 (64.3%)	3/31 (9.6%)	<0.001
Level in positive cases: pg/ml	6.2-19000* 159.3	1.1, 8.1, 80.01**	
IL10: No (%)	7/14 (50%)	6/31 (19.3%)	<0.05
Level in positive cases: pg/ml	9.5-858.6 128	14-359.0 45.39	

*Range, Median of cases with detectable level
**Levels of the 3 cases

Table 3: Frequency and level of IFN γ and IL10 in MLC supernatant in patients with and without GVHD after allogeneic PBSCT from a sibling.

develop GVHD. Seven AML patients had detectable cytokines in their culture supernatant, four developed GVHD and 3 did not. Among the 4 who developed GVHD, 3 were transplanted in second (cases 5, 8 and 25) and one in first remission (case 42). The fifth AML case that developed grade 1 GVHD (case 38) had no detectable cytokines in the culture supernatant. Of the three cases that did not develop GVHD, one (case 20) was transplanted in second and two (cases 9 and 11) were transplanted in first remission. There was no relation between the pattern of cytokines production and age or remission status of patients at the time of transplantation. However, the single CML case that was transplanted in accelerated phase showed high level of cytokines in the culture supernatant (case 21) (Table 4).

At a cutoff level of 15.9 pg/ml, IFNγ was predictive of acute GVHD with a sensitivity of 64.3%, specificity of 96.8% and a total accuracy of 80.4%. At a cutoff of 2.27 pg/ml, IL10 showed a sensitivity of 50%, specificity of 80.6% and a total accuracy of 71.1%. At a cutoff of 1.13, IFNγ/IL10 ratio showed a sensitivity of 85.7%, specificity of 83.3% and a total accuracy of 84.6 (Figure 1).

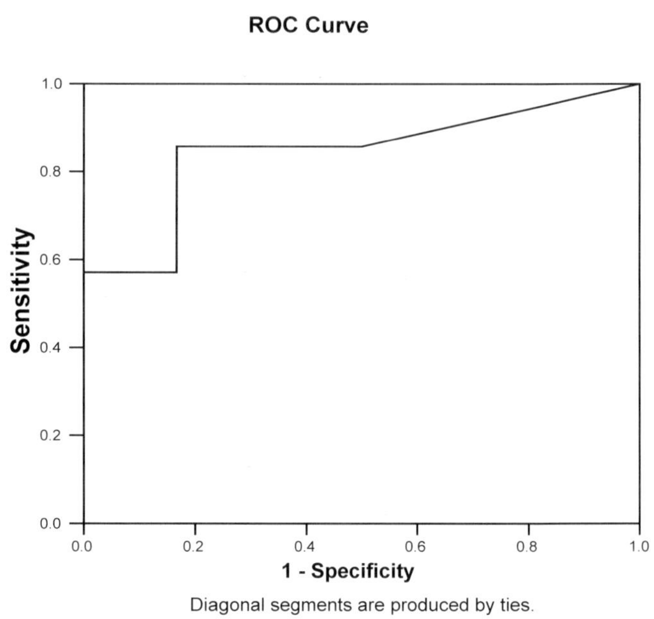

Figure 1: ROC curve for IFN/IL10 ratio in MLC supernatant in patients with and without GVHD after allogeneic PBSCT from a sibling.

Discussion

GVHD is an exaggerated, undesirable manifestation of a normal inflammatory response [15,16]. The donor CD4+ T-cell interaction with host APCs leads to the activation of the donor T cells and their differentiation into Th1, Th2, and Th17 cells, depending on the cytokine milieu [16,17]; the T helper cells then secrete a variety of cytokines to mediate GVHD inflammation [9,16,18].

The role of Th1, Th2, and Th17 cells in acute GVHD pathogenesis is still controversial. However, in general, Th1 cells play a critical role in mediating acute GVHD pathogenesis; Th2 cells can mediate acute GVHD under special circumstances but they are generally protective [16].

Case No	Age (years)	Diagnosis	IFNγ pg/ml	IL10 pg/ml	GVHD Grade
4	22	CML	<DL	9.5	G2
5	29	AML	6.2	128	G2
6	18	CML	<DL	131	G2
8	31	AML	41.66	<DL	G1
15	29	CML	651.2	22.3	G3
21	34	CML	2914	520.8	G1
24	45	CML	19000	858.6	G3
25	23	AML	23.7	7.9	G3
36	29	MDS	118.6	<DL	G2
37	41	CML	159.3	<DL	G3
42	10	AML	7.12	<DL	G1

Only cases with detectable IFNγ and/or IL10 are included
MLC: Mixed lymphocyte culture
PBSCT: Peripheral blood stem cell transplantation
<DL: Below detection limit

Table 4: IFNγ and IL10 levels in MLC culture supernatant of 11/14 cases with acute GVHD after allogeneic PBSCT from a sibling.

Case No	Age (years)	Diagnosis	IFNγ pg/ml	IL10 pg/ml
2	23	ALL	1.1	121
3	22	CML	<DL	14
7	28	CML	<DL	25
9	22	AML	<DL	46
11	30	AML	8.1	359
20	44	AML	80.01	44.78

MLC: Mixed lymphocyte culture
PBSCT: Peripheral blood stem cell transplantation
<DL: Below detection limit

Table 5: IFNγ and IL10 levels in MLC culture supernatant of 6/31 cases without acute GVHD after allogeneic PBSCT from a sibling.

Accordingly the balance between Th1 and Th2 rather than either alone might reflect the outcome in any particular immune response.

In this work, we measured IFNγ and IL10 in the supernatant of a MLC as a surrogate of the in vivo donor immune response to patient's antigens. Our data suggest that IFNγ production apparently reflects potential development of acute GVHD while IL10 production is apparently protective. When both are produced the IFNγ/IL10 ratio is more informative than either alone. To the best of our knowledge, this is the first study to address the impact of the Th1/Th2 balance, in a MLC setup, on the development of acute GVHD. Only one previous study used the MLC setup to evaluate cytokine production in the sibling transplant situation [19]. This study, however, relied on calculating the number of IFNγ, IL10 and IL4 secreting cells by the Ellispot technique and concluded that only IL10 is informative; they did not measure the actual level of the secreted cytokines [19]. Donor T-cells are the main effectors in the induction of GVHD [20]. Conversely, host B cells may attenuate GVHD by secreting IL10 [11]. The differentiation of CD4+ T cell populations into two distinct groups, Th1 and Th2 cells, is reflected on the pattern of cytokines secreted by the T cells. Th1 and Th2 mediated immune responses cross inhibit each other through the secreted cytokines [21]. In our study, the level of IFNγ was found to be significantly higher in culture supernatant of patients who developed acute GVHD; it was encountered at a higher frequency and at significantly higher levels.

In concordance with our results, serum IFNγ was reported to be increased in patients with acute GVHD [22]. Furthermore, Remberger et al. [23] had reported a significantly higher levels of IFNγ among patients who had moderate to severe acute GVHD compared to patients with little , if any, GVHD when IFNγ was measured after engraftment.

In the current study, the level of IL10 was significantly higher in patients who developed acute GVHD as compared to those who did not when it was measured in culture supernatant. Increased IL 10 level may represent a compensatory mechanism to counter-act the effect of Th1 cytokines. The same explanation was stated by Miura et al. [10] reporting high serum IL10 levels in patients with severe GVHD.

IL10 and TGF β have similar and overlapping roles in regulation by the adaptive immune system; a study suggested that GVHD that develops after allogeneic SCT is attenuated by the additive effects of donor derived TGF β and IL10 [24]. Yet we did not encounter any impact of TGF β in the current study (data not included). Macrophages, the major source of IL10, are stimulated to produce IL10 by several endogenous and exogenous factors [25]. Considering IL10 as just immunosuppressive and anti-inflammatory might be oversimplifying [12]. Considering IL10 as immune-regulatory instead of immunosuppressive might be more appropriate [26]. IL10 inhibits allo-antigen specific T cell responses through its strong endogenous anti-inflammatory effects [5]. IL10 controls inflammatory processes and inhibits IFN induced gene transcription; IL10 inhibition can be overcome by increasing IFN concentrations [27].

A strong Th1 response tends to be hostile during transplantation, playing a major role in exacerbating graft versus host reactions [9]. On the other hand, Th2 response could inhibit allo-antigen specific T cell responses through secretion of cytokines as IL10. IL 4 and IL10 are more often perceived as being anti-Inflammatory protective with respect to transplantation [28]. In the current study IL4 was detectable in two cases only; both developed GVHD and both expressed IFNγ and IL10 as well (data not presented).

Cytokine polarization is a relative definition that reflects the relative ratio of type 1 cytokines over type 2 cytokines [29]. Th1 cytokines are the main mediators in GVHD production. Generation of $CD4^+$ IL4 and IL10 producing Th2 cells inhibited GVHD and the balance between these two responses determine the outcome of an inflammatory response; hence was the idea to investigate if IFNγ/IL10 ratio could potentially predict the occurrence of acute GVHD rather than either alone. ROC curve for IFNγ, IL10 and IFNγ/IL10 ratio in MLC supernatant proved that the IFNγ/IL10 is superior to IFNγ with IL10 coming last with regards to sensitivity, specificity and total accuracy in predicting the occurrence of acute GVHD.

In the current study, there was no association between the pattern of cytokine production and age or remission status at the time of transplantation. However, it is worth mentioning that the single CML case transplanted in accelerated phase showed a high level of cytokine production; more cases are needed to verify this observation.

Conclusions

In vitro cytokine production by graft immune cells in response to host antigens is extremely variable; it may serve as a surrogate system of the immune reaction following allogeneic stem cell transplantation. IFNγ production apparently reflects potential development of acute GVHD while IL10 production is apparently protective. When both are produced the IFNγ/IL10 ratio is more informative than either alone. These conclusions, however, are drawn from a relatively small number of cases. A validation cohort is essential to verify these results.

Acknowledgement

This work was supported by USA/Egypt Fund: ID CODE: BIO8-002-002 Contract/Agreement No: 224.

References

1. Ljungman P, Bregni M, Brune M, Cornelissen J, de Witte T, et al (2010) Allogeneic and autologous transplantation for haematological diseases, solid tumours and immune disorders: current practice in Europe 2009. Bone Marrow Transplant 45: 219-234.
2. Anderson BE, McNiff J, Yan J, Doyle H, Mamula M, et al. (2003) Memory CD4+ T cells do not induce graft-versus-host disease. J Clin Invest 112: 101-108.
3. Poutsiaka DD, Munson D, Price LL, Chan GW, Snydman DR (2011) Blood stream infection (BSI) and acute GVHD after hematopoietic SCT (HSCT) are associated. Bone Marrow Transplant 46: 300-307.
4. Ferrara JL, Yanik G (2005) Acute graft versus host disease: pathophysiology, risk factors, and prevention strategies. Clin Adv Hematol Oncol 3: 415-419.
5. Holler E, Roncarolo MG, Hintermeier-Knabe R, Eissner G, Ertl B, et al. (2000) Prognostic significance of increased IL-10 production in patients prior to allogeneic bone marrow transplantation. Bone Marrow Transplant 25: 237-241.
6. Moore KW, de Waal Malefyt R, Coffman RL, O'Garra A (2001) Interleukin-10 and the interleukin-10 receptor. Annu Rev Immunol 19: 683-765.
7. Shlomchik WD (2007) Graft-versus-host disease. Nat Rev Immunol 7: 340-352.
8. Tanaka J, Imamura M, Kasai M, Hashino S, Kobayashi S, et al. (1997) The important balance between cytokines derived from type 1 and type 2 helper T cells in the control of graft-versus-host disease. Bone Marrow Transplant 19: 571-576.
9. Ferrara JL, Cooke KR, Teshima T (2003) The pathophysiology of acute graft-versus-host disease. Int J Hematol 78: 181-187.
10. Miura Y, Thoburn CJ, Bright EC, Chen W, Nakao S, et al. (2002) Cytokine and chemokine profiles in autologous graft-versus-host disease (GVHD): interleukin 10 and interferon gamma may be critical mediators for the development of autologous GVHD. Blood 100: 2650-2658.
11. Rowe V, Banovic T, MacDonald KP, Kuns R, Don AL, et al. (2006) Host B cells produce IL-10 following TBI and attenuate acute GVHD after allogeneic bone marrow transplantation. Blood 108: 2485-2492.
12. Yeh SP, Liao YM, Lo WJ, Lin CL, Bai LY, et al. (2012) Kinetics of T helper subsets and associated cytokines correlate well with the clinical activity of graft-versus-host disease. PLoS One 7: e44416.
13. Reddy P, Ferrara JL (2003) Immunobiology of acute graft-versus-host disease. Blood Rev 17: 187-194.
14. Mahmoud H, El-Haddad A, Fahmy O, El-Emary M, Nassar A, et al. (2008) Hematopoietic stem cell transplantation in Egypt. Bone Marrow Transplant 42: S76-S80.
15. Nomura S, Ishii K, Shimizu M, Inami N, Uoshima N, et al. (2009) The significance of EMAP-II after allogeneic stem cell transplantation. Transpl Immunol 21: 23-26.
16. Yi T, Chen Y, Wang L, Du G, Huang D, et al. (2009) Reciprocal differentiation and tissue-specific pathogenesis of Th1, Th2, and Th17 cells in graft-versus-host disease. Blood 114: 3101-3112.
17. Bader P, Kreyenberg H, Hoelle W, Dueckers G, Handgretinger R, et al. (2004) Increasing mixed chimerism is an important prognostic factor for unfavorable outcome in children with acute lymphoblastic leukemia after allogeneic stem-cell transplantation: possible role for pre-emptive immunotherapy? J Clin Oncol 22: 1696–1705.
18. Zeiser R, Marks R, Bertz H, Finke J (2004) Immunopathogenesis of acute graft-versus-host disease: implications for novel preventive and therapeutic strategies. Ann Hematol 83: 551-565.
19. Weston LE, Geczy AF, Briscoe H (2006) Production of IL-10 by alloreactive sibling donor cells and its influence on the development of acute GVHD. Bone Marrow Transplant 37: 207-212.
20. Welniak LA, Blazar BR, Murphy WJ (2007) Immunobiology of allogeneic hematopoietic stem cell transplantation. Annu Rev Immunol 25: 139-170.
21. Gerald B. Pier, Jeffrey B. Lyczak, Lee M. Wetzler (2004) Immunology, Infection, and Immunity merican Society for Microbiology Press, Washington, DC.
22. Niederwieser D, Herold M, Woloszczuk W, Aulitzky W, Meister B, et al. (1990) Endogenous IFN-gamma during human bone marrow transplantation. Analysis of serum levels of interferon and interferon-dependent secondary messages. Transplantation 50: 620-625.

23. Remberger M, Jaksch M, Uzunel M, Mattsson J (2003) Serum levels of cytokines correlate to donor chimerism and acute graft-vs.-host disease after haematopoietic stem cell transplantation. Eur J Haematol 70: 384-391.

24. Banovic T, MacDonald KP, Morris ES, Rowe V, Kuns R, et al. (2005) TGF-beta in allogeneic stem cell transplantation: friend or foe? Blood 106: 2206-2214.

25. Riese U, Brenner S, Döcke WD, Prösch S, Reinke P, et al. (2000) Catecholamines induce IL-10 release in patients suffering from acute myocardial infarction by transactivating its promoter in monocytic but not in T-cells. Mol Cell Biochem 212: 45-50.

26. Asadullah K, Sterry W, Volk HD (2003) Interleukin-10 therapy--review of a new approach. Pharmacol Rev 55: 241-269.

27. Ichikawa T, Nakao K, Nakata K, Yamashita M, Hamasaki K, et al. (2002) Involvement of IL-1beta and IL-10 in IFN-alpha-mediated antiviral gene induction in human hepatoma cells. Biochem Biophys Res Commun 294: 414-422.

28. Le Moine A, Goldman M, Abramowicz D (2002) Multiple pathways to allograft rejection. Transplantation 73: 1373-1381.

29. Guo H, Qiao Z, Zhu L, Wang H, Su L, et al. (2004) Th1/Th2 cytokine profiles and their relationship to clinical features in patients following nonmyeloablative allogeneic stem cell transplantation. Am J Hematol 75: 78-83.

Effects of Resveratrol and Vitamin C on the Self-Renewal Capacity of Blast Progenitors in Hematologic Malignancies

Yi Zhang[1], Yan Zhao[1], Kazuma Miyahara[2], Mai Shimada[2], Ken-ichi Tanaka[3], Hiroyuki Hayashi[4], Noriko Ihara[2] and Ikuo Murohashi[1*]

[1]*Hematology, Center for University-Wide Education, School of Health and Social Services, Saitama Prefectural University, Koshigaya-City, Saitama 343-8540, Japan*
[2]*Department of Health Sciences, School of Health and Social Services, Saitama Prefectural University, Koshigaya-City, Saitama 343-8540, Japan*
[3]*Physiology, Center for University-Wide Education, School of Health and Social Services, Saitama Prefectural University, Koshigaya-City, Saitama 343-8540, Japan*
[4]*Anatomy, Center for University-Wide Education, School of Health and Social Services, Saitama Prefectural University, Koshigaya-City, Saitama 343-8540, Japan*

Abstract

Although a large number of phytochemicals has been shown to inhibit the growth of leukemic and cancer cells, their effects on the self-renewal (SR) capacity of the malignant stem/progenitor cells were not examined. In seven hematologic malignant cell lines including U-937, Mo7e, K-562, HL-60, U-266, Raji and Daudi, the SR capacity of blast progenitors was assessed by measuring cumulative clonogenic cells in suspension, whereas the terminal division of blast progenitors was assessed by blast colony formation (BCF) in methylcellulose. Resveratrol and vitamin C (Vit-C) with mean IC_{50} values of 41 and 514 μM for inhibiting BCF were added twice per week to cells in long-term suspension at 10 and 300 μM, respectively. Vit-C induced slight increase in senescence or necrosis rates, marked G_2/M arrest and significant inhibition of telomerase activity in two, one and five cell lines, respectively. Resveratrol, but not Vit-C, induced cell cycle arrest and/or cellular stress responses such as senescence, apoptosis, and necrosis and inhibited SR in all seven cell lines. Resveratrol coordinately induced S-phase arrest and cellular stress responses, inhibited telomerase activity and abolished SR in U-937, Mo7e and K-562 cells. Resveratrol induced marked increase in *p21* and/or *p27* transcript levels and senescence rates in U-937, K-562 and U-266 cells. Taken together, resveratrol has been shown to exert multifactorial actions and inhibit SR, whereas Vit-C by inhibition of telomerase activity alone did not affect SR.

Keywords: Leukemia; Self-renewal capacity; Terminal divisions; Resveratrol; Vitamin C

Introduction

Throughout the adult life of a mammalian organism, hematopoietic stem cells (HSCs) must replicate themselves to maintain the constant HSC pool in the marrow. The process of HSC replication through mitosis is called self-renewal (SR) [1]. Acute myeloid leukemia (AML) is organized hierarchically. Non-stem leukemia cells originate from leukemia stem cells (LSC), which represent the ultimate therapeutic target for AML [2-4]. In AML and acute lymphoblastic leukemia, LSCs arise from hematopoietic stem cells or from more differentiated and committed progenitors that acquire SR potential [5,6]. Leukemic blast progenitors are characterized as stem cells; they renew themselves and/or undergo terminal divisions with limited differentiation [7]. Therefore, the target of chemotherapy for leukemia may be leukemic blast progenitors.

In recent years, interest in the use of food plants and their products for cancer prevention has grown [8]. They act through one or more signaling pathways like NF-κB, Cox-2, STAT3, Akt, MAPK/ERK, Bcl-2, Caspases, PARP, MMP-2/-9 and Cyclin D1. Resveratrol, a polyphenol found in grape skins, has also been shown to inhibit the proliferation and induce the apoptosis in leukemia [9] and cancer [10] through signaling pathways such as STAT3 [11-13], PTEN [14,15], Akt/PI3k [14-20], mTOR [17,19], telomerase activity [21], MAPK/ERK [11,15,16,20,22-24], p38-MAPK [17,18, 23-25], JNK [22,25], MTA1/HDAC [14], H2AX [25], Wnt/β-catenin [26,27], TCF4 [24,27], SIRT1 [12,28], NKG2D ligands [29] and NFκB [13]. Anti-tumor effects of vitamin C (Vit-C) in leukemia and cancer have also been reported [30-32]. In addition, telomerase activity has been shown to be limiting the growth of human AML [33,34] and transformed cells [35]. However, in the previous studies, cell viability assay or blast colony formations (BCF) have been used to assess the growth inhibition by the two agents, and none of them determined the effects of the agents on the SR capacity.

Oxidative stress is an imbalance between pro-oxidant and anti-oxidant factors that can lead to cellular damage [36]. Tumor suppressor genes regulate diverse cellular activities, including DNA damage repair, cell cycle arrest, mitogenic signaling, cell differentiation, migration, programmed cell death and senescence. Links between tumor suppressor genes and reactive oxygen species have been uncovered.

In the present study, we investigated the effects of resveratrol and Vit-C on the growth of hematologic malignant blast progenitors in liquid suspension for up to one month. The cell cycle, type and rate of cellular stress responses, *p21* and *p27* trasncript levels and telomerase activity were also assessed.

Materials and Methods

Cell lines

The HL-60 (a gift from Dr. D.W. Golde, UCLA School of Medicine, Los Angeles, CA) is a myeloid cell line derived from an acute promyelocytic leukemia patient. The Mo7e (a gift from Dr. S. Tohda, Tokyo Medical and Dental University, Tokyo, Japan) is a subclone of the human megakaryoblastic leukemia cell line Mo7, and requires interleukin (IL)-3 for growth [37]. The K-562 is a myeloid cell line derived from a patient with chronic myelogenous leukemia in myeloid

***Corresponding author:** Ikuo Murohashi, MD, Hematology, Center for University-Wide Education, School of Health and Social Services, Saitama Prefectural University, Sannomiya 820, Koshigaya-City, Saitama 343-8540, Japan, E-mail: murohashi-ikuo@spu.ac.jp crisis. Daudi and Raji are B lymphoid cell lines derived from Burkitt's lymphoma patients. The U-937 is a human histiocytic, monocyte-like cell line derived from a diffuse histiocytic lymphoma patient. K-562, Daudi, Raji and U-937 cell lines were obtained from the Japanese Collection of Research Bioresources (JCRB) Cell Bank (Osaka, Japan). The human myeloma cell line U-266 was a gift from Dr. M. Kawano (Yamaguchi University School of Medicine, Ube, Japan).

Reagents

Iscove's modified Dulbecco's medium (IMDM), fetal calf serum (FCS) and PBS were from Gibco (Grand Island, NY). Trypan blue (TB) and L-ascorbic acid (Vit-C) were from Sigma (Tokyo, Japan). Recombinant human (rh) IL-3 was a gift from Dr. S. Clark (Genetics Institute, Cambridge, MA). Resveratrol was obtained from Biomol International LP (Farmingdale, PA).

Clonogenic assay in methylcellulose culture

BCF was done as previously reported [38].

Resveratrol and Vit-C treatments in long-term suspension cultures

Cells were cultured at a concentration of 10^4 cells/ml in 35-mm Lux tissue culture dishes (Miles Lab., Naperville, IL) in 2 ml of IMDM supplemented with 10% FCS + 0.38% DMSO (Cont media), 10% FCS + 0.38% DMSO + 10 μM resveratrol (Res media), or 10% FCS + 0.38% DMSO + 300 μM Vit-C (Vit-C media) [39]. Twice a week, to determine the plating efficiency, the cells were harvested, counted, washed and plated in 96-well plates at a concentration of 2×10^3 cells per well in 0.1 ml of IMDM with 1% methylcellulose and 10% FCS. The recovery per dish was determined by multiplying the plating efficiency by the number of cells harvested from the suspension. At each subculture, the harvested cells were transferred into the same fresh media. This procedure was repeated for each round of plating and the cumulative clonogenic cell number per dish with time was calculated. Mo7e cells were cultured in methylcellulose and suspension supplemented with 10 ng/ml rh IL-3.

Calculation of kinetic parameters for cumulative clonogenic cells

The number of cumulative clonogenic cells from the start of liquid suspension culture was serially plotted on a semi-logarithmic graph (Figures 1 and 2). Linear regression analysis using Excel was performed. The line of the fitted equation describing the plots and the significance of linearity were determined [40]. The relative slope (SLP) (rSLP) of the line defined as $SLP_{agent}/SLP_{control}$ indicated the level of SR in the presence of agent.

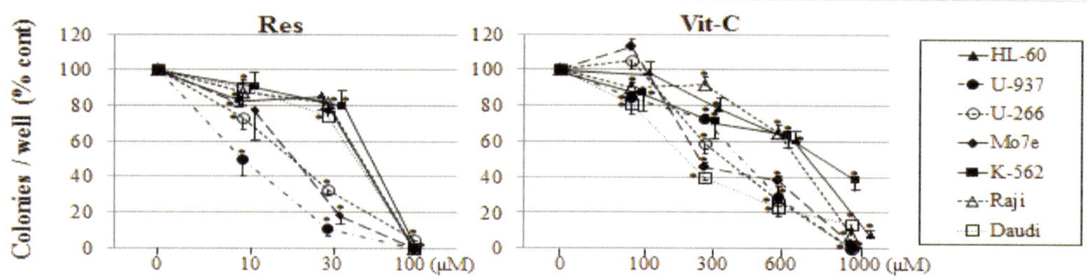

Figure 1: Effects of resveratrol and Vit-C on BCF in methylcellulose.
Full titration curves of resveratrol (Res) and Vit-C for the seven leukemia cell lines were generated. BCF per well in control culture was 100 ± 5, 68 ± 14, 125 ± 8, 129 ± 10, 115 ± 2, 70 ± 9 and 192 ± 20 in U-937, Mo7e, K-562, HL-60, U-266, Raji and Daudi cells, respectively. The data shown represent the mean ± SD of five replicate cultures. The data were normalized as the percentage of the control value in each experiment. Control medium contained 0.38% DMSO alone.
*$p < 0.05$ when compared with control cultures.

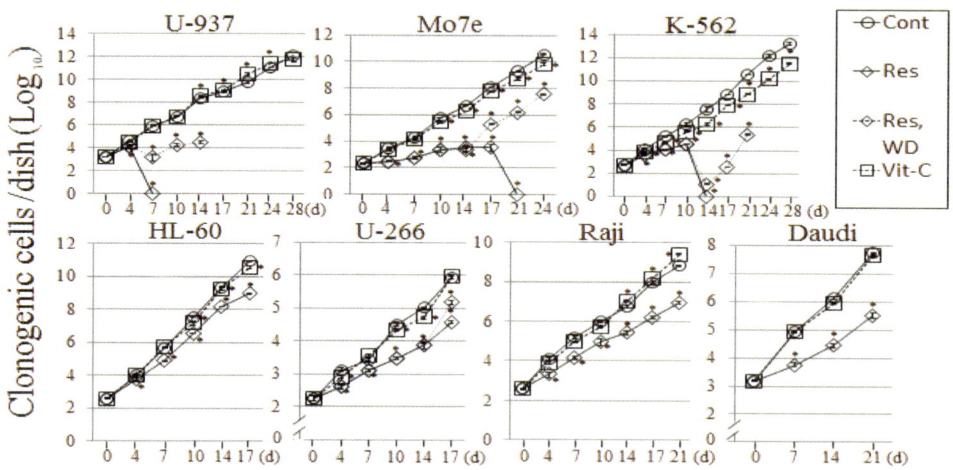

Figure 2: Effects of resveratrol and Vit-C on cumulative clonogenic cell recovery in long-term suspension cultures.
Cells were cultured in suspension with DMSO alone (Cont) or with DMSO plus resveratrol (Res) or Vit-C. Resveratrol was withdrawn at days 4, 10, 10 and 14 in U-937, Mo7e, K-562 and U-266, respectively. The data shown represent the mean ± SD of five replicate cultures. rSLP was expressed as inhibition relative to untreated cells (1.0). rSLP by Vit-C was 1.024, 0.92, 0.818, 0.963, 0.99, 1.109 and 0.967 in U-937, Mo7e, K-562, HL-60, U-266, Raji and Daudi cells, respectively. Inhibition of SR was defined as <0.8. *$p < 0.05$ when compared with control cultures. WD: withdrawal.

Telomerase activity

Telomerase activity was assessed using a Quantitative Telomerase Detection Kit (Allied Biotech, Inc., Benicia, CA). Cells were lysed and protein was isolated using the kit. The concentration of the isolated protein was determined using a NanoDrop Spectrophotometer (Thermo Scientific, Waltham, MA). The telomerase activity in a cell extract was measured from its ability to synthesize telomeric repeats onto an oligonucleotide substrate. The extended product was amplified and visualized using SYBR Green. The increase in fluorescence was monitored, and the telomerase activity was determined using real-time PCR (Chromo 4TM Real-Time PCR System; Bio-Rad, Tokyo, Japan).

Trypan blue staining

Equal volumes of a cell suspension and 0.4% TB solution in 0.85% saline were incubated for 5 min at room temperature. Cells that stained blue were counted as positive. For quantification of TB-positive cells, 100 cells were counted in three separate fields using an inverted Nikon microscope, and the proportion of blue-stained cells was determined. Cells stained with specific membrane-impermeant nucleic acid dyes such as TB and propidium iodide (PI) (data not shown) were considered to be necrotic, because loss of membrane integrity is a pathognomonic feature of necrotic cell death [41].

Senescence-associated (SA)-β-galactosidase labeling

SA-β-galactosidase was detected using a Senescence Detection Kit (BioVision Inc., Milpitas, CA). Briefly, cells were fixed for 15 min with Fixative Solution and washed once with PBS. Cells were then incubated overnight at 37°C with Staining Solution Mix containing 1 mg/ml X-Gal. For quantification of SA-β-galactosidase-positive cells, 100 cells were counted in three separate fields using an inverted Nikon microscope, and the proportion of blue-stained cells was determined.

Cell cycle analysis

DNA in permeabilized cells was stained with PI using a cell phase determination kit (Cayman Chemical Company). Flow cytometry was used to detect staining and determine the percentage of cells in each phase of the cell cycle [42]. The fluorescence of PI-stained cells (10^4 nuclei) was measured within 30 min on a FACSCanto II (BD Biosciences, Tokyo, Japan) equipped with a doublet discrimination module. The apoptotic cell fraction was also determined.

Reverse transcription-PCR (RT-PCR) assay

Total cellular RNA was extracted using a High Pure RNA Isolation Kit (Roche, Mannheim, Germany). The concentration and purity of the extracted RNA were evaluated from spectrophotometric absorbance readings at 260 and 280 nm (JASCO V-530 UV-Vis spectrophotometer, Easton, MD). RT-PCR was performed with total RNA and an mRNA Selective PCR Kit Ver. 1.1 (TaKaRa, Tokyo, Japan), which prevents amplification of genomic DNA, using a PCR system (TaKaRa). The primers were 5'-ATCCCGTGTTCTCCTTT-3' (forward) and 5'-CGACCGATCTTCGG-3' (reverse) for *p21*, 5'-AACGTGCGAGTGTCTAACGG-3' (forward) and 5'-TGCGTGTCCTCAGAGTTAGCC-3' (reverse) for *p27*, and 5'-CGATGCTGGCGCTGAGTAC-3' (forward) and 5'- CGTTCAGCTCAGGGATGACC-3' (reverse) for *GAPDH*. Samples were size-fractionated by agarose gel electrophoresis along with a 50-bp molecular weight marker (Roche), and stained with ethidium bromide (Wako, Osaka, Japan).

Densitometry

Gel images were captured using a ChemiDoc XRS (Bio-Rad). A housekeeping gene (*GAPDH*) was co-amplified under the same conditions, and the expression of each target gene relative to *GAPDH* expression was determined. Specific bands and backgrounds were enclosed within the same square, and background subtraction densitometric analysis was performed using Quality One (Bio-Rad).

Statistics

Data for BCF are shown as the mean ± SD of five replicate cultures. The other assay was done in triplicate. The statistical significance was evaluated using Student's *t*-test (two-tailed) or the chi-squared test.

Results

Growth regulation in methylcellulose

In the seven cell lines, resveratrol and Vit-C inhibited BCF in a dose-dependent manner and IC_{50} ranged from 9.9 to 68 μM and 240 to 830 μM with a mean of 41 and 514 μM, respectively (Figure 1). Thus, in subsequent experiments, we cultured cells in suspension with resveratrol and Vit-C at 10 and 300 μM, respectively. These concentrations inhibited BCF by 20% ± 15% and 34% ± 17% (mean ± SD for % inhibition relative to control in seven cell lines), respectively. Three cell lines (U-937, Mo7e and U-266) were sensitive and three (HL-60, K-562 and Raji) were resistant to the two agents, and the remaining one (Daudi) showed reversed sensitivities to the agents.

Growth regulation in liquid suspension

An exponential increase in the number of cumulative clonogenic

Table 1: Inhibition of SR and telomerase activity and induction of cellular stress response and cell cycle arrest by resveratrol and Vit-C in seven cell lines.

Variable	HL-60	U-937	U-266	Mo7e	K-562	Raji	Daudi
rSLP[a]	Res (0.787)	Res (-0.378)	Res (0.666)	Res (-0.281)	Res (-0.443)	Res (0.713)	Res (0.514)
Telomerase activity[b]	Vit-C (+)	Res (+), Vit-C (+)	(-)	Res (+), Vit-C (+)	Res (+), Vit-C (+)	Vit-C (+)	(-)
Senescence[c]	(-)	Res (+++), Vit-C (+)	Res (++)	(-)	Res (+++)	(-)	Res (+)
Necrosis[c]	(-)	Res (+++)	Res (+)	Res (+++)	(-)	(-)	Res (+), Vit-C (+)
Apoptosis[d]	Res (+)	Res (++)	Res (+)	Res (++)	Res (++)	(-)	Res (+)
G_1 arrest[e]	(-)	(-)	(-)	(-)	(-)	(-)	(-)
S-phase arrest[e]	(-)	Res (++)	(-)	Res (+++)	Res (+++)	Res (++)	(-)
G_2/M arrest[e]	(-)	(-)	(-)	Vit-C (++)	(-)	(-)	Res (+)

[a] Inhibition of SR was defined as <0.8. rSLP is shown in parenthesis.
[b] No significant inhibition compared with control (-); and significant inhibition compared with control (+) by Student's *t*-test.
[c] The percentage of positive cells <10 or not significantly higher than those of control (-); and ≥10 and <20 (+), ≥20 and <40 (++), and ≥40 (+++) with values significantly higher than those of control by Student's *t*-test.
[d] % control as ≤250: (-); >250 and ≤350: (+); and > 350: (++).
[e] % control as ≤124: (-); >124 and ≤130: (+); >130 and ≤140: (++); and >140: (+++).

cells recovered per dish was observed in each of the 21 conditions (7 cell lines treated with or without each of the two agents), except for three in which growth was abolished ($p < 0.01$, r ranged from 0.984 to 0.999 by linear regression analysis) (Figure 2). Repeated addition of 10 μM resveratrol abolished SR in U-937, Mo7e and K-562 cells at days 7, 21 and 14, respectively and reduced rSLP levels to less than 0.8 in the remaining four cell lines (Table 1). Furthermore, after washout of resveratrol, rSLP returned to the control levels in four cell lines. Repeated addition of 300 μM Vit-C reduced rSLP level to less than 0.8 in none of the seven cell lines and enhanced SR in Raji cells with an rSLP of 1.109.

The sensitivities of BCF and SR to resveratrol were high in U-937 and Mo7e cells, low in HL-60 and Raji cells, and reversed in K-562 cells (Figures 1 and 2).

Cellular stress responses such as senescence, apoptosis and necrosis in liquid suspension

In U-937 cells, repeated addition of 10 μM resveratrol markedly increased the rate of senescence and necrosis (Figure 3) and the relative apoptotic ratio, determined with flow cytometry analysis (Figure 4). Resveratrol markedly increased senescence in U-266 cells, senescence and apoptosis in K-562 cells, and necrosis and apoptosis in Mo7e cells, and slightly increased apoptosis in HL-60 cells and all three in Daudi cells. Repeated addition of 300 μM Vit-C slightly increased senescence in U-937 cells and necrosis in Daudi cells.

Resveratrol increased senescence (4/7, 57%), necrosis (4/7, 57%) and apoptosis (6/7, 86%), and Vit-C increased senescence (1/7, 14%), necrosis (1/7, 14%), and apoptosis (0/7, 0%) (Table 1). Thus, resveratrol more frequently increased apoptosis than Vit-C ($p < 0.01$ by the chi-squared test).

Resveratrol withdrawal effects

In K-562 cells in liquid suspension, withdrawal of resveratrol after 4 days or after 4 days and 7 days significantly decreased necrosis and senescence when compared with the effects of repeated addition of resveratrol for 7 days or 10 days, respectively (Figure 5). Similarly, in U-937 cells, withdrawal of resveratrol after 4 days significantly decreased necrosis and senescence when compared with the effects of repeated addition of resveratrol for 14 days.

Cell cycle analysis

Repeated addition of 10 μM resveratrol induced S-phase arrest in U-937, Mo7e, K-562 and Raji cells, and G_2/M arrest in Daudi cells (Figure 6 and Table 1). Repeated addition of 300 μM Vit-C induced G_2/M arrest in Mo7e cells. Resveratrol (5/7; 71%) induced cell cycle arrest more frequently than Vit-C (1/7; 14%) ($p < 0.05$ by the chi-squared test).

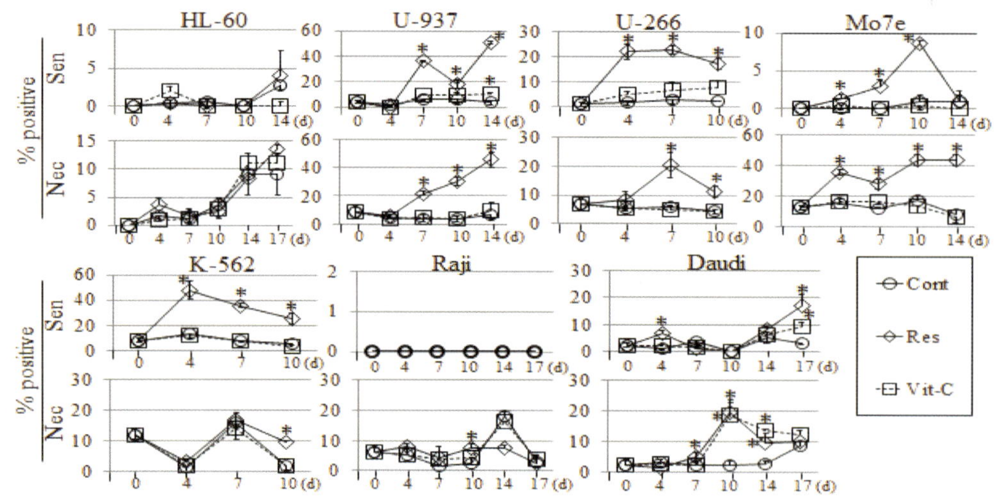

Figure 3: Senescence and necrosis in liquid suspension cultures.
Cells were treated as described in Figure 2. The percentage of cells stained with SA-β-galactosidase (Sen) or trypan blue (Nec) was determined. The data shown represent the mean ± SD of three separate measurements. *$p < 0.05$ when compared with control cultures.

Figure 4: The relative apoptotic cell fraction determined with flow cytometry analysis.
Cells were treated as described in Figure 2. The data were normalized as the percentage of the control value in each experiment. The percentage of apoptotic cells in control culture was 0.3% ± 0.7% (n = 7), 4.8% ± 5.6% (n = 7), 3.1% ± 2.6% (n = 7) and 1.1% ± 0.6% (n = 4) at day 0, 4, 7 and 10, respectively. * Induction of apoptosis was defined as >250%. ≤250%: (-) (see Table 1).

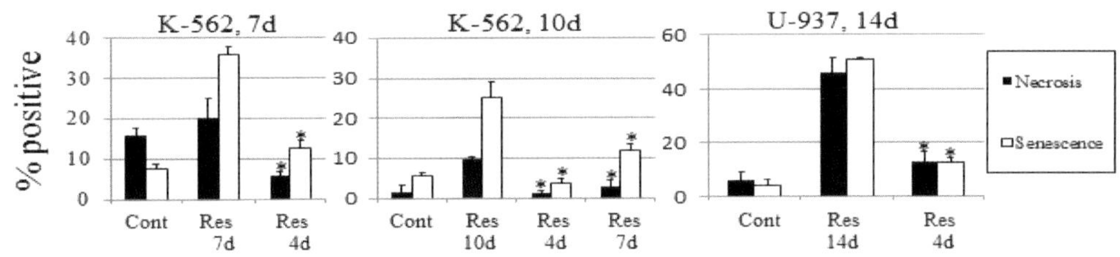

Figure 5: Effects of Resveratrol withdrawal on senescence and necrosis of leukemia cells.
K-562 and U-937 cells in liquid suspension were cultured for the indicated periods with continuous exposure to resveratrol (Res) or with exposure to resveratrol followed by resveratrol withdrawal. Control (Cont) medium contained 0.38% DMSO alone. The percentages of cells stained with SA-β-galactosidase or trypan blue were determined after culture for the indicated periods. The data shown represent the mean ± SD of three separate determinations. *$p < 0.05$ when compared with continuous exposure to resveratrol.

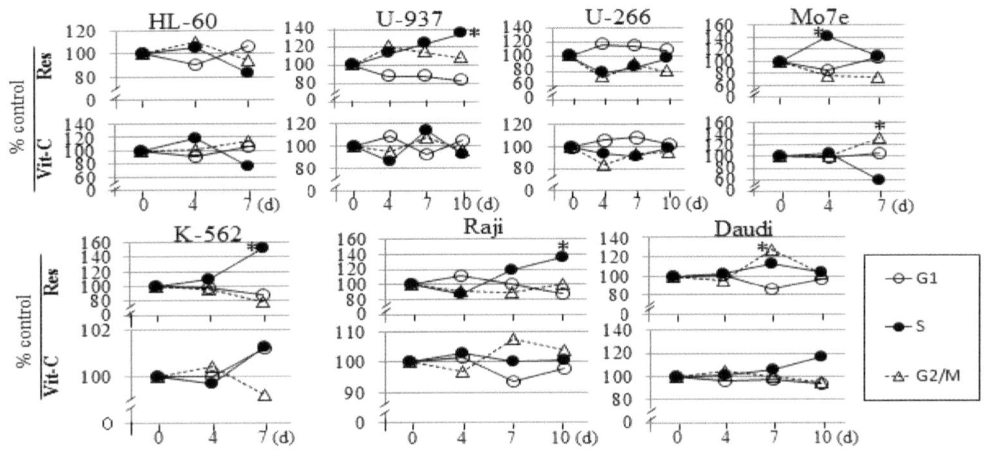

Figure 6: Cell cycle analysis.
Cells were treated as described in Figure 2. The data shown represent the mean of two or three separate measurements. The data were normalized as the percentage of the control value in each experiment. *Cell cycle arrest was defined as >124%. ≤ 124%: (-) (see Table 1).

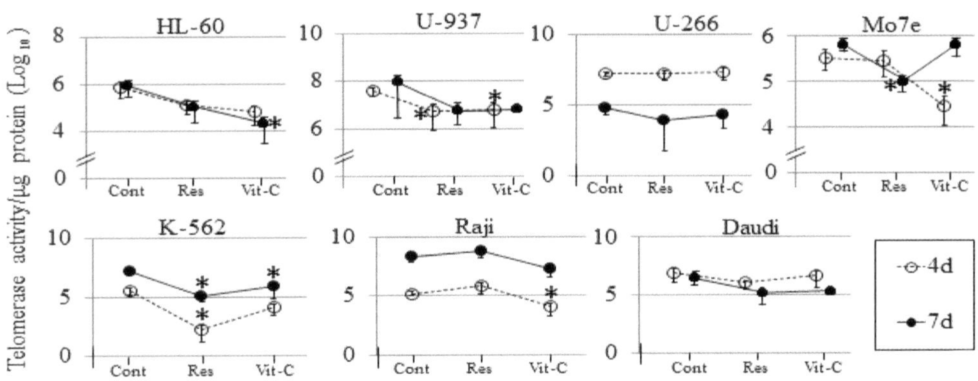

Figure 7: Effects of resveratrol and Vit-C on the telomerase activity of leukemia cells.
Cells were treated as described in Fig. 2. The data shown represent the mean ± SD of three separate measurements. *$p < 0.05$ when compared with control cultures.

Telomerase activity

Each of the two agents, by repeated addition, significantly inhibited telomerase activity in U-937, Mo7e and K-562 cells at day 4 or 7 (Figure 7). In U-266 and Daudi cells, neither of the two agents significantly inhibited telomerase activity.

CKI gene expression profiles in liquid suspension culture

In U-937 and K-562 cells, repeated addition of 10 μM resveratrol induced more than tenfold increase in *p21* levels on day 4 and the expression returned to basal level on day 7 (Figure 8). In U-266 cells, resveratrol also markedly and transiently increased *p27*, but not *p21*.

Discussion

SR inhibition by repeated addition of resveratrol was as follows:

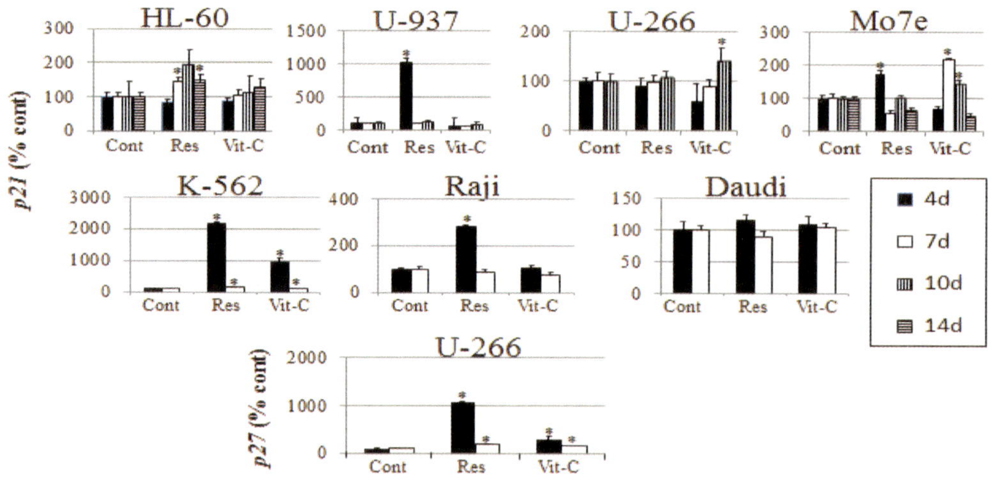

Figure 8: *p21* and *p27* gene expression profiles in liquid suspension cultures.
Cells were treated as described in Figure 2. The relative band densities were expressed as the mean ± SD of three separate determinations. * $p < 0.05$ when compared with control.

induction of S-phase arrest and cellular stress responses, inhibition of telomerase activity and abolishment of SR in U-937, Mo7e and K-562 cells; induction of G_2/M arrest and cellular stress responses, no inhibition of telomerase activity and inhibition of SR with rSLP of 0.514 in Daudi cells; and induction of either cell cycle arrest or cellular stress responses, no inhibition of telomerase activity and inhibition of SR with rSLP between 0.666 and 0.787 in the remaining three (Table 1). SR inhibition by repeated addition of Vit-C was as follows: induction of either cell cycle arrest or cellular stress responses with rSLP between 0.92 and 1.024 in three cell lines; and induction of neither cell cycle arrest nor cellular stress response with rSLP between 0.818 and 1.109 in the remaining four, including inhibition of telomerase activity in two and three cell lines, respectively.

The SR capacity of leukemic blast progenitors, assessed by measuring secondary plating efficiency or exponential growth in suspension culture [39], but not BCF, has been reported to be highly correlated with the clinical outcome in AML patients [43-45]. Competitive repopulation units (CRU) assay [46] and *in vitro* serial plating assay [47] are also available to determine the SR capacity. From this point of view, the effects of antitumor drugs on not only terminal divisions but also SR of blast progenitors should be examined to predict the effectiveness of the drugs in the therapy for malignancy. We showed that resveratrol and Vit-C preferentially inhibits SR capacity and BCF, respectively. There was no significant correlation between rSLP and % of control BCF in the seven cell lines after treatment with resveratrol (r = 0.24 by linear regression analysis) or Vit-C (r = 0.369 by linear regression analysis). This may be mainly owing to the differences in the exposure duration of the cells to the agents and the cumulative cellular damage by the agents between the two culture conditions.

In the present study, 10 μM resveratrol induced reversible inhibition of leukemia SR capacity. In HepG2 cells, lower (6.25–25 μM) and higher (≥ 50 μM) concentrations of resveratrol induced reversible S-phase arrest and irreversible apoptosis, and inhibition of PI3K and MAPK/ERK may be responsible for the induction of S-phase arrest and apoptosis, respectively [16]. However, silencing of the *p21* gene did not show any effect on resveratrol-induced S-phase arrest.

Our data indicate that the differential induction of the three types of cellular stress responses by each of the two agents depends on the type of the leukemia cell line. This may be compatible with the recent report that the cell type and the nature and intensity of the damage are the critical determinants of senescence or apoptosis induction [48].

Senescence is characterized by irreversible cell cycle arrest; overexpression of cyclin-dependent kinase inhibitors (CKIs); caspase-independent cell death; and a strong resistance to apoptosis [49]. Consistent with the notion that senescence is a tumor suppression mechanism, CKIs such as p53, pRb, p16, p19, p21 and p27 are regulators of senescence [50,51]. Resveratrol in U-937, K-562 and U-266 markedly increased *p21* and/or *p27* transcript levels and senescence rates, although *p53* and *p16* genes are absent or mutated in the cell lines [42,50,51].

Vit-C induces partial G_1/S block, inhibits telomerase activity, upregulates p53 and Bax, and inhibits Bcl-2 [52]. Resveratrol downregulates telomerase activity and cancer cell growth in vitro [21]. In cancer, the noncanonical signaling loop between telomerase reverse transcriptase (TERT) and NF-κB and between TERT and Wnt/β-catenin signaling has been proposed as a mechanism for the concomitant activation of NF-κB- and Wnt/β-catenin-dependent transcription following TERT overexpression. This drives the prolonged expression of target genes critical for the maintenance of tumor survival and proliferation [53]. However, hTERT depletion alone did not affect cancer cell survival [54].

Induction of cell cycle arrest and apoptosis, but not the inhibition of telomerase activity, was more frequent by resveratrol than Vit-C. It remains to be further clarified through which signaling pathways resveratrol, but not Vit-C, abolishes SR of blast progenitors. Compared with previous reports [39,46,47], our newly proposed assay may be quite useful to evaluate the SR capacity of blast progenitors because it indicates SR capacity as rSLP. By adding inhibitors, stimulators, ligands or siRNA to our assay, major stimulatory and inhibitory signaling pathways for SR capacity of blast progenitors may be uncovered.

Financial support

2013 Graduate Student Exchange and Grant-in-Aid for Encouragement of Scientists Research Funds, Saitama Prefectural University.

Acknowledgments

The authors are indebted to Drs. Susumu Ohshima and Masami Bessho (Saitama Medical University, Saitama) for analysis and discussion of flow cytometry data, Dr. Steven C. Clark (Genetics Institute, Cambridge, MA) for rhIL-3, Dr. Ryo Kubota (our university) for statistical analysis, and Kanae Sakate (Saitama Medical University, Saitama) for expert technical assistance.

References

1. Huang X, Cho S, Spangrude GJ (2007) Hematopoietic stem cells: generation and self-renewal. Cell Death Differ 14: 1851-1859.
2. Lapidot T, Sirard C, Vormoor J, Murdoch B, Hoang T, et al. (1994) A cell initiating human acute myeloid leukaemia after transplantation into SCID mice. Nature 367: 645-648.
3. Bonnet D, Dick JE (1997) Human acute myeloid leukemia is organized as a hierarchy that originates from a primitive hematopoietic cell. Nat Med 3: 730-737.
4. Hope KJ, Jin L, Dick JE (2004) Acute myeloid leukemia originates from a hierarchy of leukemic stem cell classes that differ in self-renewal capacity. Nat Immunol 5: 738–743.
5. Goardon N, Marchi E, Atzberger A, Quek L, Schuh A, et al. (2011) Coexistence of LMPP-like and GMP-like leukemia stem cells in acute myeloid leukemia. Cancer Cell 19: 138-152.
6. Castor A, Nilsson L, Astrand-Grundström I, Buitenhuis M, Ramirez C, et al. (2005) Distinct patterns of hematopoietic stem cell involvement in acute lymphoblastic leukemia. Nat Med 11: 630-637.
7. McCulloch EA (1986) Regulatory mechanisms affecting the blast stem cells of acute myeloblastic leukemia. J Cell Physiol Suppl 4: 27-33.
8. Khuda-Bukhsh AR, Das S, Saha SK (2014) Molecular approaches toward targeted cancer prevention with some food plants and their products: inflammatory and other signal pathways. Nutr Cancer 66: 194-205.
9. Tsan MF, White JE, Maheshwari JG, Chikkappa G (2002) Anti-leukemia effect of resveratrol. Leuk Lymphoma 43: 983-987.
10. Han G, Xia J, Gao J, Inagaki Y, Tang W, et al. (2015) Anti-tumor effects and cellular mechanisms of resveratrol. Drug Discov Ther 9: 1-12.
11. Quoc Trung L, Espinoza JL, Takami A, Nakao S (2013) Resveratrol induces cell cycle arrest and apoptosis in malignant NK cells via JAK2/STAT3 pathway inhibition. PLoS One 8: e55183.
12. Li Y, Zhu W, Li J, Liu M, Wei M (2013) Resveratrol suppresses the STAT3 signaling pathway and inhibits proliferation of high glucose-exposed HepG2 cells partly through SIRT1. Oncol Rep 30: 2820-2828.
13. Espinoza JL, Takami A, Trung LQ, Kato S, Nakao S (2012) Resveratrol prevents EBV transformation and inhibits the outgrowth of EBV-immortalized human B cells. PLoS One 7: e51306.
14. Dhar S, Kumar A, Li K, Tzivion G, Levenson AS (2015) Resveratrol regulates PTEN/Akt pathway through inhibition of MTA1/HDAC unit of the NuRD complex in prostate cancer. Biochim Biophys Acta 1853: 265-275.
15. Ghorbani A, Zand H, Jeddi-Tehrani M, Koohdani F, Shidfar F, et al. (2015) PTEN over-expression by resveratrol in acute lymphoblastic leukemia cells along with suppression of AKT/PKB and ERK1/2 in genotoxic stress. J Nat Med May 1. [Epub ahead of print].
16. Zhou R, Fukui M, Choi HJ, Zhu BT (2009) Induction of a reversible, non-cytotoxic S-phase delay by resveratrol: implications for a mechanism of lifespan prolongation and cancer protection. Br J Pharmacol 158: 462-474.
17. Ge J, Liu Y, Li Q, Guo X, Gu L, et al. (2013) Resveratrol induces apoptosis and autophagy in T-cell acute lymphoblastic leukemia cells by inhibiting Akt/mTOR and activating p38-MAPK. Biomed Environ Sci 26: 902-911.
18. Dai Z, Lei P, Xie J, Hu Y (2015) Antitumor effect of resveratrol on chondrosarcoma cells via phosphoinositide 3-kinase/AKT and p38 mitogen-activated protein kinase pathways. Mol Med Rep 12: 3151-3155.
19. Jiang H, Shang X, Wu H, Gautam SC, Al-Holou S, et al. (2009) Resveratrol downregulates PI3K/Akt/mTOR signaling pathways in human U251 glioma cells. J Exp Ther Oncol 8: 25-33.
20. Banerjee Mustafi S, Chakraborty PK, Raha S (2010) Modulation of Akt and ERK1/2 pathways by resveratrol in chronic myelogenous leukemia (CML) cells results in the downregulation of Hsp70. PLoS One 5: e8719.
21. Lanzilli G, Fuggetta MP, Tricarico M, Cottarelli A, Serafino A, et al. (2006) Resveratrol down-regulates the growth and telomerase activity of breast cancer cells in vitro. Int J Oncol 28: 641-648.
22. Xie Q, Yang Y, Wang Z, Chen F, Zhang A, et al. (2014) Resveratrol-4-O-D-(2'-galloyl)-glucopyranoside isolated from Polygonum cuspidatum exhibits anti-hepatocellular carcinoma viability by inducing apoptosis via the JNK and ERK pathway. Molecules 19: 1592-1602.
23. Liao PC, Ng LT, Lin LT, Richardson CD, Wang GH, et al. (2010) Resveratrol arrests cell cycle and induces apoptosis in human hepatocellular carcinoma Huh-7 cells. J Med Food 13: 1415-1423.
24. Jeong JB, Lee J, Lee SH (2015) TCF4 Is a molecular target of resveratrol in the prevention of colorectal cancer. Int J Mol Sci 16: 10411-10425.
25. Wu XP, Xiong M, Xu CS, Duan LN, Dong YQ, et al. (2015) Resveratrol induces apoptosis of human chronic myelogenous leukemia cells in vitro through p38 and JNK-regulated H2AX phosphorylation. Acta Pharmacol Sin 36: 353-361.
26. Fu Y, Chang H, Peng X, Bai Q, Yi L, et al. (2014) Resveratrol inhibits breast cancer stem-like cells and induces autophagy via suppressing Wnt/β-catenin signaling pathway. PLoS One 9: e102535.
27. Chen HJ, Hsu LS, Shia YT, Lin MW, Lin CM (2012) The β-catenin/TCF complex as a novel target of resveratrol in the Wnt/β-catenin signaling pathway. Biochem Pharmacol 84: 1143-1153.
28. Yang Q, Wang B, Zang W, Wang X, Liu Z, et al. (2013) Resveratrol inhibits the growth of gastric cancer by inducing G1 phase arrest and senescence in a Sirt1-dependent manner. PLoS One 8: e70627.
29. Luis Espinoza J, Takami A, Trung LQ, Nakao S (2013) Ataxia-telangiectasia mutated kinase-mediated upregulation of NKG2D ligands on leukemia cells by resveratrol results in enhanced natural killer cell susceptibility. Cancer Sci 104: 657–662.
30. Park S (2013) The effects of high concentrations of vitamin C on cancer cells. Nutrients 5: 3496-3505.
31. Wilson MK, Baguley BC, Wall C, Jameson MB, Findlay MP (2014) Review of high-dose intravenous vitamin C as an anticancer agent. Asia Pac J Clin Oncol 10: 22-37.
32. Kawada H, Kaneko M, Sawanobori M, Uno T, Matsuzawa H, et al. (2013) High concentrations of L-ascorbic acid specifically inhibit the growth of human leukemic cells via downregulation of HIF-1α transcription. PLoS One 8: e62717.
33. Röth A, Vercauteren S, Sutherland HJ, Lansdorp PM (2003) Telomerase is limiting the growth of acute myeloid leukemia cells. Leukemia 17: 2410-2417.
34. Bruedigam C, Bagger FO, Heidel FH, Paine Kuhn C, Guignes S, et al. (2014) Telomerase inhibition effectively targets mouse and human AML stem cells and delays relapse following chemotherapy. Cell Stem Cell 15: 775-790.
35. Fleisig HB, Hukezalie KR, Thompson CA, Au-Yeung TT, Ludlow AT, et al. (2015) Telomerase reverse transcriptase expression protects transformed human cells against DNA-damaging agents, and increases tolerance to chromosomal instability. Oncogene.
36. Vurusaner B, Poli G, Basaga H (2012) Tumor suppressor genes and ROS: complex networks of interactions. Free Radic Biol Med 52: 7-18.
37. Avanzi GC, Lista P, Giovinazzo B, Miniero R, Saglio G, et al. (1988) Selective growth response to IL-3 of a human leukaemic cell line with megakaryoblastic features. Br J Haematol 69: 359-366.
38. Murohashi I, Yoshida K, Kishimoto K, Takahashi T, Wakao D, et al. (2002) Differential response to stem cell factor and Flt3 ligand by the FAB subtype in acute myeloid leukemia clonogenic cells. J Interferon Cytokine Res 22: 335-341.
39. Nara N, McCulloch EA (1985) The proliferation in suspension of the progenitors of the blast cells in acute myeloblastic leukemia. Blood 65: 1484-1493.
40. Wakao D, Murohashi I, Tominaga K, Yoshida K, Kishimoto K, et al. (2002) Serum thymidine kinase and soluble interleukin-2 receptor predict recurrence of malignant lymphoma. Ann Hematol 81: 140-146.
41. Elmore S (2007) Apoptosis: a review of programmed cell death. Toxicol Pathol 35: 495-516.
42. Yoshida K, Murohashi I, Hirashima K (1996) p53-independent induction of p21 (WAF1/CIP1) during differentiation of HL-60 cells by tumor necrosis factor alpha. Int J Hematol 65: 41-48.
43. Curtis JE, Messner HA, Hasselback R, Elhakim TM, McCulloch EA (1984) Contributions of host- and disease-related attributes to the outcome of patients with acute myelogenous leukemia. J Clin Oncol 2: 253-259.

44. Nara N, Tohda S, Suzuki T, Nagata K, Yamashita Y, et al. (1990) Effects of N4-behenoyl-1-beta-D-arabinofuranosylcytosine on blast progenitors of acute myeloblastic leukemia. Cancer Res 50: 7587-7592.

45. Nara N, Chen GJ, Murohashi I, Tohda S, Imai Y, et al. (1992) The in vitro growth patterns and drug sensitivities of leukemic blast progenitors among the subtypes of acute myelocytic leukemia. Exp Hematol 20: 904-908.

46. Szilvassy SJ, Humphries RK, Lansdorp PM, Eaves AC, Eaves CJ (1990) Quantitative assay for totipotent reconstituting hematopoietic stem cells by a competitive repopulation strategy. Proc Natl Acad Sci U S A 87: 8736-8740.

47. Hegde S, Hankey P, Paulson RF (2012) Self-renewal of leukemia stem cells in Friend virus-induced erythroleukemia requires proviral insertional activation of Spi1 and hedgehog signaling but not mutation of p53. Stem Cells 30: 121–130.

48. Childs BG, Baker DJ, Kirkland JL, Campisi J, van Deursen JM (2014) Senescence and apoptosis: dueling or complementary cell fates? EMBO Rep 15: 1139-1153.

49. Ohtani N, Mann DJ, Hara E (2009) Cellular senescence: its role in tumor suppression and aging. Cancer Sci 100: 792-797.

50. Campisi J (2005) Senescent cells, tumor suppression, and organismal aging: good citizens, bad neighbors. Cell 120: 513-522.

51. Majumder PK, Grisanzio C, O'Connell F, Barry M, Brito JM, et al. (2008) A prostatic intraepithelial neoplasia-dependent p27 Kip1 checkpoint induces senescence and inhibits cell proliferation and cancer progression. Cancer Cell 14: 146-155.

52. Reddy VG, Khanna N, Singh N (2001) Vitamin C augments chemotherapeutic response of cervical carcinoma HeLa cells by stabilizing P53. Biochem Biophys Res Commun 282: 409-415.

53. Li Y, Tergaonkar V (2014) Noncanonical functions of telomerase: implications in telomerase-targeted cancer therapies. Cancer Res 74: 1639-1644.

54. Liu T, Liang X, Li B, Björkholm M, Jia J, et al. (2013) Telomerase reverse transcriptase inhibition stimulates cyclooxygenase 2 expression in cancer cells and synergizes with celecoxib to exert anti-cancer effects. Br J Cancer 108: 2272-2280.

Acidosis Sensing Receptor GPR65 Correlates with Anti-Apoptotic Bcl-2 Family Member Expression in CLL Cells: Potential Implications for the CLL Microenvironment

Ashley E Rosko[1,7], Karen S McColl[2], Fei Zhong[2], Christopher B Ryder[2], Ming-Jin Chang[2], Abdus Sattar[3], Paolo F Caimi[1,2,6], Brian T Hill[4,6], Sayer Al-Harbi[5], Alexandru Almasan[5,6] and Clark W Distelhorst[1,2,6]

[1]*Division of Hematology-Oncology, University Hospitals Case Medical Center, Cleveland, Ohio, USA*
[2]*Division of Hematology-Oncology, Case Western Reserve School of Medicine, Cleveland, USA*
[3]*Department of Epidemiology and Biostatistics, Case Western Reserve University, Cleveland, OH, USA*
[4]*Department of Hematologic Oncology and Blood Disorders, Cleveland Clinic, Cleveland, Ohio, USA*
[5]*Department of Cancer Biology, Lerner Research Institute, Cleveland Clinic, Cleveland, Ohio, USA*
[6]*Case Comprehensive Cancer Center, Case Western Reserve University School of Medicine, Ohio, USA*
[7]*Division of Hematology, Department of Medicine, Ohio State University College of Medicine, Columbus, Ohio, USA*

Abstract

The tumor microenvironment is generally an acidic environment, yet the effect of extracellular acidosis on chronic lymphocytic leukemia (CLL) is not well established. Here we are the first to report that the extracellular acid sensing G-protein coupled receptor, GPR65, is expressed in primary CLL cells where its level correlate strongly with anti-apoptotic Bcl-2 family member levels. GPR65 expression is found normally within the lymphoid lineage and has not been previously reported in CLL. We demonstrate a wide range of GPR65 mRNA expression among CLL 87 patient samples. The correlation between GPR65 mRNA levels and Bcl-2 mRNA levels is particularly strong ($r=0.8063$, $p=<0.001$). The correlation extends to other anti-apoptotic Bcl-2 family members, Mcl-1 ($r=0.4847$, $p=0.0010$) and Bcl-xl ($r=0.3411$, $p=0.0252$), although at lower levels of significance. No correlation is detected between GPR65 and levels of the pro-apoptotic proteins BIM, PUMA or NOXA. GPR65 expression also correlates with the favorable prognostic marker of 13q deletion. The present findings suggest the acid sensing receptor GPR65 may be of significance to allow CLL tolerance of extracellular acidosis. The correlation of GPR65 with Bcl-2 suggests a novel cytoprotective mechanism that enables CLL cell adaptation to acidic extracellular conditions. These findings suggest the potential value of targeting GPR65 therapeutically.

Keywords: Chronic lymphocytic leukemia; TDAG8T cell death associated gene; GPR65G protein-coupled receptor 65 Bcl-2B-cell Lymphoma 2 ; Microenvironment

Introduction

Among the adaptive hallmarks of cancer cells is the ability to survive and proliferate within a caustic tumor microenvironment [1]. Metabolic derangements that contribute to a nutrient poor, hypoxic and acidic milieu are well described in malignant proliferating tissue. Nearly 80 years ago, Warburg first described the metabolic shift from mitochondrial oxidative phosphorylation to glycolysis, a characteristic metabolic modification in cancer cells [2,3]. The upregulation of glycolysis, generating lactic acid paired with an increase in proton efflux, results in an abundance of acidic waste products within the extracellular space [4-6]. The culmination of this metabolic stress along with decreased clearance of metabolic waste products lends itself to an acidic extracellular environment [7,8]. Acidic conditions are variously implicated as contributing to drug resistance, DNA damage and repair, protein alterations, angiogenesis, and metastasis [9-11]. Acidosis has been detected in the tumor microenvironment by various methods utilizing microelectrodes or non-invasive imaging approaches, documenting a spectrum of acidic conditions that vary with each malignancy [12-14].

Cancer cells can respond to extracellular acidosis through a family of acid sensing G protein-coupled receptors, the natural ligand of which is the proton [15,16]. Members of this family include OGR1/GPR68, GPR4, G2A, and GPR65/TDAG8. Upon proton binding to histidine residues in their extracellular exposed domain, these proteins signal downstream via G proteins [17,18]. GPR65 (G protein-coupled receptor 65), also known as TDAG8 (T cell death associated gene 8), is mainly expressed in the lymphoid lineage, although its expression has also been detected in certain non-lymphoid malignancies, including those of the kidney, ovary, colon and breast [19]. The oncogenic activity of GPR65 was recently demonstrated by Ihara et al., who found that its overexpression increases survival of cancer cells in a xenograft tumor model [20]. GPR65-induced cell growth and proliferation were abrogated by mutation of the proton-binding histidine residues in its extracellular domain. How GPR65 activation by extracellular acidosis promotes cancer cell survival has not been well defined.

We recently discovered that GPR65 signaling in response to extracellular acidosis increases survival of leukemia and lymphoma cell lines by up-regulating the anti-apoptotic proteins Bcl-2 and Bcl-xL [21]. Our studies placed cells under metabolic stress by depriving them of glutamine and/or glucose to mimic the adverse conditions typical of the microenvironment. Moreover, we found that GPR65 activates signaling via the MEK/ERK pathway to up-regulate these proteins and protect

***Corresponding author:** Clark W. Distelhorst M.D., Division of Hematology and Oncology, Department of Medicine, Case Western Reserve School of Medicine 10900 Euclid Avenue Cleveland Ohio 44106 216-368-4546, USA, E-mail : cwd@case.edu against cell death. Furthermore, as a potential translational correlative, extracellular acidosis induced Bcl-2/Bcl-xl level elevation, sensitizing lymphoma/leukemia cell lines to killing by the BH3-mimetic, ABT-737 [21]. This result suggests that extracellular acidosis promotes Bcl-2-dependence.

Here we are the first to report that GPR65 is expressed in primary human Chronic Lymphocytic Leukemia (CLL) cells and that GPR65 expression levels in these cells correlate strongly with expression levels of the anti-apoptotic Bcl-2 family members Bcl-2, Mcl-1, and Bcl-xl. Evidence is also presented indicating that extracellular acidosis may contribute to the elevated Bcl-2 levels typical of CLL cells. These findings are of interest in view of abundant evidence of the importance of the tumor microenvironment in the pathogenesis of CLL [22-24]. Current understanding of the CLL tumor microenvironment, primarily in lymph nodes and bone marrow, is focused mainly on interactions of CLL cells with T-lymphocytes, endothelial cells, nurse like cells, soluble elements, and stromal factors [25,26]. However, very little is known about the metabolic stresses and modulations in pH that CLL cells encounter within their microenvironment. The present findings suggest that GPR65 signaling in response to extracellular acidosis may augment the survival of CLL cells in the microenvironment. Our data provide a strong rationale for recognizing GPR65 as a viable therapeutic target for the treatment of CLL.

Materials and Methods

Cell isolation and culture

Peripheral blood samples from 87 patients with CLL were obtained in the outpatient clinic with the patients' informed consent according to protocols approved by the University Hospital Case Medical Center Institutional Review Board and the Cleveland Clinic Institutional Review Board according to the Declaration of Helsinki. University Hospitals Case Medical Center study data were collected and managed using REDCap electronic data capture tools [27]. Lymphocytes were purified by Ficoll-Paque gradient centrifugation, washed in PBS, followed by suspension in ACK (ammonium-chloride-potassium) lysis buffer (Lonza). Samples were lysed for RNA or protein analysis. All primary CLL cells used for mRNA and protein analysis were freshly processed. CLL cells used for in vitro experiments were purified and then cultured in pH buffered DMEM –HEM (HEPES, EPPS, MES) and samples were immediately incubated after isolation where the pH was adjusted to 6.5 (low pH) or 7.5 (control pH), as recently described [21]. Cell viability was quantified based on exclusion of Trypan blue.

Quantitative RT-PCR

Total RNA was isolated using Trizol/RNEasy reagent (Invitrogen, Carlsbad, CA) according to the manufacturer's protocol. Isolated RNA was precipitated in isopropanol, washed in ethanol, and dissolved in RNase-free water. RNA concentration was determined by measuring absorbance at 260 and 280 nm. Total RNA was reverse transcribed using the TaqMan Gold RT-PCR kit (Applied Biosystems, Foster City, CA). Amplification was performed either utilizing the Universal TaqMan master mix and primer/probe sets specific for the genes of interest (Applied Biosystems) and examined on a Lightcycler 480 II (Roche), or alternatively amplified using the SYBR Green Master Mix (Applied Biosystems, N8080234 and 4309155) and examined on a 7500 Real-Time PCR system (Applied Biosystems), as previously described [28]. A purchased human B cell (CD19+) total RNA was used to establish a baseline for comparison between mRNA levels in CLL and a healthy subset (Miltenyi). Quantitative, real-time RT-PCR was performed by the relative quantification ($2^{-\Delta\Delta Ct}$) method using β-actin as the reference mRNA.

Protein analysis

Western Blotting was performed using standard laboratory methods as previously described [21]. Protein quantification was performed using Image J analysis.

Statistical analysis

Distributions of GPR65 mRNA expression, apoptotic family members, and other quantitative variables were analyzed using box plots, Q-Q plots, and Shapiro-Wilk tests for normality. Logarithmic transformations were performed on highly skewed variables. The Pearson product-moment correlation coefficient was used in studying the association between GPR65 and Bcl-2 family members. The Pearson correlation coefficient was also used in determining the relationship between GPR65 and hematologic parameters. Simple linear regression analyses were used in studying the association between GPR65 expression and patient clinical characteristics such as age, sex, and Rai stage. The two-sample t-test was used in comparing Bcl-2 expression ratio and the GPR65 expression ratio. All statistical analyses were performed using STATA 11.0 software.

Results

Clinical data

Peripheral blood samples were collected for analysis from 87 individual CLL patients. Clinical and biologic data were analyzed for 76 of these patients (Table 1). Patients were mostly early Rai Stage (76% Stage 0-2), CD38 negative (58%), and Zap-70 negative (58%). More than half (57%) were untreated and managed with observation alone. Baseline laboratory data were gathered at the time of sample collection. Cytogenetic abnormalities included trisomy 12 in 20% of patients and deletion of the long arm of chromosome 13 in 53% of patients.

No. patients	76
Sex (female/male)	44/32
Median (range)	
Age (years)	67 (43 - 99)
White blood cells (10^9/L)	40.8 (3.6 - 400)
Absolute Lymphocyte Count (10^9/L)	32.30 (0 - 394)
No. (%)	
Rai Stage	
0	27 (36)
1	24 (32)
2	6 (8)
3	5 (6)
4	12 (16)
CD38 Status (60/76 patients)	
CD38 Positive	25 (42)
CD38 Negative	35 (58)
Zap 70 Status (50/76 patients)	
Zap70 Positive	21 (42)
Zap 70 Negative	29 (58)
Trisomy 12 (48/76 patients)	9 (20)
Deletion 13q (49/76 patients)	26 (53)
No Prior Therapy	43 (57)

Table 1: Clinical and biologic characteristics of CLL patients. Most patients were early Rai stage, with favorable prognostic markers, adequate circulating lymphocytes and being managed with observation alone.

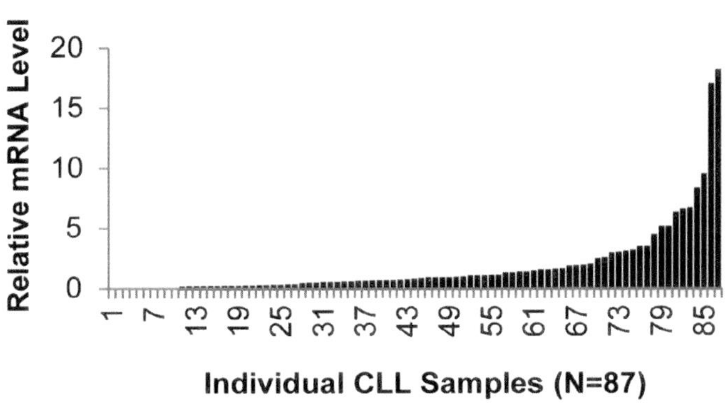

Figure 1: GPR65 mRNA expression profile in primary CLL cells. Basal GPR65 mRNA levels were measured by qRT-PCR in primary CLL cells (N=87 individual patients) relative to CD19+ healthy control cells. Levels range from 0.02 to 18.07 with a median expression of 0.71.

	No. Patients	Regression Coefficient	SE	p	95% CI
Age	76	0.0080	0.014	0.571	-0.02 - 0.04
Male	76	0.1693	0.362	0.641	-0.55 - 0.89
Stage	74	-0.1270	0.125	0.311	-0.38 - 0.12
WBC	75	0.0009	0.002	0.696	-0.004 - 0.006
ALC	75	0.0007	0.002	0.762	-.036 - 0.45
Zap 70 Positive	50	-0.6658	0.425	0.124	-1.52 - 0.19
CD38 Positive	60	0.4405	0.387	0.259	-0.33 - 1.21
Trisomy 12	48	-0.3971	0.588	0.503	-1.58 - 0.77
Deletion 13q	49	0.9739	0.431	0.029	0.11 - 1.84

Table 2: Association between clinical characteristics and GPR65 expression. Simple linear regression analysis demonstrates GPR65 expression has correlation with a favorable prognostic marker of 13q deletion. Other prognostic factors show no relationship with GPR65 expression. (ALC: Absolute Lymphocyte Count, SE: Standard Error, CI: Confidence Interval).

GPR65 expression in primary CLL cells

GPR65 mRNA expression levels were measured in primary CLL cells by qRT-PCR and normalized to corresponding levels in healthy human CD19+ B cell controls (Figure 1). Healthy CD19+ B-cell control clinical parameters include half male and half female, age distribution of 18-68 years, with a cell purity of >90%. GPR65 mRNA levels in isolated primary CLL samples range widely from 0.02 to 18.07 with a median mRNA expression of 0.71, relative to healthy human B cell controls. GPR65 levels were standardized using the respective expression of beta-actin. To investigate the potential relationship of known CLL prognostic factors to GPR65 expression, linear regression analysis was employed on all 87 samples, demonstrating that GPR65 expression correlates with 13q deletion, a favorable prognostic marker (Table 2). None of the other known CLL prognostic factors correlated with GPR65 expression.

GPR65 levels correlate with levels of anti-apoptotic Bcl-2 family members in CLL cells

In each of 87 CLL samples qRT-PCR was used to measure expression levels of GPR65 and various anti-apoptotic and pro-apoptotic Bcl-2 family members. These levels were normalized according to their respective levels in normal B-cells. GPR65 expression levels correlated quite strongly with expression levels of Bcl-2 ($r=0.8063$, $p=<0.001$) (Figure 2). GPR65 levels also correlated with levels of two other anti-apoptotic proteins known to play important roles in CLL, Mcl-1 ($r=0.4847$, $p=0.0010$) and Bcl-xl ($r=0.3411$, $p=0.0252$), although not as strongly as with Bcl-2. GPR65 mRNA expression levels did not correlate significantly with expression levels of BIM, PUMA or NOXA, three pro-apoptotic members of the Bcl-2 family typically expressed in lymphoid malignancies.

Extracellular acidosis increases Bcl-2 expression in CLL cells

To determine the influence of extracellular acidosis on levels of Bcl-2 and GPR65, CLL cells from 3 patients were cultured under either acidic conditions (pH 6.5) or non-acidic conditions (pH 7.5) for up to 24 hours. Bcl-2 and GPR65 mRNA levels were quantified by qRT-PCR at periodic time intervals. The acidic pH of 6.5 was selected since it approximates the pH at which GPR65 activity is half-maximal [29]. We find that levels of GPR65 in CLL cells are not altered by extracellular acidosis (data not shown), but average levels of Bcl-2 mRNA increase in response to reduced extracellular pH (Figure 3).

Bcl-2 protein expression was investigated by immunoblotting at baseline (i.e., before pH adjustment) and 12 hour increments in low and control pH. In low extracellular pH, Bcl-2 protein expression was either increased or stable over 36 hours (Figure 4). Under control conditions, Bcl-2 protein expression consistently declined in each patient sample by 36 hours of culture (Figure 4). Thus, from these data we conclude that extracellular acidosis favors up regulation of anti-apoptotic Bcl-2 protein compared to that of control physiologic pH conditions.

Discussion

The major findings of this study are that the extracellular acidosis sensing receptor, GPR65, is expressed in primary human CLL cells and that its expression levels correlate strongly with expression levels of the anti-apoptotic protein Bcl-2. In addition, we also observe a significant correlation between GPR65 and levels of two other anti-apoptotic proteins, Mcl-1 and Bcl-xl.

These findings raise the possibility that GPR65 signaling may contribute to elevated levels of Bcl-2, at least in a subset of CLL patient samples. We show that GPR65 expression is quite variable (Figure 1) and this may be a reflection of the microenvironment of origin from which the cells were collected: i.e. a more proliferative bone marrow or lymph node vs. a less proliferative bone marrow or lymph node. The mechanism, we postulate, is GPR65-mediated up-regulation of Bcl-2 levels in response to extracellular acidosis in the CLL microenvironment. Although we are unaware of any published, direct measurements of extracellular pH in the CLL microenvironment (i.e., involved lymph nodes or bone marrow), decreased extracellular pH is well documented in proliferative environments associated with the Warburg effect as previously outlined [2,3]. Moreover, in our experiments (Figure 2) extracellular acidosis increases Bcl-2 expression levels in primary CLL cells cultured for brief periods of time ex vivo, suggesting a potential role of acidosis in the microenvironment. In addition, we find that Bcl-2 protein expression levels in three independent CLL samples are maintained following exposure to extracellular acidosis, whereas such levels are attenuated under neutral extracellular pH conditions.

Very little is known about how GPR65 is regulated, including whether the primary mechanisms of regulation are at transcriptional or post-transcriptional levels. Moreover, our findings suggest that GPR65 mRNA levels vary widely among different CLL patient samples. Curiously, we did observe a correlation between GPR65 mRNA levels and the presence of the 13q chromosome deletion, present in more than half of CLL cases. This observation, combined with the observed correlation between GPR65 mRNA levels and Bcl-2 mRNA levels raises interest in the potential role of microRNAs in the regulation of GPR65

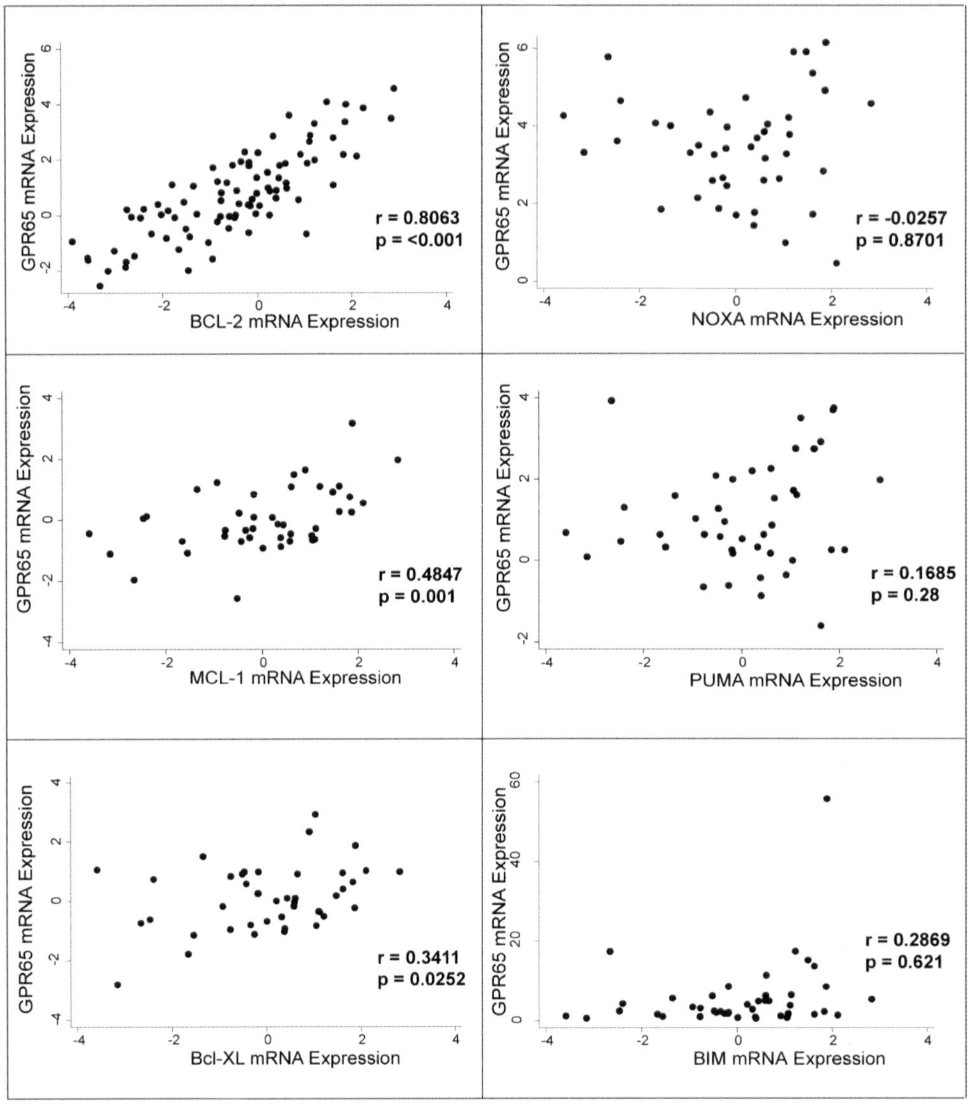

Figure 2: GPR65 correlates strongly with anti-apoptotic family members Bcl-2, Mcl-1 and Bcl-xl. Basal GPR65 mRNA levels measured by qRT-PCR in primary CLL cells were plotted versus basal expression levels of Bcl-2 protein family members, also determined by qRT-PCR (logarithmic scale). Pearson correlation coefficients (r) with associated p values are shown. GPR65 strongly correlates with anti-apoptotic members Bcl-2 (N=87 patients), and also with Mcl-1 and Bcl-xL (N=43 patients). GPR65 does not correlate with pro-apoptotic family members NOXA, PUMA or Bim (N=43 patients).

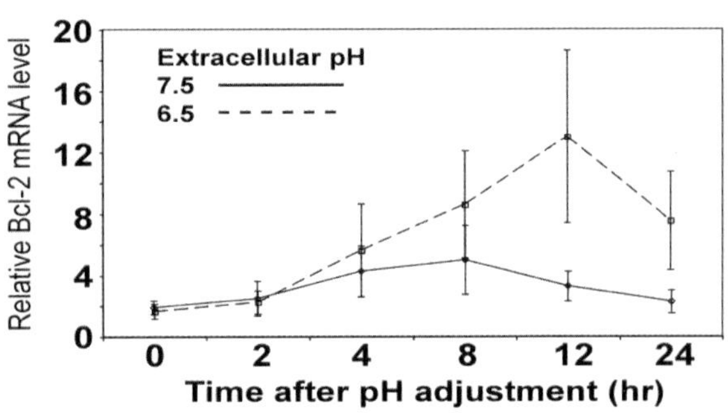

Figure 3: Extracellular acidosis upregulates Bcl-2 expression in primary CLL cells. (A) Bcl-2 mRNA levels were measured by qRT-PCR in three CLL patient samples and cultured at low pH (6.5) and high pH (7.5) for up to 24 hours. Findings indicate that Bcl-2 mRNA levels increase when exposed to extracellular acidosis.

expression, particularly in view of previous evidence that miR-15a and miR-16 are frequently deleted or down regulated in CLL samples with 13q14 deletions, contributing to elevated expression of Bcl-2 [30-34]. Utilizing publicly available microRNA databases, we find evidence that GPR65 expression may be up-regulated in response to miR-15a deficiency [35, 36]. On the other hand, another publically available microRNA database predicts GPR65 expression to be targeted by miR-155 [37]. This miR has been shown to be significantly overexpressed by greater than five-fold in patients with CLL [30]. Since miRs are generally negative regulatory elements, this finding might predict an inhibitory effect of miR-155 on GPR65 expression. Thus, the expression level of GPR65 in an individual patient sample may depend upon the relative balance between levels of miR-15a and miR-155. This possibility may explain the broad range of GPR65 levels observed among the individual patient samples included in the present study.

One of the limitations of the present study is the lack of a suitable

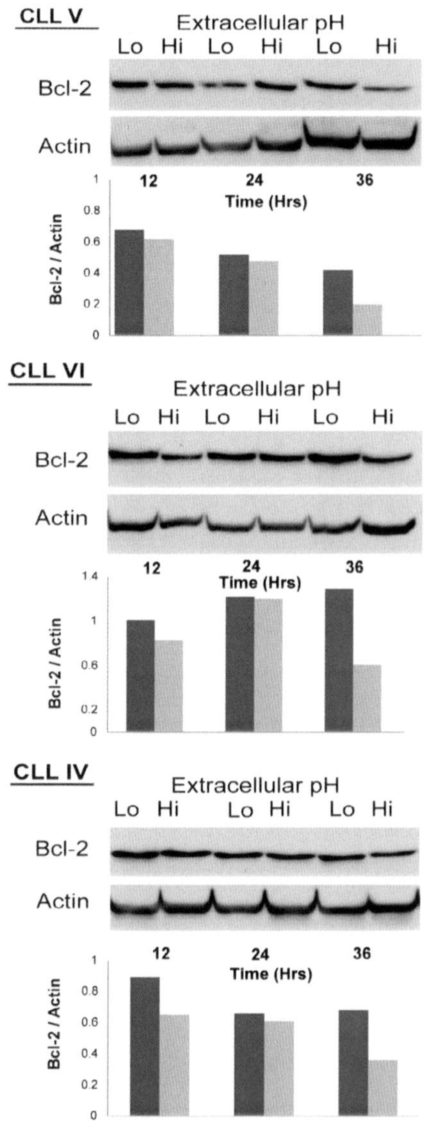

Figure 4: CLL response to extracellular acidosis maintains Bcl-2 expression. Bcl-2 protein levels were measured by immunoblotting in CLL patient samples, arbitrarily labeled by Roman numerals and cultured at low pH (6.5) and high pH (7.5) for the indicated periods of time. Below each panel showing immunoblots is a bar graph in which Bcl-2 protein levels were estimated by densitometry and normalized to actin to control for minor differences in loading at each time point. Findings indicate that the Bcl-2 level in CLL cells declines over time in ex vivo culture, and that this decline is a least partially prevented by extracellular acidosis.

quality antibody to GPR65. We have extensively tested commercial antibodies available at the time of publication and purported to react with GPR65, but have been unable to verify any of these antibodies. Thus, our measures of GPR65 expression reported here are limited to qRT-PCR estimates of mRNA levels, rather than actual protein levels. Highly sensitive and specific antibodies to GPR65 are needed for future studies to be carried out, with the long-range goal of employing GPR65 as either a novel tumor marker or novel therapeutic target. With regard to these goals, the patient population represented in this preliminary investigation included mainly low-risk, good-prognosis patients, where no significant correlation was detected between relative GPR65 expression levels and known prognostic markers, other than the 13q chromosome deletion. A larger number of patients with more aggressive CLL will likely be needed to determine if GPR65 expression has an impact on the course of this malignancy.

Regardless of these current limitations, the present findings raise the possibility that GPR65 signaling may contribute to the survival potential of CLL cells in the microenvironment. Investigation of the CLL tumor microenvironment has recently come of age. Many studies have also recognized that the poor survival of CLL cells *in vitro* has been hindered by the absence of accessory cells and/or a stromal network to support the survival and proliferation of these cells [38,39]. This observation has led investigators to further examine how the tumor microenvironment influences CLL cell survival. Our investigation focuses on extracellular acidosis as an important moderator of CLL cell survival mediated by the acid sensing receptor GPR65. The extracellular pH has classically been described in solid tumors with values that are often below 7.0 but have been reported with pH values 6.0 or less [12,40]. Although measurements of extracellular pH in the microenvironment of hematologic malignancies are limited, there is now abundant evidence of the importance of the extracellular environment in lymphoid malignancies, particularly CLL [12,41,42].

Future work is needed to characterize the role of GPR65 in more aggressive variants of CLL, where novel prognostic markers and therapeutic approaches are most applicable. It is our hope that this report will stimulate interest in the role of GPR65 in CLL and potentially other lymphoid malignancies. Understanding mechanisms by which CLL cells thrive within the acidic microenvironment may lead to future targeted agents to antagonize GPR65 signaling.

Acknowledgement

This research was supported by NIH grants RO1 CA085804 (CWD) and CA127224 (AA), and by the Biostatistics & Bioinformatics Core Facility of the Case Comprehensive Cancer Center (P30CA043703).

References

1. Hanahan D, Weinberg RA (2011) Hallmarks of cancer: the next generation. Cell 144: 646-674.
2. WARBURG O (1961) [On the facultative anaerobiosis of cancer cells and its use in chemotherapy]. Munch Med Wochenschr 103: 2504-2506.
3. Vander Heiden MG, Cantley LC, Thompson CB (2009) Understanding the Warburg effect: the metabolic requirements of cell proliferation. Science 324: 1029-1033.
4. Gatenby RA, Gillies RJ (2004) Why do cancers have high aerobic glycolysis? Nat Rev Cancer 4: 891-899.
5. Kroemer G, Pouyssegur J (2008) Tumor cell metabolism: cancer's Achilles' heel. Cancer Cell 13: 472-482.
6. Fischer K, Hoffmann P, Voelkl S, Meidenbauer N, Ammer J, et al. (2007) Inhibitory effect of tumor cell-derived lactic acid on human T cells. Blood 109: 3812-3819.
7. Gatenby RA, Gillies RJ (2008) A microenvironmental model of carcinogenesis. Nat Rev Cancer 8: 56-61.
8. Hashim AI, Zhang X, Wojtkowiak JW, Martinez GV, Gillies RJ (2011) Imaging pH and metastasis. NMR Biomed 24: 582-591.
9. Webb BA, Chimenti M, Jacobson MP, Barber DL (2011) Dysregulated pH: a perfect storm for cancer progression. Nat Rev Cancer 11: 671-677.
10. Wojtkowiak JW, Verduzco D, Schramm KJ, Gillies RJ (2011) Drug resistance and cellular adaptation to tumor acidic pH microenvironment. Mol Pharm 8: 2032-2038.
11. Izumi H, Torigoe T, Ishiguchi H, Uramato H, Yoshida Y ,et al. (2003) Cellular pH regulators: potentially promising molecular targets for cancer chemotherapy. Cancer treatment reviews. 29: 541-549.

12. Vaupel P, Okunieff P, Neuringer LJ (1989) Blood flow, tissue oxygenation, pH distribution, and energy metabolism of murine mammary adenocarcinomas during growth. Adv Exp Med Biol 248: 835-845.

13. Griffiths JR (1991) Are cancer cells acidic? Br J Cancer 64: 425-427.

14. Engin K, Leeper DB, Cater JR, Thistlethwaite AJ, Tupchong L, et al. (1995) Extracellular pH distribution in human tumours. International journal of hyperthermia: the official journal of European Society for Hyperthermic Oncology, North American Hyperthermia Group. 11: 211-216.

15. Ludwig MG, Vanek M, Guerini D, Gasser JA, Jones CE, et al. (2003) Proton-sensing G-protein-coupled receptors. Nature 425: 93-98.

16. Tomura H, Mogi C, Sato K, Okajima F (2005) Proton-sensing and lysolipid-sensitive G-protein-coupled receptors: a novel type of multi-functional receptors. Cell Signal 17: 1466-1476.

17. Im DS (2005) Two ligands for a GPCR, proton vs lysolipid. Acta Pharmacol Sin 26: 1435-1441.

18. Wang JQ, Kon J, Mogi C, Tobo M, Damirin A, et al. (2004) TDAG8 is a proton-sensing and psychosine-sensitive G-protein-coupled receptor. J Biol Chem 279: 45626-45633.

19. Sin WC, Zhang Y, Zhong W, Adhikarakunnathu S, Powers S, et al. (2004) G protein-coupled receptors GPR4 and TDAG8 are oncogenic and overexpressed in human cancers. Oncogene 23: 6299-6303.

20. Ihara Y, Kihara Y, Hamano F (2010) The G protein-coupled receptor T-cell death-associated gene 8 (TDAG8) facilitates tumor development by serving as an extracellular pH sensor. Proceedings of the National Academy of Sciences of the United States of America. 107: 17309-17314.

21. Ryder C, McColl K, Zhong F, Distelhorst CW (2012) Acidosis promotes Bcl-2 family-mediated evasion of apoptosis: involvement of acid-sensing G protein-coupled receptor Gpr65 signaling to Mek/Erk. The Journal of biological chemistry. 287: 27863-27875.

22. Zhou J, Mauerer K, Farina L, Gribben JG (2005) The role of the tumor microenvironment in hematological malignancies and implication for therapy. Front Biosci 10: 1581-1596.

23. Burger JA (2012) Targeting the microenvironment in chronic lymphocytic leukemia is changing the therapeutic landscape. Curr Opin Oncol 24: 643-649.

24. Herishanu Y, Katz BZ, Lipsky A, Wiestner A (2013) Biology of chronic lymphocytic leukemia in different microenvironments: clinical and therapeutic implications. Hematology/oncology clinics of North America. 27: 173-206.

25. Pleyer L, Egle A, Hartmann TN, Greil R (2009) Molecular and cellular mechanisms of CLL: novel therapeutic approaches. Nat Rev Clin Oncol 6: 405-418.

26. Burger JA (2013) Nurture versus nature: the microenvironment in chronic lymphocytic leukemia. Hematology / the Education Program of the American Society of Hematology American Society of Hematology Education Program. 96-103.

27. Harris PA, Taylor R, Thielke R, Payne J, Gonzalez N, et al. (2009) Research electronic data capture (REDCap)--a metadata-driven methodology and workflow process for providing translational research informatics support. Journal of biomedical informatics 42: 377-381.

28. Al-Harbi S, Hill BT, Mazumder S, Singh K, Devecchio J, et al. (2011) An antiapoptotic BCL-2 family expression index predicts the response of chronic lymphocytic leukemia to ABT-737. Blood 118: 3579-3590.

29. Ishii S, Kihara Y, Shimizu T (2005) Identification of T cell death-associated gene 8 (TDAG8) as a novel acid sensing G-protein-coupled receptor. J Biol Chem 280: 9083-9087.

30. Fulci V, Chiaretti S, Goldoni M, Azzalin G, Carucci N, et al. (2007) Quantitative technologies establish a novel microRNA profile of chronic lymphocytic leukemia. Blood 109: 4944-4951.

31. Cimmino A1, Calin GA, Fabbri M, Iorio MV, Ferracin M, et al. (2005) miR-15 and miR-16 induce apoptosis by targeting BCL2. Proc Natl Acad Sci U S A 102: 13944-13949.

32. Bonci D, Coppola V, Musumeci M, Addario A, Giuffrida R, et al. (2008) The miR-15a-miR-16-1 cluster controls prostate cancer by targeting multiple oncogenic activities. Nat Med 14: 1271-1277.

33. Calin GA, Dumitru CD, Shimizu M, Bichi R, Zupo S, et al. (2002) Frequent deletions and down-regulation of micro- RNA genes miR15 and miR16 at 13q14 in chronic lymphocytic leukemia. Proc Natl Acad Sci U S A 99: 15524-15529.

34. Pekarsky Y, Zanesi N, Croce CM (2010) Molecular basis of CLL. Semin Cancer Biol 20: 370-376.

35. Wang X (2008) miRDB: a microRNA target prediction and functional annotation database with a wiki interface. RNA 14: 1012-1017.

36. Wang X, El Naqa IM (2008) Prediction of both conserved and nonconserved microRNA targets in animals. Bioinformatics 24: 325-332.

37. Betel D, Koppal A, Agius P, Sander C, Leslie C (2010) Comprehensive modeling of microRNA targets predicts functional non-conserved and non-canonical sites. Genome Biol 11: R90.

38. Hamilton E, Pearce L, Morgan L, Robinson S, Ware V, et al. (2012) Mimicking the tumour microenvironment: three different co-culture systems induce a similar phenotype but distinct proliferative signals in primary chronic lymphocytic leukaemia cells. British journal of haematology 158: 589-599.

39. Zenz T, Mertens D, Küppers R, Döhner H, Stilgenbauer S (2010) From pathogenesis to treatment of chronic lymphocytic leukaemia. Nat Rev Cancer 10: 37-50.

40. Gerweck LE (1998) Tumor pH: implications for treatment and novel drug design. Semin Radiat Oncol 8: 176-182.

41. Ng TC, Majors AW, Vijayakumar S, Baldwin NJ, Thomas FJ, et al. (1989) Human neoplasm pH and response to radiation therapy: P-31 MR spectroscopy studies in situ. Radiology 170: 875-878.

42. Cairns R, Papandreou I, Denko N (2006) Overcoming physiologic barriers to cancer treatment by molecularly targeting the tumor microenvironment. Molecular cancer research: MCR 4:61-70.

Beta-Hydroxyisovalerylshikonin Inhibits the Growth of U266 Multiple Myeloma Cells by Triggering the Mitochondrial Pathway

Yihui He[1]*, Xiaoyan Chen[1] and Lingying Kong[2]

[1]*Department of Pathology, Fujian Provincial Hospital, Fuzhou, Fujian 350001, China*

[2]*Department of Pathology, Affiliated People's Hospital of Fujian University of Traditional Chinese Medicine, Fuzhou, Fujian 350004, P.R. China*

Abstract

Background: Beta-hydroxyisovalerylshikonin (beta-HIVS) is a compound isolated from the traditional oriental medicinal herb lithospermum radix. This drug exerts a role as an ATP non-competitive inhibitor of Protein-Tyrosine Kinases (PTKs) and shows great potential for induction of apoptosis against human cancer cells. We investigated the effect of beta-HIVS on multiple myeloma U266 cells and clarified details of the primary mechanism in its apoptosis-inducing activity.

Objective: The aim of this work was to trace the apoptosis-inducing activity of beta-HIVS on U266 cells as well as the underlying mechanisms.

Methods: Cell Counting Kit-8 (CCK-8) test and colony-forming assay were performed in estimating the effects of beta-HIVS on U266 cell viability and colony formation. Apoptosis analysis was carried out on the basis of DAPI fluorescence staining and DNA fragmentation assays. Real-time PCR was employed to evaluate changes of *Bcl-2* and *Bax* mRNA expression, while indirect immunofluorescence assay and western blotting were utilized in validating the expression of Bcl-2, Bax, caspase-3, caspase-9, PARP and cytochrome c.

Results: CCK-8 test and colony-forming assay showed that beta-HIVS treatment resulted in significantly reduced cell proliferation ($P<0.05$ or 0.01) and colony formation ($P<0.01$). Real-time PCR results indicated that the expression level of Bcl-2 mRNA was reduced at 72h following beta-HIVS co-cultivation ($P<0.01$), although *Bax* mRNA altered with no significance. Immunofluorescence assay displayed that caspase-3 was activated in beta-HIVS treated group, accompanied by an increased expression of cytochrome c. Western blotting also exhibited that the expression of Bcl-2 protein in beta-HIVS treated group decreased and cytochrome c increased at 72h after co-cultivation. Moreover, caspase-3 and -9, as well as PARP were activated, all with $P<0.01$ when compared with the two control groups.

Conclusion: Beta-HIVS revealed remarkable apoptosis-inducing activity in U266 cells, possibly by inhibiting proliferation and promoting apoptosis via the mitochondrial pathway.

Keywords: Beta-hydroxyisovalerylshikonin; Beta-HIVS; Multiple myeloma; U266 cell; Mitochondria pathway

Abbreviations: Beta-HIVS: Beta-HydroxyIsoValerylShikonin; MM:Multiple Myeloma; FBS: Fetal Bovine Serum; CCK-8: Cell Counting Kit-8; M: Mole/L

Introduction

Multiple Myeloma (MM) is a plasma cell malignancy accounts for more than 10% of hematological malignancies and is characterized by the proliferation of malignant clonal plasma cells that produce a single immunoglobulin isotype named M-protein [1,2]. At present, treatments using alkylating agents, corticosteroids, proteasome inhibitors and immunomodulatory drugs have improved the overall outcomes of MM during the past decade, and MM patients are now undergoing considerable survival rate with respect to those obtained with historical treatments. Nevertheless, MM remains in most cases an incurable disease, and novel drugs as well as therapeutic strategies are still required for continued disease control. In this regard, several new agents for MM therapy are currently receiving assessment, some of which seemed with promising on the basis of reported initial results [3-5].

Currently, a series of novel shikonin derivative analogues bearing oxygen-containing substituents were designed, synthesized or isolated [6-8], among which, beta-hydroxyisovalerylshikonin (beta-HIVS) has been highlighted for the strongest apoptosis-inducing activity among various derivatives of shikonin. This drug is an ATP non-competitive inhibitor of protein-tyrosine kinases and is capable of inducing apoptosis in various human tumor cell lines which has been documented by several publications [9-13]. It is also reported that beta-HIVS shows great promise as a potent apoptosis-inducing agent in the treatment of hematological malignancies included leukemia, although this still retains in research and development stages [14-16]. At present, the apoptosis-inducing activity of beta-HIVS on MM as well as the way in which beta-HIVS promotes cell death remains to be clarified. In consequence, the current study investigated the effect of beta-HIVS on U266 cells and traced the underlying mechanism.

Materials and Methods

Materials

The U266 cell line was purchased from the Chinese Academy of

***Corresponding author:** Yihui He, Department of Pathology, Fujian Provincial Hospital, No.134, Dongjie, Gulou, Fuzhou, Fujian 350001, P.R. China, E-mail: yihuihe2014@163.com

Sciences (Shanghai, China). The main reagents are listed as follows: beta-HIVS (Dibo Chem, Shanghai, China); RPMI-1640, fetal bovine serum (FBS) (Gibco-BRL, Carlsbad, CA, USA); DMSO, methylcellulose (Sigma-Aldrich Corporation, St. Louis, MA, USA); Cell Counting Kit-8 (Dojindo Laboratories, Kumamoto, Japan); SYBR-Green PCR Master Mix (Roche Diagnostics GmbH, Mannheim, Germany); RIPA protein lysis buffer, paraformaldehyde, DAPI dye, DNA Fragmentation kit, Cy3-conjugated anti-mouse IgG, FITC-conjugated anti-rabbit IgG, mouse anti-human β-actin, anti-cytochrome c, rabbit anticleaved PARP and anti-cleaved caspase-3 (Asp175) (Beyotime Institute of Biotechnology, Shanghai, China); rabbit antihuman Bcl-2 and anti-Bax (Abcam, Cambridge, MA,USA); rabbit anti-caspase-9 and anti-caspase-3 (Santa Cruz Biotechnology, Santa Cruz, CA, USA);

Methods

Cell culture

Human U266 cells were maintained in RPMI-1640 medium supplemented with 10% FBS, and cultured at 37°C in 5% CO_2.

Cell viability assays

Beta -HIVS was dissolved in DMSO with a stork concentration of 8000 µg/ml and the IC_{50} (1.2 µg/ml) for U266 cells was obtained by our previous study. Three groups as beta-HIVS treated group, DMSO control group and no treatment group were established. Cells were seeded in 96-well plates at a density of 5×10^3/ml and co-cultivated with beta-HIVS at a final concentration of 1.2 µg/ml. CCK-8 test was employed in the evaluation of the growth inhibitory effects of beta-HIVS on U266 cells following the manufacturer's protocol. The optical density (OD value proportional to the cell numbers) was measured using a microculture plate reader (BioTek Instruments, Winooski, VT, USA) at both 450 and 630 nm.

Colony-forming assay

Concisely, cells were suspended in a concentration of 300 cells per ml RPMI-1640 and seeded in 24-well plates. Methylcellulose dissolved in RPMI-1640 containing 30% FBS was supplied to each well at a concentration of 0.8 g/L. The colonies containing more than 50 cells were counted following incubation at 37°C in 5% CO_2 for 14 days.

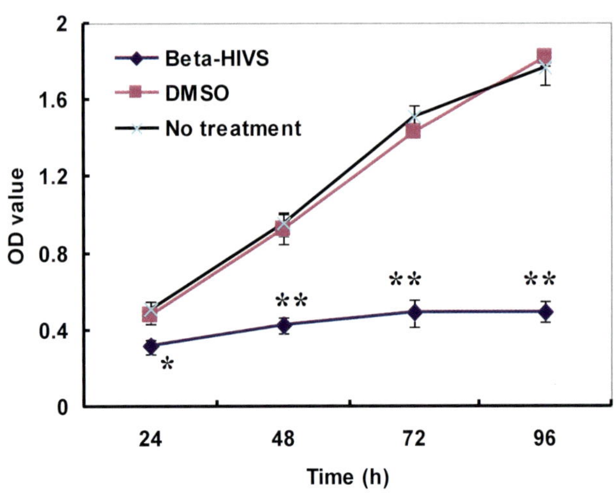

Figure 1a: Effects of beta-HIVS on the cell viability and colony formation of multiple myeloma U266 cells. (A) CCK-8 assay. The OD value proportional to the cell number was detected and plotted on the growth curve.

Apoptosis analysis

Cell apoptosis was evaluated via DAPI fluorescence staining and DNA fragmentation assays. For DAPI staining, cells were collected and washed with PBS and stained by DAPI (2 mg/ml) for 3-5 min. Morphological changes of the stained cells were examined using the fluorescence microscope (Olympus, Japan). (Non-viable apoptotic ratio) % = (cell numbers in phase IIb/200 cells) x100%. DNA fragmentation analysis was performed according to the instructions of a commercial DNA Fragmentation Kit, followed by agarose gel electrophoresis: each sample containing 2.5 µg of extracted DNA in 1.2% agarose gel and electrophoresis with a constant voltage 20 V for 4h.

Real-time PCR analysis

Real-time PCR test was carried out by utilizing the SYBR Green PCR Master Mix under the recommended conditions. The primer sequences for *Bcl-2*, *Bax* and *GAPDH* were previously described [17]. The comparative Ct method was used to calculate the relative expression level of *Bcl-2* or *Bax* as compared with *GAPDH*.

Immunofluorescence staining

The cell monolayer was fixed with 4% paraformaldehyde, and were incubated at 4°C overnight with rabbit anti-cleaved caspase-3 (Asp175) (1:300) and mouse monoclonal anti-cytochrome c (1:400) antibodies. FITC-conjugated anti-rabbit and Cy3-conjugated anti-mouse IgG were all diluted at 1:1000. DAPI was used to dye the cell nuclei. The stained cells were washed with PBS and observed with a fluorescence microscope (Olympus, Japan) at x 400 magnification.

Western blotting analysis

Cell lysates were prepared with the aid of RIPA protein lysis buffer and the protein extracts were quantified and then subjected to electrophoresis on a 10-12% SDS-PAGE gel. The proteins were transferred onto the PolyVinylidene Difluoride (PVDF) membranes and blocked in Tris-buffered saline (TBS) containing 5% non-fat milk powder. The primary antibodies and the dilutions used were: rabbit anti-Bcl-2 (1:1000), anti-caspase-9 (1:500), anti-caspase-3 (1:500) and anti-cleaved PARP (1:300). Mouse monoclonal anti-cytochrome c antibody was diluted at 1:500 and mouse anti-β-actin antibody was 1:1000.

Statistical analysis

All data are expressed as the means ± Standard Deviation (SD). One-way ANOVA, Student's t-test or the non-parametric test were performed for comparison of differences between groups using SPSS 13.0 software (SPSS Inc., Chicago, IL, USA). $P<0.05$ was considered to indicate a statistically significant difference.

Results

Beta -HIVS inhibits U266 cell viability and colony formation

As shown in (Figure 1A), the effects of beta -HIVS on the viability of U266 cells were assessed by CCK-8 assay. The results suggested that beta-HIVS treatment led to a detection of 0.312±0.035, 0.433±0.052, 0.491±0.047, and 0.489±0.076 of the OD values (proportional to the cell numbers) at 24, 48, 72 and 96 h following co- cultivation, significantly lower than those of DMSO or no treatment cells with $P<0.05$ or 0.01. For the colony formation assay, the colonies of Beta-HIVS treated group was fewer and smaller, and the colony numbers were significantly lower than those of two contrast groups ($P<0.01$) (Figure 1B).

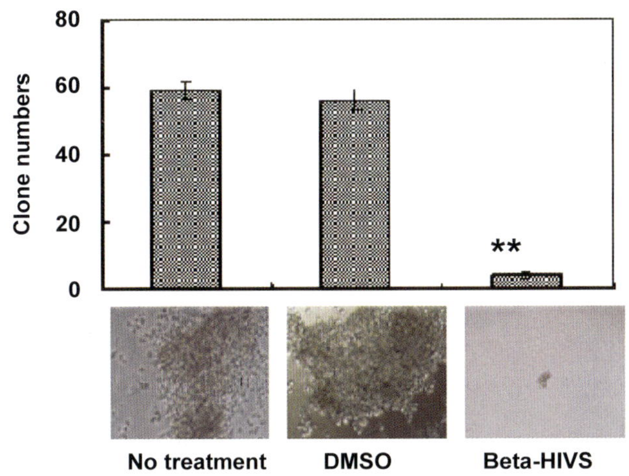

Figure 1b: Colony-forming assay. Cell colonies containing >50 cells were counted on day 14. Data shown are the means ± SD (n=15) (*: P<0.05; **: P<0.01, vs. no treatment cells).

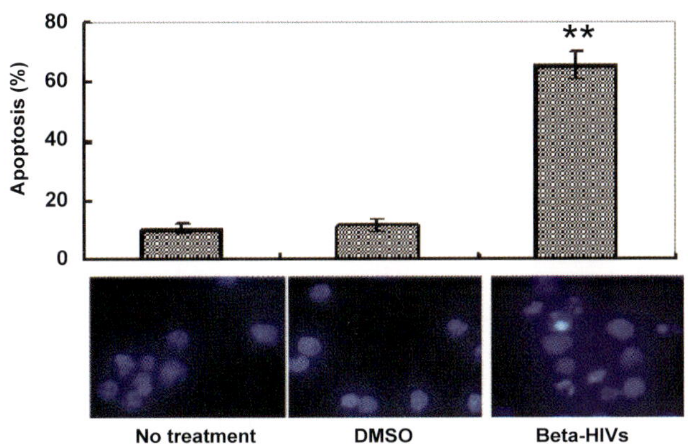

Figure 2a: Beta-HIVS promotes apoptosis in U266 multiple myeloma cells. DAPI fluorescence staining shows the microscopic changes in the nuclei of beta-HIVS treated cells observed (72h) via a fluorescence microscope, at x 400 magnification.The red arrow indicates typical morphology of the nucleus following apoptosis at phase IIb. (Non-viable apoptotic ratio) % = (phase IIb cell numbers/200 cells) x 100%. Data shown are the means ± SD (n=3) (**: P<0.01 vs. no treatment cells).

Apoptotic cell death was induced in U266 cells by beta-HIVS

The apoptosis-inducing effects were measured with the aid of DAPI staining and DNA ladder electrophoresis. As indicated in (Figure 2A), U266 cells in beta-HIVS group presented morphology of chromatin condensation and shrinkage in phase IIb of the apoptotic phase at 72 h following treatment, and the apoptotic ratio of phase IIb (%) was significantly higher than that of two control groups, with P<0.01. In contrast, cells of DMSO and no treatment groups all presented no marked apoptotic morphology. DNA degradative fragments were detected by DNA ladder electrophoresis, which also displayed typical apoptosis 'DNA ladders' in beta-HIVS treated group against that of two control groups (Figure 2B).

The intrinsic apoptotic pathway is involved in beta-HIVS induced cell apoptosis

Real-time PCR, immunofluorescence assay and western blotting were performed for the detection of apoptosis-related proteins, involved Bcl-2, Bax, PARP, cytochrome c, caspase-3 and caspase-9. Data of real-time PCR test evinced that the mRNA expression of *Bcl-2* in beta-HIVS treated group decreased, with P<0.01 vs. DMSO group, while the *Bax* mRNA expression changed unconspicuously (Figure 3A). At the same time, immunofluorescence analysis displayed that caspase-3 was activated in beta-HIVS treated group, accompanied by an increase in the levels of cytochrome c, as enhanced red fluorescence was observed in the beta-HIVS treated cells, which utilized anti-cleaved caspase-3 (Asp175) and anti-cytochrome c antibodies, combined by Cy3-conjugated anti-mouse or rabbit IgG. (Figure 3B). Similarly, western blotting showed that the expression of Bcl-2 in beta-HIVS

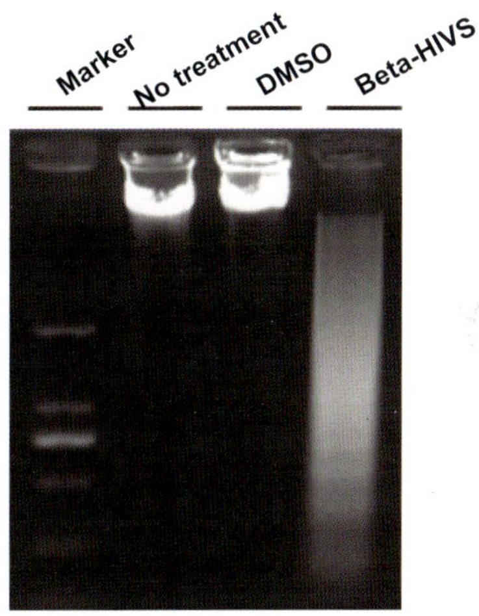

Figure 2b: DNA fragmentation analysis. DNA was extracted at 72 h following beta-HIVS treatment.

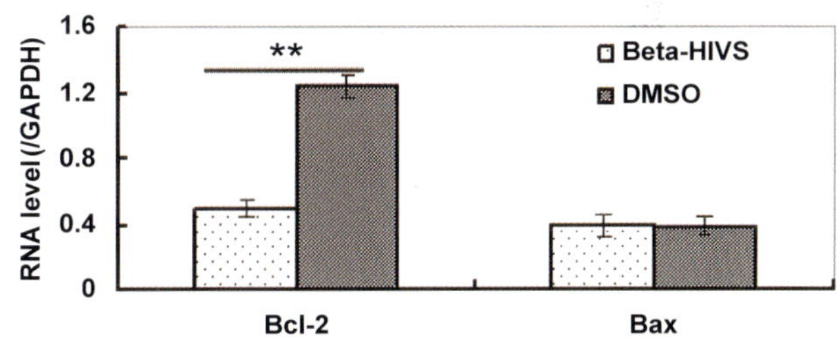

Figure 3a: Alterations of apoptosis-associated factors in different groups of U266 cells. Real-time PCR.

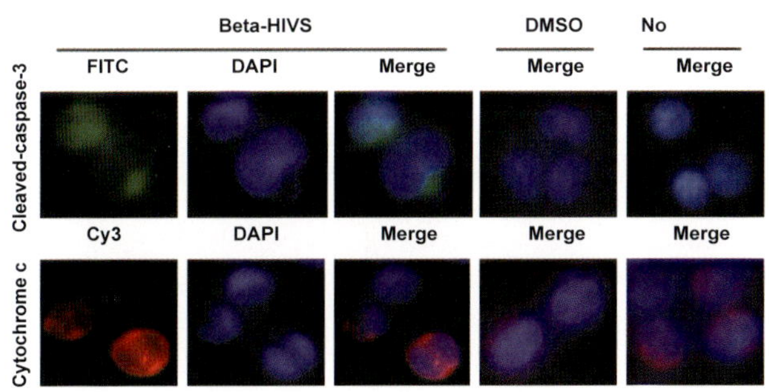

Figure 3b: Immunofluorescence staining, observed via a fluorescence microscope at 72 h after beta-HIVS treatment, at x 400 magnification. Cleaved caspase-3 was marked by green fluorescence (FITC), and cytochrome c was marked by red fluorescence (Cy3). The nucleus was stained by DAPI.

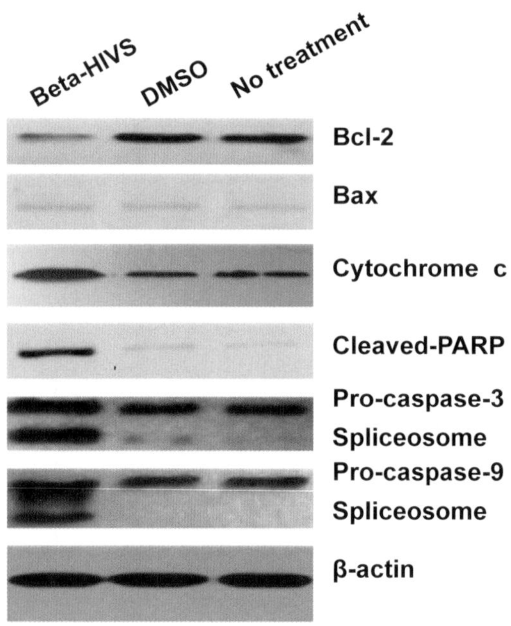

Figure 3c: Western blotting analysis of apoptosis-related proteins at 72 h after beta-HIVS treatment.

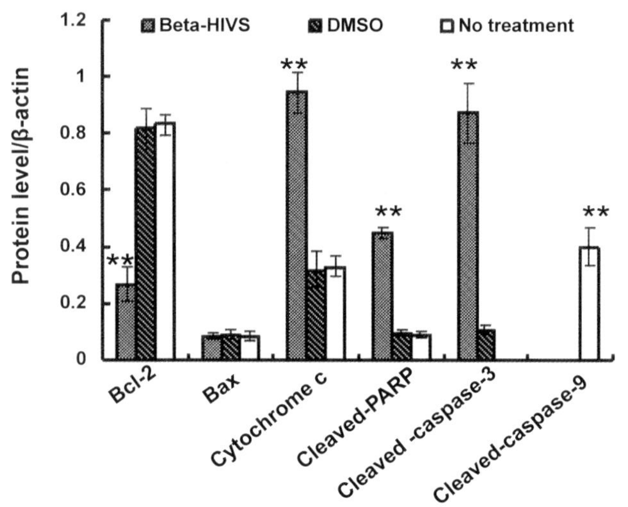

Figure 3d: Changes in expression of apoptosis-related proteins normalized to β-actin. Data shown are the means ± SD (n=3 or 5) (**: P<0.01 vs. no treatment cells).

group down-regulated, while cytochrome c expression up-regulated, all with P<0.01 when comparing the two contrast groups. Cleaved PARP was also detected in beta-HIVS treated group. Correspondingly, both cleaved caspase-3 and -9 were detected, as a 17 kDa spliceosome for pro-caspase-3 and a 37 kDa spliceosome for pro-caspase-9, were all observed in beta-HIVS treated group (Figure 3C and3D).

Discussion

In the present study, we first evaluated the apoptosis-inducing effect of beta-HIVS on U266 cells, with a result that this drug suppressed U266 cell proliferation and colony formation, and induced cell apoptosis. To further analyze the mechanism for beta-HIVS-induced apoptosis, we carried out real-time PCR, immunofluorescence staining and western blotting in the detection of changes of apoptosis-associated factors. Our data displayed that beta-HIVS treatment resulted in alterations of the expression of Bcl-2, cytochrome c, and an activation of PARP, caspase-3 and caspase-9 in U266 cells, indicating that beta-HIVS induces U266 cell death possibly by activating the mitochondria pathway.

Beta-HIVS is an ATP non-competitive inhibitor of protein-tyrosine kinases and is capable of inducing apoptosis in various lines of human tumor cells which has been documented by several publications [9-16]. Hashimoto et al, 2002 found that beta-HIVS was able to induce cell death more efficiently in DMS114 and NCI-H522 lung cancer cells [6]. Xu et al, 2004 also presented the similar results [18]. Masuda and his study group had previously validated the effects of beta-HIVS on U937 and HL-60 leukemia cells and found both two kinds of cell lines all suffered from apoptosis when treated with 10^{-6} M beta-HIVS [14]. Similarly, another proof from Hashimoto et al, 1999 also suggested that low concentrations of beta-HIVS between 10^{-8} and 10^{-6} M could inhibit the growth of various lines of cancer cells included HL-60 leukemia cells [15]. In consistant with the above findings, our data revealed that cell viability and colony formation of U266 cells were inhibited by beta-HIVS at a concentration of 1.2 μg/ml. Notably, the apoptosis-inducing effects were further validated by DAPI staining and DNA ladder electrophoresis assays, suggesting that beta-HIVS may be a potential therapeutic agent for MM treatment.

MM is considered the second most common hematological malignancy and is characterized by the clonal proliferation of neoplastic plasma cells in the bone marrow [1,2]. The improved understanding of the molecular mechanisms of MM development may provide a basis for the development of effective treatment strategies. Previous studies have demonstrated that beta-HIVS is one of the inhibitors of Protein Tyrosine Kinases (PTKs) which play important roles in a number of signal transduction pathways that are involved in cancer cell growth, differentiation, cell death, and carcinogenesis [19-22]. Particularly, beta-HIVS prohibits the activity of v-Src and EGFR in an ATP-non-competitive manner, and suppresses polo-like kinase 1 (PLK1) after inhibition of PTK activity, with resultant induction of apoptosis in human leukemia cells [23]. Correspondingly, a study from Xu et al, 2004 also indicated that beta-HIVS induced apoptosis in DMS114 cells via a PTK-dependent pathway [18]. Besides, Masuda et al, 2003 had demonstrated that beta-HIVS suppresses the growth of U937 and HL-60 leukemia cells by inhibiting the activity of a polo-like kinase 1 (PLK1) that is involved in control of the cell cycle [14].

In addition, other singling pathways are involved in beta-HIVS-mediated tumor cell death as well [15,24-27]. Early in 1999, Hashimoto et al. had reported that beta-HIVS was able to activate caspase-3 in its anti-neoplastic effect [15]. Then, Wu et al. described that shikonin inhibited cell growth in a time- and dose-dependent manner, accompanied by a decreased Bcl-2 and increased Bax expression, as well as an activation of caspase cascade [26]. Similarly, the present study showed that beta-HIVS treatment in U266 cells resulted in changes in the expression of Bcl-2, cytochrome c, PARP, caspase-3 and caspase-9, characterized by a reduced expression of Bcl-2 and increased expression of cytochrome c, although Bax expression altered with no significance. The activation of caspase-3 was further verified by western blotting and immunofluorescence assays. In addition, cleaved caspase-9 was detected by western blotting as well. Importantly, cleaved-PARP was also detected, which further provides evidence of the activation of caspase-3 and caspase-9. In short, it these data suggest that beta-HIVS suppresses cell viability and induces cell apoptosis by triggering the mitochondrial pathway in multiple myeloma. Yet, our findings are in consistent with the previous studies [15,26,27].

Taken together, the present study disclosed the apoptosis-inducing of beta-HIVS on U266 cells as well as the primary underlying mechanisms. However, the evaluation of the apoptosis status of U266 cells induced by beta-HIVS was limited due to the detection methods conducted in this study, and therefore more apoptosis evaluations are needed. Moreover, the release of cytochrome c from the mitochondria should also be validated. These experiments will be performed in our future studies.

Acknowledgement

The authors thank Professor Donghong Lin (Donghonglin65@163.com) for providing editorial assistance.

References

1. Khagi Y, Mark TM (2014) Potential role of daratumumab in the treatment of multiple myeloma. Onco Targets Ther 7: 1095-1100.

2. Kyle RA, Rajkumar SV (2008) Multiple myeloma. Blood 111: 2962-2972.

3. Lacy MQ, Hayman SR, Gertz MA, Dispenzieri A, Buadi F, et al. (2009) Pomalidomide (CC4047) plus low-dose dexamethasone as therapy for relapsed multiple myeloma. J Clin Oncol 27: 5008-5014.

4. Badros A, Burger AM, Philip S, Niesvizky R, Kolla SS, et al. (2009) Phase I study of vorinostat in combination with bortezomib for relapsed and refractory multiple myeloma. Clin Cancer Res 15: 5250-5257.

5. Alessandra Romano, Concetta Conticello, Maide Cavalli, Calogero Vetro, Cosimo Di Raimondo, et al. (2014) Salvage Therapy of Multiple Myeloma: The New Generation Drugs. Biomed Res Int 2014: 456037.

6. Hashimoto S, Xu Y, Masuda Y, Aiuchi T, Nakajo S, et al. (2002) Beta-hydroxyisovalerylshikonin is a novel and potent inhibitor of protein tyrosine kinases. Jpn J Cancer Res 93: 944-951.

7. Rao Z, Liu X, Zhou W, Yi J, Li SS (2011) Synthesis and antitumour activity of Î²-hydroxyisovalerylshikonin analogues. Eur J Med Chem 46: 3934-3941.

8. An S, Park YD, Paik YK, Jeong TS, Lee WS (2007) Human ACAT inhibitory effects of shikonin derivatives from Lithospermum erythrorhizon. Bioorg Med Chem Lett 17: 1112-1116.

9. Takai N, Ueda T, Nishida M, Nasu K, Narahara H (2008) Beta-hydroxyisovalerylshikonin has a profound anti-growth activity in human endometrial and ovarian cancer cells. Gynecol Oncol 109: 107-114.

10. Kajimoto S, Horie M, Manabe H, Masuda Y, Shibayama-Imazu T, et al. (2008) A tyrosine kinase inhibitor, beta-hydroxyisovalerylshikonin, induced apoptosis in human lung cancer DMS114 cells through reduction of dUTP nucleotidohydrolase activity. Biochim Biophys Acta 1782: 41-50.

11. Xu Y, Nakajo S, Nakaya K (2002) Synergistic inhibitory effects of transplatin and beta-hydroxyisovalerylshikon on carcinoma A431 cells involve epidermal growth factor receptor. Cancer Lett 188: 67-72.

12. Kretschmer N, Rinner B, Deutsch AJ, Lohberger B, Knausz H, et al. (2012) Naphthoquinones from Onosma paniculata induce cell-cycle arrest and apoptosis in melanoma Cells. J Nat Prod 75: 865-869.

13. Takai N, Ueda T, Nishida M, Nasu K, Narahara H (2010) Anti-neoplastic effect of Î²-hydroxyisovalerylshikonin on a human choriocarcinoma cell line. Mol Med Rep 3: 515-518.

14. Masuda Y, Nishida A, Hori K, Hirabayashi T, Kajimoto S, et al. (2003) Beta-hydroxyisovalerylshikonin induces apoptosis in human leukemia cells by inhibiting the activity of a polo-like kinase 1 (PLK1). Oncogene 22: 1012-1023.

15. Hashimoto S, Xu M, Masuda Y, Aiuchi T, Nakajo S, et al. (1999) beta-hydroxyisovalerylshikonin inhibits the cell growth of various cancer cell lines and induces apoptosis in leukemia HL-60 cells through a mechanism different from those of Fas and etoposide. Biochem 125: 17-23.

16. Nakaya K, Miyasaka T (2003) A shikonin derivative, beta-hydroxyisovalerylshikonin, is an ATP-non-competitive inhibitor of protein tyrosine kinases. Anticancer Drugs 14: 683-693.

17. Cui Z, Lin D, Cheng F, Luo L, Kong L, et al. (2013) The role of the WWOX gene in leukemia and its mechanisms of action. Oncol Rep 29: 2154-2162.

18. Xu Y, Kajimoto S, Nakajo S, Nakaya K (2004) Beta-hydroxyisovalerylshikonin and cisplatin act synergistically to inhibit growth and to induce apoptosis of human lung cancer DMS114 cells via a tyrosine kinase-dependent pathway. Oncology 66: 67-75.

19. Bertoletti F, Crespan E, Maga G (2012) Tyrosine kinases as essential cellular cofactors and potential therapeutic targets for human immunodeficiency virus infection. Cell Mol Biol (Noisy-le-grand) 58: 31-43.

20. Chiarugi P (2005) PTPs versus PTKs: the redox side of the coin. Free Radic Res 39: 353-364.

21. Katagiri K, Yokoyama KK, Yamamoto T, Omura S, Irie S, et al. (1996) Lyn and Fgr protein-tyrosine kinases prevent apoptosis during retinoic acid-induced granulocytic differentiation of HL-60 cells. J Biol Chem 271: 11557-11562.

22. Punt CJ (1992) Regulation of hematopoietic cell function by protein tyrosine kinase-encoding oncogenes, a review. Leuk Res 16: 551-559.

23. Masuda Y, Shima G, Aiuchi T, Horie M, Hori K, et al. (2004) Involvement of tumor necrosis factor receptor-associated protein 1 (TRAP1) in apoptosis induced by beta-hydroxyisovalerylshikonin. J Biol Chem 279: 42503-42515.

24. Jayasooriya RG, Lee KT, Lee HJ, Choi YH, Jeong JW et al. (2014) Anti-inflammatory effects of Î²-hydroxyisovalerylshikonin in BVmicroglia are mediated through suppression of the PI3K/Akt/NF-kB pathway and activation of the Nrf2/HO-1 pathway. Food Chem Toxicol 65: 82-89.

25. Komi Y, Suzuki Y, Shimamura M, Kajimoto S, Nakajo S, et al. (2009) Mechanism of inhibition of tumor angiogenesis by beta-hydroxyisovalerylshikonin. Cancer Sci 100: 269-277.

26. Wu Z, Wu L, Li L, Tashiro S, Onodera S, et al. (2004) p53-mediated cell cycle arrest and apoptosis induced by shikonin via a caspase-9-dependent mechanism in human malignant melanoma A375-S2 cells. J Pharmacol Sci 94: 166-176.

27. Nishida M, Nasu K, Ueda T, Yuge A, Takai N, et al. (2006) Beta-hydroxyisovalerylshikonin induces apoptosis and G0/G1 cell-cycle arrest of endometriotic stromal cells: a preliminary in vitro study. Hum Reprod 21: 2850-2856.

Crosstalk between the Smad and the Mitogen-Activated Protein Kinase Pathways is Essential for Erythroid Differentiation of Erythroleukemia Cells Induced by TGF-β, Activin, Hydroxyurea and Butyrate

Salem Akel[1,2], Daniel Bertolette[1] and Francis W Ruscetti[1]*

[1]*Leukocyte Biology Section, Laboratory of Experimental Immunology, Center for Cancer Research, NCI, Frederick, Maryland*
[2]*St. Louis Blood Bank and Cellular Therapy Laboratory, Cardinal Glennon Children's Medical Center, St. Louis, MO*

Abstract

The role of crosstalk between the Smad and the MAPK signaling pathways in activin-, transforming growth factor-β (TGF-β)-, hydroxyurea (HU) - and butyrate-dependent erythroid differentiation of K562 leukemic cells was studied. Treatment with all four inducers caused transient phosphorylation of Smad2/3 and MAPK proteins including ERK, p38 and JNK. Use of specific inhibitors of p38, ERK and JNK MAPK proteins, and TGF-β type I receptor indicated that differentiation induced by each of these agents involves activation of Smad2/3 and p38 MAPK, and inhibition of ERK MAPK. Also, treatment of cells with an inhibitor of protein serine/threonine phosphatase, okadaic acid (OA), induced phosphorylation of Smad2/3, and p38 MAPK, coincident with its induction of erythroid differentiation. Specific inhibition of TGF-β type I receptor kinase activity not only abolished TGF-β/activin effects but also prevented Smad2/3 activation and erythroid differentiation induced by OA, HU and butyrate. The TGF-β type I receptor kinase inhibitor blocked OA-induced differentiation but not p38 MAPK phosphorylation demonstrating that signals from both pathways are needed. As previously observed, addition of ERK1/2 MAPK inhibitors upregulated Smad2/3 phosphorylation and enhanced differentiation, but these effects were dependent on signals from the TGF-β type I receptor. These data indicate that activation of both Smad2/3 and p38 MAPK signaling pathways is a prerequisite to induce erythroid differentiation of erythroleukemia cells by activin, TGF-β, HU, OA and butyrate.

Keywords: Transforming Growth Factor-β; Activin; Hydroxyurea; Erythropoiesis; Smads; p38 MAP Kinase; Okadaic acid

Introduction

The transforming growth factor (TGF-β) family regulates most, if not all, mammalian cellular processes [1]. Two members, activins and TGF-βs, of the TGF-β family have many such effects on hematopoiesis, when appropriate in context, from stem cell quiescence, progenitor cell growth inhibition, stimulation of differentiation, mature cell function and cell death. Ligand binding induces phosphorylation and activation of type I receptor signaling by the type II receptor kinase. Smad2 and Smad3, the principal receptor-activated proteins involved in activin/ TGF-β signaling, are activated directly by TGF-β type I receptor kinase then translocate to the nucleus in complex with a common co-Smad, Smad4, to regulate transcription of target genes [2-4]. Smad6 and Smad7 are inhibitory Smads that interact with all TGF-β type I receptors antagonizing activin/ TGF-β signaling [1-7].

The response of TGF-β signaling is cellular type- and context-dependent [8,9]. This could involve different receptor complexes [10], cross talk with other signaling pathways, different transcription factor activities and genetic changes in cancers. Many signaling pathways interact with activin/ TGF-β signaling [1-4].The mitogen-activated protein kinase (MAPK) cascades, comprised mainly of the extracellular signal-regulated kinase (ERK), p38 MAPK, and the c-Jun N-terminal kinases (JNK) [11], have been shown to represent a major signaling pathway for TGF-β and activin independent of Smad activation [3,12-19]. In crosstalk between the Smad and MAPKs pathways, TGF-β dependent or independent induction of activated ERK MAPK can occur. Activated ERK by activation of the epidermal growth factor (EGF) receptor-Ras pathway and by Ca^{2+}- calmodulin-dependent kinase II [20,21]. Phosphorylation of Smad2/3 by ERK MAPK imposes an inhibitory effect by attenuating their nuclear translocation [18,20,21]. In contrast, activation of ERK MAPK by hepatocyte growth factor had positive effects on Smad activation [18,22]. In the nucleus, an additional crosstalk between these signaling pathways of TGF-β and activin occurs [1-4]. Reciprocal regulation (positive or negative) of activated Smads and downstream substrates of JNK and p38 MAPKs, including c-Jun and ATF-2 (components of the AP-1 complex), has been shown [1-4,23-25]. This dual ability of the TGF-β type 1 receptor (TβR1) to independently activate signaling pathways which cross-talk can have profound effects on cellular processes.

TGF-β and activin both regulate different cellular events of hematopoiesis in a lineage specific manner [26-28]. Both cytokines stimulate erythroid differentiation, accompanied by hemoglobin synthesis, and TGF-β inhibited growth of early but not late erythroid progenitor cells [26,29-32]. Although erythroid differentiation induced by erythropoietin (Epo), hydroxyurea (HU) and sodium butyrate involves p38 activation and ERK1/2 inhibition [33-37], the requirement of MAPK signaling in TGF-β- and activin-induced erythroid differentiation remains obscure. The possible integration of these two pathways in erythroid differentiation was studied. Activin/ TGF-β- dependent erythroid differentiation requires activation of both Smad and p38 MAPK signals for optimal differentiation. Chemical induction of erythro-differentiation by HU and butyrate also resulted in phosphorylation of Smad2/3 and was TRI receptor dependent.

***Corresponding author:** Dr. Francis W Ruscetti, Laboratory of Experimental Immunology, Center for Cancer Research, NCI, Frederick, MD 21702-1201, USA, E-mail: ruscettf@mail.nih.gov

Inhibition of ERK1/2 enhanced Smad2/3 phosphorylation and erythroid differentiation but this cross talk between the Smad and the ERK MAPK pathway was also TRI receptor dependent.

Materials and Methods

Cell culture and reagents

Erythroleukemia cells including K562, HEL and TF-1 were maintained in RPMI-1640 medium containing 10% fetal bovine serum (FBS). Interleukin (IL)-3 (10 ng/ml, Peprotech, Rocky Hill, NJ) was added to support the growth of TF-1 cells. To assay erythroid differentiation, cells (2×10^4/ml) were cultured in serum-free media containing 10% BIT 900 (Stem Cell Tech.) with or without the addition of rh-activin A, rh-TGF-β1 (R &D systems, Minneapolis, MN, USA), HU, sodium butyrate (Sigma, St Louis , MO) and okadaic acid (LC Laboratories, Woburn, MA). To elucidate the role of each MAPK in the regulation of cell response, specific signal transduction inhibitors in dimethyl sulfoxide (DMSO) or DMSO alone were added to cultures one hour prior to cell treatment, as indicated. Inhibitors of ERK1, -2 (PD98059 and U0126), p38 (SB203580), and JNK1, -2, -3 (SP600125) MAPK (all used at 10 μM, 0.2 DMSO) were purchased from BioSource International, Camarillo, CA, USA. SB505124, a specific inhibitor of TβR1 that inhibits activation of both activin and TGF-β type I receptors (ALK4 and ALK5 as well as ALK7 respectively, 39) was provided by GlaxoSmithKline, (King of Prussia, PA). It was used at 20 uM (0.2% DMSO) with a control (0.2% DMSO).

Evaluation of cell growth and differentiation

In the signaling studies on cells undergoing differentiation, cells were derived of serum overnight which reduces the signaling background at time zero due to factors in the serum, allowing the inhibitors to be more effective. Also, cells accumulate at G0/G1 allowing for more coordinated study on growth inhibition. A dose response of the differentiation inducers on K562 was performed to determine the optimal concentration for differentiation and cell signaling. Count of viable cells was determined using trypan blue staining. Formation of erythroid cells was monitored by flow cytometry using anti-glycophorin A (GPA) antibody (Immunotech, Marseille, France). The intracellular hemoglobin synthesis was monitored by staining of cells in suspension using 1% 2,7-diaminofluorene (DAF), 3% hydrogen peroxide and 5% acetic acid in Tris-HCl buffer (200 mmole/L; pH 7.0) [38].

Evaluation of cell apoptosis

Cells grown in the presence and absence of activin A and TGF-β1 (as indicated) were harvested at different times and analyzed for apoptosis. Whole cell lysates were evaluated for the cleavage of the nuclear poly (ADP-ribose) polymerase (PARP) by western blotting as described below, using an anti-PARP antibody (Cell Signaling Tech., Beverly, MA, USA). Cells were also were examined for early apoptosis by evaluating the expression of the mitochondrial membrane protein APO2.7 using flow cytometric analysis of cells stained with PE-conjugated anti-APO2.7 antibody (Immunotech, Marseille, France) as previously described [39].

Flow cytometric analysis

Treated cells, as indicated, were washed in 2% normal human AB serum in phosphate buffered saline (PBS), blocked with 5 μl of a mixture of normal human and mouse sera, washed, and incubated with 15 μl of either anti-GPA antibody conjugated with fluorescein isothiocyanate (FITC) (Immunotech) or an isotype control-FITC antibody (BD Laboratories, San Diego, CA) at 4°C for 30 minutes. After washing, cells were suspended in equal volumes of PBS and 4% paraformaldehyde. Analysis was carried out using a FACScan (BD laboratories) flow cytometer and FLOWJO software (Tree Star Inc., Palo Alto, CA, USA).

Western blot analysis

Relative levels of proteins were assessed in whole cell lysates using the standard immunoblotting technique [32,40,41]. Smad signaling was evaluated using anti-Smad2 (Zymed Laboratories, South San Francisco, CA), anti-phospho-Smad2 and anti-Smad2/3 (Upstate Biotech. Lake Placid, NY), and anti-phospho-Smad3 (provided by Dr. Ed Leof, Mayo Clinic, Rochester, MN). Antibodies directed against MAP kinases [anti-p44/42, anti-phospho-p44/42 (Thr202/Tyr204), anti-p38, anti-phospho-p38 (Thr180/Tyr182), anti-SAP/JNK and anti-phospho-SAP/JNK (Thr183/Tyr185)] were obtained from Cell Signaling Tech. Briefly, cells were lysed in Triton X-100 lysis buffer (25 mM HEPES at pH 7.5, 150 mM NaCl, 10% glycerol, 5 mM EDTA, 1% Triton-X 100) containing phosphatase and protease inhibitors. Cell lysates were separated by SDS-PAGE and transferred onto an Immobilon-P membrane (Millipore). After blocking with 5% non-fat dry milk and incubation (2 hrs) with phosphoprotein specific primary antibody, blots were incubated (1 hr) with an appropriate secondary antibody (horseradish peroxidase-conjugated) and detected with the ECL system (Amersham Biosciences, UK).

The gel was then stripped and incubated with an antibody that recognizes the total protein of phospho-specific protein antibody.

Statistical analysis

Results are expressed as a mean value + standard deviation (SD). The paired Student *t*-test value was used to determine the statistical significance of differences between means that was calculated from at least three independent experiments.

Results

Induction of erythroid differentiation/growth inhibition of human erythroleukemia cells by activin and TGF-β- requires activation of endogenous Smad2/3

Activin A and TGF-β1 can inhibit the growth of erythroleukemia cell lines and stimulate erythroid differentiation, in a dose dependent fashion [29,30]. Similar results were seen on differential growth inhibition and increase in the proportion of hemoglobin positive (Hb^+) DAF^+ cells [38] after treatment of K562, TF-1 and HEL cell lines with rh-activin A or rh- TGF-β1 (Figures 1A and 1B). The greater growth inhibition coincided with greater erythroid differentiation. Phosphorylation of Smad2 was strongly induced following TGF-β (Figure 1C) and activin (data not shown) treatment in the three cell lines. The activation pattern of Smad2 and Smad3 by either cytokine was similar with rapid phosphorylation (beginning at 5 min and reaching a peak at 30-60 min) that lasted for 24 hours as shown in K562 (Figure 2). Smad3 activation lasted longer than Smad2. K562 cells were then treated with 20 M of SB505124, an inhibitor of phosphorylation of the TβR1 receptors (ALK4 and ALK5) upstream of Smad2/3 activation [42] (ALK 7 is also inhibited but responds to Nodal not TGF-β, activin). SB505124 not only prevented Smad2/3 phosphorylation (Figure 3A), but also blocked growth inhibition (Figure 3B) and suppressed erythroid differentiation (Figure 3C) induced by activin and TGF-β. The differentiation activin induced was 24% and reduced to undetectable by the inhibitor. Similarly differentiation induced by TGF-β went from 35% to undetectable. Thus, TGF-β receptor/Smad

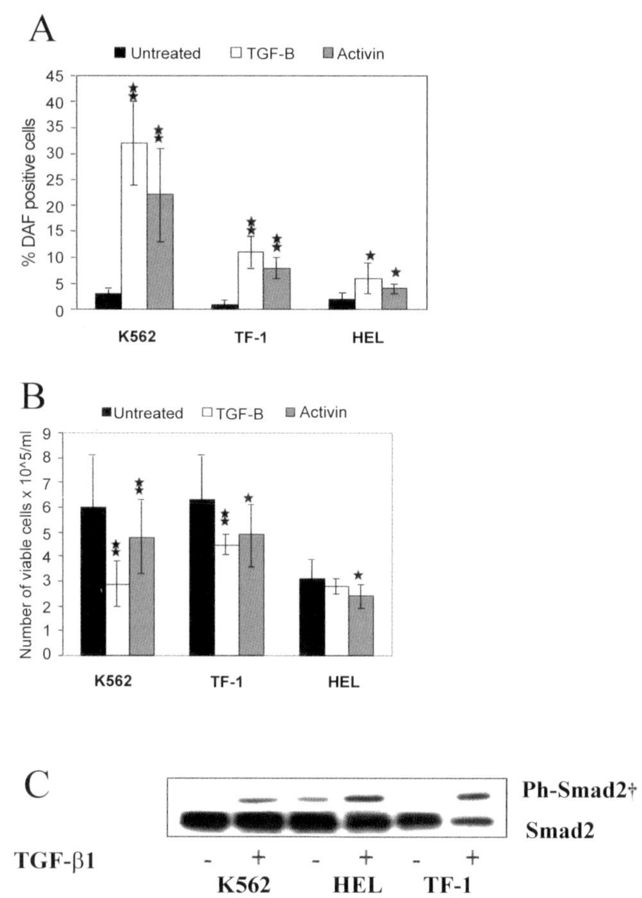

** P<0.01 and *P<0.05

Figure 1: Differentiation response of erythroleukemia cells to TGF-β and activin treatment. K562, TF-1 and HEL cells (2×10⁴/ml) were cultured in serum free conditions without (-) and with (+) the addition of rh- TGF-β1 or rh-Activin-A (5 ng/ml each). After 6 days of culture, cells were collected and evaluated for their growth and intracellular hemoglobin synthesis.
A. Percentage of Hb⁺ cells was calculated following DAF staining of cells in suspension and scoring at least 1000 cells. **B.** Total number of viable cells per ml was determined in same cultures after cell staining with trypan blue. **C.** In the same cultures, aliquots of cells were harvested after 1 hr of cytokine treatment and whole cell lysates were prepared as described in Materials and methods. Immuno-blotting with anti-phospho-Smad2 and anti-Smad2 was performed. Results are shown as the mean ± SD of four independent experiments.

signaling is not defective in these erythroleukemia cells and is required for erythroid differentiation mediated by these ligands.

Induction of erythroid differentiation precedes early apoptosis

Since the advent of treatment for acute promyelocytic leukemia (APL) [43] with all trans retinoic acid, differentiation therapy for treatment of leukemia has been a research focus. As TGF- and activin are multifunctional proteins that regulate growth, differentiation and apoptosis in various cell types [19,26,40], a relationship between activin/ TGF-β- induced erythroid differentiation/growth inhibition and the induction of apoptosis was examined. Lysates from cells treated with cytokines for different times until 72 hours, when 30-35% of TGF-β1 treated K562 cells were hemoglobinized by day 2, did not exhibit significant increases in the cleavage of PARP protein (Figure 4A), a specific marker of apoptosis in these cells [44]. The reversibility of this growth arrest mediated by activin/ TGF-β was examined. Cells were treated with 1-5 ng/ml of either agent for different periods of time, washed, recultured and their growth was compared to untreated control cells for up to 3 days. Exposure of cells to activin/ TGF-β for 2 days resulted in a reversible growth arrest (data not shown) and despite the growth inhibition of cytokine-treated cells for 2 days; cells remained largely viable and still began to accumulate hemoglobin. Moreover, FACS analysis of APO2.7, an early mitochondrial marker of apoptosis [39], at various times (1-3 days) after treatment with activin/ TGF-β revealed that a small fraction (<10%) of cells underwent apoptosis at day 2 (Figure 4B). At this time (day 2), we have noticed that the percent of Hb⁺ cells was 75% of the maximal percentage observed at the end of the culture (day 5) [45], indicating that cell apoptosis is not a feature of early differentiation. Therefore, activin/ TGF-β- mediated differentiation/growth inhibition is not preceded by the onset of apoptosis and that any delayed apoptotic response in cytokine treated cells (>20% by day3) (Figure 4B) may be the ultimate result of p38MAPK activation by activin/ TGF-β which is known to activate caspases during-terminal erythroid differentiation [36,37].

Hydroxyurea and sodium butyrate induce Smad protein phosphorylation through a TGF-β type I receptor dependent mechanism during erythroid differentiation

Since treatment with chemical inducers such as HU and sodium butyrate also stimulate Epo-independent hemoglobin synthesis in erythroleukemia cells similar to activin and TGF-β [30,34-35], the role of Smad signaling in mediating the effects of HU and butyrate was examined. Following the addition of HU (400M) and butyrate (0.6 mM) to serum-free cultures of K562 cells, both chemicals were able to induce a rapid, transient increase in phosphorylation of Smad2/3 at 15-30 min (Figure 5A), returning to base line by 60 min (by 30 min in hydroxyurea activation of Smad 3). These cellular treatments did not alter the amount of total Smad 2/3 proteins expressed in the cells, (Figure 5A). Moreover, similar regulation of phospho-Smad2/3 by HU and butyrate was found in other leukemic cell lines like TF-1 and HL60 (data not shown). Prior addition of the TβR1 signaling inhibitor, SB505124, to K562 cells treated with HU and butyrate abolished Smad2/3 phosphorylation (Figure 5B), and markedly reduced the

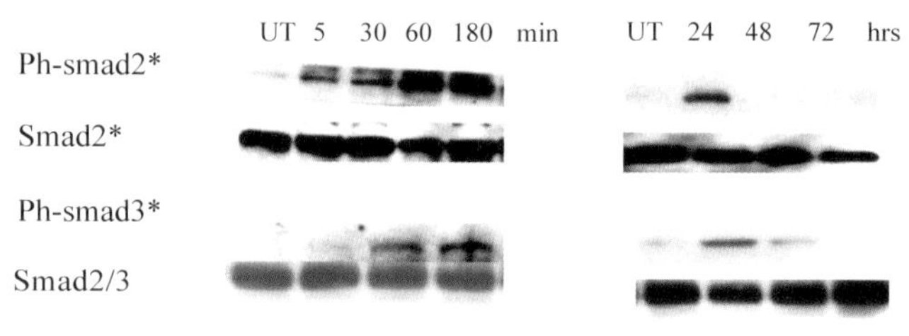

Similar results using antibodies against phospho-Smad3 and Smad2/3 proteins.

Figure 2: Time course of activation of Smad proteins by TGF-β1/activin. K562 cells were treated with 5 ng/ml of rh- **TGF-β1**, harvested at various time points (left: 5, 30, 60, and 180 minutes; right: 24, 48 and 72 hrs), lysed, and analyzed by immunoblotting. Membranes were probed with specific antibodies against the phosphorylated forms of the Smad proteins (Smad2 and Smad3). Protein-antibody reaction was detected by chemiluminescence. Same blots were stripped and hybridized with antibodies against Smad2 and Smad2/3 to evaluate the total corresponding proteins. Results are representative of 3 experiments.

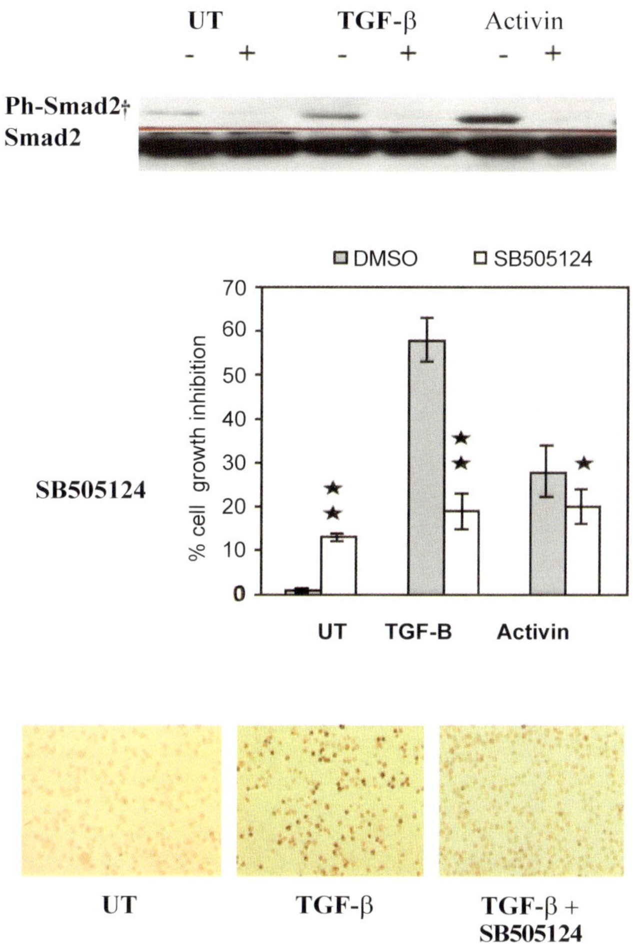

Similar results were seen in cells treated with the same dose of activin A.

Figure 3: Inhibition of TGF-β type I receptor signaling blocked the response of K562 cells to TGF-β /activin treatment. Overnight-starved K562 (5×104/ml) cells were cultured for 1 hr with SB505124 (20 μM) in DMSO (+) and with DMSO alone (-). Cultures were split and continued in the absence (UT) and the presence of **TGF-β**1 and activin A (5 ng/ml).
A. After 1 hr, 2 × 106 cells were harvested and subjected to immunoblot analysis using Anti-phospho-Smad2 antibody. Blots were stripped and reprobed with antibody that detects total Smad2 protein. **B.** Aliquots of the same treated cells were cultured for 5 more days. At this point, cells were evaluated for growth inhibition using counts of trypan blue negative viable cells and for the appearance of hemoglobinized DAF⁺ cells. **C.** Aliquots of the same treated cells were cultured for 5 more days. At this point, cells were evaluated for growth inhibition using counts of trypan blue negative viable cells. Results of A and C are representative of three experiments and results in B are mean values ± SD obtained from three independent experiments.

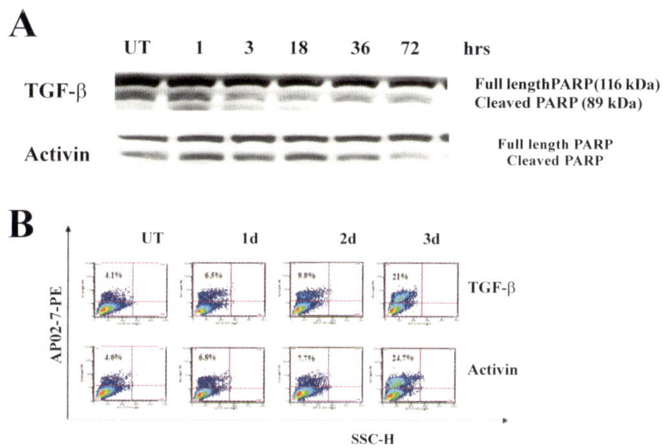

Similar results were found using anti-phospho-Smad3.
* *P*<0.05 and ** *P*<0.01.

Figure 4: Apoptotic response of K562 cells to TGF-β1 and activin A treatment does not precede differentiation
(A) K562 cells were treated with 5 ng/ml of TGF-β1 (top panel) and activin A (bottom panel) for 3 days. Time course analysis (as indicated) of PARP expression was performed using western blotting with an anti-PARP antibody that reacts with full length and cleaved PARP segments. **B.** Cells from the same cultures were evaluated for the expression of APO2.7 by flowcytometry at days 1, 2 and 3 using a PE-conjugated antibody against APO2.7. Similar results obtained in 3 independent experiments.

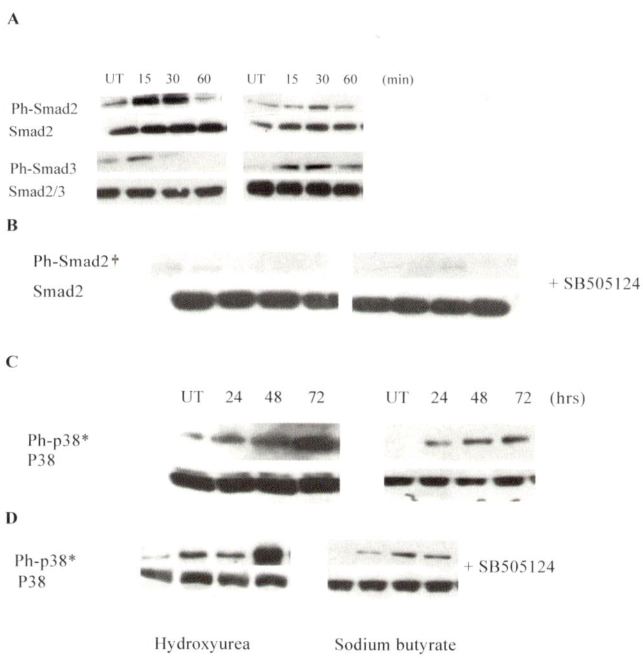

Figure 5: HU and butyrate stimulate phosphorylation of Smad2/3 and p38 MAPK. K562 cells were treated for indicated times with 400 M of HU (left) and 0.6 mM of sodium butyrate (right) without (A & C) and with (B & D) prior addition of SB505124 (20 μM). Membranes were immunoblotted with antibodies against phosphorylated Smad2, Smad3 and p38 MAPK proteins as shown in (A-D). The membranes were stripped and reprobed antibodies against total Smad2, Smad2/3, and p38 MAPK proteins (A-D). The data shown are representative of 3 independent experiments with similar results. Similar results were obtained using phospho-smad3 antibody.

development of erythroid (DAF⁺ and GPA⁺) cells (Figures 6A and 6B), compared with control cultures treated with DMSO (0.2%). These results indicate that HU and butyrate require TβR1-dependent signaling through Smads for erythroid differentiation.

JNK, p38 and ERK MAPK proteins are transiently activated during activin/ TGF-β- induced erythroid differentiation

Similar to earlier reports, HU- and butyrate-induced differentiation of K562 cells was associated with activation of p38 (Figure 5C) and inactivation of ERK MAPK (data not 8 shown) [33-37]. Since

TGF-β signaling can occur through the MAPK pathways [12-19], we investigated MAPK signaling in response to TGF-β/activin during erythroid differentiation. Unstimulated leukemic cells had basal levels of constitutively phosphorylated ERK1/2, p38 and JNK1/2 MAPK proteins despite being serum deprived overnight (Figure 7A) and stimulation by both cytokines revealed similar, rapid, transient changes in phosphorylation of all MAPK proteins studied (Figure 7A). Specific inhibitors of the MAPK proteins were effective in blocking TGF-β mediated MAPK signaling (Figure 7B) and inhibition of one MAPK pathway did not alter the phosphorylation of other tested MAPKs (data not shown), thus MAPK pathways including ERK, p38 and JNK send independent signals in K562 in response to TGF-β/activin stimulation. Prior treatment of TGF-β/activin-stimulated cells with SB505124

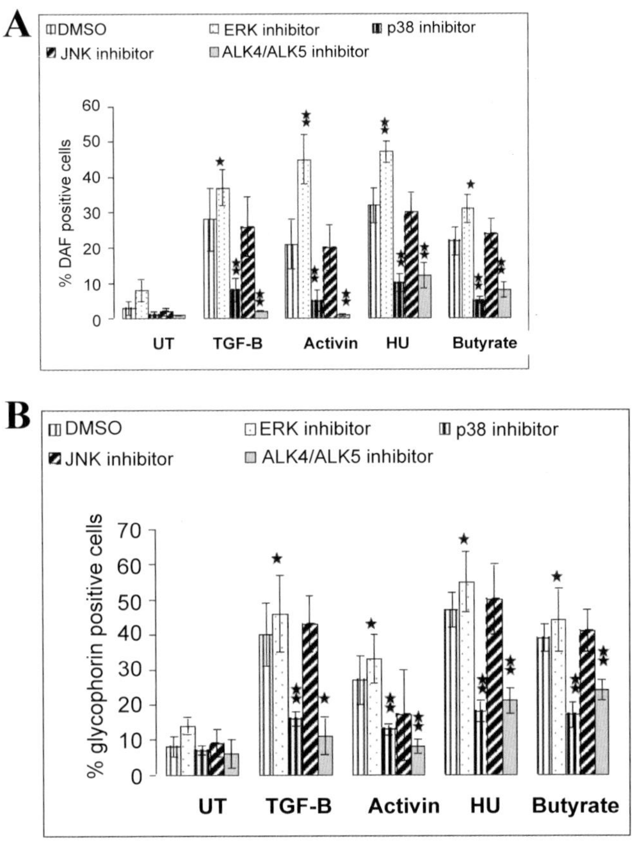

*No increase in phospho-p38 was seen earlier than 24 hrs.

Figure 6: Inhibitors of MAPK or Smad signaling pathways block erythroid differentiation.

A. K562 cells were pretreated for 1hr with and without the indicated inhibitors. Each culture was split into 5 groups. Groups were grown for 5 days in the absence and the presence of TGF-β1 (5 ng/ml), activin A (5 ng/ml), HU (150 M) and sodium butyrate (0.6 mM). Cell harvests were evaluated for the presence of Hb⁺ cells using DAF. **B**. K562 cells were pretreated for 1hr with and without the indicated inhibitors. Each culture was split into 5 groups. Groups were grown for 5 days in the absence and the presence of TGF-β1 (5 ng/ml), activin A (5 ng/ml), HU (150 M) and sodium butyrate (0.6 mM). Cell harvests were evaluated for the presence of Hb⁺ cells using DAF and for surface expression of GPA by flow cytometry. **B**. K562 cells were pretreated for 1hr with and without the indicated inhibitors. Each culture was split into 5 groups. Groups were grown for 5 days in the absence and the presence of TGF-β1 (5 ng/ml), activin A (5 ng/ml), HU (150 M) and sodium butyrate (0.6 mM). Cell harvests were evaluated for the presence of Hb⁺ cells using DAF and for surface expression of GPA by flow cytometry.

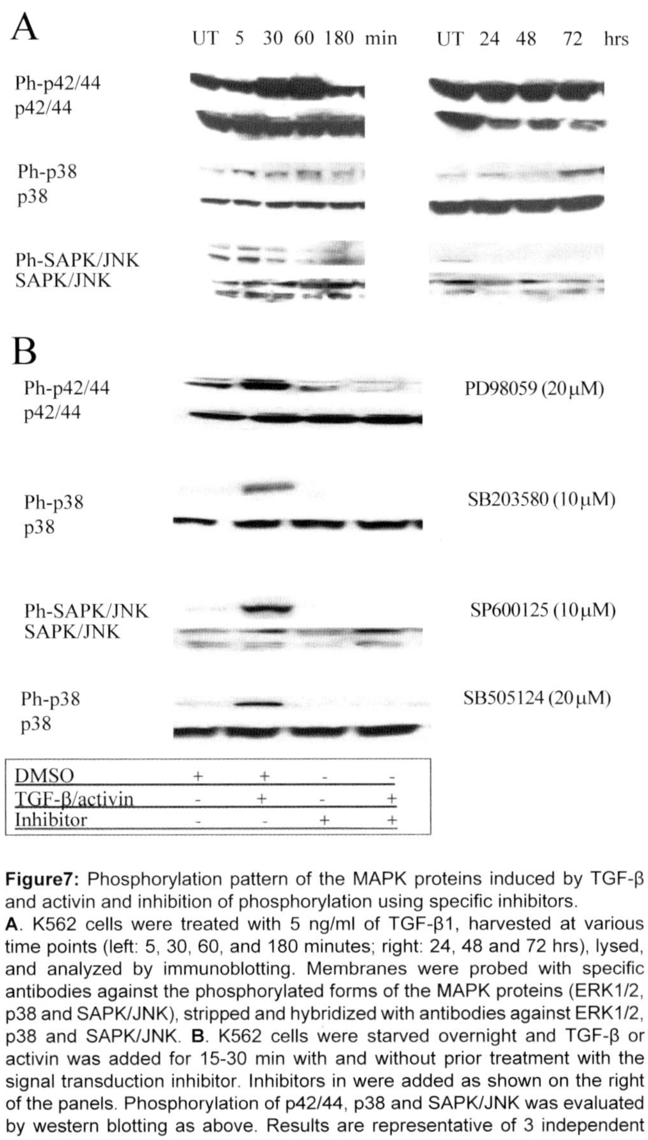

Figure7: Phosphorylation pattern of the MAPK proteins induced by TGF-β and activin and inhibition of phosphorylation using specific inhibitors.

A. K562 cells were treated with 5 ng/ml of TGF-β1, harvested at various time points (left: 5, 30, 60, and 180 minutes; right: 24, 48 and 72 hrs), lysed, and analyzed by immunoblotting. Membranes were probed with specific antibodies against the phosphorylated forms of the MAPK proteins (ERK1/2, p38 and SAPK/JNK), stripped and hybridized with antibodies against ERK1/2, p38 and SAPK/JNK. **B**. K562 cells were starved overnight and TGF-β or activin was added for 15-30 min with and without prior treatment with the signal transduction inhibitor. Inhibitors in were added as shown on the right of the panels. Phosphorylation of p42/44, p38 and SAPK/JNK was evaluated by western blotting as above. Results are representative of 3 independent experiments.

prevented the induction of phosphorylation of p38 and JNK MAPKs (Figure 7B), suggesting that these effects on MAPK kinases induced by TGF-β/activin are mediated by TβR1 signaling. Prior treatment of the TβR1 signaling inhibitor on HU/butyrate-induced MAPK activation indicated that SB505124 reduced but neither abolished p38 MAPK activation (Figures 5C and 5D) nor reversed cell growth inhibition (data not shown), suggesting that regulation of p38 MAPK by HU and butyrate is partially independent of TβR1 receptor signaling.

Crosstalk between the ERK MAPK and Smad pathways regulate erythroid differentiation

Sustained activation of ERK MAPK is required for megakaryocytic differentiation of erythroleukemia cells [45,46] and inhibition of ERKMAPK leads to erythroid differentiation [33-37]. Since ERK MAPK activation can down regulate Smad phosphorylation and Smad 7 can block erythroid differentiation and stimulate megakaryocytic differentiation in K562 cells [47,41]. ERK could mediate these effects through Smad signaling. The ERK1/2 MAPK pathway was transiently activated, after 5 to 60 minutes of cytokine treatment, returned to basal level by 3 hrs, and remained at basal level erythroid differentiation (24-72 hrs), (Figure 7A). A 1 hr pretreatment with an ERK inhibitor (PD98059), prior to cytokine stimulation deregulates ERK activation (Figure 7B) and significantly ($P<0.05$) synergizes with TGF-β/activin in erythroid differentiation (Figure 6). Prior addition of PD98059 elicited a similar effect on the differentiation of K562 cells treated with HU and butyrate, suggesting that ERK MAPK negatively regulates erythroid differentiation induced by all tested agents. Treatment of cells with the inhibitors of ERK1 (PD98059 10 μM) and ERK1/2 (U1026, 10 μM) alone resulted in a robust phosphorylation of Smad2/3 (Figure 8) and induced a slight increase in the proportion of erythroid (DAF^+ and GPA^+) cells (Figure 6). Prior addition of SB505124 prevented ERK inhibitor-induced Smad2/3 phosphorylation (Figure 8) and erythroid differentiation in a dose dependent manner (Figure 9). Hence, ERK MAPK negatively regulates Smad-mediated erythroid differentiation through TRI-dependent signaling. The ability of an inhibitor of TβR1 receptor-mediated signaling to block the erythroid differentiation of these differentiation inducers (Figure 9) indicates that TGF-β signaling is critical element needed for this differentiation.

Activation of JNK MAPK does not modulate TGF-β-, activin-, HU- and butyrate- induced erythroid differentiation

We observed here that treatment with TGF-β and activin activates JNK1/2 MAPK (Figure 7A). Using a specific inhibitor for JNK1/2/3 (SP600125, 10 μM) [48], we were able to block JNK1/2 activation induced by TGF-β/activin (Figure 7B). Inhibition of JNK1/2 MAPK activation had no significant effect ($P>0.05$) in the formation of DAF^+ and GPA^+ cells by TGF-β, activin, HU or butyrate (Figure 6). Thus, it appears that activation of JNK/1/2 is not involved in the regulation of terminal erythroid differentiation of erythroleukemia cells.

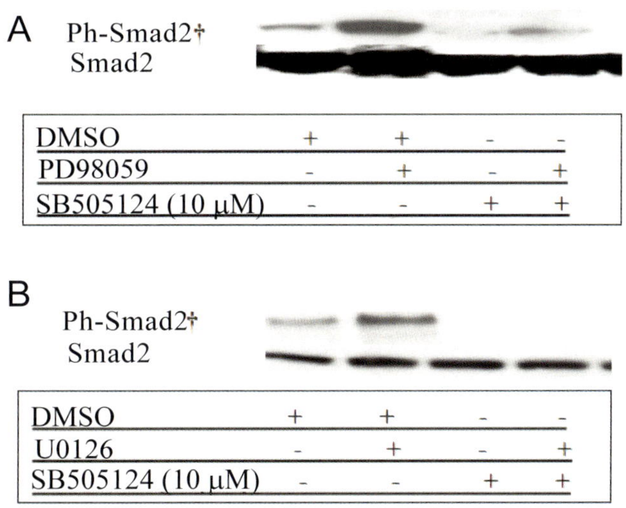

Similar results were obtained using antibodies against phophorylated ERK1/2 and SAPK/JNK proteins.

Figure 8: ERK1/2 MAPK inhibitors increase phosphorylation of Smad2/3 in presence of TGF-β receptor signaling.
A. K562 cells were treated for 1 hr with PD98059 (20 μM) or U1026 (10 μM). **B.** In the presence and absence of the inhibitor of TGF-β type I receptor, SB505124 (20 μM), as indicated. Phosphorylation of Smad2/3 and expression of endogenous Smad2/3 were evaluated by western blotting. Results are representative of 3 independent experiments.

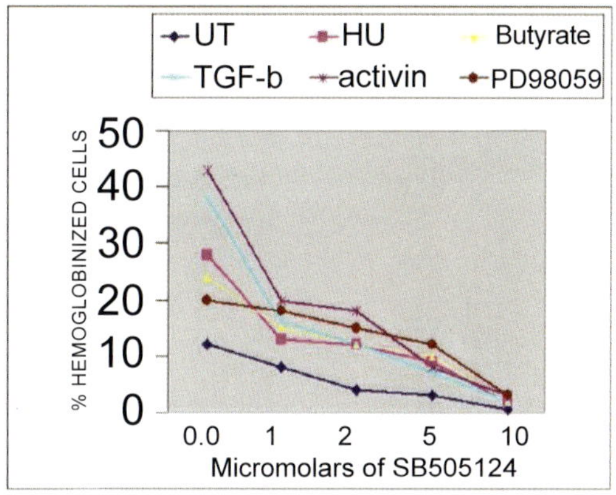

Same results were obtained using anti-phospho-Smad3 and Smad2/3 antibody.

Figure 9. Dose response of TGF-β receptor signaling inhibitor on induction of erythroid differentiation. K562 cells were pretreated for 1hr with and without the indicated concentrations of SB505124 inhibitor. Each culture was split into 6 groups. Groups were grown for 5 days in the absence and the presence of TGF-β1 (5 ng/ml), activin A (5 ng/ml), HU (150 M), sodium butyrate (0.6 mM) and PD980059 (10 uM). Cell harvests were evaluated for the presence of Hb^+ cells using DAF. Results are representative of 3 experiments.

Erythroid differentiation of erythroleukemia cells by activin, TGF-β, HU and butyrate involves activation of p38 MAPK

Activation of the p38 MAPK pathway was found to be critical for Epo-, butyrate-, and HU- induced hemoglobin synthesis [33-37]. Our data confirmed this relationship between the p38 MAPK pathway and TGF-β/activin in differentiation of K562 cells. Cytokine treatment caused transient activation of p38 MAPK (Figure 7A), and specific inhibition of p38 MAPK by SB203580 (10 M) prevented p38 phosphorylation (Figure 7B), and abrogated the appearance of DAF^+ and GPA^+ cells (Figure 6). Moreover, prior treatment of TGF-β/activin-stimulated cells with SB505124, which interferes with ligand/receptor signaling, prevented the activation of p38 MAPK and erythroid differentiation (Figure 9). Thus, p38 MAPK activation is involved in TGF-β/activin-induced erythroid differentiation.

We have observed high levels of p38 MAPK phosphorylation after 72 hrs of cytokine stimulation (Figure 7A). Similar levels of phospho-p38 MAPK were found in cells treated for more than 24-48 hrs with HU and butyrate (Figure 5C). Addition of p38 MAPK inhibitor up to 36 hrs after cell treatment with HU, butyrate, activin or TGF-β caused an inhibition of erythroid differentiation the same as when added prior to cell treatment (data not shown), which raises the probability that p38 MAPK activation is a late but essential event in erythroid differentiation. The activation of capases by p38 MAPK suggests that it is involved the apoptosis seen in late stage differentiation [35-37].

Activation of Smad2/3 and p38 MAPK by the protein phosphatases inhibitor okadaic acid alone induces erythroid differentiation

We have previously shown that okadaic acid (OA) treatment results in phosphorylation of Smad2 in HL60 cells and promotes monocytic differentiation [40]. OA is an inhibitor of the serine/threonine protein phosphatases, which can upregulate the phosphorylation of signaling intermediates and alter cell fate in the absence of added differentiation agents. Starved K562 cells were treated with various amounts of OA for 3 hrs, washed 3 times and cultured in the presence of 5% FBS and 2.5 nM of OA. Treatment of cells with 75 nM OA alone resulted in a marked increase in phospho-Smad2/3 and -p38 MAPK (Figure 10A). This change in the signaling balance by OA alone was enough to increase the proportion of cells expressing GPA (Figure 10B) and accumulating intracellular Hb (Figure 10C) in a dose dependent fashion. Consistent with this, OA enhanced erythroid differentiation induced by activin, TGF-β, HU and butyrate (data not shown). Pre-treatment of the cells with the TR I receptor signaling inhibitor, SB505124, selectively prevented OA-induced phosphorylation of Smad2/3 but only had a marginal effect on p38 MAPK activation (Figure 10D) and resulted in subsequent inhibition of formation of Hb⁺ cells (Figure 10C) and GPA⁺ cells (data not shown). These findings emphasize that activation of p38MAPK alone is not enough to promote erythroid differentiation of K562 cells, which requires activation of Smad2/3 and p38MAPK pathways.

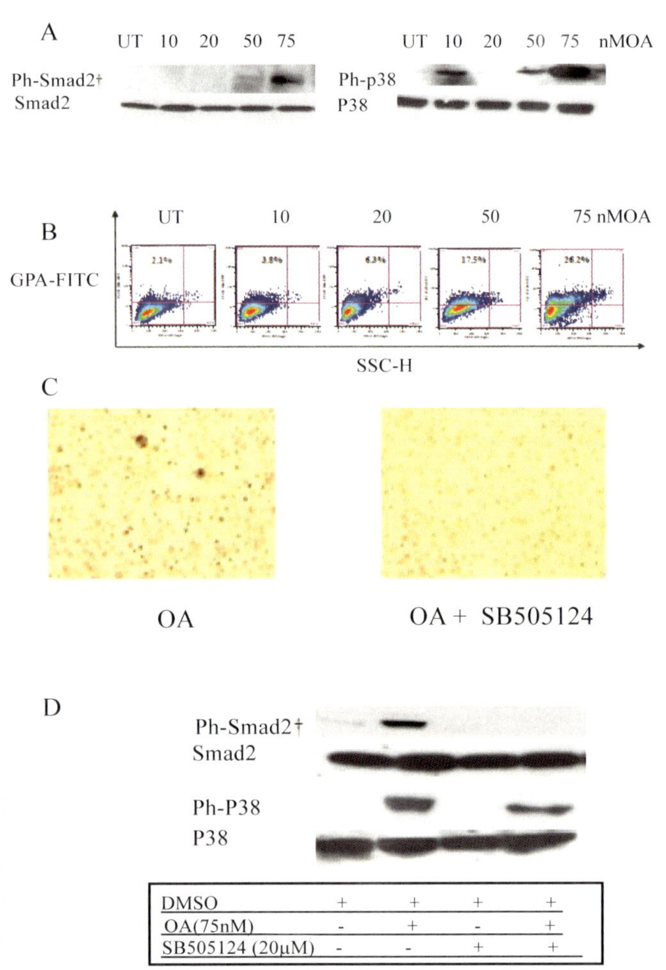

Similar results were found using anti-phospho-smad3.

Figure 10: Induction of activation of Smad2/3 and p38 MAPK, and erythroid differentiation in K562 cells treated with Okadaic acid. Cells were starved, treated with various concentrations (10-75 nM) of OA for 3 hrs then incubated with 2.5 nM OA.

Discussion

A distinct role for TGF-β and activin in erythropoiesis has been reported in studies of primary and transformed cells [16-28,30-32,36,49,50]. However, given the many stages of erythropoiesis from the stem cell quiescence to red cell enucleation and the many cytokines involved, these studies cannot be fully informative about the context in which signaling networks co-mediate TGF-β/activin effects [8,9]. In terms of leukemia, since the success of treating APL with retinoic acid [43], there has been interest in developing differentiation therapies. To study these two problems, erythroleukemia cell lines, which have the potential to give rise to erythroid and other mature hematopoietic lineages were used as a model to study the changes necessary for erythroid differentiation. Three classes of inducers were used: 1) cytokines, TGF-β and activin, 2) chemicals, HU and butyrate, and 3) a phosphatase inhibitor, OA. We have delineated the importance of cross-talk between receptor-activated Smad signaling and the MAPK pathways in the regulation of erythroid differentiation and growth inhibition seen with all of these inducers. Treatment of cells with TGF-β/activin resulted in inhibition of cell growth and led to erythroid differentiation as evidenced by a significantly increased proportion of Hb-containing cells. Changes in cell fate were preceded by cytokine/receptor-mediated intracellular signaling, which involved activation of the receptor-activated Smads; Smad2 and Smad3, and various cascades of MAPK; ERK, p38 and JNK. Direct activation of Smad2/3 by TGF-β type I receptors is well established [1-4] as well as studies describing links between MKK4/JNK and MKK3/p38 activation and TβR1 signaling involving XIAP, HPK1 and TAK1 [1-4,12-19]. Active ERK MAPK may negatively or positively modulate receptor mediated Smad activation and nuclear translocation [18,20-22]. Inhibition of TβR1 signaling abrogated TGF-β/activin-induced activation of ERK, p38 and JNK MAPKs in K562 cells. This suggests that all these MAPKs may actually be linked to TβR1-mediated Smad signaling during erythroid differentiation. Our results are in accordance with the results, showing that SB505124 interferes with TGF-β-induced activation of MAPKs [42].

There is a strong correlation between leukemic transformation and loss of sensitivity to the antiproliferative effects of TGF-β, which is frequently associated with defective Smad signaling [51,52]. The effects of TGF-β in various erythroleukemia cells showing association between Smad signaling, and suppression of cell growth and erythroid differentiation suggests that the Smad pathway is intact in these transformed cells. In K562 cells that represent leukemic human hematopoietic progenitor cells (HPC), we have explored the role of the TGF-β/activin-induced signaling in mediating cell growth arrest. TGF-β/activin-induced growth arrest was reversed in cells pre-treated with the inhibitor of TGF-β/activin type I receptors and to a lesser extent with a p38 MAPK inhibitor but not with ERK inhibitors. Also, activation of p38 MAPK mediates growth inhibition of normal HPC by TGF-β [53]; thus the suppressive effect of TGF-β in normal and leukemic human HPC involves activation of both Smad2/3 and p38MAPK.

Further evidence of cooperation between these two pathways was seen in the Epo-independent erythroid differentiation by chemicals. Cytokine-induced erythroid differentiation was dependent on the activation of p38 MAPK. Either selective inhibition of p38 by SB203580 or co-inhibition of phosphorylation of Smad2/3 and p38 MAPK by SB505124 was sufficient to prevent the formation of GPA⁺ Hb⁺ cells. Because it was not possible to achieve selective inhibition of phosphorylation of Smad2/3 without inhibition of p38 MAPK by

SB505124 in cells treated with TGF-β/activin, it remains uncertain whether activation of Smad2/3 is a prerequisite for TGF-β/activin-induced erythro-differentiation. We and others have reported that overexpression of Smad7, which interferes with TRI receptor activation of Smad2/3 phosphorylation and inhibited erythroid differentiation induced by TGF-β or activin [41]. We found that ectopic stable expression of Smad7 also prevented phosphorylation of p38 MAPK in response to TGF-β/activin treatment [45], clouding the requirement of phospho-Smad2/3 in TGF-β/activin-induced erythroid differentiation.

We have previously shown that okadaic acid stimulates phosphorylation of Smad2 in HL60 cells and promotes monocytic differentiation [40]. Okadaic acid-induced Smad2/3 and p38 MAPK activation in K562 cells resulting in the induction of erythroid differentiation and promotion of differentiation induced by various other agents. The selective inhibition by SB505124 of phosphorylation of Smad2/3 but not p38 MAPK in OA treated cells was sufficient to prevent OA-induced differentiation. Thus, activation of p38MAPK alone is insufficient for erythroid differentiation and activation of Smad2/3 is also required. This ability of TGF-β signaling through the TβRI receptor to activate both Smad and MAPK pathways ensure their cooperation in differentiation pathways [54,55]. HU and butyrate induce cytodifferentiation and growth inhibition of a variety of tumor cells, and have been used in cytoreductive and differentiation therapy of malignant disease [56-58]. The ability of these chemicals to alter gene expression is mediated in part by changes in signal transduction pathways. Butyrate caused sustained activation of JAK/ STAT signaling in murine erythroleukemia cells [59]; erythro-differentiation of K562 by HU and butyrate involved the phosphorylation of p38 and dephosphorylation of ERK MAPKs [33-37]. In this report, we have shown that the canonical signaling pathway (Smad activation) for the TGF-β family is also involved in the regulation of HU- and butyrate-induced erythroid differentiation of K562 cells. Although, no direct binding has been described between HU or butyrate and TGF-β receptors, results of SB505124 indicate that both chemicals activate the TGF-β type I receptor kinase upstream of Smad2/3. It remains unclear whether these chemicals act directly or indirectly (through autocrine TGF-β) to regulate receptor mediated Smad signaling. Attempts to block ligand induction of differentiation by anti- TGF-β antibody did not prevent HU/butyrate-induced erythroid differentiation (data not shown). Given that these agents induce phosphorylation of Smads so quickly, it is possible that they, like OA, block phosphatase activity which increases the strength of basal endogenous signaling by autocrine TGF-β/activin in K562 cells leading to erythroid differentiation. The biological effects of HU and butyrate on erythro- differentiation, growth inhibition, cell cycle arrest at G1 phase, and stimulation of fetal hemoglobin synthesis share similarity with those of TGF-β [60,61], supporting the idea that these agents may mediate their effects through common signal transduction pathways. Collectively our data suggest that activation of both Smad2/3 and p38 MAPK is required during erythroid differentiation.

For erythro-megakaryocytic differentiation several reports demonstrate that ERK MAPK negatively regulates erythroid differentiation [33-37] and that sustained activation of ERK MAPK is sufficient to induce a differentiation program along the megakaryocytic lineage [41,45-47]. Consistent with these reports, we have shown that ERK1/2 is transiently activated by TGF-β/activin but reduced below basal level during erythroid differentiation. Moreover, inhibitors of ERK1/2 enhanced erythroid differentiation in the absence and the presence of TGF-β/activin stimulation. Similar synergism was reported between ERK inhibitors and HU and butyrate, showing that ERK MAPK negatively regulate this Epo-independent hemoglobin synthesis [34,35]. We found that ERK inhibitors induced Smad2/3 phosphorylation, which was dependent on TRβ1 signaling. Similar results were seen in HL60 and TF-1 cells (data not shown), indicating that crosstalk between the Smad and ERK MAPK pathway is a modulator of cell differentiation. Inhibition of ERK MAPK in mouse embryo fibroblasts potentiates Smad signaling and activation of Smad-dependent gene targets [62]. Also, ERK inhibition increased both the basal and TGF-β-induced Smad7 promoter activity in rat fibroblasts [63]. Based on these findings, inhibition of ERK MAPK augments Smad2/3 signaling, which by itself leads to increase Smad7 transcripts as part of the negative feedback loop of TGF-β/Smad signaling [1-7,41].

Antisense oligonucleotides of JNK1 and JNK2 suppressed Epo induced hemoglobinization in SKT6 cells [33]. We showed an activation of JNK1/2 in K562 cells treated with TGF-β, but use of a specific JNK inhibitor, SP600125, did not influence the formation of Hb^+ cells. Similarly, the JNK1/2/3 inhibitor had no effect on hemoglobinization induced by HU and butyrate. Thus it seems that activation of JNK is dispensable during the development of erythroid cells by HU, butyrate and TGF-β/activin.

In summary, our data provide evidence that both TGF-β Smad and p38 MAPK signaling networks are needed during the Epo-independent erythrodifferentiation of erythroid leukemia cells stimulated with TGF-β, activin, HU, OA and butyrate. We showed that signals through the Smad and the p38 MAPK pathways are independent but integrate in erythroid differentiation while the balance between the interrelated Smad and ERK MAPK signals appear to also play a role in the ultimate differentiation outcome.

Acknowledgment

The authors thank Anita Roberts for many useful discussions in the initiation of these studies and Jonathan Keller for critical reading of the manuscript. This project has been funded whole or in part with federal funds from NCI, NIH, under Contract No. NO1-CO-56000.

References

1. Derynck, R and Miyazono, K (2008) The TGF-β Family Cold Spring Harbor Monograph.
2. Heldin CH, Miyazono K, ten Dijke P (1997) TGF-beta signalling from cell membrane to nucleus through SMAD proteins. Nature 390: 465-471.
3. Derynck R, Zhang YE (2003) Smad-dependent and Smad-independent pathways in TGF-beta family signalling. Nature 425: 577-584.
4. Shi Y, Massagué J (2003) Mechanisms of TGF-beta signaling from cell membrane to the nucleus. Cell 113: 685-700.
5. Afrakhte M, Morén A, Jossan S, Itoh S, Sampath K, et al. (1998) Induction of inhibitory Smad6 and Smad7 mRNA by TGF-beta family members. Biochem Biophys Res Commun 249: 505-511.
6. von Gersdorff G, Susztak K, Rezvani F, Bitzer M, Liang D, et al. (2000) Smad3 and Smad4 mediate transcriptional activation of the human Smad7 promoter by transforming growth factor beta. J Biol Chem 275: 11320-11326.
7. Nagarajan RP, Zhang J, Li W, Chen Y (1999) Regulation of Smad7 promoter by direct association with Smad3 and Smad4. J Biol Chem 274: 33412-33418.
8. Massagué J (2012) TGFÎ² signalling in context. Nat Rev Mol Cell Biol 13: 616-630.
9. Ikushima H, Miyazono K (2012) TGF-Î² signal transduction spreading to a wider field: a broad variety of mechanisms for context-dependent effects of TGF-Î². Cell Tissue Res 347: 37-49.
10. Santibañez JF, Quintanilla M, Bernabeu C (2011) TGF-Î²/TGF-Î² receptor system and its role in physiological and pathological conditions. Clin Sci (Lond) 121: 233-251.
11. Robinson MJ, Cobb MH (1997) Mitogen-activated protein kinase pathways. Curr Opin Cell Biol 9: 180-186.

12. Javelaud D, Mauviel A (2005) Crosstalk mechanisms between the mitogen-activated protein kinase pathways and Smad signaling downstream of TGF-beta: implications for carcinogenesis. Oncogene 24: 5742-5750.

13. Mulder KM (2000) Role of Ras and Mapks in TGFbeta signaling. Cytokine Growth Factor Rev 11: 23-35.

14. Engel ME, McDonnell MA, Law BK, Moses HL (1999) Interdependent SMAD and JNK signaling in transforming growth factor-beta-mediated transcription. J Biol Chem 274: 37413-37420.

15. Shibuya H, Yamaguchi K, Shirakabe K, Tonegawa A, Gotoh Y, et al. (1996) TAB1: an activator of the TAK1 MAPKKK in TGF-beta signal transduction. Science 272: 1179-1182.

16. Hanafusa H, Ninomiya-Tsuji J, Masuyama N, Nishita M, Fujisawa J, et al. (1999) Involvement of the p38 mitogen-activated protein kinase pathway in transforming growth factor-beta-induced gene expression. J Biol Chem 274: 27161-27167.

17. Zhou G, Lee SC, Yao Z, Tan TH (1999) Hematopoietic progenitor kinase 1 is a component of transforming growth factor beta-induced c-Jun N-terminal kinase signaling cascade. J Biol Chem 274: 13133-13138.

18. de Caestecker MP, Piek E, Roberts AB (2000) Role of transforming growth factor-beta signaling in cancer. J Natl Cancer Inst 92: 1388-1402.

19. Cocolakis E, Lemay S, Ali S, Lebrun JJ (2001) The p38 MAPK pathway is required for cell growth inhibition of human breast cancer cells in response to activin. J Biol Chem 276: 18430-18436.

20. Kretzschmar M, Doody J, Timokhina I, Massagué J (1999) A mechanism of repression of TGFbeta/ Smad signaling by oncogenic Ras. Genes Dev 13: 804-816.

21. Wicks SJ, Lui S, Abdel-Wahab N, Mason RM, Chantry A (2000) Inactivation of smad-transforming growth factor beta signaling by Ca(2+)-calmodulin-dependent protein kinase II. Mol Cell Biol 20: 8103-8111.

22. de Caestecker MP, Parks WT, Frank CJ, Castagnino P, Bottaro DP, et al. (1998) Smad2 transduces common signals from receptor serine-threonine and tyrosine kinases. Genes Dev 12: 1587-1592.

23. Wong C, Rougier-Chapman EM, Frederick JP, Datto MB, Liberati NT, et al. (1999) Smad3-Smad4 and AP-1 complexes synergize in transcriptional activation of the c-Jun promoter by transforming growth factor beta. Mol Cell Biol 19: 1821-1830.

24. Zhang Y, Feng XH, Derynck R (1998) Smad3 and Smad4 cooperate with c-Jun/c-Fos to mediate TGF-beta-induced transcription. Nature 394: 909-913.

25. Sano Y, Harada J, Tashiro S, Gotoh-Mandeville R, Maekawa T, et al. (1999) ATF-2 is a common nuclear target of Smad and TAK1 pathways in transforming growth factor-beta signaling. J Biol Chem 274: 8949-8957.

26. Fortunel NO, Hatzfeld A, Hatzfeld JA (2000) Transforming growth factor-beta: pleiotropic role in the regulation of hematopoiesis. Blood 96: 2022-2036.

27. Ruscetti FW, Bartelmez SH (2001) Transforming growth factor beta, pleiotropic regulator of hematopoietic stem cells: potential physiological and clinical relevance. Int J Hematol 74: 18-25.

28. Shav-Tal Y, Zipori D (2002) The role of activin a in regulation of hemopoiesis. Stem Cells 20: 493-500.

29. Shiozaki M, Sakai R, Tabuchi M, Nakamura T, Sugino K, et al. (1992) Evidence for the participation of endogenous activin A/erythroid differentiation factor in the regulation of erythropoiesis. Proc Natl Acad Sci U S A 89: 1553-1556.

30. Chen LL, Dean A, Jenkinson T, Mendelsohn J (1989) Effect of transforming growth factor-beta 1 on proliferation and induction of hemoglobin accumulation in K-562 cells. Blood 74: 2368-2375.

31. Zermati Y, Fichelson S, Valensi F, Freyssinier JM, Rouyer-Fessard P, et al. (2000) Transforming growth factor inhibits erythropoiesis by blocking proliferation and accelerating differentiation of erythroid progenitors. Exp Hematol 28: 885-894.

32. Akel S, Petrow-Sadowski C, Laughlin MJ, Ruscetti FW (2003) Neutralization of autocrine transforming growth factor-1 in human cord blood CD34(+)CD 38(-) lin(-) cells promotes stem cell factor-mediated erythropoietin independent early erythroid progenitor development and reduces terminal differentiation. Stem Cells 21: 557- 567.

33. Nagata Y, Takahashi N, Davis RJ, Todokoro K (1998) Activation of p38 MAP kinase and JNK but not ERK is required for erythropoietin-induced erythroid differentiation. Blood 92: 1859-1869.

34. Park JI, Choi HS, Jeong JS, Han JY, Kim IH (2001) Involvement of p38 kinase in hydroxyurea-induced differentiation of K562 cells. Cell Growth Differ 12: 481-486.

35. Witt O, Sand K, Pekrun A (2000) Butyrate-induced erythroid differentiation of human K562 leukemia cells involves inhibition of ERK and activation of p38 MAP kinase pathways. Blood 95: 2391-2396.

36. Moosavi MA, Yazdanparast R, Lotfi A (2007) ERK1/2 inactivation and p38 MAPK-dependent caspase activation during guanosine 5'-triphosphate-mediated terminal erythroid differentiation of K562 cells. Int J Biochem Cell Biol 39: 1685-1697.

37. Huang HM, Li YC, Chung MH (2010) Activin A induction of erythroid differentiation through MKK6-p38alpha/p38beta pathway is inhibited by follistatin. J Cell Physiol 223: 687-694.

38. McGuckin CP, Forraz N, Liu WM (2003) Diaminofluorene stain detects erythroid differentiation in immature haemopoietic cells treated with EPO, IL-3, SCF, TGFbeta1, MIP-1alpha and IFNgamma. Eur J Haematol 70: 106-114.

39. Koester SK, Roth P, Mikulka WR, Schlossman SF, Zhang C, et al. (1997) Monitoring early cellular responses in apoptosis is aided by the mitochondrial membrane protein-specific monoclonal antibody APO2.7. Cytometry 29: 306-312.

40. Cao Z, Flanders KC, Bertolette D, Lyakh LA, Wurthner JU, et al. (2003) Levels of phospho-Smad2/3 are sensors of the interplay between effects of TGF-beta and retinoic acid on monocytic and granulocytic differentiation of HL-60 cells. Blood 101: 498-507.

41. Akel S, Bertolette D, Petrow-Sadowski C, Ruscetti FW (2007) Levels of Smad7 regulate Smad and mitogen activated kinases (MAPKs) signaling and controls erythroid and megakaryocytic differentiation of erythroleukemia cells. Platelets 18: 566-578.

42. DaCosta Byfield S, Major C, Laping NJ, Roberts AB (2004) SB-505124 is a selective inhibitor of transforming growth factor-beta type I receptors ALK4, ALK5, and ALK7. Mol Pharmacol 65: 744-752.

43. Tallman MS, Andersen JW, Schiffer CA, Appelbaum FR, Feusner JH, et al. (1997) All-trans-retinoic acid in acute promyelocytic leukemia. N Engl J Med 337: 1021-1028.

44. Lazebnik YA, Kaufmann SH, Desnoyers S, Poirier GG, Earnshaw WC (1994) Cleavage of poly(ADP-ribose) polymerase by a proteinase with properties like ICE. Nature 371: 346-347.

45. Racke FK, Lewandowska K, Goueli S, Goldfarb AN (1997) Sustained activation of the extracellular signal-regulated kinase/mitogen-activated protein kinase pathway is required for megakaryocytic differentiation of K562 cells. J Biol Chem 272: 23366-23370.

46. Rouyez MC, Boucheron C, Gisselbrecht S, Dusanter-Fourt I, Porteu F (1997) Control of thrombopoietin-induced megakaryocytic differentiation by the mitogen-activated protein kinase pathway. Mol Cell Biol 17: 4991-5000.

47. Kitamura K, Aota Si, Sakamoto R, Yoshikawa SI, Okazaki K (2000) Smad7 selectively interferes with different pathways of activin signaling and inhibits erythroid leukemia cell differentiation. Blood 95: 3371-3379.

48. Bennett BL, Sasaki DT, Murray BW, O'Leary EC, Sakata ST, et al. (2001) SP600125, an anthrapyrazolone inhibitor of Jun N-terminal kinase. Proc Natl Acad Sci U S A 98: 13681-13686.

49. Murohashi I, Endho K, Nishida S, Yoshida S, Jinnai I, et al. (1995) Differential effects of TGF-beta 1 on normal and leukemic human hematopoietic cell proliferation. Exp Hematol 23: 970-977.

50. Dunn C, Wiltshire C, MacLaren A, Gillespie DA (2002) Molecular mechanism and biological functions of c-Jun N-terminal kinase signalling via the c-Jun transcription factor. Cell Signal 14: 585-593.

51. Dong M, Blobe GC (2006) Role of transforming growth factor-beta in hematologic malignancies. Blood 107: 4589-4596.

52. Kurokawa M, Mitani K, Imai Y, Ogawa S, Yazaki Y, et al. (1998) The t(3;21) fusion product, AML1/Evi-1, interacts with Smad3 and blocks transforming growth factor-beta-mediated growth inhibition of myeloid cells. Blood 92: 4003-4012.

53. Verma A, Deb DK, Sassano A, Uddin S, Varga J, et al. (2002) Activation of the p38 mitogen-activated protein kinase mediates the suppressive effects of type I interferons and transforming growth factor-beta on normal hematopoiesis. J Biol Chem 277: 7726-7735.

54. Yu L, Hébert MC, Zhang YE (2002) TGF-beta receptor-activated p38 MAP kinase mediates Smad-independent TGF-beta responses. EMBO J 21: 3749-3759.

55. Bakin AV, Rinehart C, Tomlinson AK, Arteaga CL (2002) p38 mitogen-activated protein kinase is required for TGFbeta-mediated fibroblastic transdifferentiation and cell migration. J Cell Sci 115: 3193-3206.

56. Tsimberidou AM, Alvarado Y, Giles FJ (2002) Evolving role of ribonucleoside reductase inhibitors in hematologic malignancies. Expert Rev Anticancer Ther 2: 437-448.

57. Zhu WG, Otterson GA (2003) The interaction of histone deacetylase inhibitors and DNA methyltransferase inhibitors in the treatment of human cancer cells. Curr Med Chem Anticancer Agents 3: 187-199.

58. Sowa Y, Sakai T (2000) Butyrate as a model for "gene-regulating chemoprevention and chemotherapy.". Biofactors 12: 283-287.

59. Yamashita T, Wakao H, Miyajima A, Asano S (1998) Differentiation inducers modulate cytokine signaling pathways in a murine erythroleukemia cell line. Cancer Res 58: 556-561.

60. Yang YM, Pace B (2001) Pharmacologic induction of fetal hemoglobin synthesis: cellular and molecular mechanisms. Pediatr Pathol Mol Med 20: 87-106.

61. Bohmer RM, Campbell TA, Bianchi DW (2000) Selectively increased growth of fetal hemoglobin-expressing adult erythroid progenitors after brief treatment of early progenitors with transforming growth factor beta. Blood 95: 2967-2974.

62. Yang YC, Piek E, Zavadil J, Liang D, Xie D, et al. (2003) Hierarchical model of gene regulation by transforming growth factor beta. Proc Natl Acad Sci U S A 100: 10269-10274.

63. Uchida K, Suzuki H, Ohashi T, Nitta K, Yumura W, et al. (2001) Involvement of MAP kinase cascades in Smad7 transcriptional regulation. Biochem Biophys Res Commun 289: 376-381.

High-dose Glucocorticoid for the Treatment of Myeloid Sarcoma

Gonul Hicsonmez*

Faculty of Medicine, Department of pediatric Hematology, Hacettepe University, Ankara 06100, Turkey

Abstract

Myeloid sarcoma is a tumor of myeloblast or poorly differentiated myeloid cells that can occur in extramedullary sites, as isolated tumor, concomitantly with or after the diagnosis of acute myeloblastic leukemia. Despite considerable improvement achieved in the outcome of patients with acute myeloblastic leukemia by using intensive chemotherapy and/or hematopoietic stem cell transplantation, it is generally considered to be poor in patients with myeloid sarcoma. The aim of this review is to indicate the potential therapeutic effects of high-dose glucocorticoid treatment which induce differentiation and apoptosis of myeloid leukemic cells, as a new treatment approach for patients with myeloid sarcoma. We have shown that short-course (3 to7 days) high-dose methylprednisolone treatment that might also induce differentiation and apoptosis of leukemic cells in the extramedullary sites resulted in dramatic decreases in the size of myeloid sarcoma in children with or without marrow infiltration. From the results of our long-term clinical studies, we suggest that to use short- course high-dose glucocorticoids combined with intensive chemotherapy protocol would be a promising treatment strategy for patients with myeloid sarcoma. However, in further studies, the prognostic significance of different localization of myeloid sarcoma and the long term effect of the addition of high-dose glucocorticoid to intensive AML chemotherapy protocols should be explored in larger series.

Keywords: Myeloid sarcoma; High-dose glucocorticoid; Methylprednisolone; Differentiation; Apoptosis; AML

Myeloid sarcoma (MS) also referred as granulocytic sarcoma or myeloblastoma is a rare extramedullary (EM) tumor of myeloblasts or poorly differentiated myeloid cells. It could be the initial presenting clinical feature with or without bone marrow infiltration in patients with acute myeloblastic leukemia (AML) and may occur in patients with myelodysplastic syndrome (MDS) or in accelerated phase of chronic myelocytic leukemia. However, diagnostic and therapeutic approach to patients presented with MS is a challenging issue as recently reviewed in detail [1,2]. Due to the lack of uniform criteria for definition of MS according to the inclusion of involved sites of EM infiltration of leukemic cells, a wide range of MS incidence has been reported both in adults (1.8-9%) [1-4] and in children (7-18%) [5,6]. In our series, among 127 previously untreated children with AML excluding the EM infiltration in gingiva, central nervous system, lymph nodes, skin and pleura, the frequency of MS was found to be 21% and the orbita is the most commonly involved site with the 10% incidence [7].

Although, the prognostic importance is controversial, the outcome of patients presented with MS is generally considered to be poor both in adults and in children [1,4,8-12] especially, in patients who developed MS after hematopoietic stem cell transplantation (HSCT) [13,14]. However, effective treatment strategy is not clear and currently recommended treatment regimen for patients with MS with or without bone marrow involvement is to use intensive AML chemotherapy protocols. Although, the role of radiotherapy on survival is not clear, the results of several studies revealed that addition of radiotherapy to chemotherapy or surgical removal of leukemic mass has no effect on the outcome, but, these may be indicated for the relief of symptomatic complications of tumor mass [1,4,5,10,12]. Some retrospective studies have shown superior outcome in adult patients with MS who underwent allogeneic or autologous HSCT [10,15,16]. Recently, an alternative therapeutic approach by using targeted therapy with thyrosine kinase inhibitor (TKI, imatinib) or anti-CD33 monoclonal antibody (gemtuzumab ozogamicin) has been reported with some beneficial effect in limited number of patients with MS [17,18]. Therefore, patients are still awaiting for development of new treatment strategies.

On the other hand, the use of agents that can induce differentiation and apoptosis of myeloid leukemic cells would be a promising treatment approach for patients with MS. Various *in vitro* studies both in mice and in human myeloid leukemic cells revealed that glucocorticoids (GCs) at high-doses can induce differentiation and/or apoptosis of leukemic cells as reviewed previously [19-21]. We first demonstrated in 1991, morphologic evidence of terminal differentiation of myeloid leukemic cells in a boy with AML-M4 who presented with orbitaocular MS treated with high-dose methylprednisolone (HDMP, 20-30 mg/kg/day, not exceeding 1 g/day) orally in a single dose. In addition to the rapid decrease of blast cells in both peripheral blood and in bone marrow short-period (4 days) after its administration, the decrease in the size of orbital mass was unexpectedly, very striking [22]. In our further studies, dramatic reductions in the size of orbital mass were also detected in non-leukemic [23] and AML children following 24 hours to 4 days after HDMP treatment [7,24]. Interestingly, remarkable decreases in the size of EM infiltration of leukemic cells in other sites (gingiva, oral cavity, spinal, soft tissues and pleura) were also noted short-period after initiation of HDMP as a single agent, in children with AML and MDS, even in patients who had no significant hematologic improvements [7,25]. Dramatic decreases in orbital, abdominal and spinal mass, following 3 to 7 days of HDMP treatment were also reported by others in a child with AML-M2 and t(8;21) and in children who had no marrow infiltration Imaging studies, computerized tomography and magnetic resonance, also disclosed the important reductions in the size of tumor mass [26,27]. Marked

***Corresponding author:** Gonul Hicsonmez, M.D, Retired Professor, Department of pediatric Hematology, Hacettepe University, Erdemkent Sitesi, Ardıc Sok. No.19, UmitkOy, Ankara 06000, Turkey, E-mail: gsonmez@hacettepe.edu.tr decrease of orbital granulocytic sarcoma and improved paraparesis due to epidural thorasic MS, 24 hours after initiation of methylprednisolone (MP, 30 mg/kg) treatment alone was also detected in a case with AML-M2 and t(8;21) translocation by Takeda et al. [28]. Although, the presence of MS is mostly occurred in patients with AML-M2 and t(8;21), it is important to note that HDMP was also effective treatment for MS when occurred in children with different subtypes of AML [7]. Moreover, in adult patient with AML or in patients without marrow infiltration, significant improvements of cutaneous leukemic infiltrations, intestinal or intracranial granulocytic sarcoma were also detected following short-course steroid treatment (without indicating dosage) alone [29-32]. More interestingly, in addition to significant improvement of respiratory disorders, we have demonstrated complete resolution of pleural effusions and marked decrease in pericardial effusion in children with chronic myelomonocytic leukemia 4 days after HDMP treatment alone, that also induced differentiation and apoptosis of malignant cells in the pleural effusion [33]. Matsushima et al. also described a case with MDS in whom pericardial and pleural effusions disappeared following HDMP (20 mg/kg/day) treatment [34]. Very recently, it has been reported that addition of dexamethasone (Dex, 10 mg/6 hours) to chemotherapy decreased early mortality rate, the incidence of respiratory deterioration and the need for ventilatory support of adult patients with AML-M5 who had lung infiltrates of leukemic cells [35].

We have shown that terminal differentiation of leukemic cells is possible in children with different subtypes of AML (AML-M1, M2, M3, M4, M7) treated with short-course (3 to 7 days) HDMP [36-38] which can also induce apoptosis of myeloid leukemic cells with or without differentiation in vivo and in vitro [39,40]. Dramatic selective blast cell reduction associated with apoptosis and improved outcome has been reported by Suzuki et al. [41] in elderly patients (63-89 years) with AML secondary to MDS treated with MP (125 mg/body) alone [41].

The use of agents that induce differentiation and/or apoptosis has also been considered to be a potential therapeutic approach for the cancer patients. Interestingly, several *in vitro* studies have also shown the growth inhibitory effects of GCs (Dex, MP) in some human malignant tumor cell lines in a dose-dependent manner and to induce apoptosis or differentiation of malignant cells [42-46]. From the results of these *in vitro* studies, the authors indicated the possible potential therapeutic effect of high-dose GC treatment for some other types of malignant tumor.

Although, the optimal dosage of MP and its duration is not clear, addition of HDMP to cytotoxic chemotherapy increased the remission rate and prolonged the duration of remission of our patients with AML [7]. Improved outcome was also observed in our small number of AML children with MS who achieved remission with HDMP and chemotherapy and received post induction therapy with high-dose cytarabine [7] and also in children with MDS and MS [25]. However, this improvement was not noted in children who initially had gingival infiltration. Bisschop et al. [6] also reported that children who presented with gingival infiltration had poor prognosis compared to those who presented with MS [6].

The translocation of t(8;21) is associated with AML-M2 phenotype and give rise to AML1-ETO fusion protein which inhibit differentiation of immature progenitors to mature neutrophils. MP has also been shown by Corsello et al. [47] *in vitro* to induce differentiation and apoptosis of AML cell lines with a t(8;21) translocation in a dose-dependent manner. They have also demonstrated that treatment of t(8;21)-positive Kasumi cells and primary patient AML cells with MP revealed dramatic decrease of AML1-ETO protein in a dose and time responsive manner [47]. In addition, it was also shown that MP had synergistic effect with either Ara-c or daunorubicin on the leukemic cell viability. More recently, Joha et al. [48] reported that restoration of GC- induced leucine zipper protein (GILZ) expression which is modulated by GCs, overcome TKI resistance in human and mouse myeloid leukemic cells expressing BCR-ABL by inhibiting mTORC2/AKT signaling pathway [48]. They have demonstrated that, treatment of TKI resistant BCR-ABL+ cells obtained from relapsed chronic myeloid leukemia patients with Dex followed by imatinib resulted in apoptosis dose-dependently. These results may suggest the possible potential effect of GCs at high doses targeting mTORC2 in other subtypes of AML. Dex has also been shown to down regulate the expression of the anti-apoptotic oncogene Bcl-2 in human and in mouse myeloid leukemic cells [47-49] and suppress the expression of c-myc protooncogene during Dex-induced differentiation of mouse myeloid leukemic cells *in vitro* [50]. Furthermore, Xu et al. [51] also demonstrated that Dex may down regulate the expression of FLT3 (FMS-like tyrosine kinase 3) receptor in some myeloid leukemic cells obtained from patients with AML, *in vitro* [51]. The results of these *in vitro* studies indicate that HDMP treatment may also suppress the expression of these apoptosis- and differentiation- inducing genes in some patients with AML. Despite, the factors involved in the exact mechanisms of GC effects at high-doses in inducing differentiation and apoptosis remains unclear, it may be effective through complex mechanisms to target several other antileukemic pathways [52-54].

In conclusion, since early response to treatment is an important prognostic factor, addition of short-course high-dose GCs as a potential targeted therapy to AML intensive chemotherapy protocols, would be a promising treatment approach for patients with MS. However, long-term effects of high-dose GCs on different localization of MS should be explored in larger randomized series.

Acknowledgement

I would like to thank to all my colleagues who made valuable contributions in these studies as seen in the list of cited references of the published papers.

I also like to thank to all doctors, nurses and technical personnel who also made contributions during the long clinical follow-up period of leukemic children.

References

1. Bakst RL, Tallman MS, Douer D, Yahalom J (2011) How I treat extramedullary acute myeloid leukemia. Blood 118: 3785-3793.
2. Avni B, Koren-Michowitz M (2011) Myeloid sarcoma: current approach and therapeutic options. Therap adv in Hematol 2: 309-316.
3. Neiman RS, Barcos M, Berard C, Bonner H, Mann R, et al. (1981) Granulocytic sarcoma: a clinicopathologic study of 61 biopsied cases. Cancer 48: 1426-1437.
4. Lan TY, Lin DT, Tien HF, Yang RS, Chen CY, et al. (2009) Prognostic factors of treatment outcomes in patients with granulocytic sarcoma. Acta Hematol 122: 238-246.
5. Jenkin RD, Al-Shabanah M, Al Nasser A, El-Solh H, Al sudairy R, et al. (2000) Extramedullary myeloid tumors in children: the limited value of local treatment. J Pediatr Hematol Oncol 22: 34-40.
6. Bisschop MM, Revesz T, Bierings M, van Verden JF, van Wering ER, et al. (2001) Extramedullary infiltrates at diagnosis have no prognostic significance in children with acute myeloid leukaemia. Leukemia 15: 46-49.
7. Hicsonmez G, Cetin M, Tuncer AM, Yenicesu I, Aslan D, et al. (2004) Children with acute myeloblastic leukemia presenting with extramedullary infiltration: the effects of high-dose steroid treatment. Leuk Res 28: 25-34.
8. Byrd JC, Weiss RB, Arthur DC, Lawrence D, Baer MR, et al. (1997)

Extramedullary leukemia adversely affects hematologic complete remission rate and overall survival in patients with t(8;21)(q22;q22): results from Cancer and Leukemia Group B 8461. J Clin Oncol 15: 466-475.

9. Paydas S, Zorludemir S, Ergin M (2006) Granulocytic sarcoma: 32 cases and review of the literature. Leuk Lyphoma 47: 2527-2541.

10. Avni B, Rund D, Levin M, Grisariu S, Ben-Yehuda D, et al. (2012) Clinical implications of acute myeloid leukemia presenting as myeloid sarcoma. Hematol Oncol 30: 34-40.

11. Cavdar AO, Babacan E ,Gozdasoglu S, Kilicturgay K, Arcasoy A, et al. (1989) High risk subgroup of acute myelomonocytic leukemia (AMML) with orbita-ocular granulocytic sarcoma (OOGS) in Turkish children. Retrospective analysis of clinical, hematological, ultrastructural and therapeutical findings of thirty-three OOGS. Acta Haematol 81: 80-85.

12. Dusenbery KE, Howells WB, Arthur DC, Alonzo T, Lee JW, et al. (2003) Extramedullary leukemia in children with newly diagnosed acute myeloid leukemia: a report from the Children's cancer group. J Pediatr Hematol Oncol 25: 760-768.

13. Harris AC, Kitko CL, Couriel DR, Braun TM, Choi SW, et al. (2013) Extramedullary relapse of acute myeloid leukemia following allogeneic hematopoietic stem cell transplantation: incidence, risk factors and outcomes. Hematologica 98:179-184.

14. Lee KH, Lee JH, Choi SJ, Lee JH, Kim S, et al. (2003) Bone marrow vs extramedullary relapse of acute leukemia after allogeneic hematopoietic cell transplantation: risk factors and clinical course. Bone Marrow Transplant 32: 835-842.

15. Pileri SA, Ascani S, Cox M, Campidelli C, Bacci F, et al. (2007) Myeloid sarcoma: Clinico-pathologic, phenotypic and cytogenetic analysis of 92 adult patients. Leukemia 21: 340-350.

16. Chevallier P, Mohty M, Lioure B, Michel G, Contentin N, et al. (2008) Allogeneic hematopoietic stem-cell transplantation for myeloid sarcoma: a retrospective study from the SFGM-TC. J Clin Oncol 26: 4940-4943.

17. Vedy D, Muehlematter D, Rausch T, Stalder M, Jotterand M, et al. (2010) Acute myeloid leukemia with myeloid sarcoma and eosinophilia: prolonged remission and molecular response to imatinib. J Clin Oncol 28: 33-35.

18. Piccaluga PP, Martinelli G, Rondoni M, Malagola M, Gaitani S, et al. (2004) Gemtuzumab ozogamicin for relapsed and refractory acute myeloid leukemia and myeloid sarcoma. Leuk Lymphoma 45:1791-1795.

19. Hicsonmez G, Ozsoylu S, Tuncer AM (1991) Differentiation of myeloid leukemic cells induced by high-dose methylprednisolone in patients with acute myeloblastic leukemia and its therapeutic potential. Leuk Res 15: 537-541.

20. Hicsonmez G (2006) The effect of steroid on myeloid leukemic cells: The potential of short-course high-dose methylprednisolone treatment in inducing differentiation, apoptosis and in stimulating myelopoiesis. Leuk Res 30: 60-68.

21. Hicsonmez G (2010) A novel approach to treatment in childhood acute myeloblastic leukemia and myelodysplastic syndrome with high-dose methylprednisolone as a differentiation- and apoptois-inducing agent of myeloid leukemic cells. Turk J Hematol 27: 1-7.

22. Hicsonmez G, Ozsoylu S, Tuncer AM, Erturk G, Ozbek N, et al. (1991) Direct morphological evidence of high-dose methylprednisolone-induced maturation of leukemic cells in children with acute nonlymphoblastic leukemia. Exp Hematol 19: 232-233.

23. Hicsonmez G, Ozbek N, Kale G, Erdem G, Bilgic S, et al. (1996) Dramatic effect of high-dose methylprednisolone on orbital granulocytic sarcoma. Pediatr Hematol Oncol 13: 187-190.

24. Hicsonmez G, Cetin M, Aslan D, Ozyurek E (2003) The role of short course of high-dose methylprednisolone in children with acute myeloblastic leukemia (FAB M2) presented with myeloid tumor. Pediatr Hematol Oncol 20: 373-379.

25. Hicsonmez G, Cetin M, Yenicesu I, Olcay L, Koc A, et al. (2001) Evaluation of Children with myelodysplastic syndrome: Importance of extramedullary disease as a presenting symptom. Leuk Lymphoma 42: 665-674.

26. Ozyurek E, Alioglu B, Coskun M, Ozbek N (2006) Successful use of short-course high-dose methylprednisolone in a child with acute myeloblastic leukemia (FAB M2) and myeloid tumor. Leuk Lymphoma 47: 923-925.

27. Isik P, Tavil B, Tunc B, Yarali N, Demir A, et al. (2011) Extramedullary orbital granulocytic sarcoma without bone marrow involvement: A report of two cases. Pediatr Hematol Oncol 28: 65-70.

28. Takeda M, Yamaguchi S, Eguchi K, Kajiume T, Nishimura S, et al. (2009) Spinal epidural granulocytic sarcoma in a child precedent to clinical manifestation of acute myeloid lymphoma: case report. Neurol Med Chir (Tokyo) 49: 221-224.

29. Benucci R, Annessi G, Signoretti S, Simoni R (1996) Minimally differentiated acute myeloid leukaemia revealed by specific cutaneous lesions. Br J Dermatol 135: 119-123.

30. Zhou L, Landa C, Zaiden R (2012) An unusual case of disseminated lymphadenopathy. Clin Adv Hematol Oncol 10: 64-66.

31. Kwan LY, Targan SR, Shih DQ (2011) A case of steroid-dependent myeloid granulocytic sarcoma masquerading as Crohn's disease. World J Gastroenterol 17: 2446-2449.

32. Nikolic B, Feigenbaum F, Abbara S, Martuza RL, Schellinger D (2003) CT changes of an intracranial granulocytic sarcoma on short-term follow-up. AJR Am J Roentgenol 180: 78-80.

33. Hiçsönmez G, Cetin M, Tunç B, Tuncer AM, Gümrük F, et al. (1998) Dramatic resolution of pleural effusion in children with chronic myelomonocytic leukemia following short-course high-dose methylprednisolone. Leuk Lymphoma 29: 617-623.

34. Matsushima T, Murakami H, Kim K, Uchiumi H, Murata N, et al. (1995) Steroid-responsive pulmonary disorders associated with myelodysplastic syndromes with der(1q;7p) chromosomal abnormality. Am J Hematol 50: 110-115.

35. Azoulay É, Canet E, Raffoux E, Lengliné E, Lemiale V, et al. (2012) Dexamethasone in patients with acute lung injury from acute monocytic leukaemia. Eur Respir J 39: 648-653.

36. Hicsönmez G, Tuncer AM, Guler E, Tan E, Tekelioglu M (1993) The potential role of high-dose methylprednisolone on the maturation of leukemic cells in children with acute promyelocytic leukemia (APL). Exp Hematol 21: 599-601.

37. Hiçsönmez G, Tuncer M, Toksoy HB, Yenicesu I, Cetin M (1999) Differentiation of leukemic cells induced by short-course high-dose methylprednisolone in children with different subtypes of acute myeloblastic leukemia. Leuk Lymphoma 33: 573-580.

38. Hiçsönmez G, Cetin M, Okur H, Erdemli E, Gürgey A (2003) The potential effect of short-course high-dose steroid on the maturation and apoptosis of leukemic cells in a child with acute megakaryoblastic leukemia. Leuk Lymphoma 44: 1037-1042.

39. Hiçsönmez G, Erdemli E, Tekelioglu M, Tuncer AM, Ozbek N, et al. (1996) Morphologic evidence of apoptosis in childhood acute myeloblastic leukemia treated with high-dose methylprednisolone. Leuk Lymphoma 22: 91-96.

40. Ozbek N, Erdemli E, Hicsonmez G, Okur H, Tekelioglu M (1999) Effects of methylprednisolone on human myeloid leukemic cells in vitro. Am J Hematol 60: 255-259.

41. Suzuki K, Ohishi K, Sekine T, Masuya M, Katayama N (2007) Selective blast cell reduction in elderly patients with acute myeloid leukemia secondary to myelodysplastic syndrome treated with methylprednisolone. Int J Hematol 85: 344-349.

42. Dobos J, Kenessey I, Tímár J, Ladányi A (2011) Glucocorticoid receptor expression and antiproliferative effect of dexamethasone on human melanoma cells. Pathol Oncol Res 17: 729-734.

43. Tan YJ, Teng E, Ting AE (2003) A small inhibitor of the interaction between Bax and Bcl-X(L) can synergize with methylprednisolone to induce apoptosis in Bcl-X(L)-overexpressing breast-cancer cells. J Cancer Res Clin Oncol 129: 437-448.

44. McLean JS, Frame MC, Freshney RI, Vaughan PF, Mackie AE, et al. (1986) Phenotypic modification of human glioma and non-small cell lung carcinoma by glucocorticoids and other agents. Anticancer Res 6: 1101-1106.

45. Xu MJ, Fang GE, Liu YJ, Song LN (2002) Effects of glucocorticoid on proliferation, differentiation, and glucocorticoid receptor expression in human ovarian carcinoma cell line 3AO. Acta Pharmacol Sin 23: 819-823.

46. Kawashima H, Ogose A, Hayami T, Yamagiwa H, Hatano H, et al. (2003) Effect of dexamethasone on growth inhibition and chondrogenic maturation of human chondrosarcoma. J Orthop Sci 8: 341-345.

47. Corsello SM, Roti G, Ross KN, Chow KT, Galinsky I, et al. (2009) Identification of AML1-ETO modulators by chemical genomics. Blood 113: 6193-6205.

48. Joha S, Nugues AL, Hétuin D, Berthon C, Dezitter X, et al. (2012) GILZ inhibits the mTORC2/AKT pathway in BCR-ABL(+) cells. Oncogene 31: 1419-1430.

49. Lotem J, Sachs L (1994) Control of sensitivity to induction of apoptosis in myeloid leukemic cells by differentiation and bcl-2 dependent and independent pathways. Cell Growth Differ 5: 321-327.

50. Kasukabe T, Okabe-Kado J, Hozumi M, Honma Y (1994) Inhibition by interleukin 4 of leukemia inhibitory factor-, interleukin 6-, and dexamethasone-induced differentiation of mouse myeloid leukemia cells: role of c-myc and junB proto-oncogenes. Cancer Res 54: 592-597.

51. Xu ZX, Xu Y, Zhu JK, Li CX, Li Y, et al. (2001) Effects of dexamethasone on Flt3 receptor expression and proliferation induced by recombinant human Flt3 ligand in malignant hematopoietic cells. Acta Pharmacol Sin 22: 534-540.

52. Reikvam H, Olsnes AM, Gjertsen BT, Ersvaer E, Bruserud O (2009) Nuclear factor-kappaB signaling: a contributor in leukemogenesis and a target for pharmacological intervention in human acute myelogenous leukemia. Crit Rev Oncog 15: 1-41.

53. Yuksel S, Saydam G, Uslu R, Sanli UA, Terzioglu E, et al. (2002) Arsenic trioxide and methylprednisolone use different signal transduction pathways in leukemic differentiation. Leuk Res 26: 391-398.

54. Kaymaz BT, Selvi N, Saydam G, Sahin F, Kosova B (2012) Methylprednisolone induces apoptosis by interacting with the JAK/STAT pathway in HL-60 and K-562 leukemic cells. Hematology 17: 93-99.

Economic Evaluations of Hematological Malignancies Compared with Solid Tumors

Nicolas Batty[1], Joseph Shatzel[2], Samuel Wiles[2], Mathew Kabalan[2], Rohit Sharma[3], Jonathan Pang[2], David Yi[2], Iris Alatovic[2*], Sana Saif[2], Deepika Narasimha[4], Joseph LaPenna[3], Anthony Troitino[2], Kristopher Attwood[3], Michael Weinstein[2], Eric Murawski[2], Mathew Valerio[2], Yong Yin[2] and Meir Wetzler[1]

[1]Department of Medicine, Roswell Park Cancer Institute, Buffalo, NY, USA
[2]State University of New York at Buffalo, Buffalo, NY, USA
[3]Erie County Medical Center, Buffalo, NY,USA

Abstract

Introduction: Cancer care costs escalated with the introduction of novel therapies. Therefore, cancer–related Cost Utility Analyses (CUAs) are used to guide policy makers. Since numerous methods (criteria) exist to evaluate CUAs, we compared these criteria between CUAs of solid tumors and those of hematological malignancies.

Methods: A systemic MEDLINE search of English-language publications between 2001 and 2012 was performed. Strict inclusion criteria were limited to CUAs examining one single intervention and one single study comparator. Standard data of 66 variables, based on the Drummond criteria, were collected to review each CUA for clarity, completeness, and health economic methodological quality.

Results: Among 8,515 screened papers on Pubmed, 177 cancer-related CUAs (2%) were eligible. Solid tumors and hematological malignancies CUAs constituted 161(91%) and 16(9%). Among the standardized methods for evaluating CUAs, those of solid tumors reported more frequently the presentation of cost-effectiveness acceptability curve (p=0.02) and the use of threshold value to interpret study results (p=0.024) than those of hematological malignancies. Further, CUAs of solid tumors were more frequently multicenter-based (p=0.014); however, CUAs of hematological malignancies listed differential quality adjusted life year separately more frequently (p=0.02). Outcomes of CUAs of solid tumors were more frequently reported as significant (p=0.014).

Conclusions: CUAs of solid tumors abided more frequently with the standardized methods (criteria) than those of hematological malignancies, which may be due in part to their multiple study sites. CUAs of hematological malignancies may warrant more methodological standardization and incorporate more study sites.

Keywords: Cost effectiveness analysis; Cost utility analyses; Solid tumors; Hematological malignancies

Abbreviations: CEA: Cost Effectiveness Analysis; CUAs: Cost Utility Analyses; ICER: Incremental Cost Effectiveness Ratio; QALY: Quality-Adjusted Life Year

Introduction

The cost of cancer care has increased tremendously in the United States and worldwide [1]. Methods to evaluate the cost of cancer care in relation to the benefit it produces are called Cost Utility Analyses (CUAs). Many variables contribute to CUAs. For this purpose, cost-effectiveness acceptability curves were used to produce confidence intervals around Incremental Cost-Effectiveness Ratios (ICERs) [2,3]. Drummond and Jefferson [4] generated a list of 35 questions to evaluate the quality of CUAs and are now used to assess systematic reviews. These criteria allow differentiation between "good" CUAs and others. On the other hand, solid tumors are common but the effect of some of the treatments on longevity is sometimes measured in months from diagnosis while hematological malignancies are rare but are associated with the potential to result in significant prolongation of life expectancy [5]. Therefore, we aimed to compare CUAs of these two groups. Moreover, considering the society perspective, the economic burden varies considerably by each type of cancer [6,7]. Hence, an increased need was recently raised to examine cost by conducting CUAs [8-14]. The purpose of our paper is to compare methodologies used to study economic evaluations using two groups: solid tumors and hematological malignancies.

Methods

A systemic MEDLINE search by the keywords: CUAs and cancer of English-language manuscripts published between 2001 and 2012 was performed. Eligibility criteria consisted of including only CUAs that examined one single intervention and one single study comparator. For example, adding rituximab to fludarabine and cyclophosphamide for the treatment of previously untreated chronic lymphocytic leukemia [15]. Exclusion criteria included CUAs that examined more than one intervention, more than one comparator or more than one study population or type of malignancy. The study population was not limited by age; therefore, CUAs examining children, adult or geriatric populations were included. Research keywords included the following words: CUAs, cost-effectiveness analysis, malignancy, leukemia, lymphoma, myeloma, tumor, genitourinary, bladder, penile, renal, prostate, gastrointestinal, stomach, esophagus, colon, duodenum,

***Corresponding author:** Meir Wetzler, Professor of Medicine, Chief, Leukemia Section, Roswell Park Cancer Institute, Elm and Carlton Streets, Buffalo, NY 14263, USA, E-mail: meir.wetzler@roswellpark.org small intestine, cecum, appendix, neuroendocrine, liver, pancreas, brain, head and neck, lung, mesothelioma, thymus, sarcoma and cancer. The number of patients was broken down by hematological malignancies or solid tumors and not by each type of cancer, as this was not the scope of our paper. Table 1 represents the workflow of the systematic approach examining all variables in each CUA. Selected CUAs incorporated studies patients of all ages and ethnic groups from the USA, Europe and developing countries. Based on the Drummond criteria [2], we examined the clarity, completeness, and health economic methodological quality of each CUA by collecting 66 variables [4]. Among the variables represented in our workflow, we examined whether CUAs performed univariate and multivariate sensitivity analyses, including the time horizon, the costs of each drug, and the transition probabilities. Additionally, we examined whether a Tornado graph (a graph to calculate the most favorable ICER by varying each parameter of interest) and a cost-effectiveness acceptability curve were used.

Pubmed ID	
Journal	
Date publication	
CUA type	
Intervention type	
Prevention Stage	
Study Theme	Disease name: cancer type
Focus study name	
Comparator name	
Funding source	
Clear Presentation of the Relevant Intervention	
Clear Presentation of the Comparator	
Clear Presentation of the Target Population	
Time Horizon	Incremental Analysis
Methods name	
Total number of patients in the study	
Number patients on focus study	
Number patients on comparator study	
Currency name of cost study	
Total/ lifetime cost of focus study	
Confidence Interval (CI) focus study cost lower value	
Confidence Interval (CI) focus study cost upper value	
Total/ lifetime cost of alternative study	
Confidence Interval (CI) comparator cost lower value	
Comparator lifetime cost	
Confidence Interval (CI) comparator cost upper value	
Incremental Cost per year of life gained- alternative	
Confidence Interval (CI) /SE of comparator intervention (lower value)	
Confidence Interval (CI) /SE of comparator intervention (upper value)	
Incremental Cost per year of life gained- focus	
Confidence Interval (CI) / Standard Error (SE) of Incremental Cost Ratio Lower Value-focus	
Confidence Interval (CI) /SE of Incremental Cost Ratio Upper Value-focus	
Confidence Interval (CI) /SE of Incremental Cost Ratio Lower Value-alternative	
Confidence Interval (CI) /SE of Incremental Cost Ratio Upper Value-alternative	
Quality-adjusted life year (QALY) unit for focus	
Quality-adjusted life year (QALY) CI for focus lower value	
Quality-adjusted life year (QALY) CI for focus upper value	
Remaining QALY for alternative	
CI for remaining QALY in alternative lower value	
CI for remaining QALY in alternative upper value	
Remaining QALY for treated	
Calculated Cost utolity analysis (CUA)	
CI/SE of CEA lower value	
CI/SE of CEA upper value	
Drug Administration Method	
Drug Combinations	
Type of therapy	
Study Institution number	
Pharmaceutical company number	
Study Site	
Cancer Type	
Outcome	
Perspective	
Continent of study	
Discounting	
ICER (incremental cost effectiveness ratio)	
Sensitivity Analysis	
Tornado Graph included	
High/Low limits Provided	
Presentation of cost-effectiveness acceptability curve	
Clinical trial based economic analysis	
Use of Threshold Value to interpret study results	

Table 1: A workflow of the systematic approach detailed examining all variables in each cost utility analysis.

Statistical Analysis

The data were reported as means, standard deviations, medians and inter-quartile ranges for continuous variables, and as frequencies and relative frequencies for categorical variables. Corresponding 95% confidence intervals were constructed when appropriate. The study variables were compared between the two groups (using the Chi Square test for categorical variables and either the ANOVA (Analysis of Variance) or Kruskal Wallis test for continuous variables. Statistical software SAS version 9.1.3 (SAS Institute, Inc., Cary, NC) was used for this analysis. The difference between the two groups was considered statistically significant if the p value was less than 0.05.

Results

After screening 8,515 published manuscripts on Pubmed, we identified 177 cancer-related CUAs (2%) that met our criteria. Consistent with the higher frequency of solid tumors compared with lymphoma, leukemia and myeloma [5], CUAs pertaining to solid tumors represented 91% of those studies. We compared the collected variables between solid tumors and hematological malignancies (Tables 2a and 2b). Our data reveal that CUAs of solid tumors reported more frequently the presentation of cost-effectiveness acceptability curve (p=0.02) and the use of threshold value to interpret study results (p=0.024) than their counterparts. In regards to the Quality-Adjusted Life Year (QALY) and the utility (numeric figure assigned for each particular health state) for that state over all the health states we found that CUAs of solid tumors were more frequently multicenter-based (p=0.014) and were more frequently reported as significant (p=0.014). On the other hand, CUAs of hematological malignancies listed more frequently differential QALYs separately (p=0.02).

Discussion

The cost of a drug is measured in monetary units while benefit is measured in health gain such as survival. However, quality of life is added to this formula. For example, if intervention A results in five

Characteristic	Hematological Malignancies	Solid Tumors	p-value of X^2 test
Number of CUA	16	161	
The relevant intervention, %	93.75	90.68	0.6833
The comparator, %	100.0	87.58	0.1344
The target population, %	100.0	99.38	0.7519
Time horizon, %			
Lifetime	37.5	41.61	0.7498
Other	62.5	53.42	0.4867
Not stated	0.0	4.97	0.3615
Time horizon stated, %	100.0	95.03	0.3615
Study perspective, %			
Societal	25.0	27.85	0.8081
Health-care payer	75.0	72.15	0.8081
Discounting, %			
Costs only	18.75	12.34	0.4670
QALYs only	0	0.65	0.7465
Both costs and QALYs	50.0	54.55	0.7284
Not needed	6.25	19.48	0.1921
Any discounting, %	68.75	70.13	0.9087
Clinical trial based economic analysis, %	56.25	71.88	0.1915
Sensitivity analysis, %			
Univariate or multivariate	50.0	44.10	0.6507
Probabilistic	37.5	44.10	0.6116
Other/Unknown	6.25	7.45	0.8603
Not performed	6.25	4.35	0.7269
Any sensitivity analysis, %	93.75	95.65	0.7269
Presentation of cost-effectiveness acceptability curve, %	18.75	49.07	**0.0204**
Use of threshold value to interpret study results, %	56.25	80.50	**0.0249**

Table 2a: Characteristics of CUAs of hematological malignancies and solid tumors.

additional years of survival compared to no intervention with a quality of life of 0.5, than the intervention results in 5×0.5=2.5 QALYs. If, on the other hand, intervention B results in seven additional years of life compared to no additional intervention but at a quality of life of 0.25, then it confers 7×0.25=1.75 QALYs. Therefore, the additional benefit of intervention A over intervention B is 0.75 QALYs even though intervention B results in longer survival.

Another way to compare the two treatments is to calculate the ICER. For that we will need to add the monetary effect of each treatment. For example, intervention A would cost $10,000 per year while intervention B would cost $5,000 per year. In the above example, ICER equals 10,000-5,000/2.5-1.75=$6,666.67 per QUALY for intervention A compared with intervention B.

Calculation of costs is complicated; for example, one can calculate only the price of a drug. However, the societal effect of an intervention has to be taken into consideration as well. If we look at intervention A that requires the patient to return to the hospital three times per week compared to intervention B that requires the patient to return to the hospital only every two weeks, the effect of the each interventions can be significantly different, especially if both interventions require that the patient be escorted. The effect of the intervention on the companion in regards to loss of working days has to be taken into account when one considers cost. Another important factor is the time horizon, that is, how long the intervention is used. In the examples above, if intervention A is used for one year while intervention B is to be administered for the lifetime of the patient, it is clear that a difference in time horizon exists between the two matological malignancies are rare and represent a distinct group of cancer. In recent years, there have been a significant number of compounds approved for the treatment of these rare tumors. Those drugs impose a substantial financial burden in regards to the US and worldwide taxpayers [15,16]. Therefore, CUAs of novel therapies either in solid tumors or hematological malignancies are particularly important to delineate their additional cost and benefit. Hence, it is imperative to evaluate whether these CUAs are strictly conducted without any contamination of a financial bias. Moreover, it is essential that these studies follow rigorous scientific rules. Therefore, we for the most part, explored if any differences existed between CUAs of solid tumors and hematological malignancies. Based on the collected variables (defined in Table 1, 2a and 2b), we found that CUAs of solid tumors abided more frequently with the standardized methods (criteria) than those of hematological malignancies. This may have been due in part to the fact that these studies were conducted in multiple sites. On the other hand, CUAs of hematological malignancies may warrant more standardization of their methodologies and incorporating more study sites. While we are quite concerned how experts would evaluate methodologies of conducting CUAs, we noted an improvement in the percentage of studies that appropriately report a calculated ICER [16] because reporting a calculated ICER is an established criterion that the CUA has been appropriately conducted. Moreover, a probabilistic sensitivity analysis has been more frequently reported in recent CUAs, again denoting an improvement in the quality of these studies. Nonetheless, while reviewing the literature we found that many of these studies still did not report time horizon. Other important deficiencies involved the quality of reporting the discount costs (the discount rate is the rate that needs to be discounted at future date and to estimate accurately the net present value of cost and benefits) or the QALYs. Another major concern was the publication bias that tackles publishing CUAs in peer-reviewed journals that are experienced in reporting such studies to the public domain [17]. As faculty in academic malignant hematology, we are concerned about the quality of CUAs in this field. After reviewing carefully the literature, we believe that applying standardized methods [2] for evaluating CUAs methodologies is essential. There are numerous ways to assess these methodologies; however, we think that the Drummond criteria may be quite sufficient to lead to an accurate reporting of CUAs [4].

Characteristic	Hematological Malignancies	Solid Tumors	p-value of X^2test
Number of CEA	16	161	
Funding source, %			
Industry/Non-Industry vs. Non-Industry	72.73	52.76	0.2021
Study Institution Number, %			
Single site	73.33	40.65	**0.0148**
More than one site	26.67	59.35	**0.0148**
Currency name, %			
USD	81.25	56.85	0.0593
Industry/ Industry &Non-Industry	62.50	44.93	0.3457
Euro	18.75	43.15	0.0593
Industry/ Industry &Non-Industry	100.0	60.87	0.1731
Outcome statistically significant, %	66.67	91.80	0.0149
ICER listed, %			
Base QALY listed	41.67	41.77	0.9943
Cost listed separately	16.67	42.41	0.0800
Differential QALY listed separately	41.67	15.82	0.0236
Tornado Graph included, %	25.00	31.06	0.6158

Table 2b: Characteristics of CUAs of hematological malignancies and solid tumors.

At the end of our discussion, it is important to state that these deficiencies of CUAs were disconcerting, as they have equally been noted in solid tumors as well as hematological malignancies [4]. Additionally, we still think that more robust criteria must be carried to conduct these CUAs especially when considering newer therapies. In this area, we have noticed an obvious pressure from pharmaceutical industry to deviate the outcome in favor of their products.

Conclusion

CUAs of hematological malignancies when compared with those of solid tumors abided less frequently with the standardized methods (criteria) as well as they were conducted in fewer study sites. Therefore, economic evaluations of hematological malignancies may warrant applying strict criteria and incorporating more study centers. However, more validation in future prospective studies is needed.

Acknowledgement

Supported partially by grants from the National Cancer Institute Grant CA16056 (NB, MW), the Szefel Foundation, Roswell Park Cancer Institute (MW), the Leonard S. LuVullo Endowment for Leukemia Research (MW), the Nancy C. Cully Endowment for Leukemia Research (MW), the Babcock Family Endowment (MW) and the Heidi Leukemia Research Fund, Buffalo, NY (MW).

References

1. Tangka FK, Trogdon JG, Richardson LC, Howard D, Sabatino SA, et al. (2010) Cancer treatment cost in the United States: has the burden shifted over time? Cancer 116: 3477-3484.
2. vanHout BA, Al MJ, Gordon GS, Rutten FF (1994) Costs, effects and C/E-ratios alongside a clinical trial. Health Econ 3: 309-319.
3. Briggs A, Fenn P (1998) Confidence intervals or surfaces? Uncertainty on the cost-effectiveness plane. Health Econ 7: 723-740.
4. Drummond MF, Sculpher MJ, Torrance GW, O'Brien BJ, Stoddart GL(2005) Methods for the economic evaluation of health care programmes. (3rdedn),Oxford: Oxford University Press,UK.
5. Siegel R, Naishadham D, Jemal A (2013) Cancer statistics, 2013. CA Cancer J Clin 63: 11-30.
6. Kasteng F, Sobocki P, Svedman C, Lundkvist J (2007) Economic evaluations of leukemia: a review of the literature. Int J Technol Assess Health Care 23: 43-53.
7. Kasteng F, Sobocki P, Svedman C, Lundkvist J (2007) Economic evaluations of leukemia: a review of the literature. Int J Technol Assess Health Care 23: 43-53.
8. Raftery J (2009) NICE and the challenge of cancer drugs. BMJ 338: b67.
9. Mason AR, Drummond MF (2009) Public funding of new cancer drugs: Is NICE getting nastier? Eur J Cancer 45: 1188-1192.
10. Rocchi A, Menon D, Verma S, Miller E (2008) The role of economic evidence in Canadian oncology reimbursement decision-making: to lambda and beyond. Value Health 11: 771-783.
11. Dalziel K, Segal L, Mortimer D (2008) Review of Australian health economic evaluation - 245 interventions: what can we say about cost effectiveness? Cost Eff Resour Alloc 6: 9.
12. Tengs TO (2004) Cost-effectiveness versus cost-utility analysis of interventions for cancer: does adjusting for health-related quality of life really matter? Value Health 7: 70-78.
13. Steinbrook R (2008) Saying no isn't NICE - the travails of Britain's National Institute for Health and Clinical Excellence. N Engl J Med 359: 1977-1981.
14. Van Lare JM, Conway PH, Sox HC (2010) Five next steps for a new national program for comparative-effectiveness research. N Engl J Med 362: 970-973.
15. Experts in Chronic Myeloid Leukemia (2013) The price of drugs for chronic myeloid leukemia (CML) is a reflection of the unsustainable prices of cancer drugs: from the perspective of a large group of CML experts. Blood 121: 4439-4442.
16. Hornberger J, Reyes C, Shewade A, Lerner S, Friedmann M, et al. (2012) Cost-effectiveness of adding rituximab to fludarabine and cyclophosphamide for the treatment of previously untreated chronic lymphocytic leukemia. Leuk Lymphoma 53: 225-234.
17. Greenberg D, Earle C, Fang CH, Eldar-Lissai A, Neumann PJ (2010) When is cancer care cost-effective? A systematic overview of cost-utility analyses in oncology. J Natl Cancer Inst 102: 82-88.

Comparative Study of Deferiprone and Silymarin versus Deferiprone and Placebo as Iron Chelators in Children with Beta Thalassemia with Iron Overload

Adel A Hagag[1]*, Mohamed S Elfrargy[1], Mokhtar Abd Elfatah[1] and Aml Ezzat Abd El-Lateef[2]

[1]*Department of Pediatrics and Clinical Pathology, Tanta University, Egypt*
[2]*Department of Medicine, Tanta University, Egypt*

Abstract

Background: Beta thalassemia is an inherited hemoglobin disorder resulting in chronic hemolytic anemia requiring life-long blood transfusion that cause iron overload. Silymarin plays a role as an iron chelator in iron overloaded patients.

The aim of this work was to compare the iron chelating efficacy of combination therapy of oral Deferiprone and silymarin with oral Deferiprone and placebo.

Patients and methods: This study was conducted on 40 children with beta thalassemia major under follow up at Hematology Unit, Pediatric Department, Tanta University Hospital in the period between October 2012 and October 2013 with their serum ferritin levels more than 1000 ng/ml and they was divided in two groups. Group I: Received oral Deferiprone and silymarin for 6 months. Group II: Received oral Deferiprone and placebo for 6 months.

Results: In the current study, there were no significant differences in the initial serum ferritin, serum iron and TIBC levels between group I and group II but after regular chelation therapy, serum ferritin and serum iron were significantly lower and TIBC was significantly higher in group I than group II. No statistically significant difference in serum creatinine, blood urea, ALT, AST and serum bilirubin levels between Group I and Group II before and after chelation therapy.

Conclusion: From this study we concluded that, Deferiprone in combination with silymarin are better iron chelators in iron-loaded thalassemic patients than Deferiprone and placebo.

Keywords: Thalassemia; Silymarin; Deferiprone; Iron overload

Introduction

Thalassemias are a heterogeneous group of inherited anemias that collectively represents the most common monogenic disorders [1]. β- thalassemias are characterized by absent or reduced synthesis of β- globin chains of hemoglobin, caused by mutations of β-globin gene cluster [2] resulting in reduced hemoglobin in Red Blood Cells (RBCs), decreased RBCs production and anemia [3]. In Egypt, β-thalassemia is the commonest cause of chronic hemolytic anemia (85%) and it represents a major public health problem. It is particularly common in populations of Upper Egypt and peoples of Delta and Red Sea Hill Region [4,5].

The most common treatment for thalassemia is blood transfusion which is necessary to provide the patients with healthy red blood cells containing normal hemoglobin. Repeated blood transfusion leads to iron overload [6].

The iron loading in thalassemia depends on the volume of blood transfused and the amount accumulated from gut absorption [7]. In β-thalassemia increased gastrointestinal iron absorption is mediated by down-regulation of hepcidin and up-regulation of ferroportin. Hepcidin regulates iron transport across the gut mucosa, thereby preventing excess iron absorption and maintaining normal iron levels within the body. Ferroportin is a transmembrane protein that transports iron from the inside of a cell to the outside it [8]. As each unit of packed cells contains approximately 200 mg of iron so a patient who receives chelation. Add to this the increased intestinal iron absorption. For that reason, patients must undergo chelation therapy [9] that has a major 25 units per year accumulates 5 gram of iron per year in the absence of impact on the treatment of thalassemia [10] as excess iron accumulates in the body and is deposited in body organs as heart, liver and endocrine glands causing organ damage [11].

Deferiprone is a bidentate oral iron chelator that began clinical trials in UK in 1980. It was first licensed for use in thalassaemia in India, followed by European Union and other countries outside US and Canada, in 1990s [12]. According to official European Licensing Agency (EMEA), Deferiprone could be used as a second line drug for removing iron in patients who are unable to use Desferrioxamine (DFO) or in whom DFO therapy has proven ineffective [13]. Some studies show no difference between deferiprone and desferrioxamine [14]. Deferiprone daily dose that had been evaluated most thoroughly is 75 mg/kg/day, given in three divided doses [15].

Silymarin is an herbal remedy used for treatment of liver and gall bladder disorders. Silymarin is a flavonolignan complex isolated from Silybin marianum. It has a strong antioxidant, hepatoprotective,

***Corresponding author:** Adel A Hagag, Faculty of Medicine, Department of Paediatrics and Clinical Pathology, Tanta University, Egypt, E-mail: adelhagag20@yahoo.com and iron chelating activities [16]. There are some studies designed to investigate the therapeutic activity of silymarin in patients with thalassemia major under conventional iron chelation therapy [17,18].

Patient and Methods

This prospective study was conducted on 40 children with beta thalassemia major under follow-up at Hematology Unit, Pediatric Department, Tanta University Hospital having serum ferritin level more than 1000 ng/ml in the period between October 2012 and October 2013 and was performed after approval from research ethical committee center in Tanta University Hospital and obtaining an informed written parental consent from all participants in this research.

Study Design

Thalassemic patients included in the study were divided into two subgroups; Group I and Group II by simple random allocation, Group I received combination of daily oral Deferiprone 75 mg/kg/day divided into three doses [15] and oral silymarin in the form of Legalon tablets 140 mg, one hour before each meal (3 times daily) for 6 months [19] while group II received daily oral Deferiprone 75 mg/kg/day divided into three doses and placebo.

Inclusion criteria

Children with β-thalassemia with serum ferritin >1000 ng/ml who did not receive any iron chelation therapy before the start of this study.

Exclusion criteria

Children with β- thalassemia with serum ferritin <1000 ng/ml or who received any iron chelation therapy before the start of this study or who uses the drugs in irregular manner during this study.

All the children in both groups were subjected to the following:

1. Complete history taking with especial account on onset of thalassemia, chelation therapy, frequency of blood transfusion.
2. Thorough clinical examination with especial account on: pallor, jaundice, mongloid facies, splenomegaly, hepatomegaly and splenectomy.
3. Investigations including:

- Complete blood count.
- Hemoglobin electrophoresis.
- Liver functions including bilirubin level, Alanine Transferase (ALT) and Aspartate Transferase (AST).
- Renal function tests including blood urea and serum creatinine.
- Assessment of serum iron status including serum ferritin, serum iron and iron binding capacity. Assessment of liver and renal functions and serum iron status were done two times in studied patients; one time before the start of chelation therapy and one time after 6 months of chelation therapy.

Specimen collection and handling

Four ml of venous blood were collected using sterile needles through gentle venipuncture after sterilization of site of puncture by alcohol, and collected samples were divided into; 2 ml in a plain glass tube that were allowed to clot for 4 minutes and then centrifuged to separate serum which was used for estimation of serum iron, ferritin and TIBC [20-23] one ml was delivered on 20 μL EDTA solution for complete blood count including reticulocyte count and differential count which was done on leishman stained peripheral blood smear with evaluation using ERMA PCE-210 N cell counter [24] one ml was added to 2 ml hemolysate for Hb electrophoresis [25].

Determination of serum iron: The iron dissociated from transferrin-iron complex by a solution of guanidine acetate and reduced by ascorbic acid reacts with ferrozine to give a pink complex (according to procedure recommended by the serum iron from Biomaghreb company) [21].

Determination of serum total iron binding capacity (TIBC): An excess of iron is added to the serum to saturate the transferrin. The unbound iron is precipitated with basic magnesium carbonate (according to procedure recommended by the serum total iron binding capacity from Biomaghreb company) [22].

Serum ferritin test: Serum level of ferritin by ELIZA [DRG® Ferritin ELISA (EIA-4292)] [23].

Statistics

Statistical presentation and analysis of the present study was conducted, using the mean, standard deviation and chi-square test by SPSS Version 16 (Tables 1 and 2) [26].

Results and Discussion

Thalassemia's are one of the most common genetic disorders worldwide. It is the commonest cause of chronic hemolytic anemia in Middle East [27]. Silymarin is a flavonoid agent with antioxidant and free radical scavenging abilities. Silymarin also acts as an iron chelator by binding Fe (III). Despite the iron chelating activity of silymarin suggests its possible application in chelation therapy of iron overload; the biological effects of silymarin are different from other iron chelators, probably due to antioxidant activity of silymarin, which causes pro-oxidant effect via iron-catalyzed oxidation with subsequent generation of reactive oxygen species [19].

This study was carried out on 40 children with β-thalassemia major under follow up in Pediatric Hematology Unit, Tanta University Hospital in the period between October 2012 and October 2013. Patients included in the study were divided into two subgroups (group I and group II); group I received combination of Deferiprone and silymarin while group II used Deferiprone and placebo for six months.

	Group I (No=20)	Group II (No=20)	Chi-Square X^2	P - value
Age (months) Range Mean ± SD	40-60 50.35 ± 6.14	42-60 50.10 ± 6.11	0.26	0.79
Sex Males Females	10 10	9 11	0.100	0.752
Age of onset of thalassemia (months) Range Mean ± SD	6-36 11.5 ± 4.3	6-36 10.45 ± 4.13	0.63	0.97
Frequency of blood transfusion Every 2 week Every 3 week Every 4 week Every 6 week	4 cases 10 cases 5 cases 1 case	5 cases 5 cases 9 cases 1 case	2.921	0.404
Hemoglobin (gm /dl) Range Mean ± SD	7-8 7.3 ± 0.32	7-8.8 7.72 ± 0.60	0.96	0.635

differences between group I and group II regarding age.

Table 1: Clinical data of studied thalassemic patients.

	Group I (No=20)	Group II (No=20)	t value	p value
Serum creatinine (mg/dl) Before (mean ± SD) After (mean ± SD) t3 value p3 value	0.63 ± 0.11 0.59 ± 0.07 1.24 0.22	0.62 ± 0.10 0.61 ± 0.07 1.55 0.13	t1. 0.07 t2. 2.0	p1. 0.94 p2. 0. 48
Blood urea (mg/dl) Before (mean ± SD) After (mean ± SD) t3 value p3 value	35.30 ± 6.25 36.95 ± 5.44 2.31 0.32	33.75 ± 6.4 35.45 ± 5.47 1.93 0.68	t1. 1.06 t2. 0.98	p1. 0.29 p2. 0.33
ALT(U/L) Before (mean ± SD) After (mean ± SD) t3 value p3 value	26.25 ± 3.64 27.50 ± 3.16 0.90 0.73	26.30 ± 2.71 28.20 ± 3.63 2.83 0.11	t1. 0.84 t2. 1.42	p1. 0.93 p2. 0.17
AST(U/L) Before (mean ± SD) After (mean ± SD) t3 value p3 value	22.65 ± 4.51 23.7 ± 3.77 0.50 0.62	23.75 ± 5.85 24 ± 9.4.05 0.47 0.64	t1. 0.84 t2. 1.14	p1. 0.40 p2. 0.26
Total bilirubin (mg/dl) Before (mean ± SD) After (mean ± SD) t3 value p3 value	3.19 ± 0.40 3.23 ± 0.51 0.54 0.44	3.15 ± 0.43 3.24 ± 0.47 0.53 0.35	t1. 0.82 t2. 0.09	p1. 0.41 p2. 0.92
Ferritin (ng/ml) Before (mean ± SD) After (mean ± SD) t3 value p3 value	1901 ± 563.38 989.5 ± 178.57 6.53 0.000	1885.2 ± 510.54 1260 ± 212.26 5.40 0.000	t1 0.41 t2. 3.99	p1. 0.68 p2 0.000
Iron (ug/dl) Before (mean ± SD) After (mean ± SD) t3 value p3 value	236.40 ± 34.68 156.55 ± 21.42 0.7.91 0. 000	227.7 ± 35.49 172 ± 40.24.51 5.72 0.000	t1. 2.20 t2. 6.33	p1. 0.40 p2. 0.04
TIBC (ug/dl) Before (mean ± SD) After (mean ± SD) t3 value p3 value	192.45 ± 10.53 275.20 ± 10.08 24.18 0.000	191.85 ± 9.81 265.9 ± 9.19 21.72 0.000	t1. 0.29 t2. 2.33	p1. 0.77 p2. 0.03

Table 2: shows no statistically significant difference in serum creatinine, blood urea, serum bilirubin, ALT and AST between Group I and Group II before and after chelation therapy. There were no statistically significant difference in serum ferritin, serum iron and TIBC levels between group I and group II before start of chelation therapy while there was statistically significant difference between group I and group II after chelation therapy with lower serum ferritin and serum iron and higher TIBC in group I than group II. t1 comparison between group I and group II before chelation therapy, t2 comparison between group I and group II after chelation therapy and t3 comparison between the same group (as group I or II before and after chelation therapy).

Table 2: Renal and hepatic functions and iron status in studied patients before and after chelation therapy.

In the current study, there were no significant differences in the initial serum ferritin, serum iron and TIBC levels between group I and group II but after regular chelation therapy, serum ferritin and serum iron were significantly lower and TIBC was significantly higher in group I than group II. This is in agreement with [17] who assessed the efficacy of silymarin and desferroxamine compared with desferroxamine alone in removing excess iron in 48 patients with beta thalassemia and found that, serum ferritin and serum iron were significantly lower and TIBC was significantly higher in patients who received silymarin and desferroxamine than patients who received desferrioxamine alone, [28] who studied the beneficial effects of silymarin in thalassemic patients and suggests that silymarin in combination with desferrioxamine can be safely and effectively used in the treatment of iron-loaded thalassemic patients and [18] who compared (silymarin and Exjade) with (Exjade and placebo) in 40 patients with thalassemia major and found that, serum ferritin and serum iron were significantly lower and TIBC was significantly higher in patients who received silymarin and Exjade than patients who received Exjade and placebo and they concluded that combined therapy of silymarin and Exjade or silymarin and desferroxamine depleted iron stores more successfully than either Exjade or desferroxamine alone and they recommended to use combination of silymarin and desferrioxamine or silymarin and Exjade in treatment of iron overload in children with thalassemia major [17,18,28].

In disagreement with the previous studies; [29] found no significant changes in liver iron concentration after silymarin use and they recommended evaluating this drug by longer course of treatment to clarify its effects on reduction of liver iron concentration.

Variation in results could be explained by different mode of evaluating iron reduction (serum ferritin in our study versus liver iron concentration in [29] study and variation in severity of iron over load in both studies.

In this study, there were no significant differences in pre and post values of renal and liver function tests in group I before and after chelation therapy. This data is in agreement with [17,18,28] who demonstrated that; thalassemic patients with severe iron overload can be safely treated with a combination of silymarin and desferrioxamine or Exjade with no detectable abnormalities in complete blood count, liver or renal functions due to silymarin use.

Stickel and Schuppan [30] found that an average daily dose of silymarin (420 mg/day for 41 months) was found to be non-toxic, relative to placebo, in clinical trials [31]. Drug-drug interaction and liver toxicity by interference with co-drugs by induction or inhibition of cytochrome- P450 is a major concern for the use of silymarin [32]. Studies were performed to investigate the potential for hepatotoxicity, cytochrome-P450 isoenzymes induction and inhibition on dry extract from S. marianum. The results indicated that interference or hepatotoxicity of the dry extract from S. marianum at the recommended daily dose of 420 mg/day of silymarin (equivalent to 210 mg silybin) is unlikely and is considered safe [33].

Conclusion

From this study we concluded that, Deferiprone in combination with silymarin are better iron chelators in iron-loaded thalassemic patients than Deferiprone and placebo.

Recommendations

Extensive multicenter studies in large number of patients with longer duration of follow up and more advanced methods of assessment of iron status is recommended to clarify the exact role of silymarin in reduction of iron over load in children with beta thalassemia.

References

1. Miccio A, Cesari R, Lotti F (2007) The cure of thalassemia by bone marrow transplantation. Blood Rev 16: 81-85.
2. Surapon T (2011) Advances in the study of genetic disorders (1st edn) Ch 6: 102-137.
3. Galanello R, Origa R (2010) Beta-thalassemia. Orphanet J Rare Dis 5: 11.
4. El Dakhakhny AM, Hesham MA, Mohamed SE (2011) Quality of life of school age thalassemic children at Zagazig City. Journal of American Science 7 :186-197.
5. Shawky RM, Kamal TM (2012) Thalassemia intermedia: An overview. Egyptian Journal of Medical Human Genetics 13: 245-255.
6. Pathare A, Taher A, Daar S (2010) Deferasirox (Exjade) significantly improves cardiac T2* in heavily iron-overloaded patients with beta-thalassemia major. Ann Hematol 89: 405-409.
7. Crisponi G, Remelli M (2008) Review: Iron chelating agents for the treatment of iron overload. Coordination Chemistry Reviews 252: 1225-1240.
8. Gardenghi S, Marongiu MF, Ramos P, Guy E, Breda L, et al. (2007) Ineffective erythropoiesis in beta-thalassemia is characterized by increased iron absorption mediated by down-regulation of hepcidin and up-regulation of ferroportin. Blood 109: 5027-5035.
9. Prabhu R, Prabhu V, Prabhu RS (2009) Iron overload in beta thalassemia-a review. J Biosci Tech 1: 20-31.
10. Kattamis A, Ladis V, Berdousi H, Kelekis NL, Alexopoulou E, et al. (2006) Iron chelation treatment with combined therapy with deferiprone and deferioxamine: a 12-month trial. Blood Cells Mol Dis 36: 21-25.
11. Aessopos A, Berdoukas V, Tsironi M (2008) The heart in transfusion dependent homozygous thalassaemia today--prediction, prevention and management. Eur J Haematol 80: 93-106.
12. Kwiatkowski JL (2008) Oral iron chelators. Pediatr Clin North Am 55: 461-482.
13. Aessopos A, Angelucci E, Businco (2008) An Iron overload. Guidelines for the clinical of thalassemia. 2nd Revised edition. Ch 3:33-40.
14. Ha SY, Chik KW, Ling SC, Lee AC, Luk CW, et al. (2006) A randomized controlled study evaluating the safety and efficacy of deferiprone treatment in thalassemia major patients from Hong Kong. Hemoglobin 30: 263-274.
15. Cappellini MD, Musallam KM, Taher AT (2009) Overview of iron chelation therapy with desferrioxamine and deferiprone. Hemoglobin 33 Suppl 1: S58-69.
16. Valenzuela A, Garrido A (1994) Biochemical bases of the pharmacological action of the flavonoid silymarin and of its structural isomer silibinin. Biol Res 27: 105-112.
17. Gharagozloo M, Moayedi B, Zakerinia M, Hamidi M, Karimi M, et al. (2009) Combined therapy of silymarin and desferrioxamine in patients with beta-thalassemia major: a randomized double-blind clinical trial. Fundam Clin Pharmacol 23: 359-365.
18. Hagag AA, Elfrargy MS, Gazar RA, El-Lateef AE (2013) Therapeutic value of combined therapy with deferasirox and silymarin on iron overload in children with Beta thalassemia. Mediterr J Hematol Infect Dis 5: e2013065.
19. Gharagozloo M, Khoshdel Z, Amirghofran Z (2008) The effect of an iron (III) chelator, silybin, on the proliferation and cell cycle of Jurkat cells: a comparison with desferrioxamine. Eur J Pharmacol 589: 1-7.
20. Dawson DW, Fish DI, Shackleton P (1992) The accuracy and clinical interpretation of serum ferritin assays. Clin Lab Haematol 14: 47-52.
21. Bishop NL, Fudy EP, Schoeff L (2000) Priniciples and correlations. W Clinical chemistry, (5th edn) Philadelphia 180-220.
22. Peters T, Giovanniello TJ, Apt L (1956) A simple improved method for the determination of serum iron. J Lab Clin Med 48:280-288.
23. Beard JL (2001) Iron biology in immune function, muscle metabolism and neuronal functioning. J Nutr 131: 568S-579S.
24. Monica C (2005) Strategy of blood safety in Africa region 268-378.
25. Schedlbauer LM, Pass KA (1989) Cellulose acetate/citrate agar electrophoresis of filter paper hemolysates from heel stick. Pediatrics 83: 839-842.
26. Levesque R (2007) SPSS programming and data management: A guide for SPSS and SAS Users, 4th edn, Chicago.
27. Khalifa AS, Baffico M, Heshmat NM (1995) Relationship between the hematological phenotype and type of beta thalassemic mutation in Egyption Children. Egy J Hematol 20: 103-137.
28. Gupta OP, Sing S, Bani S, Sharma N, Malhotra S, et al. (2000) Anti-inflammatory and anti-arthritic activities of silymarin acting through inhibition of 5-lipoxygenase. Phytomedicine 7: 21-24.
29. Adibi A, Azin SH, Behjat SM (2012) Therapeutic effects of deferoxamine and silymarin versus deferoxamine alone in ß-thalassemia major based on findings of liver MRI. Journal of Research in Medical Sciences: 73-78
30. Stickel F, Schuppan D (2007) Herbal medicine in the treatment of liver diseases. Dig Liver Dis 39: 293-304.
31. Tamayo C, Diamond S (2007) Review of clinical trials evaluating safety and efficacy of milk thistle (Silybum marianum [L] Gaertn) Integr Cancer Ther 6: 146-157.
32. Izzo AA, Ernst E (2009) Interactions between herbal medicines and prescribed drugs: an updated systematic review. Drugs 69: 1777-1798.
33. Doehmer J, Weiss G, McGregor GP, Appel K (2011) Assessment of a dry extract from milk thistle (Silybum marianum) for interference with human liver cytochrome-P450 activities. Toxicol *In Vitro* 25: 21-27.

Abl Kinase Domain Mutations in Imatinib-treated Egyptian Patients with Chronic Myeloid Leukemia

Yasser H Elnahass[1]*, Hossam K Mahmoud[2], Fahmy T Ali[3], Mohamed R Mohamed[3], Mahmoud M Said[3], Mohamad Abdel Moaty Samra[2], Mohamed AM Ali[3], Amir Salem[4] and Wafaa H ElMetnawy[5]

[1]*Department of Clinical Pathology, BMT Lab Unit, National Cancer Institute, Cairo University, Egypt*
[2]*Department of Hematology and BMT, National Cancer Institute, Cairo University, Egypt*
[3]*Department of Biochemistry, Faculty of Science, Ain Shams University, Egypt*
[4]*Department of Pathology, National Research Center, Cairo, Egypt*
[5]*Clinical Oncology Center, School of Medicine, Cairo University, Egypt*

Abstract

Background: Point mutations within *ABL* kinase domain (AKD) of the *BCR-ABL* gene are the most common cause of resistance to Imatinib Mesylate (IM) treated Chronic Myeloid Leukemia (CML) patients.

Objectives: To assess the frequency, type and impact of AKD mutations on prognosis in a cohort of Egyptian CML patients.

Patients and methods: Serial measurements of BCR-ABL transcripts level in 175 IM treated CML patients were performed using real time quantitative polymerase chain reaction (RQ-PCR). Mutation screening was performed by allele specific oligonucleotide polymerase chain reaction (ASO-PCR) in 72 patients including all 42 non-optimal responders; 28 resistant patients, 18 suboptimal responders in addition to 30 patients randomly selected with stable/ decreasing transcript level representing an optimal responder category.

Results: AKD mutations were detected in 16/28 resistant patients (57%) at time of >2-fold rise in *BCR-ABL* transcript and in none of the 44 optimal or suboptimal responders (0%) with decreasing or stable transcript levels. From 16 positive patients, P-loop mutations were detected in 9 patients; Q252H in 3 patients (19%), Y253H in 2 patients (12%), Y253F in 2 patients (12%) and E255K in 2 patients (12%). T315I was detected in 1/16 (6%) patient. Regarding non P-loop mutation; V299L was detected in one patient (6%), M351T in 4 patients (25%), F359V in 2 patients (12%). One patient had both Y253H and E255K mutations. Ten/16 (62%) patients carrying mutations experienced disease progression versus 1/56 (2%) in non mutation group (p=0.001). Median progression free survival (PFS) and overall survival (OS) of the mutation group was 13.5 months and 37.5 months, respectively versus 42.6 months in non mutation group (p=0.001). The estimated PFS and OS at 49 months in patients with mutations were 37.5% and 56.3% respectively versus 98.2% in non mutation carriers (p<0.001). Mutations detected in chronic phase (CP) were mostly non P-loop (5/6, 83%) while mutations detected in accelerated phase (AP) and acute blastic crisis (ABC) were mostly located in P-loop and gate keeper regions (8/10, 80%). Patients harboring P-loop mutations/T315I showed poorer PFS and OS; 14 months (7.5-38) and 10 months (3-40) versus 42 months (39-45) and 42 months (9-45) in non-P-loop mutations carriers, respectively (p=0.003 and p=0.017).

Conclusion: A rise in *BCR-ABL* transcript of >2-folds in IM resistant patients may signal progression that implies testing for AKD mutations and early planning for second generation tyrosine kinase inhibitors (TKIs). P-loop mutations are significantly associated with advanced CML phases and poorer OS than non-P loop mutations. ASO-PCR is a valuable tool for detection of mutations in countries where sequencing facilities are not available.

Keywords: Abl kinase domain mutation screening; BCR-ABL transcripts; IM resistance

Introduction

Chronic myeloid leukemia (CML) is characterized by a reciprocal chromosomal translocation t (9; 22) (q34; q11) resulting in the *BCR-ABL* oncogenic fusion gene, which encodes the cytoplasmic *BCR-ABL* protein. The *BCR-ABL* protein has constitutive tyrosine kinase activity that mediates cellular transformation and leukemogenic effects [1].

Imatinib Mesylate (IM) the selective inhibitor of the *BCR-ABL* tyrosine kinase, competitively targets the adenosine 5'-triphosphate (ATP) binding site of the *AKD* and blocks downstream signal transduction pathways leading to growth arrest and apoptosis [2]. Because of its excellent safety and important therapeutic benefit for patients with CML, IM has become the standard of care for the treatment of CML. However, despite high rates of hematologic, cytogenetic and molecular responses, refractoriness or acquired resistance after initial response to IM is observed in a significant proportion of patients [3].

Point mutations within the AKD are emerging as the most frequent mechanism for reactivation of *BCR-ABL* kinase activity [4]. These mutations affect amino acids involved in IM binding or in regulatory regions of the AKD and result in decreased sensitivity to the drug [5]. It is postulated that mutations within the AKD can prevent IM from binding by changing the conformation of the BCR-ABL protein [6].

***Corresponding author:** Yasser H Elnahass, Department of Clinical Pathology, BMT Lab Unit, National Cancer Institute, Cairo University, Egypt, E-mail: y_el_nahas@hotmail.com

Molecular monitoring of *BCR-ABL* transcript levels for CML patients treated with IM has proved effective in defining patient response and provides important guide for clinical management and has prognostic relevance, in addition that it can indicate timing of mutation testing. Knowing the AKD mutational status is clinically useful, since it may prompt a change in therapy [7].

Biochemical and cellular assays have demonstrated that different AKD mutations result in varying levels of resistance [8,9]. Clinical studies have shown that the site of mutation within the kinase domain may affect disease outcome. The different mutations may therefore require different strategies to overcome resistance such as dose escalation for those that confer moderate resistance, or shifting to second generation TKIs or even transplantation for more resistant mutations [10].

The aim of the current study was to perform mutation analysis in a series of IM treated CML Egyptian patients of different response category in light of serial BCR-ABL measurements by RQ-PCR. We report on their type, frequency, relation to IM response and impact on clinical outcome of the disease.

Patients and Methods

Study group

Between March 2005 and April 2011, 175 newly diagnosed adult patients with Philadelphia-positive (Ph^+) CPCML were enrolled in this study. Seventy two patients; 44 males and 28 females were selected for ABL kinase domain mutational screening representing all resistant patients (28/175, 16%) in this study with >2 fold rising BCR-ABL level in addition to all suboptimal responders (18/175, 10%) and a fraction of patients representing optimal responders (n:30) with stable/decreasing transcript level. The study was conducted in accordance with the Declaration of Helsinki and was approved by the National Cancer Institute (NCI) Institutional Review Board. Median age of patients at diagnosis was 42 years (range 18-72 years). Median Follow up period was 41.6 month (7.5-49.5).

Patient eligibility

Inclusion criteria were (1) morphologic and cytogenetic evidence of Ph^+ CML in early chronic phase (defined as less than 12 months from diagnosis); (2) age 18 years or older; (3) normal renal and hepatic functions (4) normal cardiac function. Women at childbearing age were required to have a negative pregnancy test before starting IM, and to use contraception during therapy. Exclusion criteria included previous treatment for CML (Busulfan, IFN-α, or Ara-C). Exceptions included hydroxyurea and anagrelide for the treatment of elevated WBC ($>50\times10^9$/L) and platelet count ($>700\times10^9$/L), respectively; usage was limited to 4 weeks before starting IM therapy.

Treatment

Patients received 400 mg IM orally once a day. The dose was reduced for any ≥ Grade 3 drug-related hematologic toxicity. No dose adjustments were made for Grade 1 or 2 hematologic toxicity. No dose reductions below 300 mg/day were allowed. Any toxicity had to be resolved within 28 days.

Quantitation of BCR-ABL mRNA transcript levels by RQ-PCR

Patients were monitored by RQ-PCR for *BCR-ABL* transcript levels at diagnosis and at 3-month intervals during IM therapy. The *ABL* control gene and the *BCR-ABL* target gene transcript levels were quantitated using TaqMan Universal PCR Master Mix *(Applied Biosystems, Foster City, California, USA)*, the *BCR-ABL* Mbcr FusionQuant Kit *(Ipsogen, Luminy Biotech Entreprises, Marseille, France)* and the Smart Cycler detection system *(Cepheid, USA)*. A set of reference RNA was provided from *Ipsogen* to convert results into international scale (IS).

Definition of treatment responses

Hematologic, molecular and cytogenetic responses were defined according to European Leukemia Net criteria. MMR was defined as a 3-log reduction of BCR-ABL transcripts level, corresponding to ≤ 0.1% on international scale (IS) [11]. PFS was defined as loss of hematologic or cytogenetic response, death, or development of advanced CML; OS defined by the absence of death from any reason [12].

Abl Kinases Domain (AKD) mutations screening

Mutation screening was performed using allele specific oligonucleotide - polymerase chain reaction (ASO-PCR). Genomic DNA was extracted from peripheral blood using Gentra Puregene blood kit *(QIAGEN, Hilden, Germany)*. ASO-PCR assay was established for the detection of 16 known mutations which were selected according to their frequency in IM-resistant CML patients. Mutation panel selected included M244V, L248V, G250E, Q252H (a, b) showing 2 different nucleotides substitution, Y253H, Y253F, E255K, E255V, V299L, F311L, T315I, F317L, M343T, M351T, E355G and F359V mutations. Mutated or wild-type sequences were specifically amplified in a PCR reaction to analyze the most frequently identified mutations in the AKD (amino acids 220 to 498). The strong specificity of the assay was demonstrated for each mutation by detection of wild *ABL* sequence in DNA from clinically-declared healthy controls. Sequence of forward and reverse primers for both wild and mutant types used for ASO-PCR was adapted from previous reports [13,14]. The amplified products were detected by electrophoresis on 2% ethidium bromide-stained agarose gel.

Statistical analysis

The chi-square test was used to determine the significance between variables. Kaplan-Meier survival curves were used to assess outcome of patients with and without mutations [15]. Log rank test was used to compare between groups. PFS was calculated from start of treatment until the first reported appearance of AP or ABC. OS was calculated from start of treatment until death. All analyses were performed using the statistical package for the social sciences (SPSS software 17; SPSS Inc., Chicago, USA) [16].

Results

RQ-PCR results and mutational status

Twenty eight resistant patients (18 with 1ry resistance and 10 with 2ry resistance) and all 18 suboptimal responders in addition to a group of 30 patients with optimal response to IM randomly selected (15 in CMolR and 15 in MMolR) were submitted for mutation screening. Sixteen resistant patients (16/28, 57%) showed a mutation event while none of the optimal (0/30, 0%) or suboptimal responders (0/18, 0%) with stable or decreasing transcript level showed any detectable mutation ($p<0.001$). Baseline characteristics, mutational status and disease outcome of the 28 IM-resistant patients are listed in table 1.

Frequency of AKD mutations in IM-resistant CML patients

Nine different AKD mutations were found in 16/28 (57%) patients. Mutations of the P-loop (amino acids 248-255) were detected in 9/16 (56%) patients while non-P loop mutations were detected in 7/16 (44%)

UPN	Sex	Age	Therapeutic response	Mutational status	Disease outcome
1	M	48	Primary resistance	Q252Hb (P)	AP, died
2	M	47	Primary resistance	M351 T (NP)	CP, alive
3	M	29	Primary resistance	Q252Hb (P)	CP, alive
4	F	60	Primary resistance	F359V (NP)	CP, alive
5	M	40	Primary resistance	M351T (NP)	AP, alive
6	M	49	Primary resistance	Y253H (P)	AP, alive
7	F	47	Primary resistance	T315I (G)	ABC, died
8	F	39	Primary resistance	Y253F (P)	ABC, died
9	F	65	Primary resistance	Y253F (P)	ABC, died
10	F	40	Primary resistance	E255K (P)	ABC, died
11	M	39	Primary resistance	V299Lb (NP)	CP, alive
12	M	49	Primary resistance	Y253H (P), E255K (P)	ABC, died
13	M	63	Secondary resistance	Q252Ha (P)	ABC, died
14	M	52	Secondary resistance	F359V (NP)	CP, alive
15	F	25	Secondary resistance	M351 T (NP)	CP, alive
16	M	46	Secondary resistance	M351T (NP)	ABC, alive
17	F	30	Primary resistance	NM	ABC, died
18	M	45	Primary resistance	NM	CP, alive
19	M	46	Primary resistance	NM	CP, alive
20	M	47	Primary resistance	NM	CP, alive
21	M	49	Primary resistance	NM	CP, alive
22	M	51	Primary resistance	NM	CP, alive
23	M	57	Primary resistance	NM	CP, alive
24	F	65	Primary resistance	NM	CP, alive
25	F	67	Primary resistance	NM	CP, alive
26	F	43	Secondary resistance	NM	CP, alive
27	M	44	Secondary resistance	NM	CP, alive
28	M	66	Secondary resistance	NM	CP, alive

UPN- Unique Patient Number; CP- Chronic Phase; AP- Accelerated Phase; ABC- Acute Blast Crisis; P- P Loop; NP- Non-P-Loop; G- Gatekeeper; SG-TKI- Second Generation Tyrosine Kinase Inhibitor; NM- No Mutation

Table 1: Patient Characteristics, mutational status and disease outcomes of IM-resistant patients.

patients. Q252H was detected in 3/16 patients (19%), Y253H in 2/16 patients (12%), Y253F in 2/17 (12%) and E255K in 2/17 (12%) patients. From seven non–P-loop mutations, 1/16 patient (6%) showed V299L, 4/17 patients (25%) showed M351T, and 2/16 patients (12%) showed F359V (Figure 1). One patient had both Y253H and E255K mutations (more than one mutant clone per patient). T315I was detected in 1/16 (6%) patients only.

Mutation site, frequency, and disease phase

Mutations were detected in 6/17 (35%) patients in CP and in 3/3 (100%) patients in AP and in 7/8 (87%) patients in ABC at time of rise of BCR-ABL level (Table 2). Frequency of mutations was higher in advanced phases (AP and ABC) than in CP-CML (Table 3, p=0.01). Among 6 mutations found in CP-CML patients; 5 mutations (83%) were non–P-loop and 1 mutation (17%) was located in the P-loop region. Two/3 mutations (67%) of AP were in the P-loop region. Among 7 detected mutations in ABC patients, 5 mutations (71%) were located in the P-loop region, 1 mutation (14%) non–P-loop and 1 mutation (14%) was located in gatekeeper region T315I.

Impact of mutational status on OS and PFS

Median OS of the 56 patients without detectable mutations was 42.6 months (13.5- 49.5) versus of 37.5 months (7.5-45) in the mutation positive group. The estimated OS and PFS at 49 months in the mutation positive group were 56.3% and 37.5%, respectively versus 98.2% in non-mutation group (p<0.001) (Figures 3a and 3b). Median PFS of the mutation positive group was 13.5 months (3-45) versus 42.6 months (13.5- 49.5) in the non mutation group (p<0.001). Seven/9 (78%) patients with P-loop mutation (Q252Ha, Q252Hb, Y253F, Y253H, E255K) and one patient with T315I mutation died as a result of disease progression to either AP or ABC. Median OS of P-loop/ T315I group was 14 months (7.5-39) versus 42 months (40-45) in patients with non P-loop mutations (Table 1; Figure 2). No disease related death occurred in patients with non P-loop mutations. The estimated rates of OS (Figure 3a) and PFS (Figure 3b) at 48 months for patients with P-loop/T315I mutations were 22.2% and 11% versus 100% and 71% in patients with non-P loop mutations, respectively (P = 0.003, p=0.017) (Figures 3c and 3d). Estimated OS of resistant patients with mutations detected in CP was 100% versus 30% for patients with mutations detected in AP/ABC (p=0.001) (Figure 3e).

Discussion

Measurement of *BCR-ABL* transcript levels by RQ-PCR proved to be the gold standard of identifying patients at risk of IM failure [17,18]. More recently studies focused on other predictive factors of response to IM therapy as the 10% BCR-ABL^{IS} transcript level at 3 months and the pretreatment transcript level [19-21]. However, point mutations within the AKD have been reported as the most common mechanism for IM resistance or progression in CML patients. Identification of molecular basis of IM resistance is valuable as it can provide prognostic information and contribute to determining appropriate therapy to prevent or overcome resistance [3]. It was suggested that a 2-fold increase in transcript level can be an indication of AKD mutation testing [18]. However, it is still difficult to define the extent of transcript increase that justifies mutation screening [22-24].

The choice of therapy should be guided by multiple factors including mutational analysis, disease phase, patients' characteristics and safety profile [25]. The ELN recommendations consider any rise in transcripts level a warning element requiring more stringent and careful monitoring [11] whereas fluctuations in PCR results in MMolR patients may be due to sampling effect. Since the ELN included confirmed loss of MMolR among events defining a suboptimal response to IM, in patients showing an increase in BCR-ABL transcript level, a confirmed loss of MMolR should trigger a mutation analysis as this could be a quite reproducible predictor of loss of CCyR [26].

In the present study among 28 refractory patients showing >2 fold

RQ-PCR	Consecutive *BCR-ABL* transcript levels (n=72)			
	Rise of > 2-fold (n=28, 39%)		Stable or decreasing (n=44, 61%)	
Mutational status	Mutation Positive	No mutation	Mutation Positive	No mutation
	16 (57.1%)	12 (42.9%)	0 (0%)	44 (100%)
No. of resistant patients	16 (100%)	12 (100%)	0 (0%)	0 (0%)

Table 2: Mutational status of patients with rising and stable/decreasing BCR-ABL transcripts level.

Resistant patients (n=28)		Disease phase		
		CP (n = 17)	(AP and ABC) (n = 11)	p value
Patients with mutation (n=16)		6/17 (35.3%)	10/11 (90.9%)	0.01
Location in AKD	P-loop +T315I (n=9)	1/6 (16.7%)	8/10 (80%)	0.05
	Non-P-loop (n=7)	5/6 (83.3%)	2/10 (20%)	0.01

CP- chronic phase; AP- accelerated phase; ABC- Acute Blastic Crisis; AKD- ABL Kinase Domain

Table 3: Correlation between Frequency and site of mutations and disease phase.

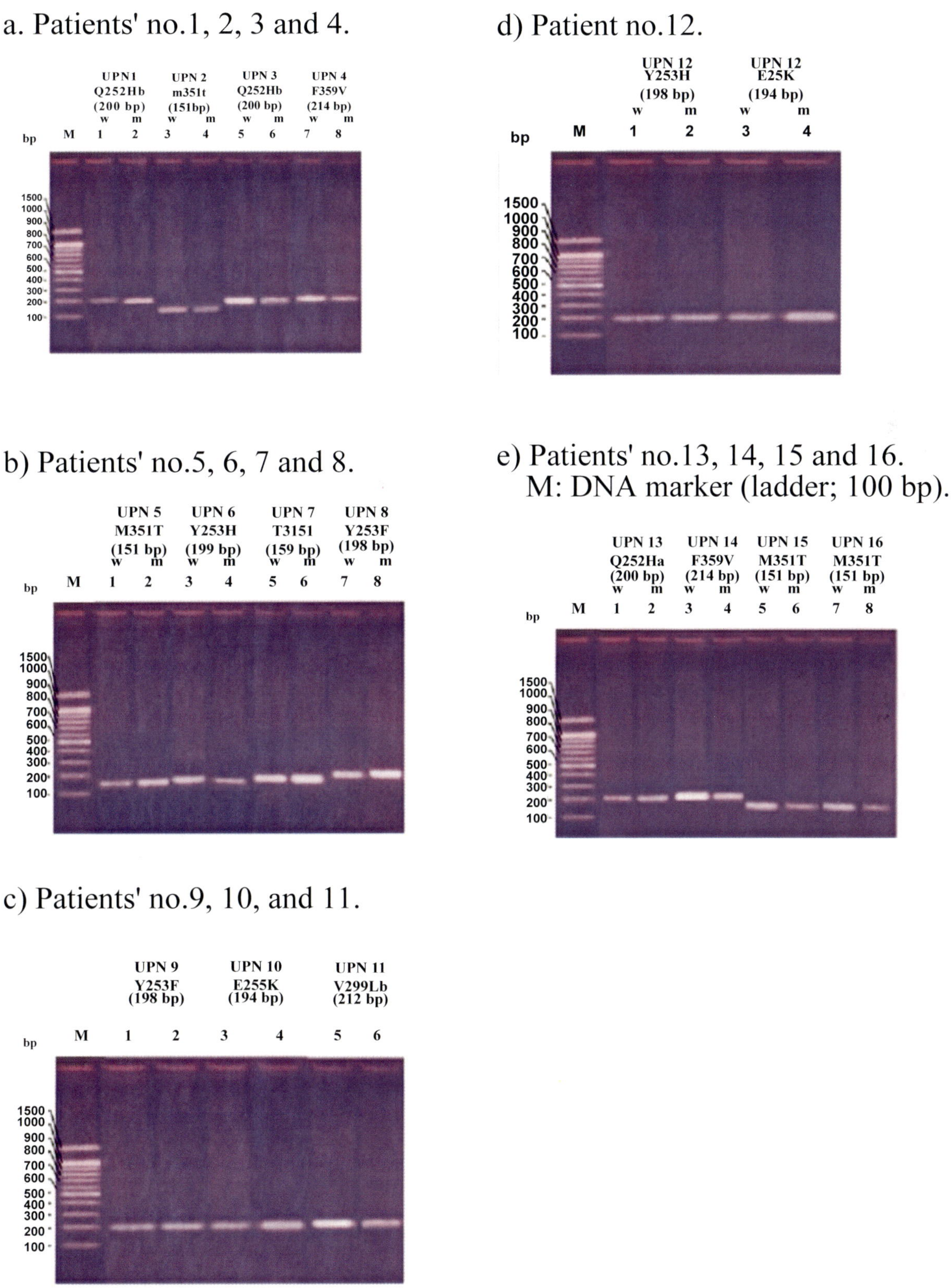

UPN: unique patient number; wt: wild type; mt: mutant type

Figure 1: ASO-PCR products on ethidium bromide-stained agarose gel.

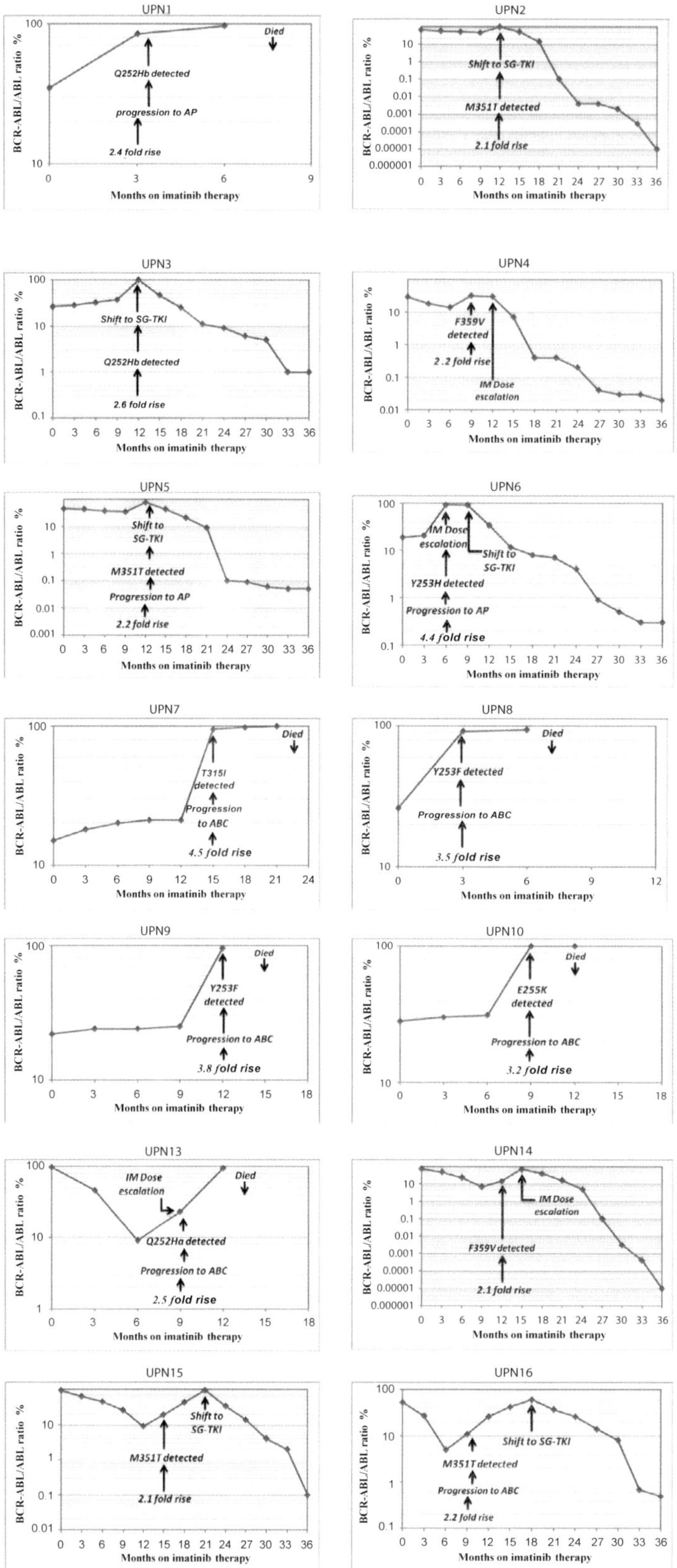

UPN, unique patient number; AP, accelerated phase; ABC, acute blast crisis; SG-TKI, second generation - tyrosine kinase inhibitor; NM, no mutation.

Figure 2: Individual patterns of BCR-ABL transcript levels in some of IM-resistant patients with mutations with > 2-fold rise in BCR-ABL transcript levels and their outcome.

(a) OS

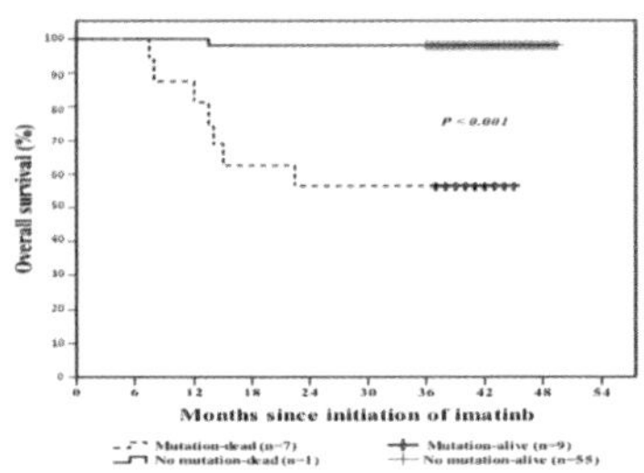

(b) PFS of mutation-screened patients according to presence (n=16) or absence (n=56) of mutations.

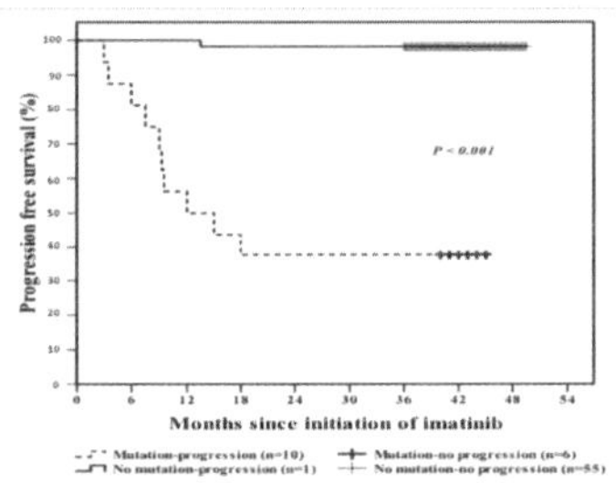

(c) OS of the 16 resistant patients with mutations according to the type of mutation.

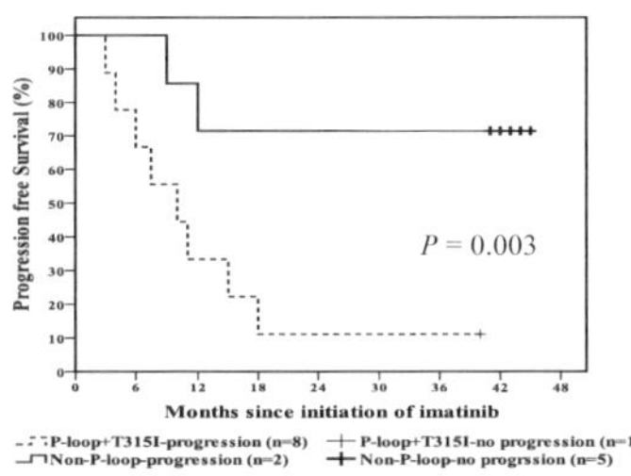

(d) PFS of the 16 resistant patients with mutations according to the type of mutation.

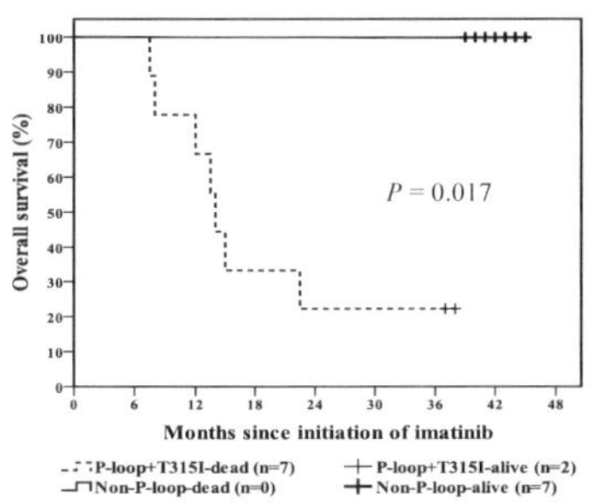

(e) OS of 16 resistant patients with mutations according to disease phase at which a mutation was detected.

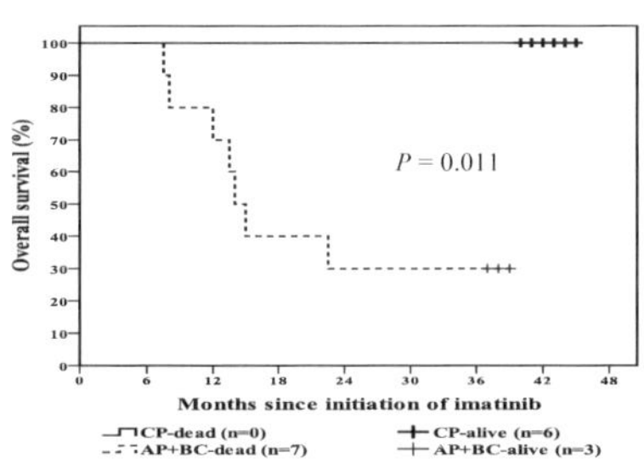

Figure 3: OS and PFS of patients.

BCR-ABL transcripts rise, 16 (57.1%) showed detectable mutations whereas no mutation was detected in optimal responders with stable or decreasing transcript level which add proof to Soverini et al. [26]. Strikingly, mutations were also undetected in suboptimal responders which raise the issue of other mechanisms of resistance as low OCT1 activity resulting in an inadequate intracellular concentration of IM [27]. All refractory patients did not achieve MMolR which explains the high mutation incidence at the time of rise of BCR-ABL. Mutation rate in this cohort was 16/28 (57%) which is relatively higher than that observed by others [28,29]. One study reported AKD mutations at a lower frequency (2 of 44 patients with relapsed or refractory disease) [30]. Differences in the frequency of mutation detection may be attributed to several factors; differences in the sensitivities of the techniques, in the time point of analysis, in phase of the disease and eventually due to differences in the genetic make-up of patient populations [31]. The frequency of *BCR-ABL* mutations in the present study was attributed to advanced phase of the disease at which mutations were detected [28]. Ten out of 16 patients with detectable mutation were in ABC (n: 7) and in AP (n:3). Seven/10 patients with detectable mutations in advanced phase died. Mutations were also detected in 6 CP patients, suggesting that this event is not restricted to patients in AP or ABC. However, none of them died due to shift to 2nd generation TKI, as early intervention that prevented progression of the disease. However, frequency of mutations was higher in advanced phases (AP and ABC) (10/11, 90.9%) compared to CP (6/17, 35.3%) indicating a cause – effect relation between disease progression and development of mutation.

OS and PFS were significantly decreased in patients harboring AKD mutations, a finding that has been stressed by others [18]. More importantly was the impact of the site of mutation on prognosis since different mutations have been associated with different degrees of resistance to IM as 7/8 patients with P loop and T315I mutations experienced disease progression. The increased kinase activity and transformation potency of several ATP binding loop mutations explain their association with poor prognosis leading to enhanced transforming capacity and associated genomic instability [30,32,33].

P-loop mutations conferred a true resistant phenotype and were not amenable to IM dose increase and implied alternative therapeutic strategies as second generation TKIs [34]. Two patients with P-loop mutations (Q252H and Y253H) were shifted to nilotinib and achieved CCyR in 1 year. T315I was detected in only one patient in the studied cohort who had no HLA identical donor for allogeneic stem cell transplantation and died in ABC. This rate was somewhat lower than that reported by Jabbour et al. [28] but higher than reported in two European studies [30].

Within our series there was also one patient harboring two known drug-resistant mutations, conferring increased oncogenic potency. On the other hand, patients with mutations that confer partial IM resistance as F359V regained clinical response with higher IM doses if the mutation was the sole abnormality [8,24]**.** In the present study, 2 patients with F359V mutation regained MMolR by increasing IM dose to 600 mg. The 4 patients harboring M351T mutation were shifted to dasatinib and 3 of them achieved MMolR within 12 months while one patient achieved CCyR. In this issue a stress on the choice of intervention with respect to the site and type of mutation should be considered [10].

In conclusion, more than 2 fold rise in BCR-ABL transcripts ratio in resistant CML patients who demonstrate molecular refractoriness to IM triggers mutation analysis as an early predictor of progression.

At this time, an early shift of therapy to appropriate 2nd generation TKI is beneficial when a positive mutation is detected in order to prevent disease acceleration. However, screening MMR patients with stable or decreasing *BCR-ABL* level for mutations is not warranted. ASO PCR is a specific and sensitive technique for mutation screening. M351T seems to be the commonest mutation in this CML Egyptian cohort. P-loop mutations are strongly associated with poor prognosis and mainly detected in advanced phases.

References

1. Baccarani M, Pileri S, Steegmann JL, Muller M, Soverini S, et al. (2012) Chronic myeloid leukemia: ESMO Clinical Practice Guidelines for diagnosis, treatment and follow-up. Ann Oncol 23: vii72-77.
2. Kantarjian HM, Cortes J, La Rosée P, Hochhaus A (2010) Optimizing therapy for patients with chronic myelogenous leukemia in chronic phase. Cancer 116: 1419-1430.
3. Bixby D, Talpaz M (2009) Mechanisms of resistance to tyrosine kinase inhibitors in chronic myeloid leukemia and recent therapeutic strategies to overcome resistance. Hematology Am Soc Hematol Educ Program.
4. Hochhaus A (2009) Dynamics of mutated clones in chronic myeloid leukemia patients. Haematologica 78-82.
5. O'Hare T, Eide CA, Deininger MW (2007) Bcr-Abl kinase domain mutations, drug resistance, and the road to a cure for chronic myeloid leukemia. Blood 110: 2242-2249.
6. Schenone S, Bruno O, Radi M, Botta M (2011) New insights into small-molecule inhibitors of Bcr-Abl. Med Res Rev 31: 1-41.
7. Hughes TP, Branford S (2009) Monitoring disease response to tyrosine kinase inhibitor therapy in CML. Hematology Am Soc Hematol Educ Program.
8. Jabbour E, Jones D, Kantarjian HM, O'Brien S, Tam C, et al. (2009) Long-term outcome of patients with chronic myeloid leukemia treated with second-generation tyrosine kinase inhibitors after imatinib failure is predicted by the in vitro sensitivity of BCR-ABL kinase domain mutations. Blood 114: 2037-2043.
9. Hughes T, Saglio G, Branford S, Soverini S, Kim DW, et al. (2009) Impact of baseline BCR-ABL mutations on response to nilotinib in patients with chronic myeloid leukemia in chronic phase. J Clin Oncol 27: 4204-4210.
10. Branford S, Melo JV, Hughes TP (2009) Selecting optimal second-line tyrosine kinase inhibitor therapy for chronic myeloid leukemia patients after imatinib failure: does the BCR-ABL mutation status really matter? Blood 114: 5426-5435.
11. Baccarani M, Cortes J, Pane F, Niederwieser D, Saglio G, et al. (2009) Chronic myeloid leukemia: an update of concepts and management recommendations of European LeukemiaNet. J Clin Oncol 27: 6041-6051.
12. Press RD, Love Z, Tronnes AA, Yang R, Tran T, et al. (2006) BCR-ABL mRNA levels at and after the time of a complete cytogenetic response (CCR) predict the duration of CCR in imatinib mesylate-treated patients with CML. Blood 107: 4250-4256.
13. Kang HY, Hwang JY, Kim SH (2006) Comparison of allele specific oligonucleotide-polymerase chain reaction and direct sequencing for high throughput screening of ABL kinase domain mutations in chronic myeloid leukemia resistant to imatinib. Haematologica 659-662.
14. Roche-Lestienne C, Soenen-Cornu V, Grardel-Duflos N, Lai JL, Philippe N, et al. (2002) Several types of mutations of the Abl gene can be found in chronic myeloid leukemia patients resistant to STI571, and they can pre-exist to the onset of treatment. Blood 100: 1014-1018.
15. Kaplan EL, Meier P (1958) Non-parametric estimation from incomplete observation. J Am Stat Assoc 457-481.
16. Norusis M (2009) SPSS 17.0 advanced statistical procedures companion. Upper Saddle-River, N.J Prentice Hall, Inc.
17. Hughes T, Branford S (2006) Molecular monitoring of BCR-ABL as a guide to clinical management in chronic myeloid leukaemia. Blood Rev 20: 29-41.
18. Branford S, Rudzki Z, Parkinson I, Grigg A, Taylor K, et al. (2004) Real-time quantitative PCR analysis can be used as a primary screen to identify patients with CML treated with imatinib who have BCR-ABL kinase domain mutations. Blood 104: 2926-2932.
19. Vigneri P, Stagno F, Stella S, Cupri A, Massimino M, Antolino A, et al. (2011) BCR-ABL (IS) Expression at Diagnosis and After 3 or 6 months of Treatment predicts CML Response to IMATINIB Therapy. Blood ASH Annu Meet 116: 3426.
20. Hanfstein B, Müller MC, Hehlmann R, Erben P, Lauseker M, et al. (2012) Early molecular and cytogenetic response is predictive for long-term progression-free and overall survival in chronic myeloid leukemia (CML). Leukemia 26: 2096-2102.
21. Marin D, Ibrahim AR, Lucas C, Gerrard G, Wang L, et al. (2012) Assessment of BCR-ABL1 transcript levels at 3 months is the only requirement for predicting outcome for patients with chronic myeloid leukemia treated with tyrosine kinase inhibitors. J Clin Oncol 30: 232-238.
22. Martinelli G, Iacobucci I, Soverini S, Cilloni D, Saglio G, et al. (2006) Monitoring minimal residual disease and controlling drug resistance in chronic myeloid leukaemia patients in treatment with imatinib as a guide to clinical management. Hematol Oncol 24: 196-204.
23. Press RD, Willis SG, Laudadio J, Mauro MJ, Deininger MW (2009) Determining the rise in BCR-ABL RNA that optimally predicts a kinase domain mutation in patients with chronic myeloid leukemia on imatinib. Blood 114: 2598-2605.
24. Kantarjian H, Schiffer C, Jones D, Cortes J (2008) Monitoring the response and course of chronic myeloid leukemia in the modern era of BCR-ABL tyrosine kinase inhibitors: practical advice on the use and interpretation of monitoring methods. Blood 111: 1774-1780.
25. Jabbour E, Soverini S (2009) Understanding the role of mutations in therapeutic decision making for chronic myeloid leukemia. Semin Hematol 46: S22-26.
26. Soverini S, Hochhaus A, Nicolini (2011) BCR-ABL kinase domain mutation analysis in chronic myeloid leukemia patients treated with tyrosine kinase inhibitors: recommendations from an expert panel on behalf of European Leukemia. Net Blood 1208-1215.
27. White DL, Saunders VA, Dang P, Engler J, Venables A, et al. (2007) Most CML patients who have a suboptimal response to imatinib have low OCT-1 activity: higher doses of imatinib may overcome the negative impact of low OCT-1 activity. Blood 110: 4064-4072.
28. Jabbour E, Kantarjian H, Jones D, Talpaz M, Bekele N, et al. (2006) Frequency and clinical significance of BCR-ABL mutations in patients with chronic myeloid leukemia treated with imatinib mesylate. Leukemia 20: 1767-1773.
29. Soverini S, Colarossi S, Gnani A, Rosti G, Castagnetti F, et al. (2006) Contribution of ABL kinase domain mutations to imatinib resistance in different subsets of Philadelphia-positive patients: by the GIMEMA Working Party on Chronic Myeloid Leukemia. Clin Cancer Res 12: 7374-7379.
30. Hochhaus A, Kreil S, Corbin A, La Rosée P, Lahaye T, et al. (2001) Roots of clinical resistance to STI-571 cancer therapy. Science 293: 2163.
31. Gorre ME, Mohammed M, Ellwood K, Hsu N, Paquette R, et al. (2001) Clinical resistance to STI-571 cancer therapy caused by BCR-ABL gene mutation or amplification. Science 293: 876-880.
32. von Bubnoff N, Schneller F, Peschel C, Duyster J (2002) BCR-ABL gene mutations in relation to clinical resistance of Philadelphia-chromosome-positive leukaemia to STI571: a prospective study. Lancet 359: 487-491.
33. Yamamoto M, Kurosu T, Kakihana K, Mizuchi D, Miura O (2004) The two major imatinib resistance mutations E255K and T315I enhance the activity of BCR/ABL fusion kinase. Biochem Biophys Res Commun 319: 1272-1275.
34. Apperley JF (2007) Part I: mechanisms of resistance to imatinib in chronic myeloid leukaemia. Lancet Oncol 8: 1018-1029.

Lenalidomide Polarizes Th1-specific Anti-tumor Immune Response and Expands XBP1 Antigen-Specific Central Memory CD3⁺CD8⁺ T cells against Various Solid Tumors

Jooeun Bae[1,2*], Derin B Keskin[1,2], Kristen Cowens[1,2], Ann-Hwee Lee[3], Glen Dranoff[1,2], Nikhil C Munshi[1,2,4] and Kenneth C Anderson[1,2]

[1]*Dana-Farber Cancer Institute, Boston, Massachusetts, USA*
[2] *Harvard Medical School, Boston, Massachusetts, USA*
[3]*Weill Cornell Medical College, New York, NY, USA*
[4]*VA Boston Healthcare System, Boston, Massachusetts, USA*

Abstract

Introduction: Effective combination immunotherapeutic strategies may be required to enhance effector cells' anti-tumor activities and improve clinical outcomes.

Methods: XBP1 antigen-specific cytotoxic T lymphocytes (XBP1-CTL) generated using immunogenic heteroclitic XBP1 US184-192 (YISPWILAV) and XBP1 SP367-375 (YLFPQLISV) peptides or various solid tumor cells over-expressing XBP1 target antigen were evaluated, either alone or in combination with lenalidomide, for phenotype and immune functional activity.

Results: Lenalidomide treatment of XBP1-CTL increased the proportion of CD45RO⁺ memory CD3+CD8+ T cells, but not the total CD3⁺CD8⁺ T cells. Lenalidomide upregulated critical T cell activation markers and costimulatory molecules (CD28, CD38, CD40L, CD69, ICOS), especially within the central memory CTL subset of XBP1-CTL, while decreasing TCRαβ and T cell checkpoint blockade (CTLA-4, PD-1). Lenalidomide increased the anti-tumor activities of XBP1-CTL memory subsets, which were associated with expression of Th1 transcriptional regulators (T-bet, Eomes) and Akt activation, thereby resulting in enhanced IFN-γ production, granzyme B upregulation and specific CD28/CD38-positive and CTLA-4/PD-1-negative cell proliferation.

Conclusions: These studies suggest the potential benefit of lenalidomide treatment to boost anti-tumor activities of XBP1-specific CTL against a variety of solid tumors and enhance response to an XBP1-directing cancer vaccine regime.

Keywords: Combination immunotherapy; Lenalidomide; XBP1; Antigen-specific cytotoxic T lymphocytes; Cancer vaccine

Introduction

Active-specific immunotherapy has the goal of inducing effector T lymphocytes with anti-tumor activities, durable immune responses with favorable side effect profile, and long-term stabilization of disease. To accomplish the goal, immunotherapy must address the tolerogenic mechanisms deployed by tumors as well as immunosuppression in cancer patients due to impaired antigen-processing ability, down-regulation of MHC class I, and increased levels of immune-suppressive cells and cytokines. Tumors often produce excessive amounts of immunosuppressive mediators such as adenosine, kynurenines, indoleamine 2,3-dixoxygenase, prostaglandin E2, TGF-β and VEGF-α [1-3]. Hence, disease-related immunosuppression is an important hurdle to overcome for immunotherapeutic strategies to be successful. Approaches including adjuvant selection have been developed to both enhance anti-tumor activities and overcome the suppressive effects within the tumor microenviroment.

Lenalidomide is an immunomodulatory drug (IMiD) with potential immune stimulatory anti-angiogenic and direct anti-tumor effects, which together act against tumor in its microenvieonment [4-6]. Studies on effector cells have found that IMiDs enhance cross-priming of naive CD8⁺ T cells by dendritic cells, activate adaptive T-cell immunity via activation of the CD28 signaling pathway, and polarize T-cell immunity toward Th1-specific response. Importantly, lenalidomide has been shown to suppress regulatory T cells, T-cell expression of CTLA-4 and PD-1, and restore T-cell immunologic synapse dysfunction [7-9]. IMiDs also inhibit the production of TNF-α and enhance innate immune responses in the bone marrow microenvironment in multiple myeloma (MM) by overcoming suppression of IFN-γ/IL-2 cytokine signaling in immune effector cells [10-12]. These findings suggest that IMiD may provide a potential adjuvant function in cancer vaccine immunotherapy. However, the ability of an IMiD to enhance or modify tumor-specific immunity in tumor directed vaccine derived CTL effector cells has not been fully explored.

XBP1 is an important transcription activator of the unfolded protein response (UPR), while activates a distinct set of genes and regulates endoplasmic reticulum (ER) stress-mediated apoptosis [13]. Previously, XBP1 has been identified as a therapeutic target in MM due to its' differential expression between plasma cells from normal donors and patients' with monoclonal gammopathy of undetermined significance (MGUS) or MM, as well as its uniform expression in all MM patient cells and cell lines [14-17]. XBP1 has also been implicated

***Corresponding author:** Jooeun Bae, Dana-Farber Cancer Institute, Harvard Medical School, Boston, USA, E-mail: jooeun_bae@dfci.harvard.edu in the proliferation of malignant plasma cells. Moreover, studies have found that XBP1 is overexpressed in a variety of solid tumors by various analyses, i.e. genome-wide profiling, flow cytometry, and immunohistochemistry; and is required for functions including tumor cell growth and survival and proliferation under hypoxic conditions [18-21]. Currently, several agents are in development to target XBP1 including Irestatin, an inhibitor of IRE1 and the UPR through inhibition of spliced XBP1 transcription activity; and Trierixin, a new member of the triene-ansamycin group which is a novel inhibitor of ER-stress induced cleavage of XBP1[22,23].

Our study examines a new selective immunotherapeutic strategy by targeting XBP1 in different types of cancers including MM [24,25], SMM [26], breast cancer, colon cancer, and pancreatic cancer [18]. Our previous studies have shown the immunotherapeutic potential of heteroclitic XBP1 $US_{184-192}$ (YISPWILAV) and XBP1 $SP_{367-375}$ (YLFPQLISV) peptides to generate XBP1 antigen-specific CTL, and we demonstrate here that lenalidomide can enhance anti-tumor activities of XBP1-CTL against a variety of solid tumors which overexpress XBP1 antigen.

Material and Methods

Cell lines

Breast cancer (MDA-MB231, MCF-7) and colon cancer (LS180, SW480) cell lines were obtained from the ATCC (Manassas, VA). The pancreatic cancer cell lines (PATU8988T, Panc1) were kindly provided by Dr. A. Kimmelman (Harvard Medical School, Boston, MA). The T2 cell line was provided by Dr. J. Molldrem (University of Texas M. D. Anderson Cancer Center, Houston, TX). MDA-MB231 and SW480 cell lines were cultured in Leibovitz's L-15 Medium (ATCC); MCF-7 and LS180 cell lines were cultured in EMEM (Gibco-Life Technologies, Rockville, MD); and Panc1, PATU8902, and T2 cell lines were cultured in DMEM (Gibco-Life Technologies) media. All media were supplemented with 10% fetal calf serum (FCS; BioWhittaker, Walkersville, MD), 100 IU/ml penicillin, and 100 µg/ml streptomycin (Gibco-Life Technologies).

Synthetic peptides

HLA-A2-specific immunogenic heteroclitic $XBP1_{184-192}$ (YISPWILAV) and heteroclitic XBP1 $SP_{367-375}$ (YLFPQLISV) peptides were synthesized by standard fmoc (9-fluorenylmethyl-oxycarbonyl) chemistry, purified to >95% using reverse-phase chromatography, and validated by mass-spectrometry for molecular weight (Biosynthesis, Lewisville, TX). Lyophilized peptides were dissolved in DMSO (Sigma, St. Louis, MO), diluted in AIM-V medium (Gibco-Life Technologies), and stored at -140°C until needed.

Reagents

Fluorochrome conjugated anti-human mAb specific to HLA-A2, CD3, CD8, CD28, CD38, CD40L, CD69, ICOS, TCRαβ, CCR7, CD45RO, CD80, CD86, ICOS ligand, IFN-γ, CTLA-4, PD-1, PD-L1, PD-L2, T-bet, granzyme B or Akt were purchased from Becton Dickinson (San Diego, CA). Fluorochrome conjugated anti-human Eomes mAb was purchased from eBioscience (San Diego, CA). Recombinant human IL-2, IL-4, IFN-α and TNF-α were purchased from R&D Systems, and human GM-CSF was obtained from Immunex (Seattle, WA). Lenalidomide (Celgene, Summit, NJ) was reconstituted in 1% DMSO and was used at a final concentration of 5 µM to treat either XBP1-CTL or various tumor cell lines.

Generation of XBP1-CTL and treatment with lenalidomide

XBP1 peptides-specific CTL (XBP1-CTL) were generated *ex vivo* by repeated stimulation of $CD3^+$ T lymphocytes obtained from HLA-$A2^+$ normal donors with a cocktail of immunogenic heteroclitic XBP1 peptides-pulsed antigen-presenting cells (APC). In brief, APC in serum-free AIM-V medium were pulsed overnight at 37°C and 5% CO_2 in humidified air with a cocktail (50 µg/ml) of heteroclitic XBP1 $US_{184-192}$ (YISPWILAV) and heteroclitic XBP1 $SP_{367-375}$ (YLFPQLISV) peptides. The peptides pulsed APC were washed, irradiated, and used to prime $CD3^+$ T cells at a 1:20 APC/peptide (stimulator)-to-$CD3^+$ T cell (responder) ratio in AIM-V medium supplemented with 10% human AB serum (BioWhittaker) and IL-2 (50 U/ml). The CTL cultures were restimulated with the heteroclitic XBP1 peptide pulsed-APC every seven days for a total of 4 cycles. After the last stimulation, XBP1-CTL were treated with lenalidomide (5 µM) for 4 days and evaluated for their phenotype and functional activities. XBP1-CTL cultured in the presence of DMSO (1% final concentration) for 4 days were used as a comparative control in these studies.

Evaluation of the effects of lenalidomide on expression of critical T cell markers on $CD3^+CD8^+$ T cells or on different T cell subtypes of XBP1-CTL

XBP1-CTL were evaluated for the frequency of $CD3^+CD8^+$ T cells and expression levels (% positive cells, mean fluorescence intensity (MFI)) of critical T cell surface markers including CD45RO, CCR7, CD28, CD38, CD40L, CD69, ICOS, TCRαβ, CTLA and PD-1. After staining with each specific antibody, the cells were washed and fixed in 2% paraformaldehyde. The cells were analyzed using a LSRII Fortessa™ flow cytometer and DIVA™ v8.0 software (BD). The XBP1-CTL were gated on non-memory or memory $CD3^+CD8^+$ T cells and central memory (CM), effector memory (EM) or terminal effector (TE) $CD3^+CD8^+$ T cell subsets.

Analysis of lenalidomide effects on the expression of surface proteins or intracellular proteins on cancer cell lines

Breast cancer (MDA-MB231, MCF-7), colon cancer (LS180, SW480), and pancreatic cancer (PATU8902, Panc1) cell lines were treated with lenalidomide (5 µm in DMSO, Celgene) for 4 days. As controls, each of the cancer cell lines was cultured in the presence of DMSO (1% final concentration) for 4 days. The cancer cell lines were evaluated with the treatment for their phenotype changes of surface markers including HLA-A2, CD80, CD86, ICOS ligand, PD-L1 and PD-L2. Separately, the lenalidomide or DMSO treated cancer cells were evaluated for intracellular expression of XBP1 unspliced or XBP1 spliced protein. In brief, each of the cancer cell lines were fixed and permeabilized using the Cytofix/Cytoperm kit (BD) and stained with rabbit anti-human XBP1 unspliced isoform monoclonal antibody (mAb) (Novus Biologicals, Littleton, CO) or mouse anti-human XBP1 spliced isoform mAb (R&D Systems, Minneapolis, MN) for 30 minutes at room temperature, washed with Perm/Wash solution (BD) and stained with donkey anti-rabbit IgG-PE (Novus Biologicals, Littleton, CO) or goat anti-mouse IgG-PE (R&D Systems, Minneapolis, MN), respectively, for 30 minutes at 4°C. The cells were washed with Perm/Wash solution and fixed in 2% formaldehyde-PBS. After staining with each specific antibody, the tumor cells were washed and analyzed using a LSRII Fortessa™ flow cytometer and DIVA™ v8.0 software (BD).

Examination of lenalidomide effects on the expression of T-bet, Eomes and Akt and anti-tumor functional activities of XBP1-CTL

The expression of transcriptional regulators and signal integrator or tumor-specific responses were evaluated in XBP1-CTL upon lenalidomide treatment. In brief, XBP1-CTL were co-incubated with each cancer cell line for 6 hours, and they were washed and stained with fluorochrome conjugated mAbs specific to surface antigens including CD3, CD8, CD45RO, and CCR7. They were further fixed and permeabilized, and stained with mAbs specific to IFN-γ, granzyme B, T-bet, Eomes and/or AKT. The cells were analyzed using a LSR Fortessa™ flow cytometer and DIVA™ v8.0 software after gating on non-memory or memory $CD3^+CD8^+$ CTL populations.

Analysis of lenalidomide effects on XBP1-CTL proliferation in response to tumor cell lines

To evaluate tumor-specific CTL proliferation, CFSE (Molecular Probes, Eugene, OR) labeled XBP1-CTLwere co-incubated with irradiated (20 Gy) cancer cell lines. On day 6, the cultures were harvested, stained with anti-CD3,CD8, CD45RO, CCR7, CD28, CD38, CTLA-4 and/or PD-1 fluorochrome conjugated mAbs, and analyzed by flow cytometry to determine their specific cell proliferation.

Statistical analysis

Results are presented as mean ± SE. Groups were compared using unpaired Student's t-test. Differences were considered significant when $*p<0.05$.

Results

Lenalidomide increases the frequency of memory $CD8^+$ T cell subsets of XBP1 antigen-specific CTL

XBP1-CTL generated using immunogenic heteroclitic XBP1 $US_{184-192}$ (YISPWILAV) and XBP1 $SP_{367-375}$ (YLFPQLISV) peptides were phenotypically evaluated, with or without treatment with Lenalidomide (5 μm, 4 days). Lenalidomide did not induce a change in the total $CD3^+CD8^+$ T cell frequency of XBP1-CTL, nor in cell viability (data not shown). However, an increase of $CD45RO^+$ memory $CD3^+$ $CD8^+$ T cells and corresponding decrease of $CD45RO^-$ non-memory $CD3^+$ $CD8^+$ T cells were observed after lenalidomide treatment in the XBP1-CTL, as compared to control XBP1-CTL (Figure 1A). The effect of lenalidomide on XBP1-CTL memory $CD3^+CD8^+$ T cells was further investigated. As compared to the EM ($CD45RO^+$ $CCR7^-$) subset, the CM ($CD45RO^+$ $CCR7^+$) subset frequency was consistently increased in XBP1-CTL (Donor 1: 95% increase, Donor 2: 292% increase, Donor 3: 50% increase), after treatment with lenalidomide (Figure 1B).

Lenalidomide regulates key activating and inhibitory molecules on XBP1-CTL

The effect of lenalidomide was next evaluated on expression of key molecules for T cell co-stimulation and cellular activation (CD28, CD38, CD40L, CD69, ICOS) and T cell inhibition (PD-1) or TCRαβ on the XBP1-CTL. Lenalidomide induced upregulation of CD28 (2/4 donors), CD38 (4/4 donors), CD40L (3/4 donors), CD69 (4/4 donors), and ICOS (3/4 donors) on the XBP1-CTL generated from different HLA-$A2^+$ donors (Figure 2A). In contrast, lenalidomide reduced the expression levels of PD-1 (3/4 donors) and TCRαβ (4/4 donors). XBP1-CTL phenotypic changes following lenalidomide treatment were further evaluated within specific memory or non-memory $CD3^+$ $CD8^+$ T cell subsets. Lenalidomide treated XBP1-CTL displayed increased levels of cellular activation, evaluated by upregulation of both CD38 and CD69. Interestingly, the central memory ($CD45RO^+$ $CCR7^+$) CTL subset, which is the main population increased by lenalidomide, also showed high upregulation of molecules involved in T cell activation/costimulation (Figure 2B). The terminal effector ($CD45RO^-$ $CCR7^-$) CTL subset showed downregulation of the CD38 cellular activation marker and decreased expression of CD28, CD40L, and ICOS post lenalidomide treatment. Importantly, the expression of T-cell inhibitory molecules, CTLA-4 and PD-1, was reduced on all XBP1-CTL memory subsets (CM. EM) after lenalidomide treatment, while their expression was increased on the non-memory subset (TE) (Figure 2B). Finally, lenalidomide consistently downregulated TCRαβ expression in all subsets of XBP1-CTL (Figures 2A and 2B).

Lenalidomide does not modify the expression of intracellular XBP1 proteins nor critical co-stimulatory or inhibitory surface antigens on breast cancer, colon cancer and pancreatic cancer cells

In contrast to its effects on antigen-specific CTL, lenalidomide treatment (5 μm, 4 days) did not significantly ($p>0.05$) change the expression of intracellular XBP1 unspliced and XBP1 spliced target antigens in breast cancer (MDA-MB231, MCF7), colon cancer (LS180, SW480) and pancreatic cancer (PATU8902, Panc1) (Figure 3A). Further analyses were performed to investigate modification of co-stimulatory and inhibitory surface antigens on these tumor cells. Our

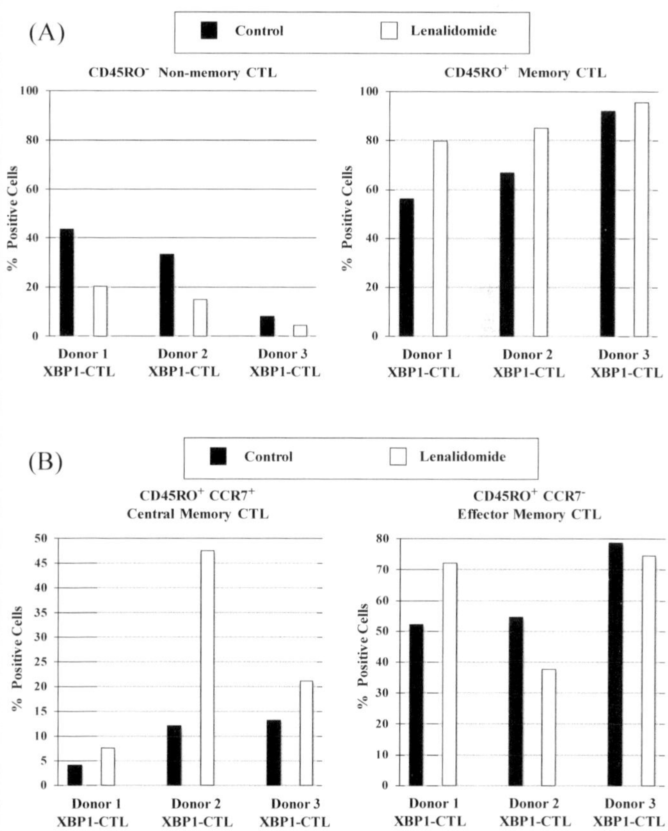

Figure 1: Lenalidomide induced $CD3^+CD8^+$ T cell memory subsets in XBP1-CTL. XBP1-CTL were generated from three respective HLA-$A2^+$ normal donors' $CD3^+$ T cells by repeated stimulation, once a week, with a cocktail of heteroclitic unspliced $XBP1_{184-192}$ (YISPWILAV) and spliced XBP1 $SP_{196-204}$ (YLFPQLISV) peptides (50 μg/ml; 25 μg/peptide). After the 4th stimulation, XBP1-CTL were treated with lenalidomide (5 μm, 4 days) and examined for their phenotypic T cell profile by flow cytometry. (A) Lenalidomide treatment induced a higher frequency of memory CTL ($CD45RO^+/CD3^+CD8^+$) and a corresponding lower frequency of non-memory CTL ($CD45RO^-/CD3^+CD8^+$) as compared to the control XBP1-CTL. (B) Lenalidomide treatment increased the percentage of central memory ($CD45RO^+CCR7^+$) $CD3^+CD8^+$ T cell subset within the memory cells of all the XBP1-CTL generated (n=3).

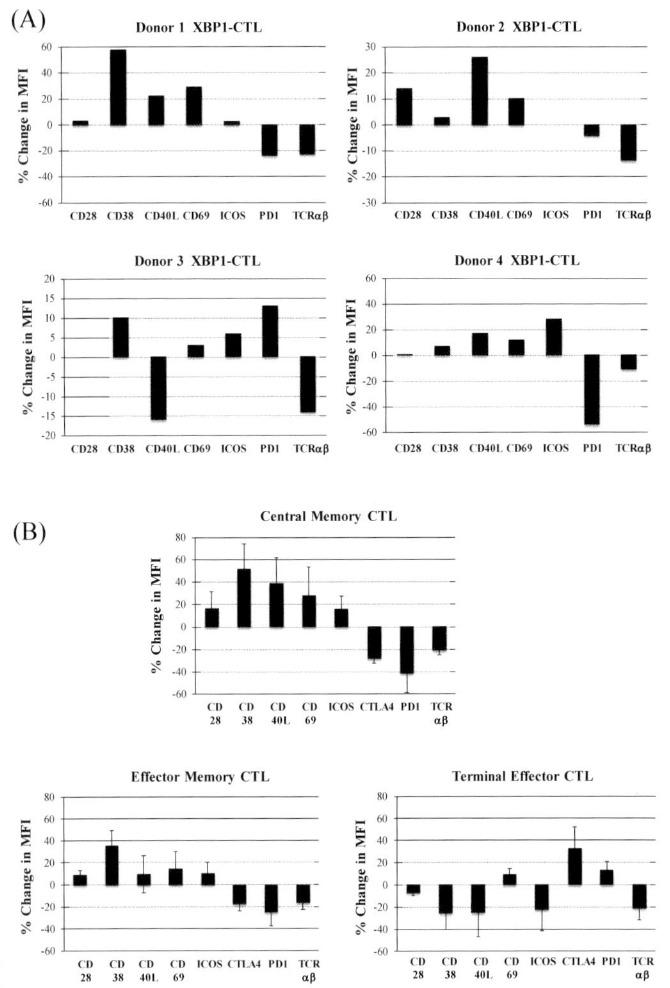

Figure 2: Lenalidomide changed T cell antigen expression on XBP1-CTL with primary modification in the central memory $CD3^+CD8^+$ T cell subset.
XBP1-CTL (n=4) were evaluated after lenalidomide (5 μm, 4 days) treatment for changes in expression of critical T cell activation markers (CD38, CD69), co-stimulatory molecules (CD28, CD40L, ICOS), inhibitory molecule (PD-1, CTLA-4) and T-cell receptor (TCRαβ). Results obtained by flow cytometric analyses are presented as the '% Change in MFI (mean fluorescence intensity)', which was calculated as [(MFI Lenalidomide treated XBP1-CTL / MFI Control XBP1-CTL) x100]' for each specific marker. (A) Lenalidomide upregulated the T cell activation markers (CD38, CD69: 4/4) and co-stimulatory molecules (CD28: 2/4, CD40L: 3/4, ICOS: 3/4) on XBP1-CTL, while down-regulating inhibitory molecule (PD-1: 3/4) and T-cell receptor (TCRαβ: 4/4). (B) The upregulation of T cell activation markers (CD38, CD69) and costimulatory molecules (CD28, CD40L, ICOS) and downregulation of inhibitory molecules (PD-1, CTLA-4) and T-cell receptor (TCRαβ) following lenalidomide treatment were mainly detected within the central memory ($CD45RO^+CCR7^+$) $CD3^+CD8^+$ T cell subset of XBP1-CTL.

results showed that lenalidomide treatment did not modify expression ($p>0.05$) of HLA-A2, a MHC class I molecule having affinity for endogenous XBP1 peptides. In addition, the expression levels of CD80 and CD86 (the B7 costimulatory molecules) and ICOS-L, which is the ligand for the T-cell-specific cell surface receptor ICOS and acts as a costimulatory signal for T-cell proliferation and cytokine secretion, were not changed ($p>0.05$) on HLA-A2$^+$ breast cancer, colon cancer and pancreatic cancer cell lines after lenalidomide treatment (Figure 3B). Similarly, no drug-related change ($p>0.05$) was noted in expression of the inhibitory program-death ligands PD-L1 or PD-L2 on tumor cells (Figure 3C).

Lenalidomide increases IFN-γ production and granzyme B upregulation by memory $CD3^+CD8^+$ T cells of XBP1-CTL in response to various solid tumor cells

In our previous studies, XBP1-CTL induced using the HLA-A2-specific XBP1 $US_{184-192}$ (YISPWILAV) and XBP1 $SP_{367-375}$ (YLFPQLISV) peptides displayed HLA-A2-restricted and antigen-specific activities against breast cancer, colon cancer and pancreatic cancer cells [18]. In current studies, we further evaluated XBP1-CTL post-lenalidomide treatment for their specific anti-tumor activity by measuring IFN-γ production and granzyme B expression against the respective HLA-A2$^+$ solid tumor cells. As compared to the XBP1-CTL control, lenalidomide-treated XBP1-CTL (n=3) showed increased IFN-γ production in response to HLA-A2$^+$ MDA-MB231 (breast cancer), Panc1 (pancreatic cancer) or SW480 (colon cancer) cells (Figure 4A). The anti-tumor response of XBP1-CTL was further investigated within the $CD45RO^+$ memory or $CD45RO^-$ non-memory $CD3^+CD8^+$ T cell populations in response to the respective tumor cell lines. Compared to non-memory cells, the memory cells of XBP1-CTL demonstrated significantly greater anti-tumor activities, measured by granzyme B upregulation and IFN-γ production. The activities of different memory cell subsets were specifically enhanced after lenalidomide treatment in XBP1-CTL (n=3) against breast cancer (MDA-MB231; Figure 4B), pancreatic cancer (Panc1; Figure 4C) and colon cancer (SW480; Figure 4D) cells.

Lenalidomide enhances tumor-specific central memory cell proliferation within XBP1-CTL

Previously, we have shown that memory $CD3^+CD8^+$ T cells are the major cell subset within XBP1-CTL that proliferate in response to various solid tumor cells [18]. Here, we further evaluated the effect of lenalidomide on XBP1-CTL proliferative capacity in CFSE-based assays. First, anti-tumor specific cell proliferation was measured by gating on the CFSE-low $CD3^+CD8^+$ T cell population, and then analyzing for the specific naïve:memory CTL subset involved. Lenalidomide treated XBP1-CTL showed a distinctive cell proliferation pattern, while was restricted mainly to the central memory ($CD45RO^+CCR7^+$) $CD3^+CD8^+$ T cell subset, in response to the respective solid tumor cells including HLA-A2$^+$ breast cancer (MDA-MB231; 89% CM proliferation), colon cancer (SW480; 92% CM proliferation) or pancreatic cancer (Panc1; 93% CM proliferation) cells (Figure 5A). Upon identification of the CM subset as the predominant proliferating population, we next investigated the specific phenotypic cell populations proliferating within the XBP1-CTL. These analyses revealed higher proliferation (Q1) of CD28-positive (Figure 5B) and CD38-positive (Figure 5C) cells within XBP1-CTL by lenalidomide treatment against breast cancer (MDA-MB231; 37% $CD28^+$, 39% $CD38^+$ proliferation), colon cancer (SW480; 24% $CD28^+$, 26% $CD38^+$ proliferation) or pancreatic cancer (Panc1; 18% $CD28^+$, 11% $CD38^+$ proliferation) cells. In contrast, control XBP1-CTL did not show any specific cell proliferation in the absence of tumor cell stimulation (Figure 5B; 5% $CD28^+$ proliferation, Figure 5C; 6% $CD38^+$ proliferation). Furthermore, lenalidomide did not trigger proliferation (Q1) of CTL expressing immune checkpoint inhibitors CTLA-4 (Figure 5D) or PD-1 (Figure 5E) in response to the various HLA-A2$^+$ tumor cells. XBP1-CTL proliferation after lenalidomide treatment was mainly restricted to CTLA-4 negative (Q3, Figure 5D) or PD-1 negative (Q3, Figure 5E) $CD3^+CD8^+$ T cells. These responses were consistent against the various solid tumors including MDA-MB231 breast cancer cells (33% CTLA-4$^-$ proliferation, 30% PD1$^-$ proliferation), SW480 colon cancer cells (14% CTLA-4$^-$ proliferation,

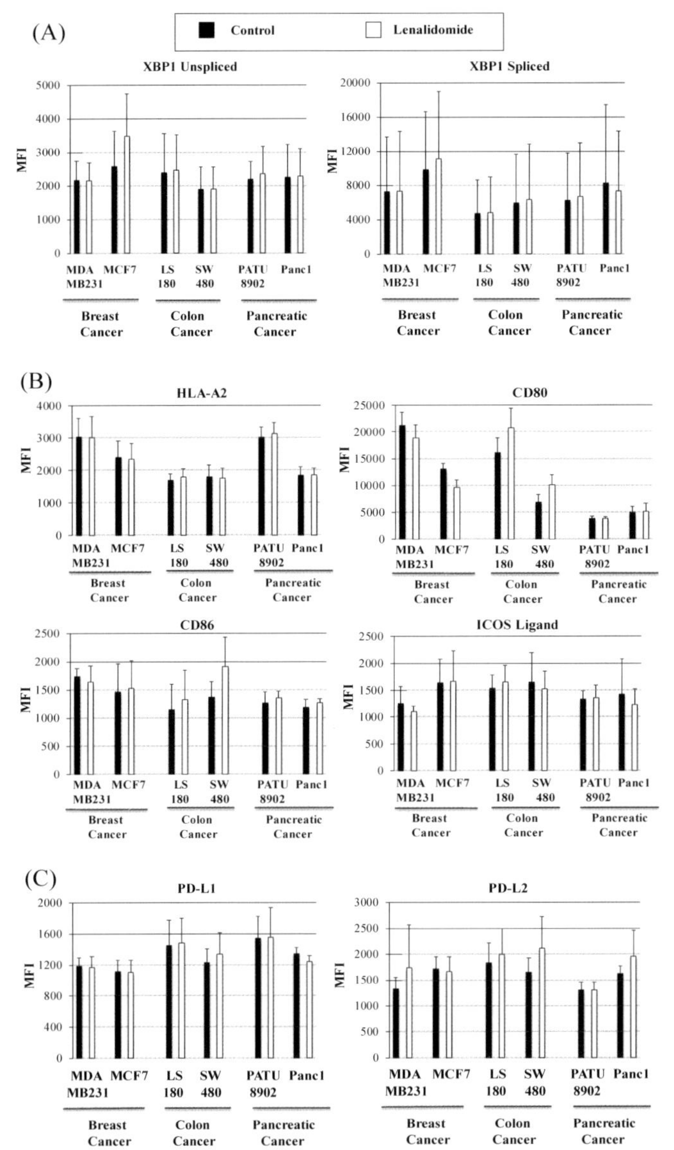

Figure 3: Lenalidomide treatment does not affect expression of intracellular XBP1 proteins and surface antigens on breast, colon and pancreatic cancer cells.

The effect of lenalidomide (5 μm, 4 days) was evaluated on the antigen expression of various cancer cells; breast cancer (MDA-MB231, MCF7), colon cancer (LS180, SW480), pancreatic cancer (PATU8902, Panc1). No major changes were detected in the expression levels of (A) intracellular XBP1 unspliced and XBP1 spliced proteins, (B) surface HLA-A2, CD80, CD86 and ICOS ligand, nor (C) surface PD-L1 and PD-L2. Results were obtained by flow cytometry analyses and shown as the MFI (mean fluorescence intensity; n=3, mean ± SE. Groups were compared using an unpaired Student's t-test and no differences ($p > 0.05$) were seen in MFI between control and lenalidomide treated tumor cells.

13% $PD1^-$ proliferation) or Panc1 pancreatic cancer cells (16% $CTLA\text{-}4^-$ proliferation, 12% $PD1^-$ proliferation).

Lenalidomide increases T-bet expression in the XBP1-CTL, along with IFN- γ production, in response to solid tumor cells

T-bet is an important transcription regulator which promotes the generation and function of effector and memory $CD8^+$ T cells. In previous studies, we have shown that XBP1 antigen-specific CTL generated with a cocktail of HLA-A2-specific heteroclitic XBP1 $US_{184-192}$ (YISPWILAV) and XBP1 $SP_{367-375}$ (YLFPQLISV) peptides express high levels of T-bet [18]. In these studies, we further evaluated the effect of lenalidomide treatment on XBP1-CTL (n=3) functional activities associated with its T-bet expression and function, in response to each type of solid tumor cells. Our results showed that the frequency of T-bet expressing and IFN-γ producing XBP1-CTL was consistently higher in total $CD3^+CD8^+$ T cells after lenalidamide treatment, as compared to untreated XBP1-CTL in response to breast cancer (MDA-MB231, Figure 6A), pancreatic cancer (Pancl, Figure 6B) or colon cancer (SW480, Figure 6C) cells. Importantly, the $T\text{-}bet^+$ $IFN\text{-}\gamma^+$ cells observed within the lenalidomide treated XBP1-CTL were confined to memory $CD3^+CD8^+$ T cells, with the greatest increase within the central memory CTL subset (Figures 6A and 6B). In contrast, lenalidomide had no affect on the frequency of $T\text{-}bet^+$ $IFN\text{-}\gamma^+$ cells within the terminal effector CTL population (Figures 6A-6C).

Lenalidomide increases Eomes expression in the XBP1-CTL, along with IFN- γ production, in response to solid tumor cells

Next, the effect of lenalidomide was evaluated on Eomes, another important transcription factor, regulating memory CTL generation. Consistent with T-bet, we observed upregulation of Eomes expression following lenalidomide treatment of XBP1-CTL. In addition, the frequency of $Eomes^+$ $IFN\text{-}\gamma^+/CD3^+$ $CD8^+$ T cells was increased in response to breast cancer (MDA-MB231, Figure 7A), pancreatic cancer (Pancl, Figure 7B) or colon cancer (SW480, Figure 7C) cells in the lenalidomide treated XBP1-CTL. In conjunction with the $T\text{-}bet^+$ CTL and their activities, we detected an increase in the frequency of $Eomes^+$ $IFN\text{-}\gamma^+$ cells within the central memory $CD3^+CD8^+$ T cell subset after lenalidomide treatment (Figures 7A-C). Finally, no or very low levels of $Eomes^+IFN\text{-}\gamma^+/CD3^+$ $CD8^+$ T cells were observed within the terminal effector subset of lenalidomide treated XBP1-CTL. Thereby, these studies demonstrate the critical immune modulatory activity of lenalidomide on memory CTL subsets within antigen-specific effector cells.

Lenalidomide increases the serine/threonine-specific protein kinase AKT expression in memory subsets of XBP1-CTL

Understanding the mechanisms that influence the differentiation of CTL memory formation is critical for development of effective peptide-based cancer vaccines. Thus, we evaluated the impact of lenalidomide on activating the serine/threonine-specific protein kinase Akt, which acts as a critical signal integrator and plays a key role in orchestrating the activation and differentiation of memory $CD8^+$ T cells. Our studies showed the specific upregulation in Akt expression within the $CD45RO^+$ memory $CD3^+$ $CD8^+$ cell population of XBP1-CTL. Increased Akt expression was confined to the memory CTL, but not to non-memory CTL, upon stimulation with breast cancer (MDA-MB231) or colon cancer (SW480) cells (Figure 8A). Lenalidomide induced Akt upregulation was seen in both central memory and effector memory XBP1-CTL subsets, but not the terminal effector subset, in response to breast cancer (MDA-MB231, Figure 8B) and colon cancer (SW480, Figure 8C) cells. Thus, these results demonstrate that lenalidomide treatment affects transcriptional regulators and the Akt signal integrator within memory $CD3^+$ $CD8^+$ T cell populations, resulting in enhanced anti-tumor activities of XBP1 antigen-specific CTL.

Discussion

Following FDA approval of lenalidomide (Revlimid®) to treat patients with del 5q myelodysplastic syndrome and its use in combination with dexamethasone to treat MM patients, there are

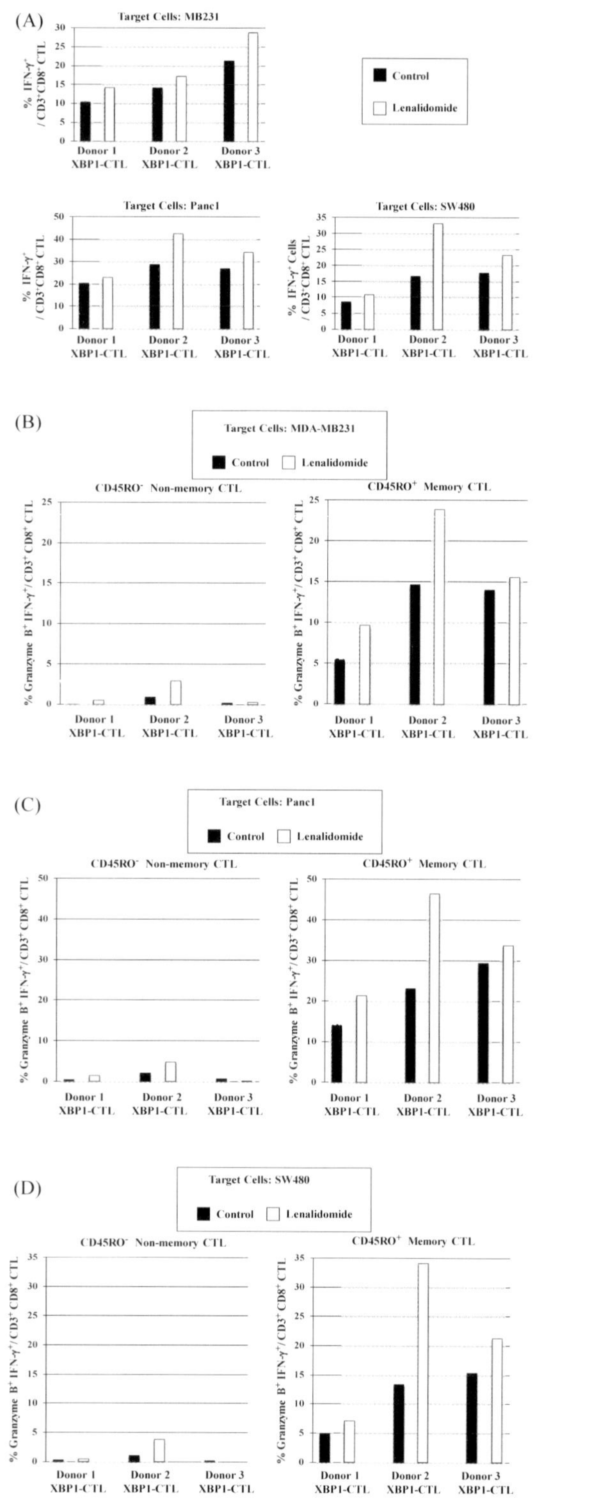

Figure 4: Lenalidomide enhanced anti-tumor activities of XBP1-CTL memory cells against solid tumor cells.
XBP1-CTL (n=3) treated with lenalidomide (5 μm, 4 days) were analyzed for their functional activities against HLA-A2⁺ breast cancer cell (MDA-MB231), pancreatic cancer cell (Panc1) or colon cancer (SW480) cells. (A) Lenalidomide increased IFN-γ production by total $CD3^+CD8^+$ T cells in response to the respective cancer cells. High levels of granzyme B upregulation and IFN-γ production were detected within the $CD45RO^+$ memory CTL population in response to (B) MDA-MB231, (C) Panc1 or (D) SW480 tumor cells. Results are expressed as '% positive cells' of the specific $CD3^+CD8^+$ T cell memory subsets for either single or poly-functional anti-tumor activity.

currently more than 220 clinical trials investigating its therapeutic role in solid tumors. As a single-agent, lenalidomide has been evaluated in patients with advanced brain, thyroid, hepatocellular, pancreatic, renal, breast, and colon cancer [27-29]. However, its ability to elicit tumor-specific immunity, especially its immunomodulatory activity in conjunction with tumor-directed vaccines, has not been well demonstrated. Our studies were designed to evaluate the potential role of an IMiD to enhance tumor-specific activities of antigen-specific CTL. We specifically investigated the effect of lenalidomide on XBP1-specific memory $CD8^+$ CTL against breast cancer, colon cancer and pancreatic cancer cells, which overexpress XBP1 unspliced and spliced antigens.

XBP1 is a critical transcription activator participating in the UPR, a cellular adaptive mechanism that occurs in majority of tumors, and it allows the tumor cell to survive under stress conditions by increasing its protein folding capacity [30,31]. XBP1 regulates a subset of ER-resident chaperone genes that are essential for protein folding and maturation; and its upregulation has been reported in various human solid tumors including breast cancer, hepatocellular carcinoma, pancreatic adenocarcinomas and colon cancer patients [32-38]. During ER stress, an ER transmembrane inositol-requiring enzyme 1 (IRE1) oligomerizes, autophosphorylates, and via its endoribonuclease activity excises a 26 nucleotide intron from unspliced XBP1 mRNA, resulting in production of a potent XBP1 transcription factor that regulates a distinct set of UPR target genes. XBP1 has been demonstrated in the setting of breast cancer, to be an estrogen-regulated gene strongly correlated with estrogen receptor alpha (ERα) expression [20,21,39]. A recent analysis of independent cohorts reported that patients with triple negative breast cancer (TNBC), a form of breast cancer in which tumor cells do not express the genes for estrogen receptor, progesterone receptor, and HER2, have a specific *XBP1* gene expression signature that is strongly associated with poor prognosis; and a demonstrated a tumorgenic function for XBP1 branch of the UPR in TNBC. Importantly, XBP1 pathway activation correlates with poor patient survival in TNBC, suggesting that its specific inhibition may enhance anti-tumor therapies and representing as alternative treatment strategies for this aggressive breast cancer subtype [19]. Additionally, XBP1 mRNA splicing processed by IRE1 causes a reading frame shift which is translated into a spliced form of XBP1 protein, which is an active transcription factor in various cancers. High spliced XBP1 expression is associated with increased tumor growth and poor patient survival [40-42]. Thus, targeting the UPR and its associated molecular components is an emerging novel anti-cancer approach with early success in clinical studies.

With the rationale of targeting XBP1 for selective cancer cell killing, we have previously shown that immunogenic heteroclitic XBP1 peptides can evoke antigen-specific CTL with anti-tumor activities against MM cells and various solid tumor cancers [18,24-26]. In the current studies, we investigated the immunomodulatory effects of lenalidomide on XBP1-specific CTL phenotype and anti-tumor activities. Consistent with our previous study [26], lenalidomide induces cellular activation (high CD69 and CD38), upregulates CD28 and CD40L co-stimulatory antigen expression, but not inhibitory CTLA-4 nor PD-1 molecules, suggesting its potential beneficial effect to enhance immune responses of XBP1-CTL against tumors. CTL phenotypic changes induced by lenalidomide treatment correlated with their enhanced anti-tumor capacity, including IFN-γ and granzyme B production against a variety of solid tumor cancers. In agreement with other studies [43,44], our results provide direct support for a combination therapy using lenalidomide to increase cancer vaccine

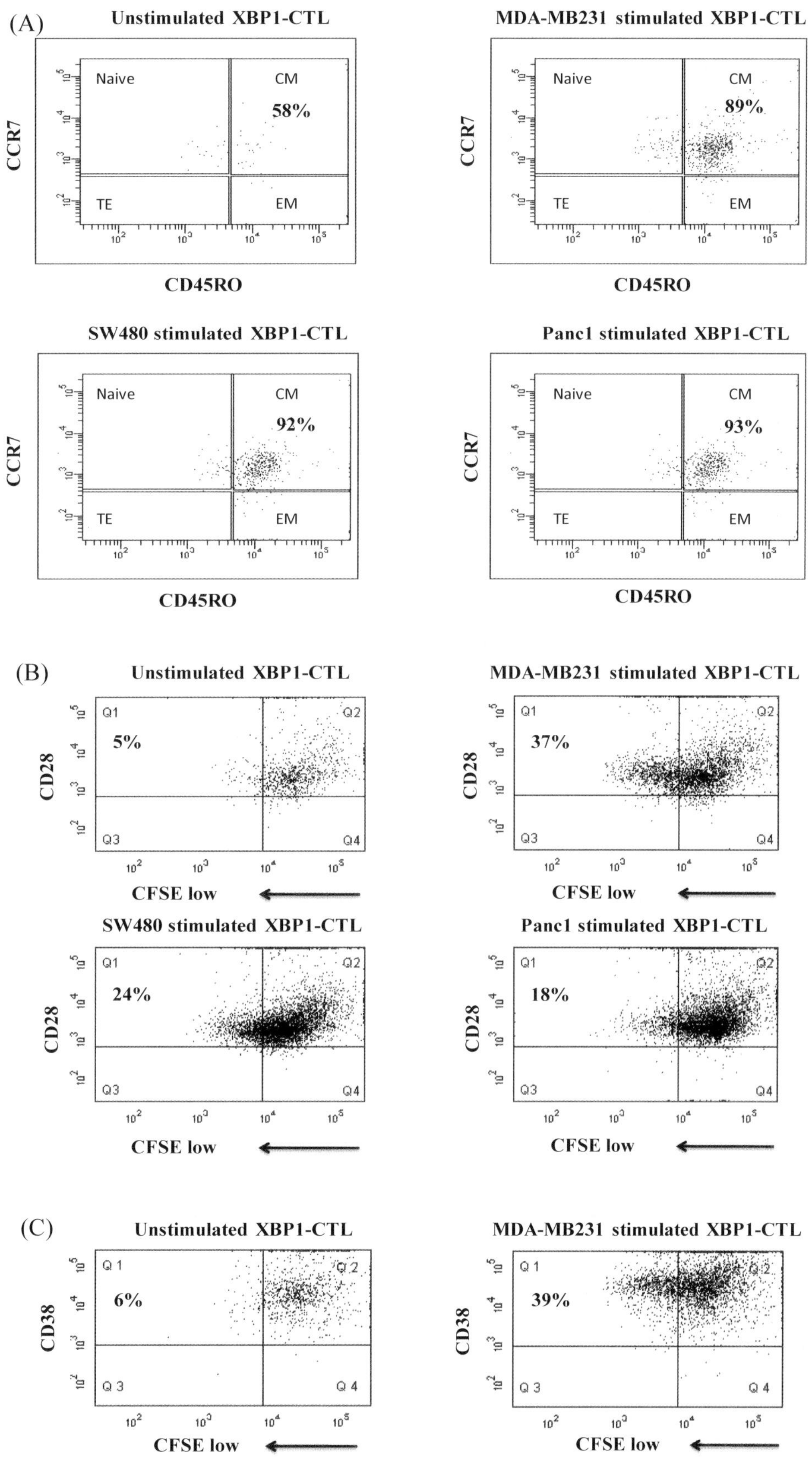
(A)
Unstimulated XBP1-CTL
Naive
CM
58%
TE
EM
CCR7
CD45RO
MDA-MB231 stimulated XBP1-CTL
89%
SW480 stimulated XBP1-CTL
92%
Panc1 stimulated XBP1-CTL
93%
(B)
Q1
Q2
Q3
Q4
5%
37%
24%
18%
CD28
CFSE low
(C)
6%
39%
CD38

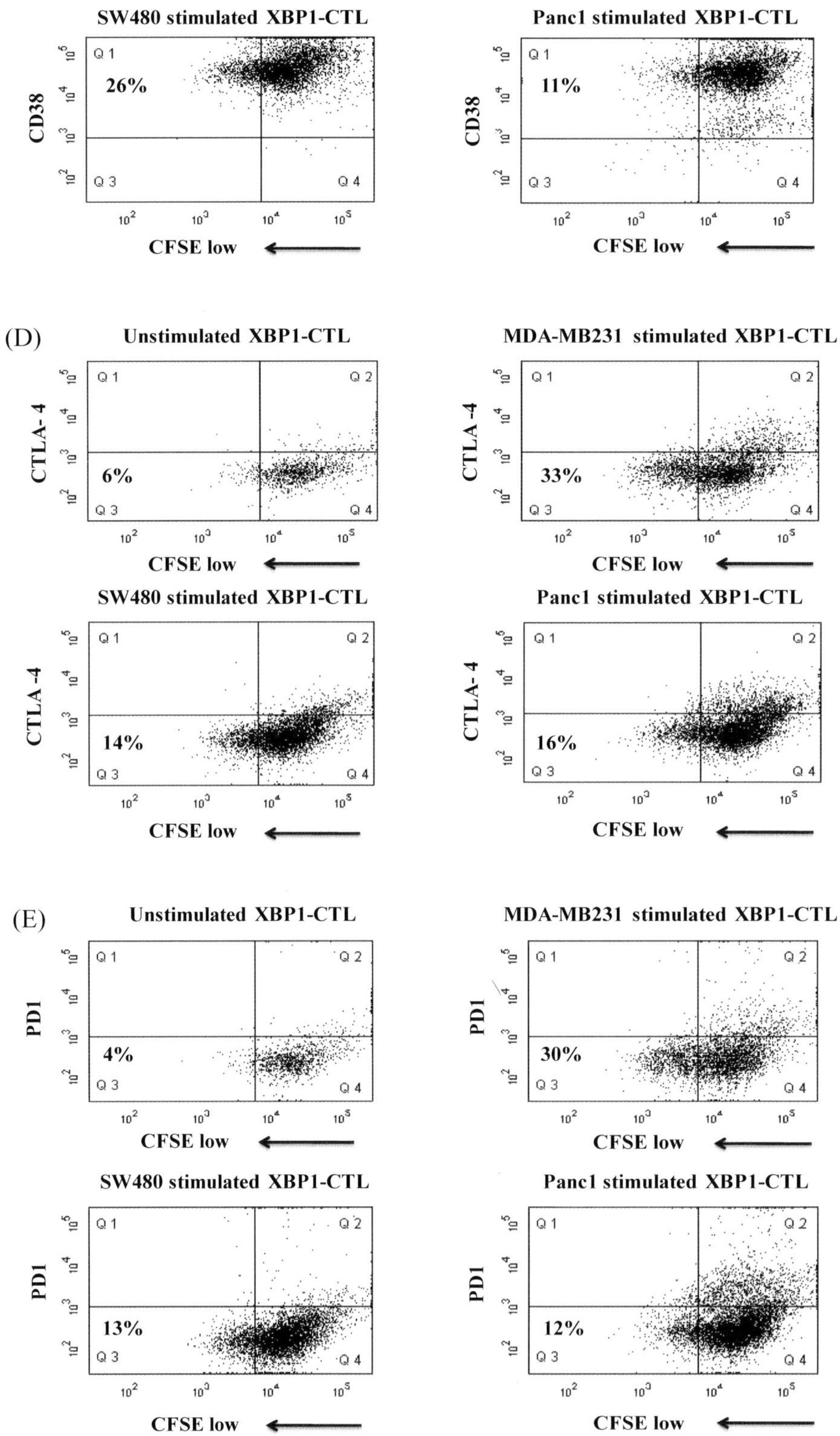

Figure 5: Lenalidomide increased specific XBP1-CTL proliferation to breast cancer, colon cancer or pancreatic cancer cells.
Specific cell proliferation was examined by flow cytometry after stimulating CFSE-labeled XBP1-CTL with tumor cells for 6 days. The proliferating $CD3^{+}CD8^{+}$T cell population was measured as the percent decrease in CFSE expression. Enhanced cell proliferation of lenalidomide treated (5 μm, 4 days) XBP1-CTL was examined in response to irradiated respective tumor cells. Background proliferation was determined using CFSE-labeled lenalidomide treated XBP1-CTL cultured in media alone. (A) The major proliferative response of XBP1-CTL after lenalidomide treatment was detected within the central memory ($CCR7^{+}CD45RO^{+}$) CTL subset against breast cancer (MDA-MB231), colon cancer (SW480) or pancreatic cancer (Panc1) cells. Phenotypic characterization demonstrates that specific cellular proliferation (Q1 gated) to HLA-A2+ breast cancer (MDA-MB231), colon cancer (SW480) or pancreatic cancer (Panc1) cells express (B) CD28 and (C) CD38, but neither (D) CTLA-4 nor (E) PD-1.

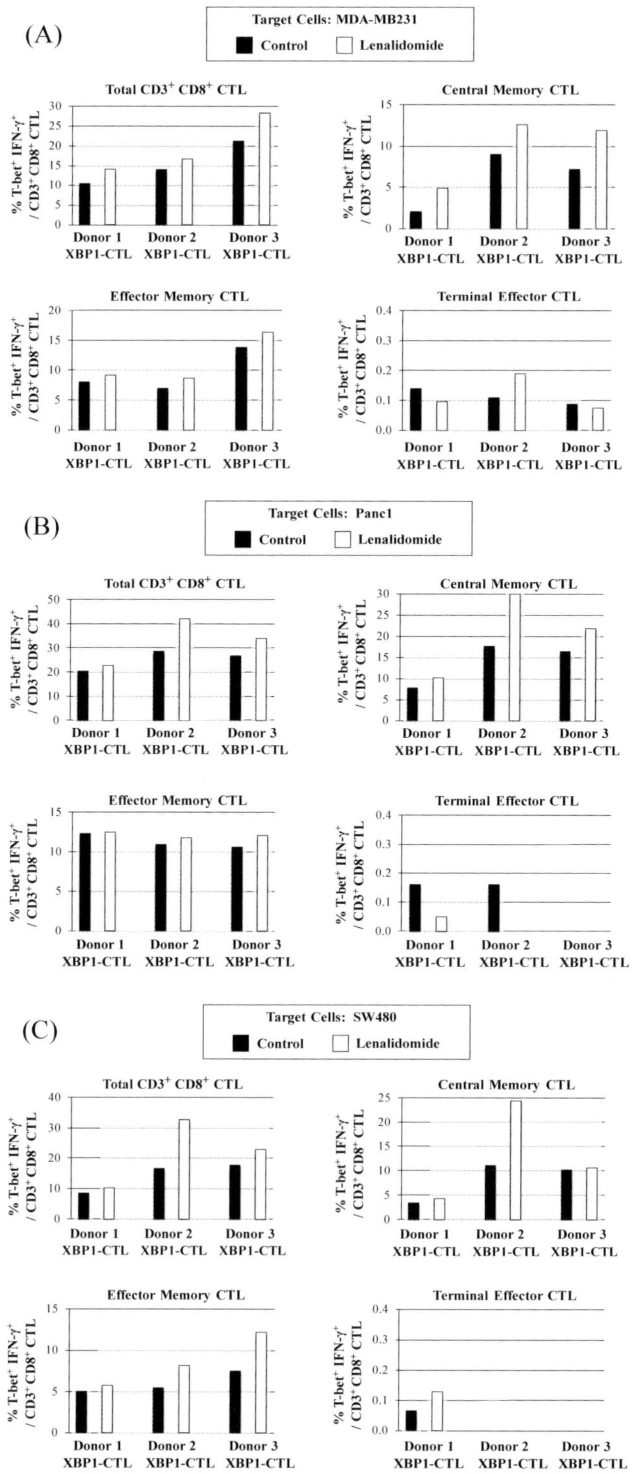

Figure 6: Lenalidomide enhanced T-bet upregulation and IFN-γ production by XBP1-CTL in response to breast cancer, colon cancer or pancreatic cancer cells.

Lenalidomide treated XBP1-CTL (n=3) were evaluated for T-bet expression and IFN-γ production in response to a variety of solid tumor cells by flow cytometric analyses. Lenalidomide increased the frequency of Tbet⁺/IFN-γ+ cells within the total CD3⁺CD8⁺ T cells or specific central (CM) and effector memory (EM) cell subsets, but not the terminal effector (TE) cell subset, by stimulation of XBP1-CTL with (A) breast cancer cells (MDA-MB231), (B) pancreatic cancer cells (Panc1) or (C) colon cancer cells (SW480).

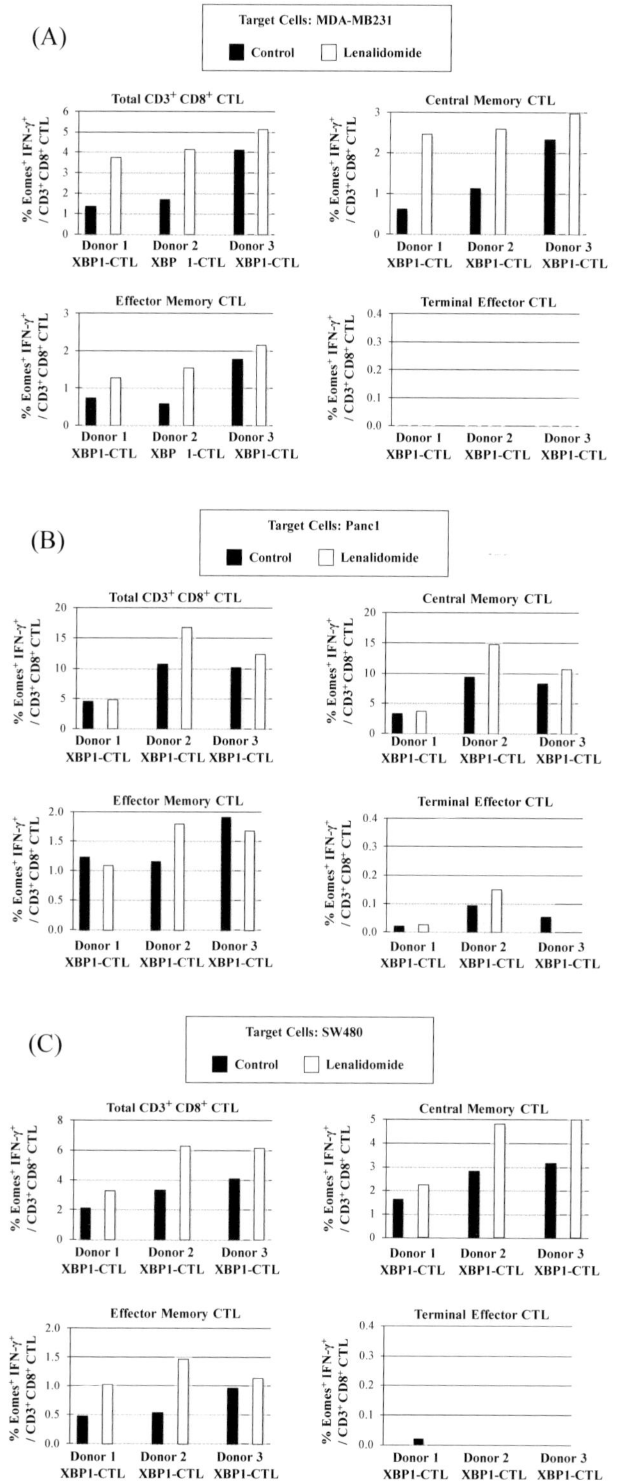

Figure 7. Lenalidomide enhanced Eomes upregulation and IFN-γ production by XBP1-CTL in response to breast cancer, colon cancer or pancreatic cancer cells.

Lenalidomide treated XBP1-CTL (n=3) were evaluated for Eomes expression and IFN- γ production in response to a variety of solid tumor cells by flow cytometric analyses. Lenalidomide increased the frequency of Eomes⁺/IFN-γ⁺ cells within the total CD3⁺CD8⁺ T cells or specific central (CM) and effector memory (EM) cell subsets, but not the terminal effector (TE) cell subset, by stimulation of XBP1-CTL with (A) breast cancer cells (MDA-MB231), (B) pancreatic cancer cells (Panc1) or (C) colon cancer cells (SW480).

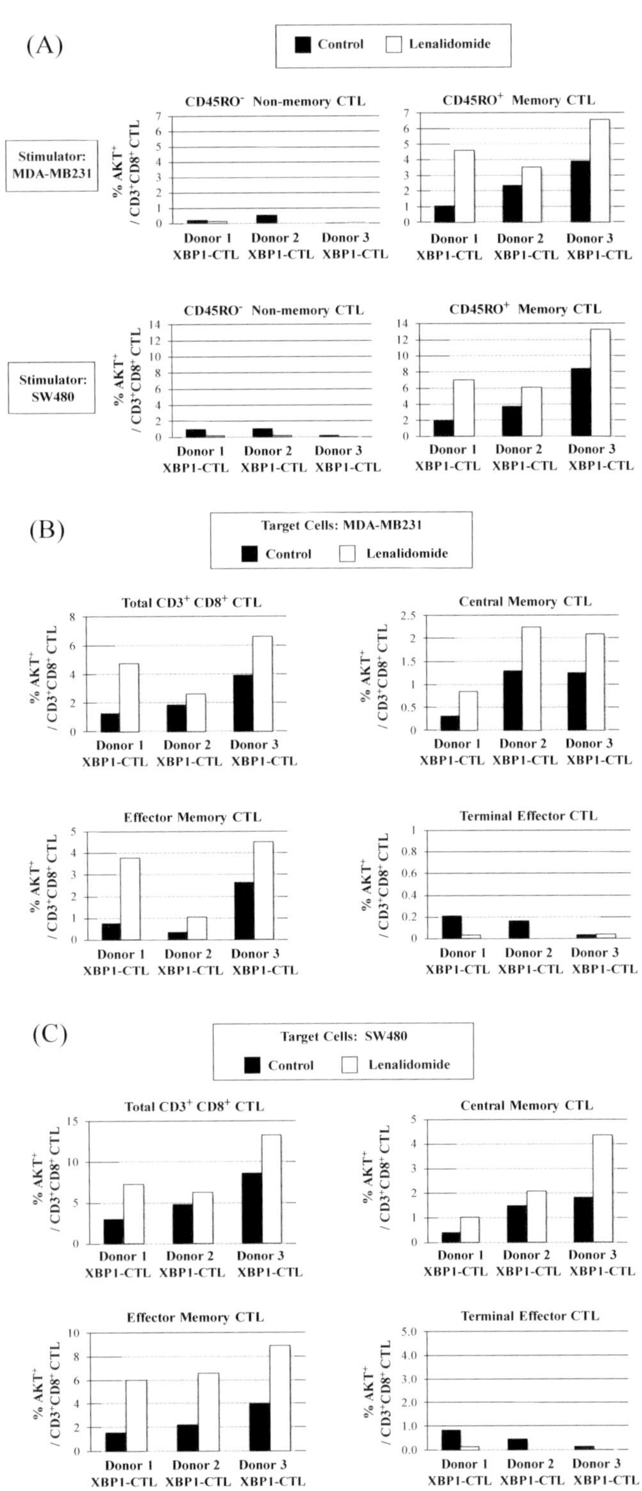

Figure 8: Lenalidomide enhanced Akt activation in memory subsets of XBP1-CTL in response to tumor cells.

Lenalidomide treated XBP1-CTL (n=3) were evaluated for Akt activation upon stimulation by flow cytometry analyses. (A) Lenalidomide treated XBP1-CTL (n=3) showed the upregulation of Akt in the CD45RO$^+$ memory CD3$^+$CD8$^+$ T cell population, but not in the CD45RO$^-$ non-memory CD3$^+$CD8$^+$ T cell population, in response to breast cancer cells (MDA-MB231) or colon cancer cells (SW480). Lenalidomide increased the frequency of Akt$^+$ cells within the total CD3$^+$CD8$^+$ T cells or specific central (CM) and effector memory (EM) cell subsets, but not the terminal effector (TE) cell subset, by stimulation of XBP1-CTL with (B) breast cancer cells (MDA-MB231) or (C) colon cancer cells (SW480).

efficacy through various mechanisms of action. Our results emphasize the impact of lenalidomide on antigen-specific central memory CD3$^+$ CD8$^+$ CTL and their tumor-specific immune responses. In contrast, these studies indicate that lenalidomide does not appear to directly affect the expression levels of the intracellular XBP1 target antigens, nor extracellular activation/inhibitory molecules on tumor cells. These observations are consistent with the effect of pomalidomide, another class of IMiD, on tumor cells, suggesting that IMiD treatment has a better potential for modifying effector T cell function than directly influencing antigen expression on tumor cells.

The transcription factors T-bet and Eomes promote the generation and function of effector and memory CD8$^+$ T cells via up-regulation of perforin/granzyme B during the early stages of CD8$^+$ T cell activation, and by inducing migration to inflamed tissues through up-regulation of key chemokine receptors [45-47]. Studies have also demonstrated the contribution of these transcription regulators on anti-tumor immunity by showing that deletion of T-bet and Eomes in CD8$^+$ T cells abrogate the persistence of effector and memory T cells [48]. Furthermore, clinical evidence showed longer patient survival with increased CD8$^+$ T cell expression of T-bet and Eomes [49-51]. A melanoma-specific peptide vaccine trial showed high levels of T-bet expression in vaccine-induced CD8$^+$ CTL, indicating that T-bet expression may be associated with CTL tumor infiltration and anti-tumor activities [52]. Results presented in these studies are consistent with our previous report of increased T-bet and Eomes expression in antigen-specific CTL generated *ex vivo* by immunogenic peptides stimulation [18]. Of particular importance in this study is the role of lenalidomide to enhance T-bet and Eomes expression, and the subsequent increase in functional anti-tumor activities of the effector cells. Specifically, we found that upregulated T-bet and Eomes expression following lenalidomide treatment of XBP1-CTL was mainly confined to the CD45RO$^+$ memory T cell population, with the highest increase observed within the CM CTL subset, which corresponded with higher levels of IFN-γ and granzyme B production and increased cell proliferation in response to the various solid tumor cells.

Successful targeted immunotherapy development requires a better understanding of the signaling pathways that regulate quantity and quality of memory CD8$^+$ T cell development, and the subsequent CTL anti-tumor activities. The serine-threonine kinase Akt has a role as a critical signal integrator that links distinct facets of antigen-specific CTL differentiation to specific signaling pathways of FOXO, mTOR and Wnt/β-catenin [53-55]. To date, how lenalidomide impacts Akt activation on effector T cell function, especially within antigen-specific CTL, is not well characterized. Thus, we investigated its effect on Akt activation within the XBP1 antigen specific-CTL. Our results demonstrated that enhanced Akt expression induced by short-term lenalidomide treatment was confined to the central memory and effector memory antigen-specific CTL subsets and corresponded with high level IFN-g production/granzyme B upregulation and T-bet/Eomes expression in response to tumor cells. The increased Akt activation by lenalidomide treated XBP1-CTL during tumor recognition may be associated with costimulatory signaling molecule CD28, a critical regulator of T cell proliferation and important for T cell activation and effector cells development [56,57]. However, sustained Akt activation might drive differentiation towards terminal effectors [58]; therefore we will investigate this aspect in future studies. Additionally, further studies using lenalidomide during CTL development are required to delineate transcriptional regulators involved, not only in generation of CD8 CTL, but also for long-term maintenance of memory/effector T cells.

In conclusion, we report on the critical role of lenalidomide to enhance anti-tumor activities (IFN-γ production, granzyme B upregulation, memory CTL proliferation) of XBP1 antigen-specific CTL through upregulation of key T cell activation markers/costimulatory molecules and downregulation of inhibitory molecules, which were associated with induction of Th1-specific transcription regulators and a signal integrator. Importantly, short-term lenalidomide exposure further increased the proportion of $CD45RO^+CCR7^+$ central memory $CD3^+CD8^+$ T cell subset within the XBP1-CTL, leading to enhanced anti-tumor activities against breast cancer, colon cancer and pancreatic cancer cells. These data provide the framework for a combination immunotherapeutic strategy encompassing both a cancer vaccine and IMiD to both enhance vaccine efficacy and promote long-lasting immune responses against cancer.

Acknowledgement

We thank Mr. John Daley and Ms. Suzan Lazo-Kallanian from the Flow Cytometry facility at Dana Farber Cancer Institute for providing flow cytometry assistance. This work was supported in part by grants from the National Institutes of Health Grants R01-124929 to Dr. Nikhil C. Munshi, P50-100007, P01-78378 and P01155258 to Drs. Kenneth C. Anderson and Nikhil C. Munshi, and R01-50947 to Dr. Kenneth C. Anderson. This research was also supported in part by a generous donation from Mr. and Mrs. Stewart Nagler. Dr. Kenneth C. Anderson is an American Cancer Society Clinical Research Professor.

References

1. Soares KC, Rucki AA, Wu AA, Olino K, Xiao Q, et al. (2015) PD-1/PD-L1 blockade together with vaccine therapy facilitates effector T-cell infiltration into pancreatic tumors. J Immunother 38: 1-11.

2. Schlößer HA, Theurich S, Shimabukuro-Vornhagen A, Holtick U, Stippel DL, et al. (2014) Overcoming tumor-mediated immunosuppression. Immunotherapy 6: 973-988.

3. Andersen MH (2014) The targeting of immunosuppressive mechanisms in hematological malignancies. Leukemia 28: 1784-1792.

4. Lopez-Girona A, Heintel D, Zhang LH, Mendy D, Gaidarova S, et al. (2011) Lenalidomide downregulates the cell survival factor, interferon regulatory factor-4, providing a potential mechanistic link for predicting response. Br J Haematol 154: 325-336.

5. Zhu YX, Braggio E, Shi CX, Bruins LA, Schmidt JE, et al. (2011) Cereblon expression is required for the antimyeloma activity of lenalidomide and pomalidomide. Blood 118: 4771-4779.

6. Kotla V, Goel S, Nischal S, Heuck C, Vivek K, et al. (2009) Mechanism of action of lenalidomide in hematological malignancies. J Hematol Oncol 2: 36.

7. Henry JY, Labarthe MC, Meyer B, Dasgupta P, Dalgleish AG, et al. (2013) Enhanced cross-priming of naive CD8+ T cells by dendritic cells treated by the IMiDs® immunomodulatory compounds lenalidomide and pomalidomide. Immunology 139: 377-385.

8. Luptakova K, Rosenblatt J, Glotzbecker B, Mills H, Stroopinsky D, et al. (2013) Lenalidomide enhances anti-myeloma cellular immunity. Cancer Immunol Immunother 62: 39-49.

9. LeBlanc R1, Hideshima T, Catley LP, Shringarpure R, Burger R, et al. (2004) Immunomodulatory drug costimulates T cells via the B7-CD28 pathway. Blood 103: 1787-1790.

10. Hsu AK, Quach H, Tai T, Prince HM, Harrison SJ, et al. (2011) The immunostimulatory effect of lenalidomide on NK-cell function is profoundly inhibited by concurrent dexamethasone therapy. Blood 117: 1605-1613.

11. Witzig TE, Wiernik PH, Moore T, Reeder C, Cole C, et al. (2009) Lenalidomide oral monotherapy produces durable responses in relapsed or refractory indolent non-Hodgkin's Lymphoma. J Clin Oncol 27: 5404-5409.

12. Görgün G, Calabrese E, Soydan E, Hideshima T, Perrone G, et al. (2010) Immunomodulatory effects of lenalidomide and pomalidomide on interaction of tumor and bone marrow accessory cells in multiple myeloma. Blood 116: 3227-3237.

13. Koong AC, Chauhan V, Romero-Ramirez L (2006) Targeting XBP-1 as a novel anti-cancer strategy. Cancer Biol Ther 5: 756-759.

14. Liou HC, Boothby MR, Finn PW, Davidon R, Nabavi N, et al. (1990) A new member of the leucine zipper class of proteins that binds to the HLA DR alpha promoter. Science 247: 1581-1584.

15. Reimold AM, Iwakoshi NN, Manis J, Vallabhajosyula P, Szomolanyi-Tsuda E, et al. (2001) Plasma cell differentiation requires the transcription factor XBP-1. Nature 412: 300-307.

16. Davies FE, Dring AM, Li C, Rawstron AC, Shammas MA, et al. (2003) Insights into the multistep transformation of MGUS to myeloma using microarray expression analysis. Blood 102: 4504-4511.

17. Bagratuni T, Wu P, Gonzalez de Castro D, Davenport EL, Dickens NJ, et al. (2010) XBP1s levels are implicated in the biology and outcome of myeloma mediating different clinical outcomes to thalidomide-based treatments. Blood 116: 250-253.

18. Bae J, Samur M, Munshi A, Hideshima T, Keskin D, Kimmelman A, et al. Heteroclitic XBP1 Peptides Evoke Tumor-Specific Memory Cytotoxic T Lymphocytes against Breast Cancer, Colon Cancer, and Pancreatic Cancer Cells. OncoImmunology (in press).

19. Chen X, Iliopoulos D, Zhang Q, Tang Q, Greenblatt MB, et al. (2014) XBP1 promotes triple-negative breast cancer by controlling the HIF1Î± pathway. Nature 508: 103-107.

20. Spiotto MT, Banh A, Papandreou I, Cao H, Galvez MG, et al. (2010) Imaging the unfolded protein response in primary tumors reveals microenvironments with metabolic variations that predict tumor growth. Cancer Res 70: 78-88.

21. Romero-Ramirez L, Cao H, Nelson D, Hammond E, Lee AH, et al. (2004) XBP1 is essential for survival under hypoxic conditions and is required for tumor growth. Cancer Res 64: 5943-5947.

22. Koong AC, Feldman D (2007) Irestatin, a potent inhibitor of IRE1 and the unfolded protein response, is a hypoxia-selective cytotoxin and impairs tumor growth. Journal of Clinical Oncology, 2007 ASCO Annual Meeting Proceedings (Post-Meeting Edition) 25:3514.

23. Futamura Y, Tashiro E, Hironiwa N, Kohno J, Nishio M, et al. (2007) Trierixin, a novel Inhibitor of ER stress-induced XBP1 activation from Streptomyces sp. II. structure elucidation. J Antibiot (Tokyo) 60: 582–585.

24. Bae J, Carrasco R, Lee AH, Prabhala R, Tai YT, et al. (2011) Identification of novel myeloma-specific XBP1 peptides able to generate cytotoxic T lymphocytes: a potential therapeutic application in multiple myeloma. Leukemia 25: 1610-1619.

25. Bae J, Smith R, Daley J, Mimura N, Tai YT, et al. (2012) Myeloma-specific multiple peptides able to generate cytotoxic T lymphocytes: a potential therapeutic application in multiple myeloma and other plasma cell disorders. Clin Cancer Res 18: 4850-4860.

26. Bae J, Prabhala R, Voskertchian A, Brown A, Maguire C, et al. (2015) A multiepitope of XBP1, CD138 and CS1 peptides induces myeloma-specific cytotoxic T lymphocytes in T cells of smoldering myeloma patients. Leukemia 29: 218-229.

27. Segler A, Tsimberidou AM (2012) Lenalidomide in solid tumors. Cancer Chemother Pharmacol 69: 1393-1406.

28. Fine HA, Kim L, Albert PS, Duic JP, Ma H, et al. (2007) A phase I trial of lenalidomide in patients with recurrent primary central nervous system tumors. Clin Cancer Res 13: 7101-7106.

29. Liu WM, Henry JY, Meyer B, Bartlett JB, Dalgleish AG, et al. (2009) Inhibition of metastatic potential in colorectal carcinoma in vivo and in vitro using immunomodulatory drugs (IMiDs). Br J Cancer 101: 803-812.

30. Luo B, Lee AS (2013) The critical roles of endoplasmic reticulum chaperones and unfolded protein response in tumorigenesis and anticancer therapies. Oncogene 32: 805-818.

31. Suh DH, Kim MK, Kim HS, Chung HH, Song YS (2012) Unfolded protein response to autophagy as a promising druggable target for anticancer therapy. Ann N Y Acad Sci 1271: 20-32.

32. Sengupta S, Sharma CG, Jordan VC (2010) Estrogen regulation of X-box binding protein-1 and its role in estrogen induced growth of breast and endometrial cancer cells. Horm Mol Biol Clin Investig 2: 235-243.

33. Fujimoto T, Onda M, Nagai H, Nagahata T, Ogawa K, et al. (2003) Upregulation

and overexpression of human X-box binding protein 1 (hXBP-1) gene in primary breast cancers. Breast Cancer 10: 301-306.

34. Malhi H, Kaufman RJ (2011) Endoplasmic reticulum stress in liver disease. J Hepatol 54: 795-809.

35. Shuda M, Kondoh N, Imazeki N, Tanaka K, Okada T, et al. (2003) Activation of the ATF6, XBP1 and grp78 genes in human hepatocellular carcinoma: a possible involvement of the ER stress pathway inhepatocarcinogenesis. J Hepatol 38: 605-614.

36. Hess DA, Humphrey SE, Ishibashi J, Damsz B, Lee AH, et al. (2011) Extensive pancreas regeneration following acinar-specific disruption of Xbp1 in mice. Gastroenterology 141: 1463-1472.

37. Um HJ, Bae JH, Park JW, Suh H, Jeong NY, et al. (2010) Differential effects of resveratrol and novel resveratrol derivative, HS-1793, on endoplasmic reticulum stress-mediated apoptosis and Akt inactivation. Int J Oncol 36: 1007-1013.

38. Protiva P, Hopkins ME, Baggett S, Yang H, Lipkin M, et al. (2008) Growth inhibition of colon cancer cells by polyisoprenylated benzophenones is associated with induction of the endoplasmic reticulum response. Int J Cancer 123: 687-694.

39. Lee AH, Iwakoshi NN, Glimcher LH (2003) XBP-1 regulates a subset of endoplasmic reticulum resident chaperone genes in the unfolded protein response. Mol Cell Biol 23: 7448-7459.

40. Mori K (2003) Frame switch splicing and regulated intramembrane proteolysis: key words to understand the unfolded protein response. Traffic 4: 519-528.

41. Calfon M, Zeng H, Urano F, Till JH, Hubbard SR, et al. (2002) IRE1 couples endoplasmic reticulum load to secretory capacity by processing the XBP-1 mRNA. Nature 415: 92-96.

42. Gomez BP, Riggins RB, Shajahan AN, Klimach U, Wang A, et al. (2007) Human X-box binding protein-1 confers both estrogen independence and antiestrogen resistance in breast cancer cell lines. FASEB J 21: 4013-4027.

43. Sakamaki I, Kwak LW, Cha SC, Yi Q, Lerman B, et al. (2014) Lenalidomide enhances the protective effect of a therapeutic vaccine and reverses immune suppression in mice bearing established lymphomas.Leukemia 28: 329-337.

44. Noonan K, Rudraraju L, Ferguson A, Emerling A, Pasetti MF, et al. (2012) Lenalidomide-induced immunomodulation in multiple myeloma: impact on vaccines and antitumor responses. Clin Cancer Res 18: 1426-1434.

45. Joshi NS, Cui W, Dominguez CX, Chen JH, Hand TW, et al. (2011) Increased numbers of preexisting memory CD8 T cells and decreased T-bet expression can restrain terminal differentiation of secondary effector and memory CD8 T cells. J Immunol 187: 4068-4076.

46. Zhu Y, Ju S, Chen E, Dai S, Li C, et al. (2010) T-bet and eomesodermin are required for T cell-mediated antitumor immune responses. J Immunol 185: 3174-3183.

47. Lord GM, Rao RM, Choe H, Sullivan BM, Lichtman AH, et al. (2005) T-bet is required for optimal proinflammatory CD4+ T-cell trafficking. Blood 106: 3432-3439.

48. Li G, Yang Q, Zhu Y, Wang HR, Chen X, et al. (2013) T-Bet and Eomes Regulate the Balance between the Effector/Central Memory T Cells versus Memory Stem Like T Cells. PLoS One 8: e67401.

49. Pipkin ME, Sacks JA, Cruz-Guilloty F, Lichtenheld MG, Bevan MJ, et al. (2010) Interleukin-2 and inflammation induce distinct transcriptional programs that promote the differentiation of effector cytolytic T cells. Immunity 32: 79-90.

50. Intlekofer AM, Takemoto N, Kao C, Banerjee A, Schambach F, et al. (2007) Requirement for T-bet in the aberrant differentiation of unhelped memory CD8+ T cells. J Exp Med 204: 2015-2021.

51. Chen LJ, Zheng X, Shen YP, Zhu YB, Li Q, et al. (2013) Higher numbers of T-bet(+) intratumoral lymphoid cells correlate with better survival in gastric cancer. Cancer Immunol Immunother 62: 553-561.

52. Clancy-Thompson E, King LK, Nunnley LD, Mullins IM, Slingluff CL Jr, et al. (2013) Peptide vaccination in Montanide adjuvant induces and GM-CSF increases CXCR3 and cutaneous lymphocyte antigen expression by tumor antigen-specific CD8 T cells. Cancer Immunol Res 1: 332-339.

53. Rao RR, Li Q, Gubbels Bupp MR, Shrikant PA (2012) Transcription factor Foxo1 represses T-bet-mediated effector functions and promotes memory CD8(+) T cell differentiation. Immunity 36: 374-387.

54. Araki K, Turner AP, Shaffer VO, Gangappa S, Keller SA, et al. (2009) mTOR regulates memory CD8 T-cell differentiation. Nature 460: 108-112.

55. Kerdiles YM, Beisner DR, Tinoco R, Dejean AS, Castrillon DH, et al. (2009) Foxo1 links homing and survival of naive T cells by regulating L-selectin, CCR7 and interleukin 7 receptor. Nat Immunol 10: 176-184.

56. Cheng J, Hamilton KS, Kane LP (2014) Phosphorylation of Carma1, but not Bcl10, by Akt regulates TCR/CD28-mediated NF-Î°B induction and cytokine production. Mol Immunol 59: 110-116.

57. Kane LP, Andres PG, Howland KC, Abbas AK, Weiss A (2001) Akt provides the CD28 costimulatory signal for up-regulation of IL-2 and IFN-gamma but not TH2 cytokines. Nat Immunol 2: 37-44.

58. Kim EH, Sullivan JA, Plisch EH, Tejera MM, Jatzek A, et al. (2012) Signal integration by Akt regulates CD8 T cell effector and memory differentiation. J Immunol 188: 4305-4314.

Lenalidomide Therapy of Myelodysplastic Syndromes

Ota Fuchs[1]*, Anna Jonasova[2] and Radana Neuwirtova[2]

[1]*Institute of Hematology and Blood Transfusion, Prague, Czech Republic*
[2]*Department of Medicine, Department of Hematology, General University Hospital, Charles University, Prague, Czech Republic*

Abstract

Partial or complete deletion of the long arm of chromosome 5 [del(5q)], with or without additional karyotypic abnormalities, is present in 10-15% of myelodysplastic syndromes (MDS). Anemia in these MDS responds less often to erythroblastic stimulating agents. However, immunomodulatory, anti-cytokine, and anti-angiogenic agent Lenalidomide (CC5013, Revlimid®) leads to red blood cells transfusion independence of low risk MDS with del(5q). The low risk del(5q) MDS is now recognized as a distinct pathologic subtype of MDS with markedly better clinical responses with lenalidomide treatment compared to non del(5q) MDS patients. Several mechanisms of action are believed to contribute to the therapeutic effect of lenalidomide. They include the effect on the immune system, with cytokine production, T- and natural killer cells co-stimulation, stimulation of erythropoiesis, substantional improvement in the hematopoiesis-supporting potential of bone marrow stroma and significant decrease in the adhesion of bone marrow CD34+ cells, and anti-inflammatory effects and angiogenesis inhibition. The exact mechanism of action of lenalidomide on del(5q) clones is not known, but there appears to be several candidate (tumor suppressor) genes whose expression may be modulated by lenalidomide treatment. The addition of lenalidomide inhibited the *in vitro* proliferation of erythroblasts harboring del(5q) while the proliferation of cells from normal controls and cells without 5q deletion was not affected. Patients with mutated *TP53* were shown to have poorer erythroid and cytogenetic responses to lenalidomide and a higher potential for acute myeloid leukemia (AML) evolution. The mechanism of lenalidomide action is different in non-del(5q) MDS, where lenalidomide restores and promotes effective erythropoiesis without direct cytotoxic effect. Recent trials have focused on combining lenalidomide with other agents active in MDS.

Keywords: del(5q) MDS; MDS without 5q Deletion; Lenalidomide; Erythropoiesis; Cell cycle; Apoptosis; Adhesion; SPARC; Phosphatases; p53

Abbreviations: AML: Acute Myeloid Leukemia; AP1: Activator Protein 1; CD: Cluster of Differentiation; DIAPH1: Diaphanous-Related Formin; FISH: Fluorescence In Situ Hybridization; EPO: Erythropoietin; HRQL-Health-Related Quality of Life; ICAM1: Intracellular Adhesion Molecule 1; IFN: Interferon; IL: Interleukin; IPSS: International Prognostic Scoring System; IRAK1: Interleukin-1 Receptor-Associated Kinase; MDS: Myelodysplastic Syndrome; NF-κb: Nuclear Factor κb; RBC: Red Blood Cell; RPS14: Protein of Small Ribosomal Subunit 14; SDF-1: Stromal Cell-Derived Factor 1; SNP: Single Nucleotide Polymorphism; SPARC: Secreted Protein Acidic and Rich in Cysteine; STAT: Signal Transducer and Activator of Transcription; TIRAP: Toll-Interleukin-1 Receptor Domain-Containing Adaptor Protein; TNF: Tumor Necrosis Factor; TRAF6: Tumor Necrosis Factor Receptor-Associated Factor-6; VEGF: Vascular Endothelial Growth Factor

Introduction

Interstitial deletions involving long (q) arm of chromosome 5 are one of the common cytogenetic abnormalities in MDS patients [1-14]. The presence of del(5q), either as the sole karyotype abnormality or as part of a more complex karyotype, is present in 10-15% of patients with *de novo* MDS and has distinct clinical implications for MDS [1]. Outcomes among MDS patients with deletion 5q vary greatly, both in terms of overall survival (OS) and risk of transformation to AML. The presence of additional chromosomal abnormalities or an excess of blasts shortens OS and increases risk of transformation to AML. Del(5q) MDS patients frequently have symptomatic anemia, and its treatment has traditionally consisted of red blood cell (RBC) transfusions and, for some, iron chelation therapy. The 5q- syndrome, a subtype of low risk MDS, is characterized by an isolated 5q deletion. Although the length of the deleted area varies from case to case, deletion in the band 5q32-33 is common. The 5q- syndrome is characterized by a female predominance, severe refractory macrocytic anemia, normal or elevated platelet counts, abnormal hypolobulated megakaryocytes, stable clinical course with relatively rare progression to acute myeloid leukemia (AML). MDS with isolated del(5q) in which the sole cytogenetic abnormality is del(5q) is a distinct entity with the risk of evolution into AML of approximately 10% [11,15]. It is characterized by macrocytic anemia with or without other cytopenias and/or thrombocytosis. Myeloblasts comprise less than 5% of bone marrow and less than 1% of peripheral blood.

Lenalidomide [3-(4-amino-1-oxo1,3-dihydro-2H-isoindol-2-yl)piperidine-2,6-dione; Revlimid; Celgene Corporation, Summit, NJ, USA] is 4-amino-glutarimide analog of thalidomide with potent immunomodulatory, antiangiogenic and direct neoplastic cell inhibitory activity [16-23]. Thalidomide was synthesized in Germany, in 1954, from α-phtaloylisoglutamine, to be used as a sedative and antimetic drug. In 1957, after a short period of preclinical studies, thalidomide was approved for first trimester gestational sickness in humans. The appearance of malformations, such as phocomelia in the newborn, resulted in its ban three years later [21-23]. The US Food and Drug Administration (FDA) approved thalidomide in 1998 for the

***Corresponding author:** Ota Fuchs, PhD, U Nemocnice 1, 128 20 Prague 2, Czech Republic, E-mail: Ota.Fuchs@uhkt.cz treatment of erythema nodosum leprosum [24]. A small but consistent fraction of transfusion-dependent MDS patients achieved transfusion independence by treatment with thalidomide [25-27].

Lenalidomide was developed in order to avoid thalidomide side effects (sedation and neuropathy), and to increase efficacy [16-21]. Lenalidomide shares a number of structural and biological properties with thalidomide but it is safer and more potent than thalidomide. Lenalidomide was first studied in a single- center trial [28]. Erythroid and cytogenetic responses were achieved in a study of 43 patients with MDS, particularly in patients with isolated del(5q31-33) [28]. Lenalidomide was administered in three different dosing schedules: 25 mg daily, 10 mg daily, and 10 mg daily for 21 days of each 28-day cycle [28]. The erythroid response rates were highest in patients with the International Prognostic Scoring System (IPSS) low or intermediate-1 risk MDS. Transfusion independence was achieved in 20 of 32 patients (63%), and three additional patients had reduced red blood cells transfusion needs [28]. Ten of 12 patients (83%) with del(5q31) experienced major erythroid responses, defined as sustained transfusion independence, compared with a 57% response rate in patients with a normal karyotype and a 12% response rate in patients with other cytogenetic abnormalities. Complete cytogenetic remissions were achieved in 75% of the del(5q31) patients (9 of 12 of these patients), with one additional patient achieving at least a 50% decreases in abnormal metaphases [28]. Myelosuppression (neutropenia and/or thrombocytopenia) was the most common adverse event, but it was dose-dependent, favoring the 10 mg daily dose for 21 days of each 28-day cycle.

Multicenter Phase II Trials of Lenalidomide

After encouraging results of a single-center trial (MDS-001) [28] (Table 1), the effect of lenalidomide on red blood cell (RBC) transfusion-dependent del(5q) MDS cases of low and intermediate-1 IPSS risk assessment was investigated in a large multicenter phase II study (MDS-003). This trial led to FDA approval of lenalidomide in the USA as well as to approval in several other countries for treatment of RBC transfusion-dependent anemia due to low or intermediate-1 risk MDS associated with a chromosome 5q deletion with or without additional cytogenetic abnormalities [29]. The initial schedule was 10 mg of lenalidomide for 21 days every 4 weeks, but the treatment schedule was subsequently amended so that the 10 mg dose was given every day because of the shorter interval between initiation of treatment and a response in the pilot study. Of the 148 transfusion-dependent patients who were included in the study, 46 were treated on the 21-day schedule and 102 received continuous daily dosing. Overall, 112 (76%) patients responded to treatment with a median time to response 4.6 weeks. Among these, 99 no longer needed transfusions by week 24, while the remaining 13 patients had a reduction of 50% or greater in the number of transfusions required. There was no significant difference in response rate between the two treatment schedules. Response rate was independent of additional chromosomal aberrations. Patients with pretreatment thrombocytopenia had an inferior outcome. Almost half of the patients, including some with complex karyotypes, had a complete cytogenetic response. Neutropenia and thrombocytopenia were the most common treatment-associated adverse events. Most other adverse events were of low or moderate severity and included pruritus, rash, diarrhea, and fatigue. Adjustment of the lenalidomide dose due to intolerance was required in 124 patients, including 93 of those receiving continuous daily dosing and 31 of those receiving 21-day dosing. Thirty patients discontinued lenalidomide treatment because of adverse events including thrombocytopenia or neutropenia, rash AML, anemia, facial edema, congestive heart failure, urticaria, diarrhea, weight loss, renal insufficiency, cerebrovascular accident, dementia, dyspnea, pyrexia, and pneumonia.

However, the European Medicine Agency (EMA) did not approve lenalidomide for this indication. Their concern, based on results of the MDS-003 trial, was that lenalidomide may trigger progression to AML in some patients with del(5q). Data comparing long-term outcomes in lenalidomide-treated and untreated patients with MDS with del(5q) are limited but it is now clear that the concern of the EMA has not been confirmed by a recent study [30].

Kuendgen et al. [30] have evaluated clinical outcomes of 295 lenalidomide-eated patients from two clinical trials (MDS-003 and MDS-004, Table 1) and 125 untreated red blood cell transfusion-dependent patients with del(5q) low- or intermediate-1-risk MDS from a large multicenter registry. Median follow-up was 4.3 years from first dose for lenalidomide-treated patients and 4.6 years from diagnosis for untreated patients. Risk factors for AML progression and mortality were assessed. In conclusion, lenalidomide treatment did not increase AML progression risk, but instead confered a survival benefit in red blood cell transfusion-dependent patients with del(5q) low- or intermediate-1-risk MDS.

The long term effect of lenalidomide on the 5q-syndrome was investigated retrospectively in 168 patients treated in four MDS trials [31]. For those patients who achieved transfusion-independency, the median duration of response was 2.2 years. In multivariate analysis cytogenetic response, lower bone marrow blast percentage, and lower baseline transfusion burden were independent predictors of prolonged overall survival.

Current recommendation state that treatment with lenalidomide in del(5q) MDS should be continued until disease progression [32]. The question whether interrruption of lenalidomide treatment for patients in remission would be beneficial has been also addressed [33]. It is important for several reasons: 1) it could reduce costs and side effects; 2) it could facilitate disease progression to AML. Different mechanisms have been discussed to explain AML progression. Evidence that pre-therapeutic telomere length was significantly shorter in those patients who ultimately transformed to AML than in those who did not, was presented [34]. Transformation to AML is occasionally observed, paticularly in patients without a cytogenetic response to lenalidomide. Jädersten et al. [35] performed molecular studies in a patient with classical 5q- syndrome with complete erythroid and partial cytogenetic response to lenalidomide, who evolved to high-risk MDS with complex karyotype. Immunohistochemistry of pretreatment marrow biopsies revealed a small fraction of progenitors with overexpression of p53 and sequencing confirmed a *TP53* mutation. *TP53* mutated subclones have not previously been detected in 5q- syndrome and indicates heterogeneity of this disease. Subsequently, *TP53* mutations with a median clone size of 11% (range, 1% to 54%) were detected in 10 from 55 (18%) low-risk MDS or intermediate-1 risk patients with del(5q) by next-generation sequencing [36]. *TP53* mutations are associated with strong nuclear p53 protein expression. Patients with mutation had significantly worse outcome. *TP53* mutations may lead to genetic instability and disease progression. This clonal heterogeneity in low-risk MDS patients with del(5q) may be of importance when assessing the prognosis and selecting the therapy in these patients. It has been speculated that continuous administration of lenalidomide may lead to selective pressure on stem cells that induces genomic instability, resulting in acute leukemia transformation [37].

Trial	Lenalidomide dose	Number of patients	Results	Comments
MDS-001 phase I/II study	Varying doses of oral lenalidomide, ranging from 25 mg daily down to 10 mg for 21 days of every 28-day cycles [28].	43 patients with MDS and transfusion-dependency or symptomatic anemia. All patients were refractory to erythropoietin or had high endogenous erythropoietin levels. 88% of patients had low- or intermediate-1 risk IPSS risk assessment. 60% of patients had del(5q) chromosomal aberration.	This study showed the potential of lenalidomide in erythropoietin-resistant del(5q) MDS but also a role of lenalidomide in erythropoietin-refractory non-del(5q) MDS patients. 83% of patients with del(5q31) MDS responded compared to 53% of patients with a normal karyotype and 12% of patients with other karyotype abnormalities [28].	Responses were definied according to the modified International Working Group (IWG) criteria [61]. Neutropenia and thrombocytopenia were common side effects.
MDS-002 phase II study	10 mg of lenalidomide orally either for 21 of 28 days, or with continuous dosing [42].	215 patients at a median age of 71 years with low or intermediate-1 risk MDS with or without non-del(5q) chromosomal abnormalities.	26 patients were identified as transfusion-independent with a median hemoglobin rise of 3.2 g/dL. A further 17% achieved a reduction of pretreatment transfusion requirements. The duration of response was at least 24 weeks.	Ebert et al. [59] identified a set of erythroid-specific genes with decreased expression in non-del(5q) MDS responders on patient samples from this trial.
MDS-003 phase II study	10 mg of lenalidomide orally for 21 of 28 days with possible dose reductions in case of adverse events to 5 mg daily and 5 mg daily every other day [29].	148 transfusion-dependent, lower-risk, del(5q) patients. 111 had a single del(5q) chromosomal abnormality, and 37 patients had additional chromosomal abnormalities.	64% of patients became transfusion-free (at least 56 days of transfusion independence) and at least 1 g/dL increase in hemoglobin. 44% of patients achieved a complete cytogenetic remission (absence of the del(5q) cytogenetic abnormality).	MDS-003 was a single-arm study. Factors predicting response to lenalidomide in del(5q) MDS were a platelet count decrease by at least 50% in non-thrombocytopenic patients at base-line (before starting with lenalidomide treatment).
MDS-004 phase III study	10 mg of lenalidomide orally for 21 of 28 days, 5 mg of lenalidomide on days 1 to 28, or placebo on days 1 to 28 of 28-day cycles [65].	205 del(5q) MDS patients were randomized 1:1:1 to lenalidomide 10 mg/day, lenalidomide 5 mg/day, or placebo in the double-blind treatment phase.	56.1% of patients treated with 10 mg of lenalidomide, 42.6% of patients treated with 5 mg lenalidomide and 5.9% of patients with placebo achieved red blood cell transfusion independence for at least 26 weeks. Median time to response was about 4 weeks, median maximum of hemoglobin increase was 6.3 g/dL. Complete cytogenetic response rates were 29.4%, 15.6%, and 0% for lenalidomide 10 mg, lenalidomide 5 mg, or placebo.	52 patients (25.4%) progressed in this phase III study to AML with almost 3 years of follow-up.
MDS-005 phase III study	10 mg of lenalidomide orally once daily (administered as one 10 mg lenalidomide capsule and 2 placebo capsules) or placebo (3 placebo capsules) once daily for up to 4 years (see Steensma DP-The Hematologist March 1, 2011 and Celgene MDS 005).	375 low risk (low- or intermediate 1-risk) MDS patients without del(5q) who do not respond to erythropoiesis-stimulating agent therapy and require regular red blood cell transfusions.	Study start date: November 2009; estimated study completion date: December 2018; estimated primary completion date: April 2016 (final data collection date for primary outcome measure).	clinicaltrials.gov Identifier: NCT01029262 (A servise of the U.S. National Institutes of Health). This international a phase III trial, double-blind is being conducted at more than 70 medical centers in 14 countries, including 9 centers in the United States and Canada.

Table 1: Trials in lenalidomide approved for use in MDS by the United States Food and Drug Administration (FDA).

Longest transfusion-free intervals are achieved in patients low-risk MDS patients with del(5q) who are exposed to lenalidomide 6 months beyond complete cytogenetic remission [33,38-41]. Lenalidomide should not be withdrawn prematurely in patients who achieve transfusion independence as partial cytogenetic remission patients seem to have a higher relapse rate than complete cytogenetic remission patients.

Response rate to lenalidomide in low- or intermediate-1-risk MDS without a 5q deletion was investigated also in a multicenter, phase II study (MDS-002) [42] (Table 1). 214 patients received 10 mg oral lenalidomide daily or 10 mg on days 1 to 21 of a 28-day cycle. The most common grade 3/4 adverse events were neutropenia (30%) and thrombocytopenia (25%). 56 (26%) patients achieved transfusion independence after a median of 4.8 weeks of treatment with a median duration of transfusion independence of 41.0 weeks. A 50% or greater reduction in transfusion requirements occured in 37 additional patients, yielding a 43% overall rate of hematologic improvement (in comparison with 76% in the case of low- or intermediate-1-risk MDS patients with del(5q)). Responding karyotypes included trisomy 8 (n=3), -Y (n=3), deletion 11q (n=2), and deletion 17p (n=1). While clonal suppression represents the main mechanism of lenalidomide action in MDS patients with del(5q), the restoration and promotion of effective erythropoiesis is the main mechanism in non-del(5q) MDS patients [43].

Sibon et al. [44] have recently reported 31 lower-risk non-del(5q) MDS patients with anemia refractory to erythropoiesis-stimulating agents (ESA) and treated with lenalidomide. Twenty patients from this group also received an ESA. An erythroid response was obtained in 15 patients (48%), including 10 of the 27 (37%) previously transfusion-dependent patients, who became transfusion-independent. Nine of responders relapsed, whereas 6 (40%) were still responding and transfusion free after 11 months. Median response duration was 24 months.

These studies were based on scientific knowledge because small deletions in several ribosomal genes, including *RPS14*, were found in CD34+ cells not only in patients with del(5q) but also in patients with non-del(5q) MDS. This observation suggested that deregulated ribosomal biogenesis may not be limited to del(5q) MDS [45-47]. Czibere et al. [48] showed that lower risk non-del(5q) MDS patients with *RPS14* haploinsufficiency tend to have prolonged survival. Defective ribosomal biogenesis has a lead role in disrupting erythropoiesis in a variety of anemias. Disruption of ribosomal biogenesis has been clearly demonstrated in multiple ribosomopathies to greatly perturb p53 signaling [49-58].

Bone marrow aspirates of patients who responded to lenalidomide showed before treatment decreased expression of the set of the genes needed for erythroid differentiation. Lenalidomide seems to overcome differentiation block in del(5q) patients with decreased expression of these genes compared to the non-responders [58]. Thus, lenalidomide restored erythroid differentiation potential by upregulation of the suppressed erythroid gene signature (genes for α- and β-globin, ankyrin 1, band 3, band 4.2, carbonic anhydrase, ferrochelatase and glycophorin B) [59].

The "Groupe Francophone des Myélodysplasies" conducted a multicenter phase 2 trial with lenalidomide in intermediate-2 (19 patients) and high-risk MDS (28 patients) with del(5q) [60]. Forty seven patients (24 males and 23 females, with a median age of 69 years, range, 36-84 years) were treated. Forty three patients of 47 patients had transfusion-dependent anemia. Patients received 10 mg lenalidomide once daily orally during 21 days every 4 weeks. In patients without response after 8 weeks, the lenalidomide dose was increased to 15 mg/day in the same time schedule during an additional 8 weeks. If no response was found in this additional time of treatment, lenalidomide was discontinued. Thirteen of the 47 patients (27%) achieved response according to International Working Group (IWG) 2006 criteria [61]. Median duration of overall response was 6.5 months, 11.5 months in patients who achieved the complete remission. Grade 3 and 4 neutropenia and thrombocytopenia were seen in most patients.

Möllgård et al. [62] hypothesized that increasing doses of lenalidomide may be successfully used in high-risk MDS and AML with chromosome 5 abnormalities. They tested this hypothesis in prospective phase II multicenter trial with 28 patients (12 with intermediate-risk 2 or high-risk MDS and 16 with AML). Oral lenalidomide was given at a dose of 10 mg/day in weeks 1 to 5. The dose was increased to 20 mg/day in weeks 6 to 9, and to 30 mg/day in weeks 10 to 16. In the case of suspected drug-related toxicity the dose was lowered to 5 mg/day. The overall response rate in treated patients with MDS was 36% (4/11) and that for AML patients was 20% (3/15). Seven patients stopped therapy due to progressive disease and nine because of complications, most of which were disease-related. Patients with *TP53* mutations responded less well than those without mutations. No responses were observed among 11 cases with deleterious *TP53* mutation [62].

Randomized Phase III Placebo-controlled Study of Lenalidomide in del(5q) Patients

This study [63-67] (Table 1) examined the safety of lenalidomide in a randomized phase III trial (MDS-004) in low-/int-1-risk myelodysplastic syndromes (MDS) with a del(5q) abnormality.

Similar criteria to those used in the MDS-003 study were chosen. Two hundred five patients were randomized to receive treatment with either lenalidomide 10 mg orally daily for 21 days of each 28-day cycle, lenalidomide 5 mg orally daily for 28 days of each 28-day cycle, or placebo. Erythroid responses were assessed at 16 weeks. Nonresponders were then in open-label treatment and they were excluded from the efficacy analysis. Red blood cell transfusion independence was achieved in 53.6% of patients treated on 10 mg arm, 33.3% on 5 mg arm and 6% on the placebo arm. Cytogenetic response rates were also highest in the 10 mg arm (41.5% of patients), while in 5 mg arm (17.4%) and in the placebo arm (0%). The median rise in hemoglobin at the time of the best response was also higher in patients treated with the 10 mg lenalidomide. No difference in the rate of AML transformation among three arms was found. This study confirmed that the preferred starting dose of lenalidomide in patients with del(5q) low-/int-1-risk MDS remains 10 mg.

Health-related quality of life (HRQL) outcomes were assessed using the Functional Assessment of Cancer Therapy-Anemia in 167 RBC transfusion-dependent patients with IPSS low- or intermediate-1-risk del5q31 MDS treated with lenalidomide versus placebo in a randomized phase III clinical trial, MDS-004 [67]. Clinically important changes in HRQL from baseline were observed at weeks 12, 14, 36, and 48 among responders in both treatment groups (5 mg and 10 mg lenalidomide). Lenalidomide treatment may be effective in improving HRQL outcomes [67].

Further Clinical Studies of Lower Risk MDS Patients with Del(5q) Treated with Lenalidomide

Many of the initial clinical and laboratory observations obtained in the MDS-003 trial were confirmed in the study of Le Bras et al. [68]. Ninety five lower risk MDS patients (low and intermediate 1 risk in IPSS, 25 males and 70 females with a median age of 70.4 years) with del(5q) were treated with 10 mg of lenalidomide daily, 21 days every 28 days for at least 16 weeks. Patients with at least a minor erythroid response after 16 weeks were treated in the same way until disease progression, treatment failure or treatment-limiting toxicity.

Erythroid response was evaluated according to IWG 2000 criteria [69]. Sixty two of the 95 patients (65%) achieved erythroid response according to IWG 2006 criteria [61]. In these 62 patients, 60 patients (63% from 95 patients) achieved red blood cell transfusion independence. Median time to transfusion independence was 16 weeks (range 8-33 weeks). Fifteen patients who achieved transfusion independence were analyzed for cytogenetic response (20% of complete and 40% of partial cytogenetic response). The rest of these 15 patients (40%) had no cytogenetic response. Six (6.3%) patients progressed to AML and 15 patients died, including 6 patients who had achieved transfusion independence. In the MDS-003 trial, the primary endpoint was hematological response, while in the study of Le Bras et al. transfusion independence. The cytogenetic remission rate was higher in the MDS-003 trial (73% versus 60% in the study of Le Bras et al. [68]). Neutropenia and thrombocytopenia were the most common adverse events in both studies [70].

A Japanese multiinstitutional study MDS-007 in MDS patients with del(5q) treated with lenalidomide has been recently performed [71,72]. This study was targeted on morphologic analysis and evaluation of the relationship among erythroid response, change of morphologic findings and cytogenetic response. MDS-007 trial was a single-arm, open-label study. Eleven patients were enrolled in this study, including 5 patients with transfusion-dependent anemia and 6 patients with transfusion-independent symptomatic anemia. Nine patients showed less than 25% of bone marrow erythroblasts before therapy with lenalidomide and no patient had more than 40% of bone marrow erythroblasts at that time. Eight patients showed a rapid increase of bone marrow erythroblasts to more than 40% on day 85. All patients except one achieved a major erythroid response as defined by either transfusion independence or by rapid increase of hemoglobin level in most patients on day 169 of lenalidomide therapy. One patient without any hematologic response by day 169, achieved a major erythroid response on day 218. Erythroid response could be achieved even without a cytogenetic response. No patient in this analysis showed a hematological relapse prior to cytogenetic one. These findings suggested that lenalidomide can improve anemia by more than one mechanism of action and also through mechanism different from del(5q) elimination.

Treatment of del(5q) Patients with Relapse during Lenalidomide Exposure

At the time of relapse of transfusion dependence, bone marrow aspiration would be performed in order to evaluate the patient for morphological or cytogenetic progression. If there is no progression, the patient is without drug next 3 to 4 monthes. Thereafter, the patient is re-exposed to lenalidomide. Second responses are regularly seen, probably by epigenetic mechanism [73]. In the case of progressive disease, salvage therapies including demethylating agents or allogeneic bone marrow transplantation are necessary [74].

Therapy with Lenalidomide in Combination with another Drug in MDS

In order to maximize the potential benefit from lenalidomide therapy combination strategies were developed. Lenalidomide in attempt to improve outcome of patients can be combined with erythropoiesis-stimulating agents (ESA), such as erythropoietin or darbepoietin alpha. This therapy is based on preclinical observations showing that lenalidomide significantly potentiated erythropoietin receptor signaling. The addition of erythropoietin (40,000 U/week) for an additional 8-week course had the beneficial effect in low and intermediate-1 risk MDS patients who had failed prior treatment with lenalidomide monotherapy for 16 weeks [75]. To evaluate the potential benefit of the combination of lenalidomide and ESA, Park et al. [76] tried the association in three del5q MDS patients, who were resistant or partially responding to lenalidomide alone. Lenalidomide had two different actions, one on the disapperance of the 5q-clone and the other one on the stimulation of the erythroid production in combination with ESA.

In low to intermediate-1 risk non-del(5q) MDS, lenalidomide treatment is less effective with a lower response rate (25%) and shorter response duration than in the same risk MDS with del(5q) [41]. Combination of lenalidomide with another drug could improve outcome of patients with low to intermediate-1 risk non-del(5q) MDS. Ezatiostat hydrochloride (Telintra, TLK199), a tripeptide glutathione analog is a reversible inhibitor of the enzyme glutathione S-transferase P1-1 (GSTP1-1) inhibitor [77-83]. This inhibitor was developed for the treatment of cytopenias associated with lower risk MDS. Ezatiostat activates jun-N-terminal kinase (JNK), promoting the growth and maturation of hematopoietic progenitors, while inducing apoptosis in human leukemia blasts [77]. The ability of ezatiostat to activate the caspase-dependent pathway may help eliminate or inhibit the emergence of malignant clones. Alternatively, ezatiostat increases reactive oxygen species in dysplastic cells and contibutes by this effect also to apoptotic death [77]. Based on these mechanisms of action, response rates, non-overlapping toxicities, and tolerability observed in a single agent ezatiostat phase 1 and 2 studies in MDS [79-81,84], a study of the combination of ezatiostat and lenalidomide was conducted to determine the safety and efficacy of ezatiostat with lenalidomide in non-del(5q) low to intermediate-1 risk MDS. Eighteen patients (median age 73 years; range 57-82; 72% male) were enrolled in the study [81]. Thirteen patients (72%) were intermediate-1 risk and 5 patients (28%) were low risk. Four patients had abnormal cytogenetics. Twelve patients (67%) were red blood cell transfusion-dependent and 2 patients (11%) were platelet transfusion-dependent. Three of 8 (38%) patients achieved transfusion independence including 1 responder who did not respond to prior lenalidomide. Ezatiostat caused clinically significant reduction in red blood cell and platelet transfusions. Since ezatiostat is non-myelosuppressive, it is a good candidate for combination with lenalidomide. The recommended doses of this combination regimen for future studies is the ezatiostat.

Lenalidomide and azacitidine are active in patients with lower- and higher-risk MDS. These agents may complement each other by targeting both the bone marrow microenvironment and hypomethylating action on the malignant clone. Phase I combination trial of lenalidomide and azacitidine in patients with higher-risk MDS was a multicenter, single-arm, open-label study [85]. Twenty five patients were screened and enrolled in this therapy and their response was assessed after four and seven cycles of the tretment. Azacitidine was administered at 75 mg/m^2 daily for five consecutive days, and lenalidomide 10 mg daily for 21 days, of a 28-day cycle. Of 18 evaluable patients, 12 (67%) responded to therapy; 8 (44%) achieved complex response, 3 (17%) had hematologic improvement and one (6%) had bone marrow complex response. Of those who responded, eight experienced relapse or disease progression at a median 7.5 months from initial response (range, 3 to 17 months). Two patients transformed to AML, one patient at 7 and one patient at 11 months from initial response. Another report from the same research group on three MDS patients with normal cytogenetics who relapsed on monotherapy and achieved a complete response with combination of lenalidomide and azacitidine has been recently published [86]. This combination was also studied by the other American, French, German and Australian groups [87-90]. The combination of lenalidomide and azacitidine is feasible and seems to be effective in lower risk MDS with del(5q) [88] and even in a very high risk patient groups with advanced MDS or AML and a del(5q) [85-87,89,90].

Romiplostim (AMG 531, Nplate) is an Fc-peptide fusion protein (peptibody) that acts as a thrombopoietin receptor agonist. It has no amino acid sequence homology with endogenous thrombopoietin. Romiplostim stimulates megakaryopoiesis and thrombopoiesis by binding to and activating the thrombopoietin receptor and downstream signaling [91-94]. Romiplostim appeared well tolerated in patients with lower risk MDS and thrombocytopenia [95]. Low platelet counts in patients with MDS may be due to the underlying disease or due to treatment with disease-modifying agents, and platelet transfusions are often the only treatment for clinically significant thrombocytopenia or bleeding. Randomized phase II study evaluating the efficacy and safety of romiplostim treatment of patients with low or intermediate-1 risk MDS receiving lenalidomide was performed [96]. This was double-blind, placebo controlled, dose finding study that evaluated the effect of romiplostim on the incidence of clinically significant thrombocytopenia events (grade 3 or 4 thrombocytopenia and/or receipt of platelet transfusions) and the safety of romiplostim in patients with low or intermediate-1 risk MDS receiving lenalidomide. Thirty nine patients (median age 74 years; range, 39 to 90) were randomized into treatment groups receiving placebo, 500 μg romiplostim, or 750 μg romiplostim by weekly subcutaneous injections in combination with lenalidomide (one 10 mg capsule by mouth daily for each 28-day cycle). Fifteen patients (39%) had platelet counts$<50\times10^9$/L and 7 (18%) had del(5q). Treatment continued for a total of four cycles. Twelve patients (31%) discontinued the study. Disease progression to AML was reported in 1 patient in the romiplostim 500 μg group. Response was 8% for the placebo, 36% for 500 μg romiplostim, and 15% for 750 μg romiplostim groups. Romiplostim appeared to be well tollerated in low or intermediate-1 risk MDS patients receiving lenalidomide.

It is possible that the effect of lenalidomide could be augmented by addition of another immunomodulation agent, cyclosporine A. A single-arm, open-label study of the efficacy and safety of lenalidomide in combination with cyclosporine A in red blood cell transfusion-dependent both 5q- and non 5q- MDS patients started at Weill Cornell Medical College in New York.

Other drugs are tried and will be probably used in combinations with lenalidomide in the treatment MDS patients with del(5q) in the future. Dexamethasone and lenalidomide rescue erythropoiesis, alone and in combination, in RPS14- and RPS19- (ribosomal proteins of small ribosomal subunit) deficient cells [97]. L-leucine was also studied in RPS14- and RPS19- deficient cells [98-101]. The combined use of L-leucine and lenalidomide might be considered for therapy in MDS patients with the del(5q) since there is evidence to suggest that these two drugs act through different mechanism and their effect may be synergistic.

Mechanisms of Action of Lenalidomide

Lenalidomide shares a number of structural and biological properties with thalidomide, but it is safer and more potent than thalidomide. Both drugs appear to function through four mechanisms: immunomodulatory, anti-inflammatory, anti-angiogenic and direct neoplastic cells inhibitory [102,103]. Lenalidomide has a direct erythropoiesis stimulating effect. Shortly, Wei et al. [104] demonstrated that the haplodeficient enzymatic targets of lenalidomide within the commonly deleted region are two dual-specificity phosphatases, the cell division cycle 25C (Cdc25C) and the protein phosphatase 2A (PP2A). These phosphatases are coregulators of G2-M checkpoint in the cell cycle and thus, their inhibition by lenalidomide leads to G2 arrest and apoptosis of del(5q) specimens. The mechanism of action is different in non-del(5q), where lenalidomide restores and promotes effective erythropoiesis with no direct cytotoxic effect [104]. Lenalidomide promotes erythropoiesis and fetal hemoglobin production in human CD34+ cells [105]. The increased fetal hemoglobin expression was associated with epigenetic effect on chromatin (an increase in histone 3 acetylation on the γ-globin gene promoter).

In MDS patients with del(5q), allelic deletion of the *RPS 14* gene is a key effector of the hypoplastic anemia. Impairment of ribosomal biogenesis liberates free ribosomal proteins to bind to and trigger degradation of HDM2 (human homologue of the mouse double minute 2 protein /MDM2/) with consequent p53 transactivation in response to nucleolar stress independently of DNA damage [106,107]. Overexpression of p53 is typical for erythroid precursors of primary bone marrow of MDS patients with with del(5q). Lenalidomide inhibits the haplodeficient PP2A resulting in hyperphosphorylation of inhibitory serine 166 and serine 186 residues on MDM2, and displaces binding of RPS14 to suppress MDM2 autoubiquitation whereas PP2A overexpression promotes drug resistance. Lenalidomide promotes p53 degradation by inhibiting HDM2 autoubiquitination in erythroid precursors of MDS patients with with del(5q) bone marrow [108].

The similar epigenetic modulation of gene for p21(CIP1/WAF1) by lenalidomide was described in both lymphoma and multiple myeloma [109]. A potent cyclin-dependent kinase inhibitor p21(CIP1/WAF1) decreases activity of cyclinE-CDK2 or cyclinD-CDK4/6 complexes, and thus functions as a regulator of cell cycle progression. The p21 protein can mediate cellular senescence and also interact with proliferating cell nuclear antigen (PCNA), a DNA polymerase accessory factor, and plays a regulatory role in S phase DNA replication and DNA damage repair.

Most MDS patients including those with del(5q) become refractory to erythropoietin (EPO). EPO is an essential glycoprotein that facilitates red blood cell maturation from erythroid progenitors and mediates erythropoiesis [110]. EPO acts through EPO-receptor (EPO-R) and the signal transducer and activator of transcription 5 (STAT5) [43,111]. Disruption of STAT5 results in a variety of cell-specific effects, one of which is the impaired erythropoiesis [108]. Lenalidomide relieves repression of ligand-dependent activation of the EPO-R/STAT5 pathway. Ebert et al. [59] showed that target genes of this pathway are underexpressed in lenalidomide-responsive MDS patients wihout del(5q). Lenalidomide promotes erythropoiesis in MDS by CD45 protein tyrosine phosphatase inhibition [112]. CD45 phosphatase is overactivated in MDS and may inhibit phosphorylation of STAT5 stimulated by EPO-R. Lenalidomide is able to restore EPO-R/STAT5 signaling that is essential for hematopoiesis. Lenalidomide restores and promotes effective erythropoiesis in non-del(5q) without direct cytotoxic effect.

A deregulated immune system plays the important role in pathogenesis of MDS. Deregulation is caused by the alteration of cytokines in the bone marrow microenvironment, deffective T-cell regulation and diminished natural killer (NK) cell activity. Deficiences in T cells, NK cells and interferon-γ (IFN-γ) production were described in the bone marrow and peripheral blood of MDS patients [113,114]. Lenalidomide exhibits potent T-cell costimulatory properties and augmented production of IL-2 and IFN-γ [16,115]. Akt (proteinase B) signaling pathway and transcription factor AP1 (activator protein 1) are involved in T-cell activation [115]. Increased numbers and activation of NK and NK T-cell populations were also observed in peripheral blood cells cultured with lenalidomide [116,117].

Anti-inflammatory effects of lenalidomide is based on inhibition of proinflammatory cytokines and chemokines, such as TNF-α, IL-1β, IL-6, IL-12, monocyte chemotactic protein-1 and macrophage inflammatory protein-1α. On the other hand, lenalidomide elevates anti-inflammatory cytokine IL-10. Interestingly, haploinsuficiency of miR-145 and miR-146a in 5q - syndrome increases IL-6 levels by elevation of interleukin-1 receptor-associated kinase 1 (IRAK1), Toll-interleukin-1 receptor domain-containing adaptor protein (TIRAP), tumor necrosis factor receptor-associated factor-6 (TRAF6), and NF-κB [118-120]. RPS14, miR-145, and miR-146 were significantly increased and TNF-α, IL-1β and IL-10 significantly downregulated during the treatment with lenalidomide [121-123].

Angiogenesis, the formation of new blood vessels, plays an important role in the growth and progression of MDS. The vascular endothelial growth factor (VEGF) and to a lesser extent IL-6 are cytokines that stimulate the formation of blood vessels. Increased levels of these cytokines have been shown in MDS [124]. Anti-angiogenic effects of lenalidomide are independent of immunomodulatory effects and are mediated through endothelial cell migration inhibition [125-128]. The mechanism by which lenalidomide inhibited VEGF-induced endothelial cell migration may be related to VEGF-induced inhibition of Akt phosphorylation. Furthermore, loss of anti-angiogenic effect of lenalidomide predicted disease progressionand an increased risk of transformation to AML [129].

Lenalidomide does not affect DNA synthesis but inhibits cytokinesis of MDS cells. Cytokinesis occurs as the final stage of cell division after mitosis. A contractile ring, made of non-muscle myosin and actin filaments assembles in the middle of the cell adjacent to the cell membrane. Formins are Rho-GTPase effector proteins that are involved in the polymerization of actin and effects microtubule during meiosis, mitosis, the maintenance of cell polarity, vesicular trafficking and signaling to the nucleus [130,131]. Diaphanous (mDia)-related formin mDia1 is encoded by *DIAPH1* located on the long arm of chromosome 5 (5q31.3) and lies between the two commonly deleted regions in MDS patients with 5q- syndrome. It is not clear whether mDia1 plays a role in lenalidomide effect on cytokinesis. Knock-out of *DIAPH1* in mice has T cell responses and myelodysplastic phenotype [132-134].

The clinical effect of lenalidomide is associated with significant increases in the numbers of erythroid, myeloid and megakaryocytic colony-forming cells and a substantial improvement in the hematopoiesis-supporting capacity of bone marrow stroma. Lenalidomide induces significant alterations in the adhesion profile of hematopoietic progenitor cells, including over-expression of membrane ligands (CXCR4/CD184, CD54/ICAM1, CD11a and CD49d where CD is cluster of differentiation) and overproduction of soluble stromal cell-derived factor-1 (SDF-1) and of ICAM1 in the bone marrow microenvironment. CXC4 is C-X-C chemokine receptor type 4 also known as fusin or CD184. ICAM1 (intracellular adhesion molecule 1 also known as CD54) is a cell surface glycoprotein. All these effects favor the maintenance of CD34+ cells in the bone marrow [135]. Lenalidomide-mediated induction of the SLAM antigen CD48 on patients' CD34+ cells may be associated with the drug's apoptosis-inducing effect through co-stimulatory interactions between CD34+ cells and cytotoxic lymphocytes in the bone marrow microenvironment.

Conclusion and Perspectives

Lenalidomide is currently the treatment of choice for lower risk transfusion-dependent del(5q) MDS patients, and remains a treatment alternative for the management of anemia in lower risk MDS without 5q deletion MDS patients with adequate neutrophil and platelet counts [136]. Lenalidomide has also activity in higher risk MDS and AML with del(5q) and even in non(del5q) MDS.

Though the mechanism of lenalidomide action has not been definitively determined, it is clear that there is a difference between mechanisms in MDS with del(5q) and MDS with non-del(5q).

In MDS with del(5q), lenalidomide acts through inhibition of phosphatase activity in the commonly deleted region of the long arm of chromosome 5. This phosphatases play a key role in cell cycle regulation. The inhibition of these phosphatases by lenalidomide leads to G2 arrest, followed by apoptosis of del(5q) specimens. The direct cytotoxic effects of lenalidomide on the del(5q) clone are also very important. Lenalidomide inhibits the malignant clone and up-regulates the *SPARC* (secreted protein acidic and rich in cysteine) gene mapping to the commonly deleted region in 5q- syndrome patients [137]. However, SPARC is dispensable for murine hematopoiesis [138]. While haploinsufficiency of the *RPS14* gene appears to be a key contributor to erythropoietic failure associated with del(5q) MDS, the critical genes responsible for clonal dominance in del(5q) high-risk MDS and AML are less well-defined. It is known that this deleted region is different in del(5q) high-risk MDS and AML [139]. The effect of lenalidomide in these cases needs to identify further biologic features accounting for the response, thereby allowing rational use of this drug, both alone and in combination with another agents.

In MDS with non-del(5q), an increased expression of adhesion molecules caused by lenalidomide treatment leads to recovery and maintenance of the CD34+ cells through interactions between the hematopoietic and stromal cells. This effect of lenalidomide on the bone marrow microenvironment causes abrogation of the function of pro-apoptotic and pro-inflammatory cytokines. Lenalidomide is capable to increase red blood cell production independently of ribosome dysfunction. Lenalidomide restores and promotes effective erythropoiesis without direct cytotoxic effect. Lenalidomide activates the EPO-R/STAT5 pathway.

New cytogenetic tools such as fluorescence in situ, hybridization (FISH) or single nucleotide polymorphism array (SNP-A)-based karyotyping, increased the diagnostic yield over metaphase cytogenetics. Sugimoto et al. [140] have recently found with help of these new cytogenetic tools that normal karyotype and gain of chromosome 8 were predictive of response to lenalidomide in non-del(5q) patients with myeloid malignancies.

The presence of multiple cellular and genetic abnormalities in MDS is common and suggests that combination therapy targeting different mechanisms of action may be beneficial, particularly in higher-risk disease, for which both microenvironment and cell regulatory mechanisms play a role. The optimal dose, schedule and duration of treatment is still an area of active investigation, especially in the use of lenalidomide combinations with other drugs.

Acknowledgments

This work was supported, by PRVOUK-27/LF 1/2. The research grant NT/13836-4/2012 from the Ministry of Health of the Czech Republic and by the project (Ministry of Health, Czech Republic) for conceptual development of research organization (Institute of Hematology and Blood Transfusion, Prague).

References

1. Haase D, Germing U, Schanz J, Pfeilstöcker M, Nösslinger T, et al. (2007) New insights into the prognostic impact of the karyotype in MDS and correlation with subtypes: evidence from a core dataset of 2124 patients. Blood 110: 4385-4395.
2. Van den Berghe H, Cassiman JJ, David G, Fryns JP, Michaux JL, et al. (1974) Distinct haematological disorder with deletion of long arm of no. 5 chromosome. Nature 251: 437-438.
3. Van den Berghe H, Vermaelen K, Mecucci C, Barbieri D, Tricot G (1985) The 5q-anomaly. Cancer Genet Cytogenet 17: 189-255.
4. Nimer SD, Golde DW (1987) The 5q- abnormality. Blood 70: 1705-1712.
5. Mathew P, Tefferi A, Dewald GW, Goldberg SL, Su J, et al. (1993) The 5q-syndrome: a single-institution study of 43 consecutive patients. Blood 81: 1040-1045.
6. Boultwood J, Lewis S, Wainscoat JS (1994) The 5q-syndrome. Blood 84: 3253-3260.
7. Giagounidis AA, Germing U, Wainscoat JS, Boultwood J, Aul C (2004) The 5q-syndrome. Hematology 9: 271-277.
8. Mohamedali A, Mufti GJ (2009) Van-den Berghe's 5q- syndrome in 2008. Br J Haematol 144: 157-168.
9. Boultwood J, Fidler C, Lewis S, Kelly S, Sheridan H, et al. (1994) Molecular mapping of uncharacteristically small 5q deletions in two patients with the 5q-syndrome: delineation of the critical region on 5q and identification of a 5q-breakpoint. Genomics 19: 425-432.
10. Boultwood J, Fidler C, Strickson AJ, Watkins F, Gama S, et al. (2002) Narrowing and genomic annotation of the commonly deleted region of the 5q- syndrome. Blood 99: 4638-4641.
11. Giagounidis AA, Germing U, Haase S, Hildebrandt B, Schlegelberger B, et al. (2004) Clinical, morphological, cytogenetic, and prognostic features of patients with myelodysplastic syndromes and del(5q) including band q31. Leukemia 18: 113-119.
12. Nimer SD (2006) Clinical management of myelodysplastic syndromes with interstitial deletion of chromosome 5q. J Clin Oncol 24: 2576-2582.
13. Boultwood J, Pellagatti A, McKenzie AN, Wainscoat JS (2010) Advances in the 5q- syndrome. Blood 116: 5803-5811.
14. Mallo M, Cervera J, Schanz J, Such E, García-Manero G, et al. (2011) Impact of adjunct cytogenetic abnormalities for prognostic stratification in patients with myelodysplastic syndrome and deletion 5q. Leukemia 25: 110-120.
15. Hasserjian RP, Le Beau MM, List AF, Thiele J (2008) "WHO Classification of Tumors of Haematopoietic and Lymphoid Tissues," International Agency for Research on Cancer Press, Lyon, France 102-103.
16. Corral LG, Haslett PA, Muller GW, Chen R, Wong LM, et al. (1999) Differential cytokine modulation and T cell activation by two distinct classes of thalidomide analogues that are potent inhibitors of TNF-alpha. J Immunol 163: 380-386.

17. Davies FE, Raje N, Hideshima T, Lentzsch S, Young G, et al. (2001) Thalidomide and immunomodulatory derivatives augment natural killer cell cytotoxicity in multiple myeloma. Blood 98: 210-216.

18. Richardson PG, Schlossman RL, Weller E, Hideshima T, Mitsiades C, et al. (2002) Immunomodulatory drug CC-5013 overcomes drug resistance and is well tolerated in patients with relapsed multiple myeloma. Blood 100: 3063-3067.

19. Vallet S, Palumbo A, Raje N, Boccadoro M, Anderson KC (2008) Thalidomide and lenalidomide: Mechanism-based potential drug combinations. Leuk Lymphoma 49: 1238-1245.

20. Quach H, Ritchie D, Stewart AK, Neeson P, Harrison S, et al. (2010) Mechanism of action of immunomodulatory drugs (IMiDS) in multiple myeloma. Leukemia 24: 22-32.

21. Cives M, Milano A, Dammacco F, Silvestris F (2012) Lenalidomide in multiple myeloma: current experimental and clinical data. Eur J Haematol 88: 279-291.

22. Bartlett JB, Dredge K, Dalgleish AG (2004) The evolution of thalidomide and its IMiD derivatives as anticancer agents. Nat Rev Cancer 4: 314-322.

23. Kotla V, Goel S, Nischal S, Heuck C, Vivek K, et al. (2009) Mechanism of action of lenalidomide in hematological malignancies. J Hematol Oncol 2: 36.

24. Teo S, Resztak KE, Scheffler MA, Kook KA, Zeldis JB, et al. (2002) Thalidomide in the treatment of leprosy. Microbes Infect 4: 1193-1202.

25. Musto P (2004) Thalidomide therapy for myelodysplastic syndromes: current status and future perspectives. Leuk Res 28: 325-332.

26. Raza A, Meyer P, Dutt D, Zorat F, Lisak L, et al. (2001) Thalidomide produces transfusion independence in long-standing refractory anemias of patients with myelodysplastic syndromes. Blood 98: 958-965.

27. Strupp C, Germing U, Aivado M, Misgeld E, Haas R, et al. (2002) Thalidomide for the treatment of patients with myelodysplastic syndromes. Leukemia 16: 1-6.

28. List A, Kurtin S, Roe DJ, Buresh A, Mahadevan D, et al. (2005) Efficacy of lenalidomide in myelodysplastic syndromes. N Engl J Med 352: 549-557.

29. List A, Dewald G, Bennett J, Giagounidis A, Raza A, et al. (2006) Lenalidomide in the myelodysplastic syndrome with chromosome 5q deletion. N Engl J Med 355: 1456-1465.

30. Kuendgen A, Lauseker M, List AF, Fenaux P, Giagounidis AA, et al. (2012) Lenalidomide does not increase AML progression risk in RBC transfusion-dependent patients with Low- or Intermediate-1-risk MDS with del(5q): a comparative analysis. Leukemia.

31. List AF, Wride K, Dewald G, Bennett JM, Giagounidis A, et al. (2007) C028 Cytogenetic response to lenalidomide is associated with improved survival in patients with chromosome 5q deletion. Leuk Res 31: S38-S38.

32. Giagounidis A, Fenaux P, Mufti GJ, Muus P, Platzbecker U, et al. (2008) Practical recommendations on the use of lenalidomide in the management of myelodysplastic syndromes. Ann Hematol 87: 345-352.

33. Giagounidis AA, Kulasekararaj A, Germing U, Radkowski R, Haase S, et al. (2012) Long-term transfusion independence in del(5q) MDS patients who discontinue lenalidomide. Leukemia 26: 855-858.

34. Göhring G, Lange K, Hofmann W, Nielsen KV, Hellström-Lindberg E, et al. (2012) Telomere shortening, clonal evolution and disease progression in myelodysplastic syndrome patients with 5q deletion treated with lenalidomide. Leukemia 26: 356-358.

35. Jädersten M, Saft L, Pellagatti A, Göhring G, Wainscoat JS, et al. (2009) Clonal heterogeneity in the 5q- syndrome: p53 expressing progenitors prevail during lenalidomide treatment and expand at disease progression. Haematologica 94: 1762-1766.

36. Jädersten M, Saft L, Smith A, Kulasekararaj A, Pomplun S, et al. (2011) TP53 mutations in low-risk myelodysplastic syndromes with del(5q) predict disease progression. J Clin Oncol 29: 1971-1979.

37. Tehranchi R, Woll PS, Anderson K, Buza-Vidas N, Mizukami T, et al. (2010) Persistent malignant stem cells in del(5q) myelodysplasia in remission. N Engl J Med 363: 1025-1037.

38. Melchert M, Kale V, List A (2007) The role of lenalidomide in the treatment of patients with chromosome 5q deletion and other myelodysplastic syndromes. Curr Opin Hematol 14: 123-129.

39. List AF (2007) Lenalidomide--the phoenix rises. N Engl J Med 357: 2183-2186.

40. Kurtin SE, List AF (2009) Durable long-term responses in patients with myelodysplastic syndromes treated with lenalidomide. Clin Lymphoma Myeloma 9: E10-13.

41. Komrokji RS, List AF (2010) Lenalidomide for treatment of myelodysplastic syndromes: current status and future directions. Hematol Oncol Clin North Am 24: 377-388.

42. Raza A, Reeves JA, Feldman EJ, Dewald GW, Bennett JM, et al. (2008) Phase 2 study of lenalidomide in transfusion-dependent, low-risk, and intermediate-1 risk myelodysplastic syndromes with karyotypes other than deletion 5q. Blood 111: 86-93.

43. Hoefsloot LH, van Amelsvoort MP, Broeders LC, van der Plas DC, van Lom K, et al. (1997) Erythropoietin-induced activation of STAT5 is impaired in the myelodysplastic syndrome. Blood 89: 1690-1700.

44. Sibon D, Cannas G, Baracco F, Prebet T, Vey N, et al. (2012) Lenalidomide in lower-risk myelodysplastic syndromes with karyotypes other than deletion 5q and refractory to erythropoiesis-stimulating agents. Br J Haematol 156: 619-625.

45. Sohal D, Pellagatti A, Zhou L, Mo Y, Opalinska JB, et al. (2008) Downregulation of ribosomal proteins is seen in non 5q- MDS. ASH Meeting, USA.

46. Ebert BL, Pretz J, Bosco J, Chang CY, Tamayo P, et al. (2008) Identification of RPS14 as a 5q- syndrome gene by RNA interference screen. Nature 451: 335-339.

47. Pellagatti A, Hellström-Lindberg E, Giagounidis A, Perry J, Malcovati L, et al. (2008) Haploinsufficiency of RPS14 in 5q- syndrome is associated with deregulation of ribosomal- and translation-related genes. Br J Haematol 142: 57-64.

48. Czibere A, Bruns I, Junge B, Singh R, Kobbe G, et al. (2009) Low RPS14 expression is common in myelodysplastic syndromes without 5q- aberration and defines a subgroup of patients with prolonged survival. Haematologica 94: 1453-1455.

49. Dutt S, Narla A, Lin K, Mullally A, Abayasekara N, et al. (2011) Haploinsufficiency for ribosomal protein genes causes selective activation of p53 in human erythroid progenitor cells. Blood 117: 2567-2576.

50. Zhang Y, Lu H (2009) Signaling to p53: ribosomal proteins find their way. Cancer Cell 16: 369-377.

51. Fumagalli S, Di Cara A, Neb-Gulati A, Natt F, Schwemberger S, et al. (2009) Absence of nucleolar disruption after impairment of 40S ribosome biogenesis reveals an rpL11-translation-dependent mechanism of p53 induction. Nat Cell Biol 11: 501-508.

52. Pellagatti A, Marafioti T, Paterson JC, Barlow JL, Drynan LF, et al. (2010) Induction of p53 and up-regulation of the p53 pathway in the human 5q-syndrome. Blood 115: 2721-2723.

53. Danilova N, Kumagai A, Lin J (2010) p53 upregulation is a frequent response to deficiency of cell-essential genes. PLoS One 5: e15938.

54. Fumagalli S, Thomas G (2011) The role of p53 in ribosomopathies. Semin Hematol 48: 97-105.

55. Cazzola M (2008) Myelodysplastic syndrome with isolated 5q deletion (5q-syndrome). A clonal stem cell disorder characterized by defective ribosome biogenesis. Haematologica 93: 967-972.

56. Barlow JL, Drynan LF, Trim NL, Erber WN, Warren AJ, et al. (2010) New insights into 5q- syndrome as a ribosomopathy. Cell Cycle 9: 4286-4293.

57. Ebert BL (2009) Deletion 5q in myelodysplastic syndrome: a paradigm for the study of hemizygous deletions in cancer. Leukemia 23: 1252-1256.

58. Narla A, Ebert BL (2010) Ribosomopathies: human disorders of ribosome dysfunction. Blood 115: 3196-3205.

59. Ebert BL, Galili N, Tamayo P, Bosco J, Mak R, et al. (2008) An erythroid differentiation signature predicts response to lenalidomide in myelodysplastic syndrome. PLoS Med 5: e35.

60. Adès L, Boehrer S, Prebet T, Beyne-Rauzy O, Legros L, et al. (2009) Efficacy and safety of lenalidomide in intermediate-2 or high-risk myelodysplastic syndromes with 5q deletion: results of a phase 2 study. Blood 113: 3947-3952.

61. Cheson BD, Greenberg PL, Bennett JM, Lowenberg B, Wijermans PW, et al.

(2006) Clinical application and proposal for modification of the International Working Group (IWG) response criteria in myelodysplasia. Blood 108: 419-425.

62. Möllgård L, Saft L, Treppendahl MB, Dybedal I, Nørgaard JM, et al. (2011) Clinical effect of increasing doses of lenalidomide in high-risk myelodysplastic syndrome and acute myeloid leukemia with chromosome 5 abnormalities. Haematologica 96: 963-971.

63. Fenaux P, Giagounidis A, Selleslag, Beyne-Rauzy O, Mufti GJ, et al. (2009) RBC transfusion independence and safety profile of lenalidomide 5 or 10 mg in pts with low- or int-1-risk MDS with del5q: results from a randomized phase III trial (MDS-004). ASH Abstract, USA.

64. Fenaux P, Giagounidis A, Selleslag D, Beyne-Rauzy O, Mittelman M, et al. (2010) Safety of lenalidomide (LEN) from a randomized phase III trial (MDS-004) in low-/int-1-risk myelodysplastic syndromes (MDS) with a del(5q) abnormality. J Clin Oncol 28: 6598.

65. Fenaux P, Giagounidis A, Selleslag D, Beyne-Rauzy O, Mufti G, et al. (2011) A randomized phase 3 study of lenalidomide versus placebo in RBC transfusion-dependent patients with Low-/Intermediate-1-risk myelodysplastic syndromes with del5q. Blood 118: 3765-3776.

66. Sekeres MA (2011) Lenalidomide in MDS: 4th time's a charm. Blood 118: 3757-3758.

67. Revicki DA, Brandenburg NA, Muus P, Yu R, Knight R, et al. (2013) Health-related quality of life outcomes of lenalidomide in transfusion-dependent patients with Low- or Intermediate-1-risk myelodysplastic syndromes with a chromosome 5q deletion: results from a randomized clinical trial. Leuk Res 37: 259-265.

68. Le Bras F, Sebert M, Kelaidi C, Lamy T, Dreyfus F, et al. (2011) Treatment by lenalidomide in lower risk myelodysplastic syndrome with 5q deletion--the GFM experience. Leuk Res 35: 1444-1448.

69. Cheson BD, Bennett JM, Kantarjian H, Pinto A, Schiffer CA, et al. (2000) Report of an international working group to standardize response criteria for myelodysplastic syndromes. Blood 96: 3671-3674.

70. Tiu RV, Sekeres MA (2011) Lenalidomide in del 5q MDS: responses and side effects revisited. Leuk Res 35: 1440-1441.

71. Harada H, Watanabe M, Suzuki K, Yanagita S, Suzuki T, et al. (2009) Lenalidomide is active in Japanese patients with symptomatic anemia in low- or intermediate-1 risk myelodysplastic syndromes with a deletion 5q abnormality. Int J Hematol 90: 353-360.

72. Matsuda A, Taniwaki M, Jinnai I, Harada H, Watanabe M, et al. (2012) Morphologic analysis in myelodysplastic syndromes with del(5q) treated with lenalidomide. A Japanese multiinstitutional study. Leuk Res 36: 575-580.

73. Sharma SV, Lee DY, Li B, Quinlan MP, Takahashi F, et al. (2010) A chromatin-mediated reversible drug-tolerant state in cancer cell subpopulations. Cell 141: 69-80.

74. Giagounidis AA (2012) Lenalidomide for del(5q) and non-del(5q) myelodysplastic syndromes. Semin Hematol 49: 312-322.

75. List AF, Lancet JE, Melchert M, Saba H, Lush R, et al. (2007) Two-stage pharmacokinetic & efficacy study of lenalidomide alone or combined with recombinant erythropoietin (EPO) in lower risk MDS EPO-failures [PK-002]. ASH Meeting 110: 4626.

76. Park S, Vassilieff D, Bardet V, Viguié F, Dreyfus F (2010) Efficacy of the association of lenalidomide to erythropoiesis-stimulating agents in del (5q) MDS patients refractory to single-agent lenalidomide. Leukemia 24: 1960-1962.

77. Emanuel PD, Wang Z, Cai D, Sofega MR, Keck JG, et al. (2004) TLK199 (TelintraTM), a novel glutathione analog inhibitor of GST P1-1, causes proliferation and maturation of bone marrow precursor cells and correlates with clinical improvement in myelodysplastic syndrome (MDS) patients in a phase 2a study. Blood 104: ASH Meeting Abstract 2372.

78. Galili N, Tamayo P, Botvinnik OB, Mesirov JP, Brooks MR, et al. (2012) Prediction of response to therapy with ezatiostat in lower risk myelodysplastic syndrome. J Hematol Oncol 5: 20.

79. Raza A, Galili N, Smith S, Godwin J, Lancet J, et al. (2009) Phase 1 multicenter dose-escalation study of ezatiostat hydrochloride (TLK199 tablets), a novel glutathione analog prodrug, in patients with myelodysplastic syndrome. Blood 113: 6533-6540.

80. Raza A, Galili N, Callander N, Ochoa L, Piro L, et al. (2009) Phase 1-2a multicenter dose-escalastion study of ezatiostat hydrochloride liposomes for injection (Telintra, TLK199), a novel glutathione analog prodrug in patients with myelodysplastic syndrome. J Hematol Oncol 2: 20.

81. Quddus F, Clima J, Seedham H, Sajjad G, Galili N, et al. (2010) Oral Ezatiostat HCl (TLK199) and Myelodysplastic syndrome: a case report of sustained hematologic response following an abbreviated exposure. J Hematol Oncol 3: 16.

82. Raza A, Galili N, Mulford D, Smith SE, Brown GL, et al. (2012) Phase 1 dose-ranging study of ezatiostat hydrochloride in combination with lenalidomide in patients with non-deletion (5q) low to intermediate-1 risk myelodysplastic syndrome (MDS). J Hematol Oncol 5: 18.

83. Lyons RM, Wilks ST, Young S, Brown GL (2011) Oral ezatiostat HCl (Telintra®, TLK199) and idiopathic chronic neutropenia (ICN): a case report of complete response of a patient with G-CSF resistant ICN following treatment with ezatiostat, a glutathione S-transferase P1-1 (GSTP1-1) inhibitor. J Hematol Oncol 4: 43.

84. Raza A, Galili N, Smith SE, Godwin J, Boccia RV, et al. (2012) A phase 2 randomized multicenter study of 2 extended dosing schedules of oral ezatiostat in low to intermediate-1 risk myelodysplastic syndrome. Cancer 118: 2138-2147.

85. Sekeres MA, List AF, Cuthbertson D, Paquette R, Ganetzky R, et al. (2010) Phase I combination trial of lenalidomide and azacitidine in patients with higher-risk myelodysplastic syndromes. J Clin Oncol 28: 2253-2258.

86. Sekeres MA, O'Keefe C, List AF, Paulic K, Afable M 2nd, et al. (2011) Demonstration of additional benefit in adding lenalidomide to azacitidine in patients with higher-risk myelodysplastic syndromes. Am J Hematol 86: 102-103.

87. Garcia-Manero G, Daver NG, Borthakur G, Konopleva M, Ravandi F, et al. (2011) Phase I study of the combination of 5-azacitidine sequentially with high-dose lenalidomide in higher-risk myelodysplastic syndrome (MDS) and acute myelogenous leukemia (AML). Blood 118: ASH Meeting Abstract 2613.

88. Bally C, Itzykson R, Gruson B, Dreyfus F, Siguret V, et al. (2011) Azacitidine (AZA) after failure of lenalidomide (LEN) in low/int-1 risk MDS with del 5q. Blood 118: ASH Meeting Abstract 2786.

89. Platzbecker U, Ganster C, Neesen J, Kuendgen A, Götze K, et al. (2011) Safety and efficacy of a combination of 5-azacitidine followed by lenalidomide in high-risk MDS or AML patients with del(5q) cytogenetic abnormalities-results of the "AZALE" trial. Blood 118: ASH Meeting Abstract 3799.

90. Wei AH, Tan PT, Walker PA, Avery S, Patil SS, et al. (2011) A phase Ib dose escalation safety analysis of lenalidomide and azacitidine maintenance therapy for poor risk AML. Blood 118: ASH Meeting Abstract 3625.

91. Broudy VC, Lin NL (2004) AMG531 stimulates megakaryopoiesis in vitro by binding to Mpl. Cytokine 25: 52-60.

92. Wang B, Nichol JL, Sullivan JT (2004) Pharmacodynamics and pharmacokinetics of AMG 531, a novel thrombopoietin receptor ligand. Clin Pharmacol Ther 76: 628-638.

93. Frampton JE, Lyseng-Williamson KA (2009) Romiplostim. Drugs 69: 307-317.

94. Keating GM (2012) Romiplostim: a review of its use in immune thrombocytopenia. Drugs 72: 415-435.

95. Kantarjian H, Fenaux P, Sekeres MA, Becker PS, Boruchov A, et al. (2010) Safety and efficacy of romiplostim in patients with lower-risk myelodysplastic syndrome and thrombocytopenia. J Clin Oncol 28: 437-444.

96. Wang ES, Lyons RM, Larson RA, Gandhi S, Liu D, et al. (2012) A randomized, double-blind, placebo-controlled phase 2 study evaluating the efficacy and safety of romiplostim treatment of patients with low or intermediate-1 risk myelodysplastic syndrome receiving lenalidomide. J Hematol Oncol 5:71.

97. Narla A, Dutt S, McAuley JR, Al-Shahrour F, Hurst S, et al. (2011) Dexamethasone and lenalidomide have distinct functional effects on erythropoiesis. Blood 118: 2296-2304.

98. Cmejlova J, Dolezalova L, Pospisilova D, Petrtylova K, Petrak J, et al. (2006) Translational efficiency in patients with Diamond-Blackfan anemia. Haematologica 91: 1456-1464.

99. Pospisilova D, Cmejlova J, Hak J, Adam T, Cmejla R (2007) Successful treatment of a Diamond-Blackfan anemia patient with amino acid leucine. Haematologica 92: e66-67.

100. Payne EM, Virgilio M, Narla A, Sun H, Levine M, et al. (2012) L-Leucine improves the anemia and developmental defects associated with Diamond-Blackfan anemia and del(5q) MDS by activating the mTOR pathway. Blood 120: 2214-2224.

101. Yip BH, Pellagatti A, Vuppusetty C, Giagounidis A, Germing U, et al. (2012) Effects of L-leucine in 5q- syndrome and other RPS14-deficient erythroblasts. Leukemia 26: 2154-2158.

102. Heise C, Carter T, Schafer P, Chopra R (2010) Pleiotropic mechanisms of action of lenalidomide efficacy in del(5q) myelodysplastic syndromes. Expert Rev Anticancer Ther 10: 1663-1672.

103. Voutsadakis IA, Cairoli A (2012) A critical review of the molecular pathophysiology of lenalidomide sensitivity in 5q - myelodysplastic syndromes. Leuk Lymphoma 53: 779-788.

104. Wei S, Chen X, Rocha K, Epling-Burnette PK, Djeu JY, et al. (2009) A critical role for phosphatase haplodeficiency in the selective suppression of deletion 5q MDS by lenalidomide. Proc Natl Acad Sci U S A 106: 12974-12979.

105. Moutouh-de Parseval LA, Verhelle D, Glezer E, Jensen-Pergakes K, Ferguson GD, et al. (2008) Pomalidomide and lenalidomide regulate erythropoiesis and fetal hemoglobin production in human CD34+ cells. J Clin Invest 118: 248-258.

106. Fuchs O (2012) Important genes in the pathogenesis of 5q- syndrome and their connection with ribosomal stress and the innate immune system pathway. Leuk Res Treatment 2012: 179402.

107. Bursac S, Brdovak MC, Pfannkuchen M, Orsolic I, Golomb L, et al. (2012) Mutual protection of ribosomal proteins L5 and L11 from degradation is essential for p53 activation upon ribosomal biogenesis stress. Proc Natl Acad Sci U S A 109: 20467-20472.

108. Wei S, Chen X, McGraw K, Zhang L, Komrokji R, et al. (2013) Lenalidomide promotes p53 degradation by inhibiting MDM2 auto-ubiquitination in myelodysplastic syndrome with chromosome 5q deletion. Oncogene 32: 1110-1120.

109. Escoubet-Lozach L, Lin IL, Jensen-Pergakes K, Brady HA, Gandhi AK, et al. (2009) Pomalidomide and lenalidomide induce p21 WAF-1 expression in both lymphoma and multiple myeloma through a LSD1-mediated epigenetic mechanism. Cancer Res 69: 7347-7356.

110. Fisher JW (2003) Erythropoietin: physiology and pharmacology update. Exp Biol Med (Maywood) 228: 1-14.

111. Hennighausen L, Robinson GW (2008) Interpretation of cytokine signaling through the transcription factors STAT5A and STAT5B. Genes Dev 22: 711-721.

112. List A, Estes M, Williams A, Sekharam M, Ozawa U, et al. (2006) Lenalidomide (CC-5013; Revlimid) promotes erythropoiesis in myelodysplastic syndromes by CD45 protein tyrosine phosphatase inhibition. Blood 108: ASH Meeting Abstract 1360.

113. Epling-Burnette PK, List AF (2009) Advancements in the molecular pathogenesis of myelodysplastic syndrome. Curr Opin Hematol 16: 70-76.

114. Epling-Burnette PK, Painter JS, Rollison DE, Ku E, Vendron D, et al. (2007) Prevalence and clinical association of clonal T-cell expansions in Myelodysplastic Syndrome. Leukemia 21: 659-667.

115. Schafer PH, Gandhi AK, Loveland MA, Chen RS, Man HW, et al. (2003) Enhancement of cytokine production and AP-1 transcriptional activity in T cells by thalidomide-related immunomodulatory drugs. J Pharmacol Exp Ther 305: 1222-1232.

116. Zhu D, Corral LG, Fleming YW, Stein B (2008) Immunomodulatory drugs Revlimid (lenalidomide) and CC-4047 induce apoptosis of both hematological and solid tumor cells through NK cell activation. Cancer Immunol Immunother 57: 1849-1859.

117. Chang DH, Liu N, Klimek V, Hassoun H, Mazumder A, et al. (2006) Enhancement of ligand-dependent activation of human natural killer T cells by lenalidomide: therapeutic implications. Blood 108: 618-621.

118. Starczynowski DT, Kuchenbauer F, Argiropoulos B, Sung S, Morin R, et al. (2010) Identification of miR-145 and miR-146a as mediators of the 5q- syndrome phenotype. Nat Med 16: 49-58.

119. Starczynowski DT, Karsan A (2010) Deregulation of innate immune signaling in myelodysplastic syndromes is associated with deletion of chromosome arm 5q. Cell Cycle 9: 855-856.

120. Starczynowski DT, Karsan A (2010) Innate immune signaling in the myelodysplastic syndromes. Hematol Oncol Clin North Am 24: 343-359.

121. Oliva EN, Cuzzola M, Nobile F, Ronco F, D'Errigo MG, et al. (2010) Changes in RPS14 expression levels during lenalidomide treatment in Low- and Intermediate-1-risk myelodysplastic syndromes with chromosome 5q deletion. Eur J Haematol 85: 231-235.

122. Oliva EN, Cuzzola M, Aloe Spiriti MA, Poloni A, Laganà C, et al. (2013) Biological activity of lenalidomide in myelodysplastic syndromes with del5q: results of gene expression profiling from a multicenter phase II study. Ann Hematol 92: 25-32.

123. Venner CP, Woltosz JW, Nevill TJ, Deeg HJ, Caceres G, et al. (2013) Correlation of clinical response and response duration with miR-145 induction by lenalidomide in CD34+ cells from patients with del(5q) myelodysplastic syndrome. Haematologica 98: 409-413.

124. Schecter J, Galili N, Raza A (2012) MDS: Refining existing therapy through improved biologic insights. Blood Rev 26: 73-80.

125. Dredge K, Maarriott JB, Macdonald CD, Man HW, Chen R, et al. (2002) Novel thalidomide analogues display anti-angiogenic activity independently of immunomodulatory effects. Br J Cancer 87: 1166-1172.

126. Dredge K, Horsfall R, Robinson SP, Zhang LH, Lu L, et al. (2005) Orally administered lenalidomide (CC-5013) is anti-angiogenic in vivo and inhibits endothelial cell migration and Akt phosphorylation in vitro. Microvasc Res 69: 56-63.

127. Gandhi AK, Kang J, Naziruddin S, Parton A, Schafer PH, et al. (2006) Lenalidomide inhibits proliferation of Namalwa CSN.70 cells and interferes with Gab1 phosphorylation and adaptor protein complex assembly. Leuk Res 30: 849-858.

128. Lu L, Payvandi F, Wu L, Zhang LH, Hariri RJ, et al. (2009) The anti-cancer drug lenalidomide inhibits angiogenesis and metastasis via multiple inhibitory effects on endothelial cell function in normoxic and hypoxic conditions. Microvasc Res 77: 78-86.

129. Buesche G, Dieck S, Giagounidis A, Göhring G, Schlegelberger B, et al. (2009) Anti-angiogenic in-vivo effect of lenalidomide and its impact on neoplastic and non-neoplastic hematopoiesis in MDS with del(5q) chromosome abnormality. Blood 114: ASH Meeting Abstract 3800.

130. Goode BL, Eck MJ (2007) Mechanism and function of formins in the control of actin assembly. Annu Rev Biochem 76: 593-627.

131. Aspenström P (2010) Formin-binding proteins: modulators of formin-dependent actin polymerization. Biochim Biophys Acta 1803: 174-182.

132. Peng J, Kitchen SM, West RA, Sigler R, Eisenmann KM, et al. (2007) Myeloproliferative defects following targeting of the Drf1 gene encoding the mammalian diaphanous related formin mDia1. Cancer Res 67: 7565-7571.

133. Eisenmann KM, West RA, Hildebrand D, Kitchen SM, Peng J, et al. (2007) T cell responses in mammalian diaphanous-related formin mDia1 knock-out mice. J Biol Chem 282: 25152-25158.

134. DeWard AD, Leali K, West RA, Prendergast GC, Alberts AS (2009) Loss of RhoB expression enhances the myelodysplastic phenotype of mammalian diaphanous-related Formin mDia1 knockout mice. PLoS One 4: e7102.

135. Ximeri M, Galanopoulos A, Klaus M, Parcharidou A, Giannikou K, et al. (2010) Effect of lenalidomide therapy on hematopoiesis of patients with myelodysplastic syndrome associated with chromosome 5q deletion. Haematologica 95: 406-414.

136. Komrokji RS, List AF (2011) Role of lenalidomide in the treatment of myelodysplastic syndromes. Semin Oncol 38: 648-657.

137. Pellagatti A, Jädersten M, Forsblom AM, Cattan H, Christensson B, et al. (2007) Lenalidomide inhibits the malignant clone and up-regulates the SPARC gene mapping to the commonly deleted region in 5q- syndrome patients. Proc Natl Acad Sci U S A 104: 11406-11411.

138. Siva K, Jaako P, Miharada K, Rörby E, Ehinger M, et al. (2012) SPARC is dispensable for murine hematopoiesis, despite its suspected pathophysiological role in 5q-myelodysplastic syndrome. Leukemia 26: 2416-2419.

139. Steensma DP, Stone RM (2011) Lenalidomide in AML: del(5q) or who? Blood 118: 481-482.

140. Sugimoto Y, Sekeres MA, Makishima H, Traina F, Visconte V, et al. (2012) Cytogenetic and molecular predictors of response in patients with myeloid malignancies without del[5q] treated with lenalidomide. J Hematol Oncol 5: 4.

Expression and Function of the Eph Receptor Family in Leukemia and Hematopoietic Malignancies: Prospects for Targeted Therapies

Sara Charmsaz[1*] **and Andrew W Boyd**[1,2]

[1]Leukaemia Foundation Research Unit, Queensland Institute of Medical Research, 300 Herston Road, Herston, Queensland 4006, Australia
[2]Department of Medicine, University of Queensland, Herston, Queensland 4006, Australia

Abstract

There has been considerable interest in recent years in the development of therapies, which target Eph receptors or their ephrin ligands. The Eph receptor tyrosine kinases and their membrane bound ephrin ligands are cell surface molecules involved in many biological functions and cell behaviors during embryogenesis and in adult life. However, they are also expressed in an aberrant fashion on many tumors and are re-expressed on normal cells in non-malignant pathological states. Some of the eph/ephrins including EphA7 and EphA1 protein are thought to function as tumor suppressors in particular cancers. In tumors where Eph/ephrin proteins are expressed at high levels, being expressed on the cell surface these proteins are readily accessible to antibody-mediated therapies several of which are in advanced pre-clinical or early clinical evaluation, including antibodies specific for EphA2, EphA3, and EphB4 which are expressed on many different tumors. We will review the general features of the Eph/ephrin system and discuss the role of this system in normal hematopoiesis before focusing on the role of Eph proteins in leukemia and other hematological malignancies and possible avenues for therapy.

Keywords: Eph receptor; Ephrin; Receptor Tyrosine Kinase; Hematopoiesis; Hematopoietic Stem Cells; Leukemia

Classification, Structure and Binding of Eph/ephrin

The Eph receptors and their membrane bound ephrin ligands represent the largest family of receptor tyrosine kinases (RTK's). The first member, EphA1, was originally termed Eph, as it was first identified in an Erythropoietin-Producing Hepatocellular (Eph Nomenclature committee, 1997) carcinoma cell line [1]. Fourteen members of the Eph family of RTK have been identified in mammals, which are divided into two groups, the EphA and EphB family. This is based on their sequence homology, ligand specificity and structural features. In mammals there are nine members of the EphA subgroup (EphA1-8 and EphA10) and five EphB receptors (EphB1-4 and EphB6) [2,3].

Eph receptors are type I transmembrane proteins composed of extracellular region including a ligand binding domain with two distinct ligand-binding interfaces (N terminal β jelly roll domain) determining the ephrin binding, and a cysteine-rich region containing an epidermal growth factor (EGF)-like motif that is involved in receptor dimerization followed by two fibronectin type-III domains [4,5]. The intracellular region comprised of a conserved juxtamembrane domain, a tyrosine kinase domain and a sterile alpha motif (SAM) domain, the latter having a potential role in receptor clustering [6,7]. Most of the Eph receptors, possess a C-terminal PDZ (Postsynaptic density protein, Disc large, Zona occludens tight junction protein) binding motif that is involved in signaling at a sub-cellular level and in the assembly of large molecular complexes [3,5,8] (Figure 1a).

The ephrin ligands of Eph receptors are also membrane bound proteins and like the Ephs they are divided into two groups based on their structural features and preferential binding to either EphA or EphB receptors. The two classes of ephrin ligands are the A-class (ephrinA1-5) and B-class (ephrinB1-3) [3]. The two classes of the ephrin ligands have homology at their N-terminus region while their C-terminal amino acid sequence differs, the ephrin-A ligands that are bound to the plasma membrane by a glycosylphosphatidylinositol (GPI)-linker and the ephrin-B ligands, which possess a transmembrane–spanning region and a highly conserved cytoplasmic tail with a number of highly conserved tyrosine residues and a PDZ-binding motif. The conserved tyrosine residues have been shown to serve as a docking site for proteins, which mediate downstream ephrin signaling [2,9] (Figure 1b).

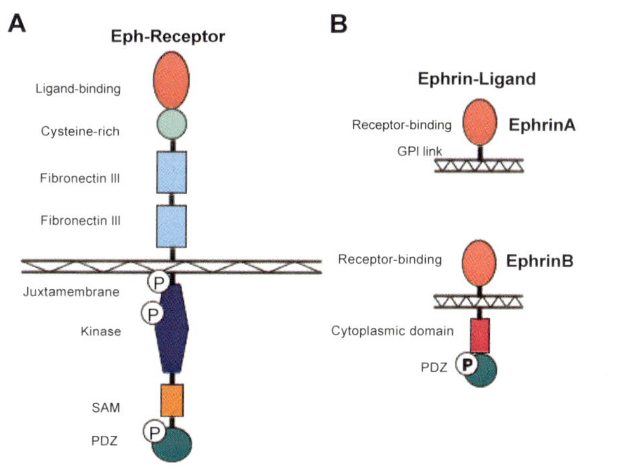

Figure 1: Schematic representation of Eph receptors and ephrin ligand structure. (A) The structure of the Eph receptor. (B) The structure of the ephrin-A and ephrin-B ligand.

***Corresponding author:** Sara Charmsaz, Leukaemia Foundation Research Unit, Queensland Institute of Medical Research, P.O. Royal Brisbane Hospital, Queensland, 4029, Brisbane, Australia, E-mail: sara.charmsaz@qimr.edu.au

Generally, the EphA receptors will preferentially bind to members of the ephrin-A ligands (ephrinA1-5) while the EphB receptors will preferentially bind to the ephrin-B ligands (ephrinB1-3) [3,10]. There is a high level of binding promiscuity between the Eph receptors and the ephrin ligands, however for an individual Eph receptor there is a distinct order of affinity of ephrin interactions with affinity constants ranging from 5-500 nM [11]. For instance the EphA1 receptor binds with a high affinity to ephrin-A1 and a lower affinity to other members of the ephrin-A family, including ephrin-A3 and ephrin-A4, and shows essentially no binding to ephrin-A5 [12]. Similarly EphA3 and EphB4 have a higher affinity for ephrin-A5 and ephrin-B2 respectively than for other members of the ephrin family [11,13]. High affinity interaction is also possible between the classes, for example EphA4 binds to both ephrin-B and -A ligands and some of its most important functions depend on interaction with ephrin-B3. Another example is EphB2, which binds to ephrin-A5 as well as ephrin-B ligands [14,15] (Figure 2).

Eph/ephrin Activation and Signaling

Eph/ephrin interactions have the capacity to initiate bidirectional signaling. In other words both Ephs and ephrins can act as a ligand as well as a receptor and they both have the ability to initiate signaling. Signaling initiated by the Eph receptor is referred to as forward signaling whereas signaling initiated by the ephrin ligand is termed reverse signaling.

Eph receptor activation occurs following the physical association of the receptor and an ephrin ligand on adjacent cell surfaces mediated by the high affinity binding site (dimerization), this is followed by interaction with a second Eph/ephrin complex, mediated by separate low affinity (tetramerization) binding site to create a hetero-tetrameric complex [16]. The tetramers are then assembled into higher order clusters, which appear to be required for effective forward signaling [17,18]. The clustering of Eph receptors results in ligand-dependent auto-phosphorylation of several tyrosine residues within the cytoplasmic kinase domain and juxtamembrane region of the receptor, which serve as docking sites for downstream signaling proteins including the small GTPases of the Rho and Ras family, focal adhesion kinase (FAK), the Janus kinase/signal transducers and activators of transcription (Jak/Stat) and phosphatidylinositol 3-kinase (P13K) pathways [19].

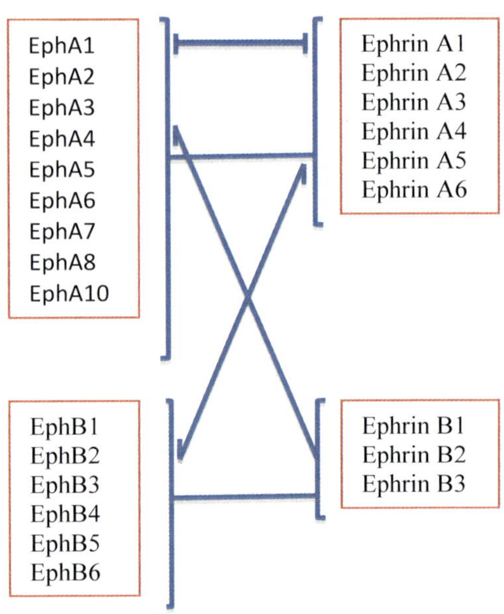

Figure 2: Schematic of Eph receptor and ephrin binding preference.

Eph receptor activation influence cell shape and motility through the regulation of the Rho GTPases, including RhoA, Cdc42, Rac and Ras, via interactions with specific Rho GTPase activating (Rho GAP) and exchange (Rho GEF) factors. The interaction with individual Rho GTPases, mediated via direct binding to the cytoplasmic domain of Eph proteins of Rho GAP and Rho GEF or their recruitment via adaptor proteins, thereby mediating different effects on actin dynamics and cell process formation thus regulating cell shape and movement. For example, activation of EphA4 receptor results in recruitment of ephexin (Rho GEF), leading to activation of RhoA, and α-chimaerin (Rho GAP), leading to inactivation of Rac, jointly resulting in actin depolymerization and retraction of cell processes [15]. Activation through EphB plays a role in actin filament extension, morphogenesis and maturation of dendritic spines. Ras family of GTPases (H- and R- Ras) are also activated through Eph receptors however, unlike the Rho GTPases, the majority of Eph receptors negatively regulate the Ras/Mitogen-activated protein kinase (Ras/MAPK) pathway, with activation normally resulting in regulation of proliferation and migration [15].

Eph receptors are also important in mediating a number of other molecules involved in cell migration and adhesion due to their ability to regulate signal transduction molecules including integrin signaling pathway elements paxillin, FAK, P130 (Cas) and integrins themselves. The effect of Eph signaling on integrins is complex as they can mediate either promoting or suppressing effects. FAK is important in mediating integrin signaling and Eph receptors can down-regulate this pathway [20].

The Jak/Stat pathway, involved in cell growth and viability, is regulated by EphA receptor activation [21]. EphB receptors mediate cell migration and proliferation through P13K pathway and the protein kinase B/phosphatidylinositol 3-kinase (Akt/ PI3K) pathway is involved in the regulation of cell proliferation and viability. Eph/ephrin also regulates other signaling pathways including Abl/Arg and p53-family of tumor suppressor proteins [19]. A recent study in glioblastoma multiforme (GBM) shows that loss of EphA3 results in elevated MAPK signaling thereby inducing differentiation and reducing proliferation and self-renewal. This study showed that regulation of extracellular signal-regulated kinases/mitogen-activated protein kinases (ERK/ MAPK) signaling by EphA3 is kinase independent of the upstream activators of MAPK signaling [22]. A similar finding has been made for GBM which express EphA2 at high levels [23].

In the ephrin-expressing cells reverse signaling can be induced after Eph/ephrin interaction [19,24]. Ephrin-B reverse signaling partly depends on the tyrosine phosphorylation of conserved residues in the cytoplasmic region, where phosphorylation is mediated by associated tyrosine kinases, most notably members of the Src family (Src, Fyn, Lyn, Yes) of tyrosine kinases. When the ephrin-B ligand is phosphorylated it can bind to cytosolic adaptor molecules via (Src Homology-2) SH-2 and SH-3 domains or PDZ domains [8]. The protein tyrosine phosphatase basophil-like (PTP-BL) has been identified as a negative regulator of ephrin-B signaling and it binds to ephrin-B through its C-terminal PDZ binding motif. De-phosphorylation of the ephrin-B cytoplasmic domain can inactivate the Src family of kinase and therefore cause termination of reverse signaling [25]. In the activated ephrin-B ligand, the PDZ motif plays an important role in assembly of other signaling molecules. Ephrin-B binds to cytoplasmic protein PDZ-RGS3, which contains a PDZ domain and a regulator of G-protein signaling (RGS) domain. Activation of the ephrin-B ligand by EphB receptor via the PDZ-RGS interferes with signaling of the stromal derived factor (SDF)-1 via its G-protein coupled receptor and the chemokine receptor-4 (CXCR4). Ephrin-B reverse signaling has thus been implicated with regulation of migration in cerebellar development [26].

The ephrin-A reverse signaling mechanism is not well understood, however it is likely that the signaling response is initiated by activity of the Src family of RTK in which transmembrane adaptor molecules, associating with the lipid anchor of the ephrin-A proteins, transmit the signal across the membrane. For example ephrin-A5 induces signaling within the ephrin-A expressing cell when bound to its cognate Eph receptor [27-29].

Expression and Function of the Eph and Ephrin Genes

Eph signaling controls cell adhesion, migration, invasion and morphology by influencing integrin and intercellular adhesion molecule activity and by modification of actin cytoskeleton organization as described above. Through these mechanisms Eph function effects not only the processes of embryogenesis but also specialized cellular function in adult tissues, including bone remodeling, immune function and synaptic plasticity as well as cell proliferation and survival specific tissue stem cells as described further below [27,30].

Both Eph and ephrin proteins are important in regulating cell-cell interactions and their interaction can initiate either cell adhesion or repulsion. Cell repulsion occurs when bidirectional signaling triggers cytoskeletal contraction, loss of focal adhesions, cell rounding and cell detachment, whereas cell attachment occurs when signals are in favor of cell adhesion and migration [31]. This interaction influence many different cell behaviors during embryogenesis and in adult life [27]. Eph/ephrin interactions mediate formation of tissue boundaries (e.g. hindbrain rhombomeres) [32], control axon guidance during development and also tissue morphogenesis and patterning [33,34]. Eph/ephrin interactions are also involved in development of vascular system [35], stem cell biology [36], hematopoiesis, erythropoiesis, immune function and in tumor invasion and metastasis [27,30,37-39].

Many members of the Eph/ephrin family are expressed at high levels in some cancer cells and also elements of the tumor microenvironment, where they influence tumor growth and spread. Specific examples include lung, breast and prostate cancer, as well as melanoma, sarcomas and leukemias [40,41]. There is evidence that the Eph receptors can have either tumor suppressing or tumor promoting activity, depending on the tissue and their expression pattern [27]. Thus, the role and function of Eph/ephrins in cancer is not yet fully elucidated as some tumors show an elevated level of Eph expression while others show a decrease in Eph expression and as yet no single model of their function encompasses all cancers. For example EphA2 is up regulated in many cancers including breast and prostate and its expression is linked to an increase in malignancy [42,43] but it is down regulated in colon cancer [44]. Similarly, EphA1 expression is up-regulated in ovarian cancer [40] but down-regulated in advanced skin and colorectal cancers [45,46]. Studies have also shown the role of EphA7 as a tumor suppressor in follicular lymphoma [47], tumor suppressor function has also been reported for EphB receptors, including EphB2 and EphB3 in colorectal cancer [30,48]. EphB4 is another important example as this gene can act as either a tumor suppressor or an oncogene in different facets of breast cancer progression [49,50]. Table 1 represents the expression of Eph receptors in normal and malignant tissues [51-82].

The Eph/ephrin in HSC and Leukemia

Eph/ephrin expression in HSC and progenitors

The expression of Eph/ephrin has been detected on purified population of hematopoietic stem cells (HSCs) in both human and mouse. Gene expression analysis of HSC showed expression of ephrin-B2, indicating that it may be involved in signaling between HSC and their microenvironment. Other array based studies on primary human HSC ($CD34^+$ hematopoietic cells) shows expression of the EphA1 protein and its ligands ephrin-A3 and ephrin-A4 suggesting that their interaction may play a role in hematopoietic stem and progenitor cell positioning and function [83,84]. Further analysis of $CD133^+$ and $CD34^+$ hematopoietic stem cells in peripheral blood showed expression of EphA2 in all $CD34^+$ cells and the majority of $CD133^+$ cells however EphB2 was expressed in all $CD133^+$ cells and fifty percent of $CD34^+$ cells, these data suggest that a number of elements of the Eph/ephrin system may have a role in HSC function through regulatory effects on cell adhesion, migration and differentiation but also that there may be a degree of functional redundancy between several Eph proteins [85].

Real-time quantitative PCR of mouse $Lin^-ckit^+sca1^+$ (KLS) showed detectable expression of all EphA receptors except EphA6 and EphA8, along with ephrin-A ligands, with ephrin-A4 and ephrin-A5 being the most highly expressed ligands on purified HSCs in the mouse bone marrow [86]. Flow cytometric analysis of EphA2, A3, A4 and A5 along with ephrinA1-5 showed that EphA2 and EphA3 were the highest expressing EphA receptors. Expression of EphA2, A3, A4 and A5 was also detected in the mouse stromal cell lines however human stromal cell line showed only EphA2 expression at moderate levels [86]. Whilst the function has not been fully investigated, a role in HSC trafficking was demonstrated by treatment of mice with an Eph/ephrin inhibitor, EphA3-Fc, which resulted in mobilization of bone marrow progenitor cells into peripheral blood [86].

Some of the members of the Eph/ephrin family are also involved in development and regulation of mature hematopoietic cells. For example, EphA4 and EphB1 receptors along with ephrin-B1 ligand are expressed on human platelets [87], these studies also shows that EphA4 is involved in regulation of platelet aggregation and adhesion to fibrinogen, a process dependent on integrin $\alpha IIb\beta 3$ engagement [39].

EphB4 was originally identified on human bone marrow $CD34^+$ cells and its expression has been reported on erythroid progenitor cells in early stages of red blood cell development. Significantly, the EphB4 ligand, ephrin-B2, is expressed on bone marrow stromal cells [88] where it has been reported to be involved with regulating erythropoiesis via interaction with EphB4 [89]. Studies by Suenobu et al. [89] showed co-culturing hematopoietic progenitor cells expressing EphB4 with stromal cells expressing ephrin-B2 results in hematopoietic progenitor cells detachment from stromal layer and differentiation into a mature erythroid cells accompanied by EphB4 down regulation, however co-culturing these cell with ephrin-B2-negative stromal cells resulted in less maturation of erythroid cells and no change to EphB4 expression [89]. Ephrin-B2 ectopic expression in stromal cells increased adhesion of hematopoietic cells to stromal calls and decreased transmigration of hematopoietic cells beneath a stromal cell monolayer. These findings strongly support a role for the EphB4/ephrin-B2 interaction in migration and colonization of stem/progenitors cells in the bone marrow microenvironment [90].

Some of the Eph/ephrin molecules are also involved in lymphoid development. The expression of Eph/ephrin has been studied

Eph	Tissue expression	Expression in cancer	References
EphA1	Widely expressed in mouse epithelial tissues evidence of expression in hematopoietic progenitors	Over expressed in many different cancers including hepatocellular, prostate, lung, gastric and colon cancer Down regulated in non-melanoma skin cancer, colorectal cancer	1,12,24,45,46,51-55
EphA2	Expressed highly in adult human epithelial cells and endothelium	Over expressed in prostate, breast, melanoma, lung and ovarian cancers Up-regulated in glioblastoma Down-regulated in colon cancer	23,24,42,43,54-61
EphA3	Expressed in various stages of embryonic development and in adult central nervous system	Expressed in neural cancers, leukemia, lymphomas and sarcomas Up-regulated in lung, brain, liver and kidney Over expressed in melanoma	24,54,55,62-66
EphA4	Expressed in development, final stages of embryogenesis and central nervous system	Expressed in prostate, pancreatic cancer Up-regulated in lung cancer Down-regulated kidney Over expressed in gastric cancer	24,54,55,62,67-70
EphA5	Expressed in nervous system	Expressed in neuroblastomas and neural cancer Down-regulated in breast cancer	24,54,55,70-72
EphA6	Expressed more prominently in adult tissues than in embryonic tissues	Down-regulated in colon cancer and renal carcinoma Up-regulated in lung and liver cancer	24,54,55
EphA7	Expressed in developing neural tubes, thymus, lymphoid tissues and fetal bone marrow	Expressed in colorectal cancer, lung and follicular lymphoma Up-regulated in ALL1 leukemia	24,44,47,54,55,73-75
EphA8	Expressed in spinal cord and neuronal cells	Expressed in colon cancer Down-regulated in glioblastoma	24,54,55
EphA10	Expressed in testis	Over expressed in breast cancer	76,77
EphB1	Expressed in Brain and colon	Expressed in lung cancer Down-regulated in colon carcinoma and in kidney cancer	24,46,54
EphB2	Expressed in epithelial cells, thymus, lymphoid, osteoblastic and osteoclastic cells	Over expressed in gastrointestinal Expressed in colon, ovarian and lung cancer Up-regulated in colorectal, kidney and hepatocellular cancer	24,54,78
EphB3	Expressed in various tissues	Expressed in prostate, lung and melanoma	24,54
EphB4	Expressed in placenta and in range of primary tissues including brain, endothelium, hematopoietic cells	Expressed in colon, endometrial, breast, neuroblastoma, glioblastoma and leukemia and lymphoma cancer	24,54,79-81
EphB6	Expressed in various tissues including brain, pancreas, thymus and T-cells	Expressed in T cell tumors and leukemia Up-regulated in colon cancer Down-regulated in breast, lung and kidney cancer	24,54,82

Table 1: Eph expression in normal and malignant tissues.

extensively in T-lymphocytes and expression of some of the members of this family including EphA1, EphA2, EphA3, EphA4, EphA7, EphB2, EphB6, ephrin-A1 ephrin-A3, ephrin-A5 and ephrin-B1 has been reported in the thymus, both on thymic stroma and lymphoid cells suggesting a role in T-cell development [91-93]. Interestingly, there are no reports of defective T lineage development in knockout mice, perhaps a result of there being multiple Eph receptors with overlapping functions in the T cell compartment.

As well as T-lymphocytes the expression of Eph/ephrin gene has been also reported in B-lymphocytes [38,94,95]. EphA7 and EphA4 transcripts were found in human fetal bone marrow pro-B and pre-B cells. EphA4 expression is found in both adult and fetal pro-B and pre-B lineage cells with high levels of expression in peripheral blood. The full length EphA7 transcript, however, was not found in mature fetal B-lineage and adult B-lineage cells. This suggests that EphA7 may be involved in expansion and /or differentiation of pre/pro B-cell but is lost on mature B cells [95]. Further studies show that there are different types of EphA7 mRNA, one of which encodes the full length EphA7 and another splice variant encodes a truncated, soluble protein that lacks the cytoplasmic domain. Studies by Dawson et al. [74] showed that normal lymphocytes express and secrete the truncated form of EphA7 [74], which have been shown to have tumor suppressive effects in lymphoma [47].

Eph/Ephrin in vascular development

In the context of hematopoiesis, the vascular system is crucial in development of blood cells within the bone marrow and also in the function and migration of mature hematopoietic cells. The vascular system arises from two distinct processes known as vasculogenesis and angiogenesis. Vasculogenesis is an early event in embryonic development involving mesodermal cells differentiation to form a vascular plexus in embryonic tissues and angiogenesis is a process in which new blood vessels are formed from existing blood vessels. Angiogenesis has a role both in early development and in the adult hematopoietic system, it also promotes sprouting of new blood vessels in embryonic and postnatal vasculature and it has been shown to be important in development and metastasis of solid tumors [96]. Some members of Eph/ephrin family have established roles in vasculogenesis and angiogenesis. The expression analysis of Eph/ephrin using real-time polymerase chain reaction (RT-PCR) has shown expression of EphB2, EphB3, EphB4, ephrin-B1 and ephrin-B2 in the yolk sac [97]. Ephrin-B1 expression has been detected on both arteries and veins while the high affinity ligand for EphB4, ephrin-B2, is only detected on arteries and EphB4 expression is only detected on veins. Knock out ephrin-B2 mice and some of the EphB2 and EphB3 double mutants mice have defects in embryonic vasculature and therefore these mice are embryonically lethal. EphB2 and ephrin-B2 expression in mesenchyme adjacent to vessels and the vascular defects in EphB2/EphB3 double mutants indicate a requirement for Eph/ephrin signaling between endothelial cells and surrounding mesenchymal cells [97]. EphA2 has also been reported to have a role in angiogenesis and the expression of EphA2 and its ligand ephrin-A1 has been reported in both human and mouse tumor vasculature [61].

Eph/Ephrin on bone remodeling and formation

The bone marrow is the principal site of hematopoiesis in adult animals and requires both vascular and other stromal cell types to create the hematopoietic niche. Important amongst these are the osteoblasts and osteoclasts, which mediate bone formation and remodeling. Bone is constantly remodeled through resorption of mineralized bone by osteoclast and formation of new bone by osteoblast. Coupling of bone resorption and formation is critical during normal bone remodeling and it is necessary for bone growth, any deregulation in this process will result in pathological bone disease [19,78].

Eph receptors and ephrin ligands are important in bone remodeling and homeostasis during this process Eph/ephrin bidirectional signaling regulates differentiation and function of the bone cells. Real time PCR (RT-PCR) analysis of the Eph/ephrin showed mRNA expression of ephrin ligands, ephrin-B1, ephrin-B2 and ephrin-A1, A2, A4 and A5, as well as Eph receptors including EphB2-4, EphB6, EphA2-4 and EphA7 receptors on osteoblastic and osteoclastic cells [98-100]. Expression of EphB4 is observed on the osteoblasts and forward signaling through EphB4 results in bone formation and reverse signaling through ephrin-B2 inhibit bone resorption therefore ephrin-B2/EphB4 act as coupling stimulator [98]. Expression of ephrin-A2 was observed during early osteoclastogenesis and unlike the ephrin-B2 it acts as coupling inhibitor as reverse signaling through ephrin-A2 result osteoclastogenesis and EphA2 forward signaling into osteoblast inhibit osteoblastic bone formation and mineralization [99]. Ephrin-A2/EphA2 bidirectional signaling facilitates bone remodeling at initiation phase, forward signaling through EphA2 receptor on osteoblast inhibit osteoblastic differentiation and bone formation and reverse signaling into osteoclast through ephrin-A2 promote osteoclast differentiation [78,99]. Ephrin-B1 full knockout mice are prenatally lethal and they have skeletal defects. Studies on disruption of ephrin-B1 on collagen I producing cells result in reduced bone formation and skull defect and studies on ephrin-B1 conditional knockout mice shows defects in osteoblastic mediated bone formation with no increase in osteoclastic bone resorption and this condition results in reduction in bone size and density [101,102].

The importance of Eph/ephrin interactions has also been shown in various stem cell niches, including neural, dental and intestinal stem cell compartments [103,104]. More recent studies show their involvement in bone homeostasis and mesenchymal stem cell (MSC) regulation. Arthur et al. [104] showed increase in osteogenic differentiation upon ephrin-B1 and/or ephrin-B2 expression by MSC. They also showed that ephrin-B1 activation promoted chondrogenic differentiation; therefore EphB/ephrin-B interactions may be involved in recruitment, migration and differentiation of MSC during bone repair [104]. Studies by Ting et al. [86] shows that ephrin-A signaling interact with stem/progenitor cells in the bone marrow niche as it's signaling mediates the release of progenitor cells from hematopoietic niche [86].

Interestingly, Eph/ephrin interactions are also involved in bone malignancies and tumors, osteocarcinoma is a malignant bone tumor in adolescence and microarray analysis studies show increased expression of EphA2, EphA4, ephrin-B1 and ephrin-A1 in osteosarcoma cells [105,106].

Eph/Ephrin expression in leukemia and other hematopoietic tumors

Both chronic and acute myeloid leukemia are malignant diseases of the hematopoietic system which in most cases are believed to arise through the abnormal proliferation of either uncommitted or partially committed HSC [107]. The origin of other types of leukemia such as promyelocytic leukemia, pre-B acute lymphoblastic leukemia (ALL) and T-ALL and chronic lymphoblastic leukemia (CLL) are more likely due to malignant transformation of more mature progenitor cells. Expression of elements of the Eph/ephrin system has been detected on many types of human leukemia. One of the best studied is EphA3, which was originally identified in the LK63 pre-B ALL cell line and further investigations revealed its expression in T-cell leukemia cell lines such as Jurkat, JM and HSB-2 [65,108]. It has been shown that EphA3 can induce both adhesive and cell repulsive responses in different cell types [109]. In analyzing ephrin induced cell adhesion in LK63 cells, a critical role was identified for protein phosphatase activity, which prevented EphA3 phosphorylation and hence maintained the Eph/ephrin adhesive bond and prevented initiation of the signaling mechanisms leading to cell repulsion [31]. In leukemia, EphA3 is expressed at significantly higher levels compared to normal blood cells, elevated expression of EphA3 being detected in a proportion of clinical samples from cases of lymphoid and myeloid leukemias [111]. Elevated EphA3 expression has also been detected on other cancers such as lung cancer, melanoma and brain tumors [22,64,65,109], whereas expression was found to be absent or low in corresponding normal tissues [54,65,110]. Recent array based studies also showed EphA3 as one of the genes with copy number alteration (CNA) in the genome of acute myeloid leukemia (AML) patients [111]. Further studies by Guan et al. [112] showed copy number variation (CNV) of EphA3 to be associated with various types hematological malignancies and therefore CNV of EphA3 could be used as a diagnostic indicator for different types of leukemia [112]. Many cancers, including leukemia, require multiple cooperative oncogene mutations for malignant cell transformation. Specific sets of synergistically dysregulated by cooperative oncogenes are known as cooperative response gene (CRGs), which regulate leukemia stem cell (LSC) growth and survival. Studies by Ashton et al. [113], where stem cells were retrovirally transduced with two fusion genes found in human myeloid leukemias. NUP98-HOXA9 and BCR-ABL, have identified EphA3 as a common CRG. They showed that shRNA knock down of EphA3 in leukemic stem cells reduced leukemic cell engraftment, concluding that this gene may be responsible for leukemia stem cell growth and survival in bone marrow microenvironment [113]. With the involvement of EphA3 in many different types of leukemia a high affinity monoclonal antibody to EphA3 (IIIA4) [65] has been fully humaneered by Kalabios and the resulting antibody, KB004, is now in phase I clinical trial in leukemia and other hematological cancers [114].

As mentioned previously EphB4 was originally identified in human bone marrow CD34$^+$ cells and its expression been reported in erythroid progenitor cells, however it's ligand ephrin-B2 is expressed in bone marrow stromal cells [88]. Co-expression of EphB4 and ephrin-B2 is found in the yolk sac, which is the first site of hematopoiesis and vascular development during embryogenesis. EphB4/ephrin-B2 expression has been shown in the majority of leukemia and lymphoma cell lines although expression in clinical samples appears less prominent [81]. Antibodies to EphB4 have undergone extensive pre-clinical evaluation and shown good anti-tumor effects in solid tumors, which over-express EphB4 and by inhibition of angiogenesis, although no efficacy has been shown in hematopoietic tumors to date [115]. Nevertheless, these antibodies may have the potential to be developed to target EphB4 in leukemia and related blood cancers.

Studies by Nakanishi et al. [75] shows EphA7 up regulation in the ALL1 associated leukemia (ALL1/AF4 and ALL1/AF9). They also showed that EphA7 up-regulation was associated with phosphorylation

Eph	Targeted therapy	References
EphA1	Tumor suppressor in colorectal cancer	44
EphA2	EphA2 targeting reagents in ovarian cancer therapy	119
EphA3	Therapeutic target in leukemia and glioblastoma	22,110
EphA7	Tumor suppressor in T-LBL and follicular lymphoma	47,120
EphB4	EphB4 antibody to inhibit solid tumor growth	115

Table 2: Eph receptors as a therapy target for cancer.

of ERK and treatment with a phosphorylated ERK blocking drug resulted in apoptotic cell death in ALL1/AF4 leukemic blast cells [75]. Thus, anti-EphA7 antibodies or other inhibitors may well have a role in leukemia associated with this translocation. In contra-distinction to this positive role in leukemia, EphA7 is lost in lymphomas, where the gene is hypermethylated and repressed in germinal center B-cell non-Hodgkins lymphomas and this has a potential to influence tumor progression and spread [74]. In this study a soluble form of EphA7 was shown to inhibit lymphoma in a mouse model, a chimeric protein consisting of soluble EphA7 and CD20 antibody had still greater therapeutic effect. Further studies show EphA7 as targeted tumor suppressor gene in T-cell lymphoblastic leukemia and lymphoma (T-LBL) and follicular B cell lymphoma [47,116].

EphB6 expression has been observed in normal human tissue and over-expression of EphB6 has also been reported in both myeloid [117] and lymphoid leukemias [82,118]. The expression level of EphB6 decreases with maturation of the cells in T-cell derived leukemia-cells, therefore suggesting that EphB6 expression regulates T-cell development but has less significant role in mature T cells [82]. To date there are no reports of experimental therapies targeting EphB6. Table 2 [110,119,120] represents the summary of Eph receptors used as therapy target in various malignancies.

Summary

In summary, the aberrant expression of Eph receptors in hematopoietic tumors reflects the spectrum of functions of these receptors in all cancers. In some cancers these genes act as tumor suppressor, examples being EphA1 in colorectal cancer and EphA7 in follicular lymphomas. On the other hand these proteins can also have oncogenic effects, examples being the expression of EphA2 and EphA3 in glioma and the over-expression of EphA3 in leukemia. In terms of therapy, the over-expression in certain tumors, taken together with the surface expression of these proteins, makes a strong case for targeted therapies. This is particularly the case when expression on normal tissues is minimal; this is exemplified by EphA3 and EphB4 where no toxicity was evident in pre-clinical testing of potential therapeutic antibodies. These studies reveal the therapeutic potential of targeting components of the Eph/ephrin system in leukemia and other cancers. These results should prompt further research into the specific roles of these proteins in different cancers as a prelude to designing and optimizing the therapeutic targeting of these proteins.

References

1. Hirai H, Maru Y, Hagiwara K, Nishida J, Takaku F (1987) A novel putative tyrosine kinase receptor encoded by the eph gene. Science 238: 1717-1720.
2. Himanen JP, Nikolov DB (2003) Eph signaling: a structural view. Trends Neurosci 26: 46-51.
3. Pasquale EB (2005) Eph receptor signalling casts a wide net on cell behaviour. Nat Rev Mol Cell Biol 6: 462-475.
4. Pasquale EB (1997) The Eph family of receptors. Curr Opin Cell Biol 9: 608-615.
5. Himanen JP, Nikolov DB (2003) Eph receptors and ephrins. Int J Biochem Cell Biol 35: 130-134.
6. Holland SJ, Gale NW, Gish GD, Roth RA, Songyang Z, et al. (1997) Juxtamembrane tyrosine residues couple the Eph family receptor EphB2/Nuk to specific SH2 domain proteins in neuronal cells. EMBO J 16: 3877-3888.
7. Stapleton D, Balan I, Pawson T, Sicheri F (1999) The crystal structure of an Eph receptor SAM domain reveals a mechanism for modular dimerization. Nat Struct Biol 6: 44-49.
8. Torres R, Firestein BL, Dong H, Staudinger J, Olson EN, et al. (1998) PDZ proteins bind, cluster, and synaptically colocalize with Eph receptors and their ephrin ligands. Neuron 21: 1453-1463.
9. Cerretti DP, Vanden Bos T, Nelson N, Kozlosky CJ, Reddy P, et al. (1995) Isolation of LERK-5: a ligand of the eph-related receptor tyrosine kinases. Mol Immunol 32: 1197-1205.
10. Boyd AW, Lackmann M (2001) Signals from Eph and ephrin proteins: a developmental tool kit. Sci STKE 2001: re20.
11. Lackmann M, Mann RJ, Kravets L, Smith FM, Bucci TA, et al. (1997) Ligand for EPH-related kinase (LERK) 7 is the preferred high affinity ligand for the HEK receptor. J Biol Chem 272: 16521-16530.
12. Coulthard MG, Lickliter JD, Subanesan N, Chen K, Webb GC, et al. (2001) Characterization of the Epha1 receptor tyrosine kinase: expression in epithelial tissues. Growth Factors 18: 303-317.
13. Blits-Huizinga CT, Nelersa CM, Malhotra A, Liebl DJ (2004) Ephrins and their receptors: binding versus biology. IUBMB Life 56: 257-265.
14. Mosch B, Reissenweber B, Neuber C, Pietzsch J (2010) Eph receptors and ephrin ligands: important players in angiogenesis and tumor angiogenesis. J Oncol 2010: 135285.
15. Lackmann M, Boyd AW (2008) Eph, a protein family coming of age: more confusion, insight, or complexity? Sci Signal 1: re2.
16. Himanen JP, Rajashankar KR, Lackmann M, Cowan CA, Henkemeyer M, et al. (2001) Crystal structure of an Eph receptor-ephrin complex. Nature 414: 933-938.
17. Wimmer-Kleikamp SH, Janes PW, Squire A, Bastiaens PI, Lackmann M (2004) Recruitment of Eph receptors into signaling clusters does not require ephrin contact. J Cell Biol 164: 661-666.
18. Smith FM, Vearing C, Lackmann M, Treutlein H, Himanen J, et al. (2004) Dissecting the EphA3/Ephrin-A5 interactions using a novel functional mutagenesis screen. J Biol Chem 279: 9522-9531.
19. Edwards CM, Mundy GR (2008) Eph receptors and ephrin signaling pathways: a role in bone homeostasis. Int J Med Sci 5: 263-272.
20. Miao H, Burnett E, Kinch M, Simon E, Wang B (2000) Activation of EphA2 kinase suppresses integrin function and causes focal-adhesion-kinase dephosphorylation. Nat Cell Biol 2: 62-69.
21. Lai KO, Chen Y, Po HM, Lok KC, Gong K, et al. (2004) Identification of the Jak/Stat proteins as novel downstream targets of EphA4 signaling in muscle: implications in the regulation of acetylcholinesterase expression. J Biol Chem 279: 13383-13392.
22. Day BW, Stringer BW, Al-Ejeh F, Ting MJ, Wilson J, et al. (2013) EphA3 maintains tumorigenicity and is a therapeutic target in glioblastoma multiforme. Cancer Cell 23: 238-248.
23. Binda E, Visioli A, Giani F, Lamorte G, Copetti M, et al. (2012) The EphA2 receptor drives self-renewal and tumorigenicity in stem-like tumor-propagating cells from human glioblastomas. Cancer Cell 22: 765-780.
24. Surawska H, Ma PC, Salgia R (2004) The role of ephrins and Eph receptors in cancer. Cytokine Growth Factor Rev 15: 419-433.
25. Palmer A, Zimmer M, Erdmann KS, Eulenburg V, Porthin A, et al. (2002) EphrinB phosphorylation and reverse signaling: regulation by Src kinases and PTP-BL phosphatase. Mol Cell 9: 725-737.
26. Lu Q, Sun EE, Klein RS, Flanagan JG (2001) Ephrin-B reverse signaling is mediated by a novel PDZ-RGS protein and selectively inhibits G protein-coupled chemoattraction. Cell 105: 69-79.
27. Pasquale EB (2008) Eph-ephrin bidirectional signaling in physiology and disease. Cell 133: 38-52.
28. Davy A, Gale NW, Murray EW, Klinghoffer RA, Soriano P, et al. (1999) Compartmentalized signaling by GPI-anchored ephrin-A5 requires the Fyn tyrosine kinase to regulate cellular adhesion. Genes Dev 13: 3125-3135.

29. Davy A, Robbins SM (2000) Ephrin-A5 modulates cell adhesion and morphology in an integrin-dependent manner. EMBO J 19: 5396-5405.

30. Pasquale EB (2010) Eph receptors and ephrins in cancer: bidirectional signalling and beyond. Nat Rev Cancer 10: 165-180.

31. Wimmer-Kleikamp SH, Nievergall E, Gegenbauer K, Adikari S, Mansour M, et al. (2008) Elevated protein tyrosine phosphatase activity provokes Eph/ephrin-facilitated adhesion of pre-B leukemia cells. Blood 112: 721-732.

32. Dahmann C, Oates AC, Brand M (2011) Boundary formation and maintenance in tissue development. Nat Rev Genet 12: 43-55.

33. Scicolone G, Ortalli AL, Carri NG (2009) Key roles of Ephs and ephrins in retinotectal topographic map formation. Brain Res Bull 79: 227-247.

34. Coulthard MG, Duffy S, Down M, Evans B, Power M, et al. (2002) The role of the Eph-ephrin signalling system in the regulation of developmental patterning. Int J Dev Biol 46: 375-384.

35. Adams RH, Eichmann A (2010) Axon guidance molecules in vascular patterning. Cold Spring Harb Perspect Biol 2: a001875.

36. Murai KK, Pasquale EB (2010) Restraining stem cell niche plasticity: a new talent of Eph receptors. Cell Stem Cell 7: 647-648.

37. Rivera J, Lozano ML, Navarro-Núñez L, Vicente V (2009) Platelet receptors and signaling in the dynamics of thrombus formation. Haematologica 94: 700-711.

38. Ting MJ, Boyd AW (2008) The Role of Eph Receptor Tyrosine Kinases and Ephrin Ligands in Hematopoietic Cell Development and Function. The Open Hematology Journal 2: 103-110.

39. Prévost N, Woulfe DS, Jiang H, Stalker TJ, Marchese P, et al. (2005) Eph kinases and ephrins support thrombus growth and stability by regulating integrin outside-in signaling in platelets. Proc Natl Acad Sci U S A 102: 9820-9825.

40. Herath NI, Spanevello MD, Sabesan S, Newton T, Cummings M, et al. (2006) Over-expression of Eph and ephrin genes in advanced ovarian cancer: ephrin gene expression correlates with shortened survival. BMC Cancer 6: 144.

41. Noberini R, Pasquale EB (2009) Proliferation and tumor suppression: not mutually exclusive for Eph receptors. Cancer Cell 16: 452-454.

42. Walker-Daniels J, Coffman K, Azimi M, Rhim JS, Bostwick DG, et al. (1999) Overexpression of the EphA2 tyrosine kinase in prostate cancer. Prostate 41: 275-280.

43. Zelinski DP, Zantek ND, Stewart JC, Irizarry AR, Kinch MS (2001) EphA2 overexpression causes tumorigenesis of mammary epithelial cells. Cancer Res 61: 2301-2306.

44. Herath NI, Spanevello MD, Doecke JD, Smith FM, Pouponnot C, et al. (2012) Complex expression patterns of Eph receptor tyrosine kinases and their ephrin ligands in colorectal carcinogenesis. Eur J Cancer 48: 753-762.

45. Hafner C, Becker B, Landthaler M, Vogt T (2006) Expression profile of Eph receptors and ephrin ligands in human skin and downregulation of EphA1 in nonmelanoma skin cancer. Mod Pathol 19: 1369-1377.

46. Herath NI, Doecke J, Spanevello MD, Leggett BA, Boyd AW (2009) Epigenetic silencing of EphA1 expression in colorectal cancer is correlated with poor survival. Br J Cancer 100: 1095-1102.

47. Oricchio E, Nanjangud G, Wolfe AL, Schatz JH, Mavrakis KJ, et al. (2011) The Eph-receptor A7 is a soluble tumor suppressor for follicular lymphoma. Cell 147: 554-564.

48. Schneikert J, Behrens J (2007) The canonical Wnt signalling pathway and its APC partner in colon cancer development. Gut 56: 417-425.

49. Noren NK, Foos G, Hauser CA, Pasquale EB (2006) The EphB4 receptor suppresses breast cancer cell tumorigenicity through an Abl-Crk pathway. Nat Cell Biol 8: 815-825.

50. Noren NK, Pasquale EB (2007) Paradoxes of the EphB4 receptor in cancer. Cancer Res 67: 3994-3997.

51. Nakamoto M, Bergemann AD (2002) Diverse roles for the Eph family of receptor tyrosine kinases in carcinogenesis. Microsc Res Tech 59: 58-67.

52. Robinson D, He F, Pretlow T, Kung HJ (1996) A tyrosine kinase profile of prostate carcinoma. Proc Natl Acad Sci U S A 93: 5958-5962.

53. Kao HW, Chen HC, Wu CW, Lin WC (2003) Tyrosine-kinase expression profiles in human gastric cancer cell lines and their modulations with retinoic acids. Br J Cancer 88: 1058-1064.

54. Hafner C, Schmitz G, Meyer S, Bataille F, Hau P, et al. (2004) Differential gene expression of Eph receptors and ephrins in benign human tissues and cancers. Clin Chem 50: 490-499.

55. Böhme B, Holtrich U, Wolf G, Luzius H, Grzeschik KH, et al. (1993) PCR mediated detection of a new human receptor-tyrosine-kinase, HEK 2. Oncogene 8: 2857-2862.

56. Coulthard MG, Morgan M, Woodruff TM, Arumugam TV, Taylor SM, et al. (2012) Eph/Ephrin signaling in injury and inflammation. Am J Pathol 181: 1493-1503.

57. Hess AR, Seftor EA, Gardner LM, Carles-Kinch K, Schneider GB, et al. (2001) Molecular regulation of tumor cell vasculogenic mimicry by tyrosine phosphorylation: role of epithelial cell kinase (Eck/EphA2). Cancer Res 61: 3250-3255.

58. Kinch MS, Moore MB, Harpole DH Jr (2003) Predictive value of the EphA2 receptor tyrosine kinase in lung cancer recurrence and survival. Clin Cancer Res 9: 613-618.

59. Thaker PH, Deavers M, Celestino J, Thornton A, Fletcher MS, et al. (2004) EphA2 expression is associated with aggressive features in ovarian carcinoma. Clin Cancer Res 10: 5145-5150.

60. Easty DJ, Herlyn M, Bennett DC (1995) Abnormal protein tyrosine kinase gene expression during melanoma progression and metastasis. Int J Cancer 60: 129-136.

61. Ogawa K, Pasqualini R, Lindberg RA, Kain R, Freeman AL, et al. (2000) The ephrin-A1 ligand and its receptor, EphA2, are expressed during tumor neovascularization. Oncogene 19: 6043-6052.

62. Kilpatrick TJ, Brown A, Lai C, Gassmann M, Goulding M, et al. (1996) Expression of the Tyro4/Mek4/Cek4 gene specifically marks a subset of embryonic motor neurons and their muscle targets. Mol Cell Neurosci 7: 62-74.

63. Dottori M, Down M, Hüttmann A, Fitzpatrick DR, Boyd AW (1999) Cloning and characterization of EphA3 (Hek) gene promoter: DNA methylation regulates expression in hematopoietic tumor cells. Blood 94: 2477-2486.

64. Chiari R, Hames G, Stroobant V, Texier C, Maillère B, et al. (2000) Identification of a tumor-specific shared antigen derived from an Eph receptor and presented to CD4 T cells on HLA class II molecules. Cancer Res 60: 4855-4863.

65. Boyd AW, Ward LD, Wicks IP, Simpson RJ, Salvaris E, et al. (1992) Isolation and characterization of a novel receptor-type protein tyrosine kinase (hek) from a human pre-B cell line. J Biol Chem 267: 3262-3267.

66. Salvaris E, Novotny JR, Welch K, Campbell L, Boyd AW (1992) Characterization of two novel pre-B-cell lines (LK63 and LiLa-1): potential models of pre-B-cell differentiation. Leuk Res 16: 655-663.

67. Iiizumi M, Hosokawa M, Takehara A, Chung S, Nakamura T, et al. (2006) EphA4 receptor, overexpressed in pancreatic ductal adenocarcinoma, promotes cancer cell growth. Cancer Sci 97: 1211-1216.

68. Dottori M, Hartley L, Galea M, Paxinos G, Polizzotto M, et al. (1998) EphA4 (Sek1) receptor tyrosine kinase is required for the development of the corticospinal tract. Proc Natl Acad Sci U S A 95: 13248-13253.

69. Oki M, Yamamoto H, Taniguchi H, Adachi Y, Imai K, et al. (2008) Overexpression of the receptor tyrosine kinase EphA4 in human gastric cancers. World J Gastroenterol 14: 5650-5656.

70. Olivieri G, Miescher GC (1999) Immunohistochemical localization of EphA5 in the adult human central nervous system. J Histochem Cytochem 47: 855-861.

71. Fu DY, Wang ZM, Wang BL, Chen L, Yang WT, et al. (2010) Frequent epigenetic inactivation of the receptor tyrosine kinase EphA5 by promoter methylation in human breast cancer. Hum Pathol 41: 48-58.

72. Szabó PM, Pintér M, Szabó DR, Zsippai A, Patócs A, et al. (2012) Integrative analysis of neuroblastoma and pheochromocytoma genomics data. BMC Med Genomics 5: 48.

73. Vergara-Silva A, Schaefer KL, Berg LJ (2002) Compartmentalized Eph receptor and ephrin expression in the thymus. Mech Dev 119 Suppl 1: S225-229.

74. Dawson DW, Hong JS, Shen RR, French SW, Troke JJ, et al. (2007) Global DNA methylation profiling reveals silencing of a secreted form of Epha7 in mouse and human germinal center B-cell lymphomas. Oncogene 26: 4243-4252.

75. Nakanishi H, Nakamura T, Canaani E, Croce CM (2007) ALL1 fusion proteins induce deregulation of EphA7 and ERK phosphorylation in human acute leukemias. Proc Natl Acad Sci U S A 104: 14442-14447.

76. Aasheim HC, Patzke S, Hjorthaug HS, Finne EF (2005) Characterization of a novel Eph receptor tyrosine kinase, EphA10, expressed in testis. Biochim Biophys Acta 1723: 1-7.

77. Fox BP, Kandpal RP (2011) A paradigm shift in EPH receptor interaction: biological relevance of EPHB6 interaction with EPHA2 and EPHB2 in breast carcinoma cell lines. Cancer Genomics Proteomics 8: 185-193.

78. Matsuo K, Otaki N (2012) Bone cell interactions through Eph/ephrin: bone modeling, remodeling and associated diseases. Cell Adh Migr 6: 148-156.

79. Andres AC, Reid HH, Zürcher G, Blaschke RJ, Albrecht D, et al. (1994) Expression of two novel eph-related receptor protein tyrosine kinases in mammary gland development and carcinogenesis. Oncogene 9: 1461-1467.

80. Stephenson SA, Slomka S, Douglas EL, Hewett PJ, Hardingham JE (2001) Receptor protein tyrosine kinase EphB4 is up-regulated in colon cancer. BMC Mol Biol 2: 15.

81. Steube KG, Meyer C, Habig S, Uphoff CC, Drexler HG (1999) Expression of receptor tyrosine kinase HTK (hepatoma transmembrane kinase) and HTK ligand by human leukemia-lymphoma cell lines. Leuk Lymphoma 33: 371-376.

82. Shimoyama M, Matsuoka H, Tamekane A, Ito M, Iwata N, et al. (2000) T-cell-specific expression of kinase-defective Eph-family receptor protein, EphB6 in normal as well as transformed hematopoietic cells. Growth Factors 18: 63-78.

83. Ivanova NB, Dimos JT, Schaniel C, Hackney JA, Moore KA, et al. (2002) A stem cell molecular signature. Science 298: 601-604.

84. Steidl U, Bork S, Schaub S, Selbach O, Seres J, et al. (2004) Primary human CD34+ hematopoietic stem and progenitor cells express functionally active receptors of neuromediators. Blood 104: 81-88.

85. Lazarova P, Wu Q, Kvalheim G, Suo Z, Haakenstad KW, et al. (2006) Growth factor receptors in hematopoietic stem cells: EPH family expression in CD34+ and CD133+ cell populations from mobilized peripheral blood. Int J Immunopathol Pharmacol 19: 49-56.

86. Ting MJ, Day BW, Spanevello MD, Boyd AW (2010) Activation of ephrin A proteins influences hematopoietic stem cell adhesion and trafficking patterns. Exp Hematol 38: 1087-1098.

87. Prevost N, Woulfe D, Tanaka T, Brass LF (2002) Interactions between Eph kinases and ephrins provide a mechanism to support platelet aggregation once cell-to-cell contact has occurred. Proc Natl Acad Sci U S A 99: 9219-9224.

88. Wang Z, Cohen K, Shao Y, Mole P, Dombkowski D, et al. (2004) Ephrin receptor, EphB4, regulates ES cell differentiation of primitive mammalian hemangioblasts, blood, cardiomyocytes, and blood vessels. Blood 103: 100-109.

89. Suenobu S, Takakura N, Inada T, Yamada Y, Yuasa H, et al. (2002) A role of EphB4 receptor and its ligand, ephrin-B2, in erythropoiesis. Biochem Biophys Res Commun 293: 1124-1131.

90. Okubo T, Yanai N, Obinata M (2006) Stromal cells modulate ephrinB2 expression and transmigration of hematopoietic cells. Exp Hematol 34: 330-338.

91. Muñoz JJ, Alonso-C LM, Sacedón R, Crompton T, Vicente A, et al. (2002) Expression and function of the Eph A receptors and their ligands ephrins A in the rat thymus. J Immunol 169: 177-184.

92. Yu G, Mao J, Wu Y, Luo H, Wu J (2006) Ephrin-B1 is critical in T-cell development. J Biol Chem 281: 10222-10229.

93. Shimoyama M, Matsuoka H, Nagata A, Iwata N, Tamekane A, et al. (2002) Developmental expression of EphB6 in the thymus: lessons from EphB6 knockout mice. Biochem Biophys Res Commun 298: 87-94.

94. Trinidad EM, Zapata AG, Alonso-Colmenar LM (2010) Eph-ephrin bidirectional signaling comes into the context of lymphocyte transendothelial migration. Cell Adh Migr 4: 363-367.

95. Aasheim HC, Terstappen LW, Logtenberg T (1997) Regulated expression of the Eph-related receptor tyrosine kinase Hek11 in early human B lymphopoiesis. Blood 90: 3613-3622.

96. Brantley DM, Cheng N, Thompson EJ, Lin Q, Brekken RA, et al. (2002) Soluble Eph A receptors inhibit tumor angiogenesis and progression in vivo. Oncogene 21: 7011-7026.

97. Adams RH, Wilkinson GA, Weiss C, Diella F, Gale NW, et al. (1999) Roles of ephrinB ligands and EphB receptors in cardiovascular development: demarcation of arterial/venous domains, vascular morphogenesis, and sprouting angiogenesis. Genes Dev 13: 295-306.

98. Zhao C, Irie N, Takada Y, Shimoda K, Miyamoto T, et al. (2006) Bidirectional ephrinB2-EphB4 signaling controls bone homeostasis. Cell Metab 4: 111-121.

99. Irie N, Takada Y, Watanabe Y, Matsuzaki Y, Naruse C, et al. (2009) Bidirectional signaling through ephrinA2-EphA2 enhances osteoclastogenesis and suppresses osteoblastogenesis. J Biol Chem 284: 14637-14644.

100. Allan EH, Häusler KD, Wei T, Gooi JH, Quinn JM, et al. (2008) EphrinB2 regulation by PTH and PTHrP revealed by molecular profiling in differentiating osteoblasts. J Bone Miner Res 23: 1170-1181.

101. Xing W, Kim J, Wergedal J, Chen ST, Mohan S (2010) Ephrin B1 regulates bone marrow stromal cell differentiation and bone formation by influencing TAZ transactivation via complex formation with NHERF1. Mol Cell Biol 30: 711-721.

102. Cheng S, Zhao SL, Nelson B, Kesavan C, Qin X, et al. (2012) Targeted disruption of ephrin B1 in cells of myeloid lineage increases osteoclast differentiation and bone resorption in mice. PLoS One 7: e32887.

103. Lathia JD, Rao MS, Mattson MP, Ffrench-Constant C (2007) The microenvironment of the embryonic neural stem cell: lessons from adult niches? Dev Dyn 236: 3267-3282.

104. Arthur A, Zannettino A, Panagopoulos R, Koblar SA, Sims NA, et al. (2011) EphB/ephrin-B interactions mediate human MSC attachment, migration and osteochondral differentiation. Bone 48: 533-542.

105. Kiyokawa E, Takai S, Tanaka M, Iwase T, Suzuki M, et al. (1994) Overexpression of ERK, an EPH family receptor protein tyrosine kinase, in various human tumors. Cancer Res 54: 3645-3650.

106. Varelias A, Koblar SA, Cowled PA, Carter CD, Clayer M (2002) Human osteosarcoma expresses specific ephrin profiles: implications for tumorigenicity and prognosis. Cancer 95: 862-869.

107. McKenzie (1996). Textbook of Hematology. (2ndedn), Williams & Wilkins Publishers, USA.

108. Wicks IP, Wilkinson D, Salvaris E, Boyd AW (1992) Molecular cloning of HEK, the gene encoding a receptor tyrosine kinase expressed by human lymphoid tumor cell lines. Proc Natl Acad Sci U S A 89: 1611-1615.

109. Lawrenson ID, Wimmer-Kleikamp SH, Lock P, Schoenwaelder SM, Down M, et al. (2002) Ephrin-A5 induces rounding, blebbing and de-adhesion of EphA3-expressing 293T and melanoma cells by CrkII and Rho-mediated signalling. J Cell Sci 115: 1059-1072.

110. Vearing C, Lee FT, Wimmer-Kleikamp S, Spirkoska V, To C, et al. (2005) Concurrent binding of anti-EphA3 antibody and ephrin-A5 amplifies EphA3 signaling and downstream responses: potential as EphA3-specific tumor-targeting reagents. Cancer Res 65: 6745-6754.

111. Walter MJ, Payton JE, Ries RE, Shannon WD, Deshmukh H, et al. (2009) Acquired copy number alterations in adult acute myeloid leukemia genomes. Proc Natl Acad Sci U S A 106: 12950-12955.

112. Guan M, Liu L, Zhao X, Wu Q, Yu B, et al. (2011) Copy number variations of EphA3 are associated with multiple types of hematologic malignancies. Clin Lymphoma Myeloma Leuk 11: 50-53.

113. Ashton JM, Balys M, Neering SJ, Hassane DC, Cowley G, et al. (2012) Gene sets identified with oncogene cooperativity analysis regulate in vivo growth and survival of leukemia stem cells. Cell Stem Cell 11: 359-372.

114. Hagey A, et al. (2011) A recombinant antibody to EPHA3 for the treatment of hematologic malignancies: research update and interim Phase 1 study results. ASH Annual Meeting Abstracts.

115. Krasnoperov V, Kumar SR, Ley E, Li X, Scehnet J, et al. (2010) Novel EphB4 monoclonal antibodies modulate angiogenesis and inhibit tumor growth. Am J Pathol 176: 2029-2038.

116. López-Nieva P, Vaquero C, Fernández-Navarro P, González-Sánchez L, Villa-Morales M, et al. (2012) EPHA7, a new target gene for 6q deletion in T-cell lymphoblastic lymphomas. Carcinogenesis 33: 452-458.

117. Müller-Tidow C, Schwäble J, Steffen B, Tidow N, Brandt B, et al. (2004) High-throughput analysis of genome-wide receptor tyrosine kinase expression in human cancers identifies potential novel drug targets. Clin Cancer Res 10: 1241-1249.

Properties of the Bone Marrow Stromal Microenvironment in Adult Patients with Acute Lymphoblastic Leukemia before and After Allogeneic Transplantation of Hematopoietic Stem Cells

Irina Shipounova, Natalia Petinati, Alexey Bigildeev, Nina Drize*, Tamara Sorokina, Larisa Kuzmina, Elena Parovichnikova, Valery Savchenko

FGBU Hematological Scientific Center, Ministry of Health, Russia

Abstract

The bone marrow stromal microenvironment that regulates normal hematopoiesis suffers during leukemia development and its treatment. In this study, we examined Multipotent Mesenchymal Stromal Cells (MMSCs) and fibroblast colony-forming units (CFU-F) derived from the Bone Marrow (BM) of 15 adult patients with acute lymphoblastic leukemia (ALL) before and after allogeneic hematopoietic stem cell transplantation (allo-HSCT). The time points assessed after allo-HSCT were defined by the treatment protocol. The analogous cells obtained from the BM of 64 healthy donors were used as controls. The ability of MMSCs to proliferate, concentration of CFU-F in BM, and gene expression in both cell types were assessed. The data indicate that MMSCs of ALL patients before allo-HSCT did not differ from MMSCs of healthy donors either in cumulative cell production or in gene expression except for SDF1. The SDF1 expression was decreased 2-fold in the MMSCs of ALL patients. The MMSC cumulative cell production from ALL patients was significantly decreased during 1 year after allo-HSCT. The expression level of SDF1 was also downregulated during the observation period. We identified changes in the FGF2 and PDGF signaling pathways. The CFU-F analysis revealed that its concentration in the BM of ALL patients had been profoundly decreased for the whole year after allo-HSCT. This decrease was accompanied by the downregulation of FGFR1 and slight upregulation of differentiation marker gene expression. Thus the number of stromal precursor cells decreased and their ability to regenerate was depressed after allo-HSCT. These changes were accompanied by an increase of more mature precursor cells with reduced proliferative potential.

Keywords: Acute lymphoblastic leukemia (ALL); Allogeneic hematopoietic stem cell transplantation (allo-HSCT); Stromal microenvironment; Multipotent mesenchymal stromal cells (MMSCs); Fibroblast colony-forming units (CFU-F); Gene expression

Introduction

Hematopoiesis is supported in adults by a stromal microenvironment consisting of mesenchymal stem cells (MSCs) and their descendants that include fibroblast Colony-Forming Unit (CFU-F) progenitors of intermediate maturity and specialized differentiated cells. MSCs are stem cells with the capacity to differentiate into all elements of the stromal microenvironment [1]. More mature descendants of MSCs such as CFU-F are able to maintain hematopoiesis by differentiating into osteogenic and adipogenic lineages [2,3]. The stromal microenvironment has higher radio- and chemoresistance than hematopoietic cells because of its low self-renewal frequency [4].

The stromal microenvironment is often damaged in patients with hematological diseases [5-8]. The following changes in the stromal microenvironment of acute leukemia patients were previously described: disturbances of signaling pathways [9], genetic abnormalities [10-12] and functional changes [13-15]. Alterations in the stromal microenvironment were also observed in chronic leukemia patients [16,17], myelodysplastic syndrome patients [18,8,12,19], and multiple myeloma patients [7]. However, other investigators have not found pathological changes in the stromal microenvironment of acute and chronic leukemia patients [20,21]. The treatments for patients with hematological malignancies include high doses of cytotoxic drugs and allogeneic hematopoietic stem cell transplantation (allo-HSCT). Both chemotherapy and pretransplant conditioning affect stromal progenitor cells [22-25]. A damaged stromal microenvironment may impair hematopoiesis in patients after allo-HSCT [26-28].

Acute lymphoblastic leukemia (ALL) is the most common neoplastic disease in children [29] and is well characterized in this age group. Stromal precursor cells of ALL patients have also been studied and their functional changes were previously identified [14,15]. However, the state of the stromal microenvironment in adult ALL patients has not been studied in detail.

This study examines the elements of the MSCs compartment including the multipotent mesenchymal stromal cells (MMSCs) [30] and CFU-F in patients with ALL before and after allo- HSCT.

Materials and Methods

ALL patients and healthy donors

This study included 15 ALL patients (Table 1) with the following immunophenotypes: Pro-B (1 patient), Pre-B (4 patients), B common (5 patients), Mature B (2 patients), T (1 patient), and Pro -T (2 patients). The age of the patients ranged from 18 to 39 years (median age 28.6 years). Bone marrow (BM) was obtained during routine diagnostic aspiration after receiving the patients' informed consent. The routine

***Corresponding author:** Nina Drize, Head of laboratory, FGBI Hematological Scientific Center MH Russia, Physiology of hematopoiesis,NovoZykovskiy, 4 Moscow, 125167, Russian Federation, E-mail: ndrize@yandex.ru

Patient	Age/gender	Diagnosis	Treatment before allo-HSCT	Conditionoing regimen
1 Sch	36/female	Pre-B*	ALL-2009+ glivek	Busulfan+cyclophosphan
2 Elm	22/male	T	ALL-2009	Busulfan+cyclophosphan
3 Gor	35/male	T	ALL-2009	Busulfan+cyclophosphan
4 Nic	39/male	B *	ALL-2009+ glivek	Busulfan+cyclophosphan
5 Vas	24/male	B com	ALL-2009	Busulfan+cyclophosphan
6 Zey	37/male	B com	ALL-2009	FLAMSA mod
7 Tes	18/male		ALL-BFM-90m	Busulfan+flurad+ATG
8 Bor	29/male	Pre-B	ALL-2009	Busulfan+cyclophosphan
9 Che	28/male	Pre-B	ALL-2009	Busulfan+cyclophosphan
10 Isi	22/male	Pro-B	ALL-2009	Busulfan+cyclophosphan
11 Chr	33/female	Pre-B	ALL-2009	Busulfan+cyclophosphan
12 Bul	24/male	B com*	Hoeltzer95	Busulfan+cyclophosphan +ATG
13 Kor	25/female	B with myeloid markers	ALL-2009	Busulfan+cyclophosphan
14 Rak	38/male	Pro-T	ALL-2009	Busulfan+cyclophosphan
15 Vor	24/male	B com	ALL-2009	Busulfan+cyclophosphan

Table 1: Characteristics of acute lymphoblastic leukemia (ALL) patients
*Indicate Ph+ positive patients; FLAMSA (consisting of one dose of fudarabine, amsacrine and ara-C for four days), ATG (Anti-thymocyte globulin), Flurad (fluradabine).

diagnostic aspiration was performed prior to conditioning and at +30, 60, 90, 120, 180 and 365 days after allo- HSCT.

BM samples were analyzed from 64 healthy donors and included 34 men and 30 women aged from 18 to 59 years (median-34 years). All BM samples were obtained during exfusion for allo-HSCT in the FGBU Hematological Scientific Center after receiving the patients' signed informed consent. These samples were used as controls. Characteristics of ALL patients are shown in (Table 1).

MMSCs cultivation

MMSCs were derived from 5-10 ml of the BM cells. To obtain mononuclear cells the BM was mixed with an equal volume of alpha-MEM (ICN, Costa Mesa, USA) media containing 0.2% methylcellulose (1500 cP, Sigma-Aldrich, St. Louis, USA). After 40 min, the erythrocytes and granulocytes had precipitated and the mononuclear cells remained in suspension. The suspended (upper) fraction was aspirated and centrifuged for 10 minutes at 450 × g.

The cells from the sediment were resuspended in a standard cultivation medium composed of alfa-MEM supplemented with 10% fetal calf serum (Hyclone, Waltham, USA), 2 mM L-glutamine (ICN), 100 U/ml penicillin (Ferein, Moscow, Russia) and 50 mg/ml streptomycin (Ferein). The cells were cultured at 3×10^6 cells per T25 cm^2 culture flask (Corning-Costar, Tewksbury, USA). When a confluent monolayer of cells had formed (passage 0), the cells were washed with 0.02% EDTA (ICN) in a physiologic solution (Sigma-Aldrich) and then trypsinized (ICN) with 0.25% trypsin (ICN). The cells were seeded at 4×10^3 cells per cm^2 in culture flasks. The cultures were maintained at 37°C in 5% CO^2. MMSCs were cultured until the second passage.

All MMSCs were immunophenotyped as described [31] with the following markers: CD105, CD73, CD45, CD34, CD14, and HLA-DR using standard protocols. The antibodies were purchased at BD Pharmingen, Franklin Lakes, USA (CD105, CD59, CD73, CD90, CD31, CD34 and CD14), Sigma, St. Louis, USA (CD45, FSP) and DAKO, Glostrup, Denmark (HLA-DR). The level of nonspecific antibody binding was analyzed using a mouse immunoglobulin IgG1 isotype control (BD Pharmingen, Franklin Lakes, USA). To assess viability the cells were stained with 7 -aminoactinomycin D (7-AAD), (Sigma). The analysis was performed on a FACSCanto II (BD Biosciences, Franklin Lakes, USA) and the results were analyzed with BD FACSDiva 6.1.3 software (Franklin Lakes, USA).

Analysis of CFU-F

Mononuclear BM cells were seeded at 10^6 and 5×10^5 per T25 flask in alpha -MEM with 20% fetal calf serum (Hyclone), 2 mM L- glutamine (ICN), 100 U/ml penicillin (Ferein), 50 mg/ml streptomycin (Ferein) and analyzed after 14 days. The colony count was performed using a microscope (Opton, Oberkochen , Germany) after staining the cells with 1% crystal violet in 20% methanol.

RNA isolation and quantitative reverse transcription-polymerase chain reaction

Total RNA was extracted from the MMSCs at passage 1 using the standard guanidine isothiocyanate method [32]. The cDNA was synthesized using a mixture of random hexamers and oligo(dT) primers. Gene expression levels were quantified by real-time quantitative PCR (qRT-PCR) using hydrolysis probes (Taqman) on a Rotor-Gene 6000 (Corbett Research, Concorde, USA). The gene-specific primers were designed by the authors and synthesized by Syntol R&D (Moscow, Russia). The primers and probes are provided in (Table 2). The relative gene expression levels were determined by normalizing the expression of each target gene to the levels of *BACT* (beta- actin) and *GAPDH* (glyceraldehyde -3- phosphate dehydrogenase) and calculated using the $\Delta\Delta C_t$ method [33] for each MMSC sample. The reaction was conducted using the following PCR protocol: initial denature at 95 °C for 10 min, cyclic denaturation at 95 °C for 20 sec, hybridization with primers and template extension at 60 °C for 60 sec.

Statistical analysis

All values are expressed as the means ± SEM. The data were analyzed using independent Student's t-tests in Microsoft Excel.

Results and Discussion

Cell production in MMSC cultures from ALL patients

The total cell production of MMSCs derived from ALL BM prior to allo-HSCT conditioning was not significantly different than BM from healthy donors (Figure 1). At the moment of allo-HSCT, 14 of 15 studied patients were in remission after treatment with the standard protocol ALL-2009 and 1 patient was in relapse. There were 2 patients with Ph+ ALL that received additional tyrosine kinase inhibitor therapy. Thus, the treatment protocol used did not inhibit MMSC proliferation. Notably the total MMSCs cell production from the patient in relapse

Gene		Sequence
b-ACTIN	Forward primer	CAA CCG CGA GAA GAT GAC C
	Reverse primer	CAG AGG CGT ACA GGG ATA GC
	Probe	ROX-AGACCTTCAACACCCCAGCCATGTACG-RTQ2
GAPDH	Forward primer	GGT GAA GGT CGG AGT CAA CG
	Reverse primer	TGG GTG GAA TCA TAT TGG AAC A
	Probe	ROX CTC TGG TAA AGT GGA TAT TGT TGC CAT CA RTQ2
BMP-4	Forward primer	ACAGCACTGGTCTTGAGTATC
	Reverse primer	TGGGATGTTCTCCAGATGTTC
	Probe	FAM- AACACCGTGAGGAGCTTCCACCA -RTQ1
IL6	Forward primer	ACCTGAACCTTCCAAAGATG
	Reverse primer	CTCCAAAAGACCAGTGATGA
	Probe	FAM-ATTCAATGAGGAGACTTGCCTGGTG-RTQ1
CFH	Forward primer	TTACCCTTACAGGAGGAAATGT
	Reverse primer	GCTGTCACTGGTAAACACTTC
	Probe	FAM-CTTCACATATAGGAATATCATTGGTCCAT-RTQ1
IDO1	Forward primer	AGCGTCTTTCAGTGCTTTG
	Reverse primer	GGATTTGACTCTAATGAGCACA
	Probe	FAM-ACATGCTGCTCAGTTCCTCCAGG-RTQ1
PTGES	Forward primer	CTGGTCATCAAGATGTACGTG
	Reverse primer	CTCCGTGTCTCAGGGCAT
	Probe	FAM- CTTCTTCCGCAGCCTCACTTGG-RTQ1
CSF1	Forward primer	AGGAACTCTCTTTGAGGCTG
	Reverse primer	CATTCTTGACCTTCTCCAGCA
	Probe	FAM-CTTGTCATGCTCTTCATAATCCTTGG-RTQ1
FABP4	Forward primer	ATGATAAACTGGTGGTGGAAT
	Reverse primer	TCAATGCGAACTTCAGTCC
	Probe	FAM-TGGCTTATGCTCTCTCATAAACTCTCG-RTQ1
PPARG	Forward primer	TACTGTCGGTTTCAGAAATGC
	Reverse primer	CAACAGCTTCTCCTTCTCG
	Probe	FAM-CCATCAGGTTTGGGCGGATGCC-RTQ1
SPP1	Forward primer	ATAGTGTGGTTTATGGACTGAG
	Reverse primer	ATTCAACTCCTCGCTTTCC
	Probe	FAM-CCAGTACCCTGATGCTACAGACGAG-RTQ1
BGLAP	Forward primer	GCAGCGAGGTAGTGAAGAG
	Reverse primer	GAAAGCCGATGTGGTCAG
	Probe	FAM-CTCCCAGCCATTGATACAGGTAGC-RTQ1
JAG1	Forward primer	ATAAAGTCCTTCCCGCTG
	Reverse primer	TTATCTTCTCCCATCATTAAG
	Probe	FAM-AGACAACAGACAAATCACCATTCGT-RTQ1
FGFR1	Forward primer	CAGAATTGGAGGCTACAAGG
	Reverse primer	TGATGCTGCCGTACTCATTC
	Probe	FAM- CATCATAATGGACTCTGTGGTGC-RTQ1
FGFR2	Forward primer	GCAGCGAGGTAGTGAAGAG
	Reverse primer	GAAAGCCGATGTGGTCAG
	Probe	FAM-CTCCCAGCCATTGATACAGGTAGC-RTQ1
LGALS1	Forward primer	CCAGCAACCTGAATCTCA
	Reverse primer	CGAAGCTCTTAGCGTCAG
	Probe	FAM-CACTCGAAGGCACTCTCCAGGT-RTQ1
Il1B	Forward primer	ATTCTCTTCAGCCAATCTTCA
	Reverse primer	AAGGAGCACTTCATCTGTTTA
	Probe	FAM-AGAACAAGTCATCCTCATTGCCAC-RTQ1
IL1R1	Forward primer	CTAATGAGACAATGGAAGTAGAC
	Reverse primer	AGCACTGGGTCATCTTCATC
	Probe	FAM- CAGTTGAGTGACATTGCTTACTGGAA -RTQ1
PDGFRA	Forward primer	TGGCTAAGAATCTCCTTGGA
	Reverse primer	ACCAGGACAATAAGTGAGATG
	Probe	FAM-CAATCACCAACAGCACCAGGACT-RTQ1
PDGFRB	Forward primer	CTCCCTTATCATCCTCATCA
	Reverse primer	TCCACGTAGATGTACTCATG
	Probe	FAM-TCACAGACTCAATCACCTTCCATC-RTQ1

IL8	Forward primer	ACCATCTCACTGTGTGTAAAC
	Reverse primer	GTTTGGAGTATGTCTTTATGC
	Probe	FAM-CAGTTTTGCCAAGGAGTGCTAAAG-RTQ1
SOX9	Forward primer	AGCAAGACGCTGGGCAAG
	Reverse primer	GTTCTTCACCGACTTCCTC
	Probe	FAM-CTGGAGACTTCTGAACGAGAGC-RTQ1
VEGFA	Forward primer	AGG CGA GGC AGC TTG AGT TA
	Reverse primer	ACC CTG AGG GAG GCT CCT T
	Probe	FAM-CCT CGG CTT GTC ACA TCT GCA AGT ACG T-RTQ1
FGF2	Forward primer	GAAGAGCGACCCTCACATCAAG
	Reverse primer	TCCGTAACACATTTAGAAGCCAGTA
	Probe	FAM-TCATAGCCAGGTAACGGTTAGCACACACTCCT-RTQ1
SDF	Forward primer	CTACAGATGCCCATGCCGAT
	Reverse primer	TAGCTTCGGGTCAATGCACA
	Probe	FAM-CAGTTTGGAGTGTTGAGAATTTTGAG-RTQ1

Table 2: Primers and probes.

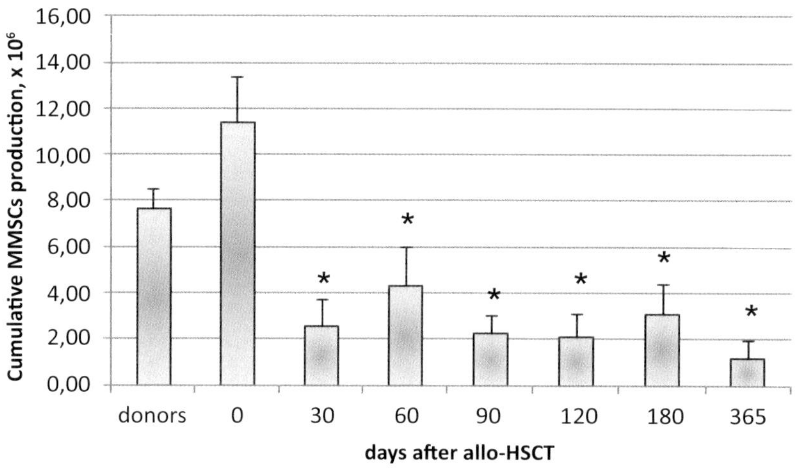

Figure 1: Alterations in cumulative cell production in MMSC cultures from ALL patients before and after allo-HSCT. Cumulative MMSC production after 3 passages is presented as the mean ± SEM. The data summarize the results of MMSCs production from 64 BM donors and 15 patients with ALL before and after allo-HSCT. *indicates a significant difference ($p<0.05$) between MMSC production after allo-HSCT and MMSC production both from donors and patients before allo-HSCT. Time point "0" indicates MMSC samples obtained before the start of pretransplant conditioning, and time points "30-365" indicate samples of MMSCs derived from BM of ALL patients obtained on corresponding days after allo-HSCT.

Number of passage	**Donors**	**ALL patients, days after allo-HSCT**						
		0	30	60	90	120	180	365
Po	12.9 ± 0.9	13.9 ± 1.3	18.6 ± 1.5*	19.2 ± 1.2*	17.7 ± 1.1*	17.0 ± 1.8	19.1 ± 1.9*	16.4 ± 0.6*
P1	4.1 ± 0.2	5.0 ± 0.7	8.7 ± 2.1	4.5 ± 0.5	6.1 ± 0.7*	7.3 ± 1.7	6.5 ± 1.0	5.8 ± 1.1
P2	4.3 ± 0.1	4.4 ± 0.6	4.0 ± 0.5	7.4 ± 0.3*	6.4 ± 0.9	4.0 ± 0.5	5.7 ± 1.1	7.0 ± 0.7
P3	4.5 ± 0.4	5.5 ± 0.8	7.3 ± 0.9	8.0 ± 1.0	7.5 ± 1.3	3.8 ± 0.1	5.5 ± 0.8	5.7 ± 0.6
P4	5.4 ± 0.4	5.5 ± 0.6	6.0 ± 0. 5	7.0 ± 0.6	7.5 ± 1.3	6.0 ± 0.5	9.5 ± 1.6	4.7 ± 0.5
P5	5.4 ± 0.5	4.7 ± 0.4	4.3 ± 0.6	6.0 ± 0.5	6.7 ± 0.7	5.0 ± 0.5	5.0 ± 0.4	5.7 ± 0.6

Table 3: Time needed to achieve confluence of the layer of MMSCs
P_0 is the time since seeding of $3x10^6$ BM cells in a flask to confluent monolayer. P1 – P5 is the time between passages. (*) significant differences with donor MMSCs ($p<0.05$) Data presented as M ± SEM.

was substantially reduced. These results are consistent with the data on cell production in MMSC cultures from newly diagnosed ALL patients [34]. However, studies of ALL in children at the time of diagnosis [35] and after chemotherapy [14,15] demonstrated that MMSCs were strongly suppressed. This result might occur because in children the disease developed simultaneously with the formation and growth of the hematopoietic microenvironment. In adults with acute myeloid leukemia (AML) [36], chronic myeloid leukemia (CML) [20] and B-cell chronic leukemia (B-CLL) [13] growth characteristics of MMSCs were not changed.

The pretransplant conditioning significantly reduced the proliferative potential of MMSCs (Figure 1). There was no recovery of MMSCs proliferation observed during the year after allo- HSCT. There was a significant increase in the time needed to reach a confluent monolayer of MMSCs from ALL patients compared with cultures of control MMSCs. However, in the subsequent passages there were no significant differences in the time to confluence (Table 3).

These data suggested that in the BM of ALL patients the number of MMSCs had been reduced after allo-HSCT. It was previously shown that the total cell production of MMSCs was also reduced in patients with various hematological malignancies after allo-HSCT [31]. Therefore, the observed decline in proliferative potential of MMSCs was not associated with the disease itself and was caused by the pretransplant conditioning. The standard conditioning protocol included busulfan and cyclophosphamide. Studies using an animal model demonstrated that busulfan impaired stromal progenitor cells (CFU-F) and their function was not subsequently restored. However, the mesenchymal stem cells were insensitive to cytostatic treatments [23]. The data indicating that human MMSCs were sensitive to high doses of cytotoxic drugs used in transplantation once again confirmed that the population of MMSCs was not the population of true stem cells. Thus, MMSCs consist of more mature stromal precursor cells [37]. The growth characteristics of MMSCs from ALL patients in remission

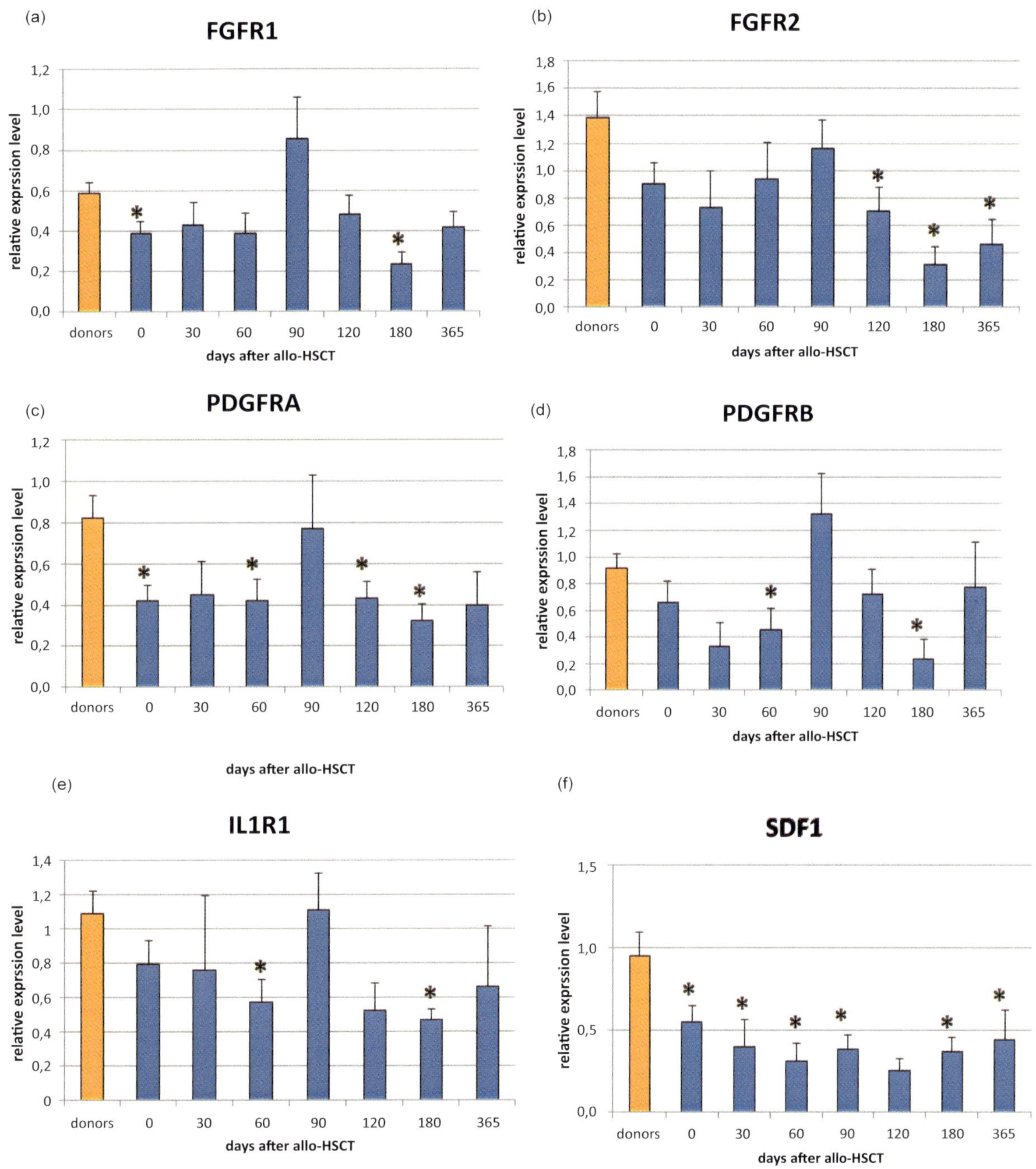

Figure 2: a,b,c,d,e,f: Relative expression level of genes in MMSCs from donors and ALL patients before and after allo-HSCT. Gene expression was analyzed by qRT-PCR with TaqMan probes. The relative expression level was calculatedusing the ΔΔCt method. The results were normalized according to the expression of BACT and GAPDH. Genes analyzed are shown as follows: A-*FGFR1*, B-*FGFR2*, C- *PDGFRA*, D-*PDGFRB*, E-*IL1R1*, F-*SDF1*.

* indicates a significant difference ($p<0.05$) between MMSC production before and after allo-HSCT and MMSC production from donors.

Time point "0" indicates MMSC samples obtained before the start of pretransplant conditioning, and time points "30-365" indicate samples of MMSCs derived from BM of ALL patients obtained on corresponding days after allo-HSCT.

Genes	ALL patients, days after allo-HSCT						
	0	30	60	90	120	180	365
IL1b	0.8 ± 1.0	30.2 ± 56.1	1.5 ± 2.6	0.4 ± 0.6	6.3 ± 10.8	7.0 ± 12.1	0.4 ± 0.6
VEGF	1.3 ± 0.4	2.5 ± 1.4	1.4 ± 0.6	2.1 ± 0.9	0.7 ± 0.3	1.2 ± 0.5	1.1 ± 0.5
FGF2	0.7 ± 0.4	4.1 ± 4.1	1.1 ± 0.8	0.8 ± 0.5	1.2 ± 0.9	1.9 ± 1.6	0.8 ± 0.5
TGFB1	0.9 ± 0.2	0.9 ± 0.3	0.8 ± 0.3	0.6 ± 0.2	0.6 ± 0.2	1.1 ± 0.4	1.4 ± 0.6
TGFB2	2.0 ± 1.2	4.9 ± 4.4	2.0 ± 1.8	1.5 ± 1.3	2.7 ± 2.8	2.0 ± 1.6	0.6 ± 0.5

Table 4: Alterations of relative expression level of gene expression in MMSCs of ALL patients compared to donor's MMSCs.

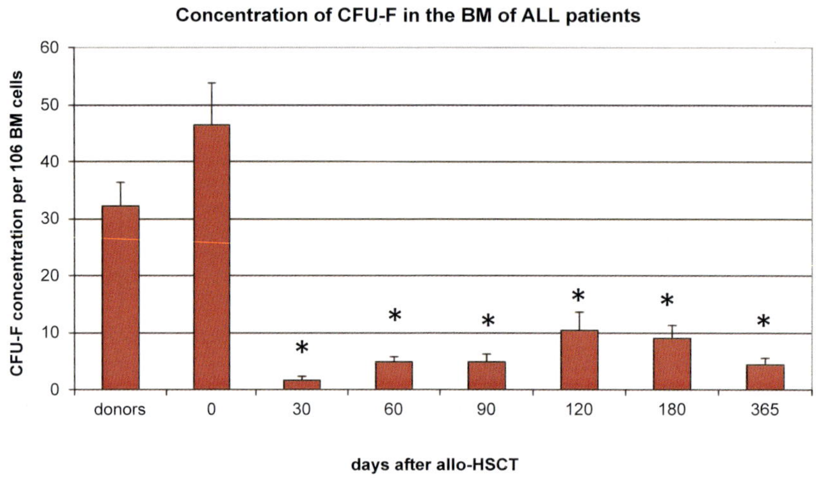

Figure 3: Alterations in CFU-F concentration in BM of donors and ALL patients before and after allo-HSCT
* indicates the significant difference (p<0.05) between CFU-F concentration after allo-HSCT and CFU-F concentration both from donors and patients before allo-HSCT.
Time point "0" indicates MMSCs samples obtained before the start of pretransplant conditioning and time points "30-365" indicate samples of CFU-F derived from BM of ALL patients obtained on corresponding days after allo-HSCT.

before allo-HSCT were slightly changed. So one can conclude that the pretransplant conditioning led to prolonged damage to MMSCs proliferation and reduced MMSCs number in the BM of patients.

Gene Expression

We next examined the expression levels of several genes regulating stromal cell division in the MMSCs of ALL patients because of the observed changes in their ability to proliferate. Prior to allo-HSCT, we observed reduced expression levels of *FGFR1, FGFR2, PDGFRA* and *PDGFRB* genes (Figure 2 A,B,C,D). However, in some cases the reduction was not significant. After allo-HSCT the expression level of these genes remained significantly reduced. These genes encode receptors for growth factors regulating the proliferation of MMSCs. It has been shown that the inhibition of at least one of these signaling pathways leads to MMSC growth reduction [38]. The reduction of gene expression in MMSCs of ALL patients indicates a possible dysregulation of signal transduction in the *FGF2* and *PDGF* pathways. This result may explain the observed decline in total cellular production of MMSCs. The expression level of *FGF2* did not vary significantly between the donors and ALL patients before and after allo-HSCT (Table 4). It is known that IL-1 beta is involved in the growth regulation of stromal progenitor cells [39-41]. Moreover, IL-1 beta is expressed by fibroblasts [42]. The expression level of the IL-1 beta receptor in MMSCs from ALL patients was reduced during the entire observation period. However, the changes were significant only at 60 and 180 days after allo-HSCT (Figure 2E). The expression of IL -1 beta itself was not altered significantly (Table 4).

A reduction in gene expression of receptors for growth factors, but not growth factors themselves, was identified. This result suggested that autocrine secretion of these growth factors did not determine the proliferative ability of MMSCs from ALL patients. These pathways could be important for the proliferation of MMSCs due to the coincident reduction in receptor expression and cells proliferation. Conversely, the expression of all these genes tended to decrease in MMSCs before allo-HSCT, while total cell production in these cultures was not reduced. Probably the genes we examined were not vital for the proliferation of MMSCs, and there still were some other regulatory mechanisms of their division that had not been included in this study.

The expression level of the chemokine *SDF1* was significantly reduced in MMSCs of ALL patients before and after allo-HSCT (Figure 2F). A similar effect was also described in patients with AML [43]. This chemokine plays a key role in the homing of hematopoietic cells to the BM niche [44]. Following autologous and allogeneic HSCT both hematopoietic dysfunction and long-term cytopenia are often observed in patients [45–47]. We predict that these disorders are associated with the changes in the interaction between hematopoietic stem cells and the elements of the stromal microenvironment. These changes may be specifically related to the decrease in *SDF1* expression.

Characteristics of CFU-F in ALL patients

The concentration of CFU-F in the BM of ALL patients before allo-HSCT slightly but insignificantly increased (p=0.15) compared to donors (Figure 3). This result might be caused by the mild differences in the mean age as ALL patients which ranged from 18 to 39 years (median - 28.6 years), whereas the donors ranged from 18 to 59 years (median - 34 years). It is known that the CFU-F concentration decreases significantly with the age of the donor [48,49]. Several authors have analyzed BM before chemotherapy and did not find differences in CFU-F concentration between patients and healthy donors [50,51]. Other studies have revealed a decline or complete exhaustion in CFU-F concentration in the BM of patients with acute leukemia [52-54,24]. The same result was observed in mice injected with acute leukemia cells [55,56]. However, it is unclear whether chemotherapy treatment occurred in the human studies and the protocol followed was not described. This information is crucial when analyzing the changes in the stromal microenvironment [25,57,58].

After allo-HSCT the concentration of CFU-F in the BM ALL patients was reduced by more than 10-fold and was not restored during the subsequent year (Figure 3). The results were consistent with the changes in the concentration of CFU-F caused by the transplantation protocol and are likely not reparable in patients more than 5 years old [48]. The effect could be associated with the significant decrease in the expression level of *FGFR1* in CFU-F of ALL patients after allo-

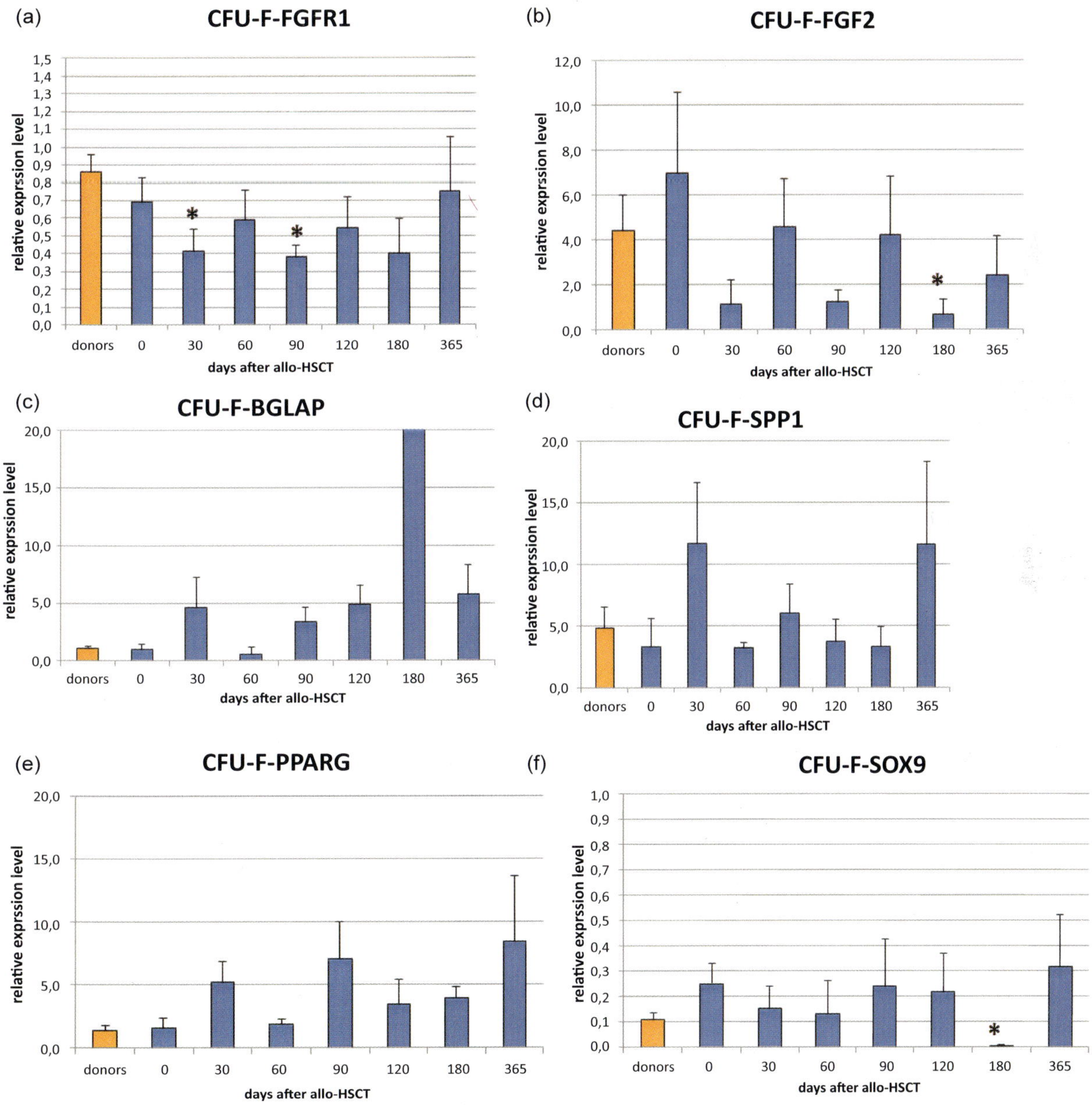

Figure 4: a,b,c,d,e,f: Relative expression level of genes in CFU-F derived colonies from donors and ALL patients before and after allo-HSCT. Gene expression was analyzed by qRT-PCR with TaqMan probes. The relative expression level was calculated using the ΔΔCt method. The results were normalized by the expression of BACT and GAPDH.

Genes analyzed are shown as follows: A-FGFR1, B-FGF2, C- BGLAP, D-SPP1, E-PPARG, F-SOX9.

*indicates a significant difference ($p<0.05$) between gene expression levels in CFU-F colonies before and after allo-HSCT and in CFU-F from donors.

Time point "0" indicates CFU-F samples obtained before the start of pretransplant conditioning, and time points "30-365" indicate samples of CFU-F derived from BM of ALL patients obtained on corresponding days after allo-HSCT.

HSCT (Figure 4A). The autocrine expression of *FGF2* was significantly upregulated before allo-HSCT, but it was not reduced significantly after transplantation (Figure 4B). We found a range of expression levels for this gene in the MMSCs from different patients. Due to the low total number of patients we cannot make a straightforward conclusion. The observed effect was consistent with the finding that *FGF2* was described as the growth factor for stromal progenitor cells [59,60]. We found the simultaneous decrease in the expression of *FGF2* and its receptors in CFU-F cells. This result suggests the reduced concentration of CFU-F in the BM after allo-HSCT was associated with impaired *FGF2* signaling. The reduced number of stromal precursor cells could be caused by the changes in their proliferative potential. The decrease in proliferative capacity reflected the loss of undifferentiated status of precursor cells and was accompanied by increased expression of differentiation-associated genes. In this study, we analyzed 2 markers for osteogenic differentiation (*BGLAP, SPP1*) and one for each of adipogenic (*PPARG*) and chondrogenic (*SOX9*) lineages. The expression of *SOX9* only was changed in CFU-F from BM of ALL patients before allo-HSCT. We found that *SOX9* was increased, but the changes were not significant (Figure 4F). The expression level of this gene remained slightly and non-significantly increased up to 120 days after allo-HSCT. The expression then decreased to nearly zero before returning to baseline one year after allo-HSCT. The expression level of osteogenic and adipogenic markers of differentiation tended to increase with time after allo-HSCT (Figure 3 C, D, E). The non-significant changes were associated with a range of values in CFU-Fs from ALL patients. Nevertheless, we suppose a shift towards more differentiated cells had occurred in the population of CFU-F derived colonies after allo-HSCT. It was shown that the conditioning before allo-HSCT was accompanied by the accumulation of reactive oxygen species in the cells of the organism [61,62], which could cause premature "aging" of the cells and tissues [63]. The reduction of the MMSCs and CFU-F number in BM of ALL patients after allo-HSCT suggest the damage to those stromal precursor cells that were attributed to the top of the mesenchymal stem cells hierarchy. It is known that the HSCT patients suffer from disorders of the musculoskeletal system including bone loss and osteoporosis [45,46,64]. The results of this study revealed possible mechanisms of bone marrow stroma damage after allo-HSCT in ALL patients. The number of stromal precursors was reduced and their growth and regeneration were inhibited after allo-HSCT. These changes were accompanied by an increased number of more differentiated progenitors with decreased proliferative potential. The damage to stromal cells by different protocols for treatment of leukemia should be taken into consideration.

Acknowledgement

The authors thank the staff of the Bone Marrow Transplantation Department. This study was supported by grant from the Russian Foundation for Basic Research (12-04-00457a).

1. Pittenger MF, Mackay AM, Beck SC, Jaiswal RK, Douglas R, et al. (1999) Multilineage potential of adult human mesenchymal stem cells. Science 284: 143-147.
2. Caplan AI (1991) Mesenchymal stem cells. J Orthop Res 9: 641-650.
3. Kuznetsov SA, Friedenstein AJ, Robey PG (1997) Factors required for bone marrow stromal fibroblast colony formation in vitro. Br J Haematol 97: 561-570.
4. Patt HM, Maloney MA (1975) Bone marrow regeneration after local injury: a review. Exp Hematol 3: 135-148.
5. Devine SM, Hoffman R (2000) Role of mesenchymal stem cells in hematopoietic stem cell transplantation. Curr Opin Hematol 7: 358-363.
6. Frisch BJ, Ashton JM, Xing L, Becker MW, Jordan CT, et al. (2012) Functional inhibition of osteoblastic cells in an in vivo mouse model of myeloid leukemia. Blood 119: 540-550.
7. Corre J, Mahtouk K, Attal M, Gadelorge M, Huynh A, et al. (2007) Bone marrow mesenchymal stem cells are abnormal in multiple myeloma. Leukemia 21: 1079-1088.
8. Lopez-Villar O, Garcia JL, Sanchez-Guijo FM, Robledo C, Villaron EM, et al. (2009) Both expanded and uncultured mesenchymal stem cells from MDS patients are genomically abnormal, showing a specific genetic profile for the 5q- syndrome. Leuk Off J Leuk Soc Am Leuk Res Fund, UK 23: 664–72.
9. van den Berk LC, van der Veer A, Willemse ME, Theeuwes MJ, Luijendijk MW, et al. (2014) Disturbed CXCR4/CXCL12 axis in paediatric precursor B-cell acute lymphoblastic leukaemia. Br J Haematol 166: 240-249.
10. Shalapour S, Eckert C, Seeger K, Pfau M, Prada J, et al. (2010) Leukemia-associated genetic aberrations in mesenchymal stem cells of children with acute lymphoblastic leukemia. J Mol Med (Berl) 88: 249-265.
11. Menendez P, Catalina P, Rodríguez R, Melen GJ, Bueno C, et al. (2009) Bone marrow mesenchymal stem cells from infants with MLL-AF4+ acute leukemia harbor and express the MLL-AF4 fusion gene. J Exp Med 206: 3131-3141.
12. Blau O, Baldus CD, Hofmann W-K, Thiel G, Nolte F, et al. (2011) Mesenchymal stromal cells of myelodysplastic syndrome and acute myeloid leukemia patients have distinct genetic abnormalities compared with leukemic blasts. Blood 118: 5583–92.
13. Pontikoglou C, Kastrinaki M-C, Klaus M, Kalpadakis C, Katonis P, et al. (2013) Study of the quantitative, functional, cytogenetic, and immunoregulatory properties of bone marrow mesenchymal stem cells in patients with B-cell chronic lymphocytic leukemia. Stem Cells Dev 22: 1329–41.
14. Vicente López Á, Vázquez García MN, Melen GJ, Entrena Martínez A, Cubillo Moreno I, et al. (2014) Mesenchymal stromal cells derived from the bone marrow of acute lymphoblastic leukemia patients show altered BMP4 production: correlations with the course of disease. PLoS One 9: e84496.
15. Conforti A, Biagini S, Del Bufalo F, Sirleto P, Angioni A, et al. (2013) Biological, functional and genetic characterization of bone marrow-derived mesenchymal stromal cells from pediatric patients affected by acute lymphoblastic leukemia. PLoS One 8: e76989.
16. Estrada-González PK, Gómez-Ceja L, Montesinos JJ, Mayani H, Chávez-González A, et al. (2014) Decreased frequency, but normal functional integrity of mesenchymal stromal cells derived from untreated and Imatinib-treated chronic myeloid leukemia patients. Leuk Res 38: 594–600.
17. Fecteau JF, Kipps TJ (2012) Structure and function of the hematopoietic cancer niche: focus on chronic lymphocytic leukemia. Front Biosci (Schol Ed) 4: 61-73.
18. Medyouf H, Mossner M, Jann JC, Nolte F, Raffel S, et al. (2014) Myelodysplastic cells in patients reprogram mesenchymal stromal cells to establish a transplantable stem cell niche disease unit. Cell Stem Cell 14: 824-837.
19. Song LX, Guo J, He Q, Xu F, Yang LP, et al. (2011) [Cytogenetic abnormalities in bone marrow mesenchymal stem cells from patients with myelodysplastic syndrome]. Zhongguo Shi Yan Xue Ye Xue Za Zhi 19: 372-378.
20. Zhao Z, Tang X, You Y, Li W, Liu F, et al. (2006) Assessment of bone marrow mesenchymal stem cell biological characteristics and support hemotopoiesis function in patients with chronic myeloid leukemia. Leuk Res 30: 993–1003.
21. Campioni D, Bardi MA, Cavazzini F, Tammiso E, Pezzolo E, et al. (2012) Cytogenetic and molecular cytogenetic profile of bone marrow-derived mesenchymal stromal cells in chronic and acute lymphoproliferative disorders. Ann Hematol 91: 1563–77.
22. Galotto M, Berisso G, Delfino L, Podesta M, Ottaggio L, et al. (1999) Stromal damage as consequence of high-dose chemo/radiotherapy in bone marrow transplant recipients. Exp Hematol 27: 1460-1466.
23. Nifontova I, Svinareva D, Petrova T, Drize N (2008) Sensitivity of mesenchymal stem cells and their progeny to medicines used for the treatment of hematoproliferative diseases. Acta Haematol 119: 98-103.
24. Banfi A, Podestà M, Fazzuoli L, Sertoli MR, Venturini M, et al. (2001) High-dose chemotherapy shows a dose-dependent toxicity to bone marrow osteoprogenitors: a mechanism for post-bone marrow transplantation osteopenia. Cancer 92: 2419-2428.
25. Georgiou KR, Scherer MA, King TJ, Foster BK, Xian CJ (2012) Deregulation of the CXCL12/CXCR4 axis in methotrexate chemotherapy-induced damage and recovery of the bone marrow microenvironment. Int J Exp Pathol 93: 104-114.
26. Devine SM, Hoffman R (2000) Role of mesenchymal stem cells in hematopoietic stem cell transplantation. Curr Opin Hematol 7: 358-363.

27. Bemark M, Holmqvist J, Abrahamsson J, Mellgren K (2012) Translational Mini-Review Series on B cell subsets in disease. Reconstitution after haematopoietic stem cell transplantation - revelation of B cell developmental pathways and lineage phenotypes. Clin Exp Immunol 167: 15-25.

28. Storek J, Geddes M, Khan F, Huard B, Helg C, et al. (2008) Reconstitution of the immune system after hematopoietic stem cell transplantation in humans. Semin Immunopathol 30: 425-437.

29. Pui CH, Robison LL, Look AT (2008) Acute lymphoblastic leukaemia. Lancet 371: 1030-1043.

30. Horwitz EM, Le Blanc K, Dominici M, Mueller I, Slaper-Cortenbach I, et al. (2005) Clarification of the nomenclature for MSC: The International Society for Cellular Therapy position statement. Cytotherapy 7: 393-395.

31. Petinati NA, Shipunova IN, Bigil'deev AE, Kuz'mina LA, Saribekian RA, et al. (2013) [Characteristics of stromal cell precursors in patients after allogeneic bone marrow transplantation]. Ter Arkh 85: 95-99.

32. Chomczynski P, Sacchi N (1987) Single-step method of RNA isolation by acid guanidinium thiocyanate-phenol-chloroform extraction. Anal Biochem 162: 156-159.

33. Schmittgen TD, Livak KJ (2008) Analyzing real-time PCR data by the comparative C(T) method. Nat Protoc 3: 1101-1108.

34. Zhao Z-G, Liang Y, Li K, Li W-M, Li Q-B, et al. (2007) Phenotypic and functional comparison of mesenchymal stem cells derived from the bone marrow of normal adults and patients with hematologic malignant diseases. Stem Cells Dev 16: 637–48.

35. Dimitriou H, Linardakis E, Martimianaki G, Stiakaki E, Perdikogianni CH, et al. (2008) Properties and potential of bone marrow mesenchymal stromal cells from children with hematologic diseases. Cytotherapy 10: 125-133.

36. Yin WJ, Yang PD, Huang YZ, Liu XP, Gong LZ (2009) [Comparison of biological characteristics of bone marrow mesenchymal stem cells in acute myeloid leukemia with those from non-leukemia]. Zhongguo Shi Yan Xue Ye Xue Za Zhi 17: 395-399.

37. Bigildeev AE, Zhironkina OA, Shipounova IN, Sats NV, Kotyashova SY, et al. (2012) Clonal composition of human multipotent mesenchymal stromal cells. Exp Hematol 40: 847-856.

38. Ng F, Boucher S, Koh S, Sastry KS, Chase L, et al. (2008) PDGF, TGF-beta, and FGF signaling is important for differentiation and growth of mesenchymal stem cells (MSCs): transcriptional profiling can identify markers and signaling pathways important in differentiation of MSCs into adipogenic, chondrogenic, and osteogenic lineages. Blood 112: 295-307.

39. Bigildeev AE, Zhironkina OA, Lubkova ON, Drize NJ (2013) Interleukin-1 beta is an irradiation-induced stromal growth factor. Cytokine 64: 131-137.

40. Dinarello CA (2009) Immunological and inflammatory functions of the interleukin-1 family. Annu Rev Immunol 27: 519-550.

41. Glossop JR, Cartmell SH (2009) Effect of fluid flow-induced shear stress on human mesenchymal stem cells: differential gene expression of IL1B and MAP3K8 in MAPK signaling. Gene Expr Patterns 9: 381-388.

42. Holzberg D, Knight CG, Dittrich-Breiholz O, Schneider H, Dörrie A, et al. (2003) Disruption of the c-JUN-JNK complex by a cell-permeable peptide containing the c-JUN delta domain induces apoptosis and affects a distinct set of interleukin-1-induced inflammatory genes. J Biol Chem 278: 40213–23.

43. Fouillard L, Francois S, Bouchet S, Bensidhoum M, Elm'selmi A CA (2014) Innovative cell therapy in the treatment of serious adverse events related to both chemo-radiotherapy protocol and acute myeloid leukemia syndrome: the infusion of mesenchymal stem cells post-treatment reduces hematopoietic toxicity and promotes h. Curr Pharm Biotechnol 14: 842–848.

44. Park D, Sykes DB, Scadden DT (2012) The hematopoietic stem cell niche. Front Biosci (Landmark Ed) 17: 30-39.

45. Domenech J, Linassier C, Gihana E, Dayan A, Truglio D, et al. (1995) Prolonged impairment of hematopoiesis after high-dose therapy followed by autologous bone marrow transplantation. Blood 85: 3320-3327.

46. Domenech J, Roingeard F, Binet C (1997) The mechanisms involved in the impairment of hematopoiesis after autologous bone marrow transplantation. Leuk Lymphoma 24: 239-256.

47. Lin Z, Kong Y, Wang Y, Zhang X, Liu D, et al. (2014) [Analysis of risk factors for secondary cytopenia after allogeneic hematopoietic stem cell transplantation]. Zhonghua Xue Ye Xue Za Zhi 35: 4-8.

48. Galotto M, Berisso G, Delfino L, Podesta M, Ottaggio L, et al. (1999) Stromal damage as consequence of high-dose chemo/radiotherapy in bone marrow transplant recipients. Exp Hematol 27: 1460-1466.

49. Shipounova IN, Petinati NA, Bigildeev AE, Sats N V, Drize NJ, et al. (2013) Hierarchy of mesenchymal stem cells: Comparison of multipotentmesenchymal stromal cells with fibroblast colony forming units. J Biomed Sci Eng 06: 66–73.

50. Carlo-Stella C, Tabilio A, Regazzi E, Garau D, La Tagliata R, et al. (1997) Effect of chemotherapy for acute myelogenous leukemia on hematopoietic and fibroblast marrow progenitors. Bone Marrow Transplant 20: 465-471.

51. Mayani H, Guilbert LJ, Janowska-Wieczorek A (1993) Functional characterization of fibroblastic cells in long-term marrow cultures from patients with acute myelogenous leukemia. Leukemia 7: 1564-1569.

52. Cao J, Tan MH, Yang P, Li WL, Xia J, et al. (2008) Effects of adjuvant chemotherapy on bone marrow mesenchymal stem cells of colorectal cancer patients. Cancer Lett 263: 197-203.

53. Isaikina Y, Kustanovich A, Svirnovski A (2006) Growth kinetics and self-renewal of human mesenchymal stem cells derived from bone marrow of children with oncohematological diseases during expansion in vitro. Exp Oncol 28: 146-151.

54. Ben-Ishay Z, Barak V (2001) Bone marrow stromal dysfunction in mice administered cytosine arabinoside. Eur J Haematol 66: 230-237.

55. Ben-Ishay Z, Prindull G, Sharon S, Borenstein A (1985) Effects of chemotherapy on bone marrow stroma in mice with acute myelogenous leukemia. Correlation with CFU-C and CFU-D. Leuk Res 9: 1059-1067.

56. Nara N, Jinnai I, Imai Y, Bessho M, Hirashima K (1984) Reduction of granulocyte-macrophage progenitor cells (CFU-C) and fibroblastoid colony-forming units (CFU-F) by leukemic cells in human and murine leukemia. Acta Haematol 72: 171–180.

57. Li H, Koh KR, Toramoto T, Nakamae H, Yamane T, et al. (2010) Cytosine-arabinoside stimulates the capability of human marrow stromal cells to support normal hematopoiesis. Osaka City Med J 56: 11-20.

58. Tauchmanovà L, Ricci P, Serio B, Lombardi G, Colao A, et al. (2005) Short-term zoledronic acid treatment increases bone mineral density and marrow clonogenic fibroblast progenitors after allogeneic stem cell transplantation. J Clin Endocrinol Metab 90: 627–634.

59. Gospodarowicz D, Neufeld G, Schweigerer L (1987) Fibroblast growth factor: structural and biological properties. J Cell Physiol Suppl Suppl 5: 15-26.

60. Gospodarowicz D (1990) Fibroblast growth factor. Chemical structure and biologic function. Clin Orthop Relat Res : 231-248.

61. Grek CL, Townsend DM, Tew KD (2011) The impact of redox and thiol status on the bone marrow: Pharmacological intervention strategies. Pharmacol Ther 129: 172-184.

62. Davis W Jr, Ronai Z, Tew KD (2001) Cellular thiols and reactive oxygen species in drug-induced apoptosis. J Pharmacol Exp Ther 296: 1-6.

63. Urao N, Ushio-Fukai M (2013) Redox regulation of stem/progenitor cells and bone marrow niche. Free Radic Biol Med 54: 26-39.

64. Banfi A, Bianchi G, Galotto M, Cancedda R, Quarto R (2001) Bone marrow stromal damage after chemo/radiotherapy: occurrence, consequences and possibilities of treatment. Leuk Lymphoma 42: 863-870.

Utility of Multiplex Mutation Analysis in the Diagnosis of Chronic Myelomonocytic Leukemia

Daphne Ang[1], Guang Fan[1], Elie Traer[3], Tibor Kovacsovics[3], Nicky Leeborg[1], Marc Loriaux[1], Andrea Warrick[2], Carol Beadling[2,3], Susan Olson[2,4], Ken Gatter[1], Rita M. Braziel[1], Christopher L. Corless[1,2], Richard Press[1,2] and Jennifer Dunlap[1*]

[1]Department of Pathology, Oregon Health & Science University
[2]Knight Cancer Institute, Oregon Health & Science University
[3]Division of Hematology and Medical Oncology, Oregon Health & Science University
[4]Department of Molecular and Medical Genetics, Oregon Health & Science University

Abstract

Chronic myelomonocytic leukemia (CMML) is a myeloid neoplasm characterized by both myeloproliferative and myelodysplastic features in addition to persistent peripheral blood monocytosis (>1×10⁹/L) that is required for the diagnosis. Clonal cytogenetic abnormalities are identified in only 20%-30% of CMML patients and it can be diagnostically challenging to exclude reactive monocytosis in some cases. Several gene mutations have recently been implicated in the pathogenesis of CMML that involve tyrosine kinase-signaling pathways, transcriptional regulation, metabolism, splicing, and epigenetic regulatory mechanisms. This study was designed to assess recurrent mutations in CMML using a multiplex mass spectrometry based approach, and to determine the utility of mutation screening in CMML, particularly in cytogenetically normal cases. The Oregon Health and Science University (OHSU) surgical pathology database was searched from 2010-2012 to identify consecutive CMML cases fulfilling WHO diagnostic criteria. Cytogenetic analyses and molecular studies were performed on the diagnostic bone marrow specimens. DNA extracts were screened for point mutations using a multiplex PCR panel with mass-spectroscopy read out that covers 370 point mutations across 31 genes associated with leukemia. Of the 48 CMML cases identified in the OHSU files, 43 had available cytogenetic studies. Of these, 10/43 cases (23%) had cytogenetic abnormalities including: trisomy 8 (n=4), trisomy 21 (n=2), deletion 7q (n=1), del 13q (n=1), complex karyotype (n=1) and t (3;3) (n=1). Of the cases with cytogenetic data, 22 had available DNA for mutation analysis, and 11 of these genotyped cases (50%) had detectable mutations in the following genes: CBL (n=3), CKIT, JAK2, KRAS (n=2), NRAS (n=3) and NPM1. Nine cases with detected mutations had normal cytogenetics. Concomitant molecular and cytogenetic abnormalities were seen in 2 cases: one case with trisomy 8 and CBL C384Y and one case with trisomy 21 and JAK2 V617F. In the 22 cases with available cytogenetic and molecular data, performing routine multiplex molecular testing in addition to cytogenetic studies in CMML patients increased the detection of genetic abnormalities from 23% (5/22) to 64% (14/22), with frequent CBL and RAS mutations in our cohort. This study confirms that gene mutations are common events in CMML, and multiplex mutation analysis can be applied in the clinical setting to assist in diagnosis and may identify actionable mutations for targeted therapy.

Keywords: Chronic myelomonocytic leukemia; Clonal cytogenetic abnormalities; Multiplex mutation analysis

Introduction

Chronic myelomonocytic leukemia (CMML) is a clonal hematopoietic stem cell disorder characterized by both myelodysplastic and myeloproliferative features and is defined by the presence of an absolute monocytosis ($>1\times10^9$ L^{-1}) according to the 2008 World Health Organization (WHO) classification [1]. CMML is subclassified as CMML-1 with <10% bone marrow and ≤ 5% peripheral blasts, and CMML-2 with 10-19% bone marrow and/or 5-19% peripheral blasts or when Auer rods are identified. This subdivision has been shown to confer a prognostically significant survival difference, with a median survival of 20 months for CMML-1 and 15 months for CMML-2 ($p<0.005$) [2-4]. The same study showed an increased cumulative risk of evolution to AML in CMML-2 ($p<0.001$) [4].

There are recurring cytogenetic abnormalities reported in CMML which include: monosomy 7, trisomy 8, complex karyotype involving ≥ 3 abnormalities, trisomy 21, isochromosome 17, deletion 5q, and deletion 20q [5]. Such et al. [6] has previously shown cytogenetic abnormalities to be prognostic in CMML [6]. Based on their survival analysis, they defined three cytogenetic risk categories: low risk (normal karyotype and loss of Y chromosome as a single anomaly), high risk (trisomy 8 alone or with one additional abnormality, abnormalities of chromosome 7 alone or with one additional abnormality and complex karyotype), and intermediate risk (all other single or double abnormalities) [6]. However, none of these cytogenetic findings are specific for CMML and the overall incidence of chromosomal abnormalities is approximately 20-30% [1]. A significant majority of CMML cases are diagnosed without a cytogenetic abnormality to support the diagnosis or allow risk stratification.

Several gene mutations have recently been implicated in the pathogenesis of CMML and involve tyrosine kinase-signaling pathways, transcriptional regulation, epigenetic regulatory mechanisms, and genes involved in the splicing machinery [7-15,16]. In this study, we evaluated the frequency of cytogenetic abnormalities in CMML and report our single institution experience of mutational analysis with a multiplex mass spectrometry based approach.

***Corresponding author:** Jennifer Dunlap, Department of Pathology, 3181 SW Sam Jackson Park Rd, Portland, OR 97239, USA, E-mail: dunlapj@ohsu.edu

Material and Methods

Cases

After Institutional Review Board approval, pathology files of Oregon Health & Science University were searched for peripheral blood and bone marrow specimens with a diagnosis of CMML; 48 cases were identified (2010-2012). Clinical data were collected including age, sex, white blood cell count, absolute monocyte count, and CMML sub classification according to WHO 2008 criteria.

Multiplex mutation screening

DNA was extracted and purified from bone marrow aspirate specimens, or formalin-fixed, paraffin-embedded tissue using standard protocols (Qiagen Qiamp Mini kit, Valencia, CA) in 22 CMML cases. DNA extracts were screened for mutations in genes known to be associated with leukemia (Table 1) using a multiplex PCR panel with mass spectroscopy readout (Sequenom Mass Array) as previously described [17]. The mutation panel covers 370 point mutations across 31 genes encoding for the following: receptor tyrosine kinases (FLT3, KIT, FMS, PDGFRB, FGFR4, NTRK1, MET), cytoplasmic-tyrosine kinases (JAK1, JAK2, JAK3, FES, ABL1), signaling molecules (CBL, CBLB, NRAS, KRAS, HRAS, SOS1), serine/threonine kinases (AKT1, AKT2, AKT3, BRAF), receptors (MPL, NOTCH1), phosphatase (PTPN11), metabolic pathway genes (IDH1, IDH2), tumor suppressor (FBXW7), and transcription factors (GATA1, NPM1, PAX5). Point mutations identified by multiplex PCR/mass spectrometry were confirmed by direct DNA sequencing on an ABI3130 sequencer using the Big Dye terminator method.

Cytogenetics

Standard cytogenetic karyotype analysis on the diagnostic bone marrow aspirate material was performed in 35 out of 48 cases of CMML. In eight cases only fluorescent in situ hybridization (FISH) analysis was performed. The specimen was cultured for 24 to 48 hours in complete RPMI 1640 medium (Invitrogen, Carlsbad, CA) with 10% fetal bovine serum (Irvine Scientific, Santa Ana, CA). Cells were harvested, and slides were prepared according to standard laboratory protocol. Slides were treated with 10% trypsin (Invitrogen) for 40 to 55 seconds followed by Wright stain (Sigma, St Louis, MO) for 2 minutes and 30 seconds. These Trypsin Writght (GTW)-banded preparations were analyzed on a Nikon Eclipse E800 microscope (Nikon Instruments, Melville, NY) with Applied Imaging CytoVysion software (Genetix, San Jose, CA). When possible, at least 20 metaphase cells were examined for each case. In eight cases, only fluorescent in situ hybridization (FISH) analysis was performed using the following probes: 5q EGR1 (5q31), D7S486 (7q31), CEP 8 (SA), D20S108 (20q12), MLL (11q23) break-apart, TP53 (17p13.1).

Statistics

Statistical analysis was performed using Chi-square to compare the detection rate of genetic abnormalities by cytogenetic testing alone vs. combined cytogenetic and molecular testing. A p value of <0.05 was considered statistically significant.

Results

Patient demographics

Our cohort consisted of 48 patients with CMML, 17 (35%) females and 31 (65%) males. The median age was 66 (range 42-88). The white blood cell count ranged from 1.5 to $96\times10^9\,L^{-1}$ with a median value of $19\times10^9\,L^{-1}$. The median absolute monocyte count was $3.3\times10^9\,L^{-1}$ (range 1 to $40\times10^9\,L^{-1}$). Based on 2008 WHO classification criteria, 35 (73%) patients were diagnosed with CMML-1, and 13 (27%) with CMML-2 (Table 2). Six of 48 patients transformed to AML.

Frequency of chromosomal abnormalities

In the 43 of 48 cases of CMML that had an available specimen for cytogenetic/FISH studies, the karyotype was normal in 33 (77%) and abnormal in 10 (23%) cases. The most frequent cytogenetic abnormalities were trisomy 8 (n=4) and trisomy 21 (n=2). Other cytogenetic abnormalities included: deletion 7q, deletion 13q, complex karyotype, and t (3;3). If classified according to the cytogenetic risk stratification established by Such et al. [6] more than half of the cases with abnormal cytogenetic analysis (6 out of 10 cases) harbored high-risk cytogenetic abnormalities including 4 cases of trisomy 8, 1 case with deletion 7q, and 1 case with complex karyotype. Cytogenetic analysis was performed in all six cases which transformed to AML. Trisomy 8 was detected in one case and trisomy 21 identified in another; the remaining cases had a normal karyotype (Table 3).

Results of multiplex mutation screening

22 cases had available DNA for multiplex mutation screening. Of these, 11 cases (50%) had mutations in the following genes: CBL (n=3), NRAS (n=3), KRAS (n=2), CKIT, JAK2 and NPM1. Of the 11 cases with mutations, nine had normal cytogenetics and two had concomitant cytogenetic abnormalities. RAS mutations were the most commonly detected (23%, 5/22); they were all identified in cytogenetically normal cases and distributed equally amongst CMML-1 and CMML-2. None of the cases with RAS mutations transformed to AML.

Combining multiplex mutation screening and cytogenetic analysis: utility of mutation screening in cytogenetically normal CMML

There were 22 cases of CMML in which both cytogenetic analysis and multiplex mutation screening were performed (Figure 1). Of these

R-tyrosine kinase	FLT3	KIT	FMS	PDGFRB	FGFR4	NTRK1	MET
C-tyrosine kinase	JAK1	JAK2	JAK3	FES	ABL1		
Signaling molecule	CBL	CBLB	NRAS	KRAS	HRAS	SOS1	
Serine/threonine kinase	AKT1	AKT2	AKT3	BRAF			
Cytokine receptor	MPL						
Receptor	NOTCH1						
Phosphatase	PTPN11						
Metabolic pathway	IDH1	IDH2					
Tumor suppressor	FBXW7						
Transcriptional factor	PAX5	NPM1	GATA1				

Table 1: Genes tested using multiplex mass spectrometry based approach.

Case	Age	Sex	Diagnosis	WBC	AMC*	Mutated Gene	Codon	Cytogenetics
1	70	F	CMML-2	38	16	*CBL*	C404Y	Normal
2	72	M	CMML-1	36.8	40	*CBL*	R420P	Normal
3	66	F	CMML-1	53	7.9	*CKIT*	D816V	Normal
4	57	M	CMML-2	29.1	8.1	*KRAS*	A146T	Normal
5	79	M	CMML-1	16	22	NEG		Normal
6	66	M	CMML-1	39.8	14	NEG		Normal
7	67	M	CMML-1	28.5	10.3	NEG		Normal
8	72	M	CMML-1	7.2	3.6	NEG		Normal
9	NA	M	CMML-2	NA	NA	NEG		Normal
10	75	M	CMML-2	65	30	NEG		Normal
11	52	M	CMML-1	30.3	1.8	NEG		Normal
12	61	F	CMML-1	20.4	3.3	NEG		Normal
13	60	M	CMML-1	2.1	0.2	*NPM*	W288fs*12	Normal
14	56	F	CMML-1	62.5	14.4	*NRAS*	G12D	Normal
15	65	M	CMML-2	26	NA	*NRAS*	G12S	Normal
16	66	M	CMML-2	4.4	1.5	*NRAS*	G12V	Normal
17	60	M	CMML-1	8.9	1.5	*KRAS*	G13C	Normal
18	58	F	CMML-1	7.7	1.6	NEG		t(3;3)
19	67	M	CMML-2	10.9	16	*JAK2*	V617F	TRISOMY21
20	76	F	CMML-1	11.6	2.7	NEG		TRISOMY 8
21	77	M	CMML-1	1.5	0.8	*CBL*	C384Y	TRISOMY 8
22	68	F	CMML-1	23.3	7.9	NEG		COMPLEX

AMC = absolute monocyte count

Table 2: Clinical characteristics, molecular mutations and cytogenetic findings in 22 CMML patients with parallel cytogenetic and mutation testing performed.

Diagnosis	Mutation Screening	Cytogenetics
CMML-2/AML	Negative	Normal
CMML-2/AML	Not done	Normal
CMML-1/AML	CBL C384Y	Trisomy 8
CMML-1/AML	CKIT D816V	Normal
CMML-2/AML	JAK2 V617F	Trisomy 21
CMML-1/AML	Not done	Normal

Table 3: Mutation screening and cytogenetic analysis in cases with transformation to AML.

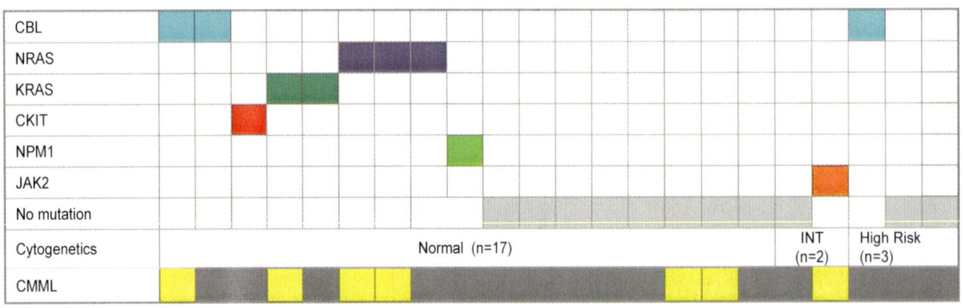

Cytogenetic risk classification based on Such et al. prognostic risk stratification. INT = Intermediate risk cytogenetics Yellow: CMML-2, Grey: CMML-1

Figure 1: Distribution of mutations in CMML across cytogenetic groups.

cases, cytogenetic analysis alone demonstrated clonal abnormalities in 23% (5/22). In comparison to cytogenetic analysis, gene mutation screening demonstrated a higher mutation frequency (11/22, 50%). Two cases had concomitant gene mutations and cytogenetic abnormalities including one case with trisomy 8 and CBL C384Y and one case with trisomy 21 and JAK2 V617F. On the other hand, 9 of 11 (22%) cases with gene mutations had normal cytogenetics. In these cases, identification of a gene mutation provided strong support for a diagnosis of CMML where otherwise no clonal abnormalities were detected by conventional cytogenetic analysis. Parallel cytogenetic and molecular testing in CMML resulted in a combined detection rate of genetic abnormalities of 64% (14/22), which was significantly higher than that identified with cytogenetic analysis alone ($p < .05$) (Figure 2).

Discussion

CMML is a heterogeneous neoplasm characterized by variable clinical presentations, disease course, hematologic findings, and genetic abnormalities [18]. The degree of heterogeneity can pose diagnostic challenges, and in some cases exclusion of reactive causes of monocytosis is difficult. Cytogenetic studies can help identify clonal abnormalities although the karyotype is frequently normal. In a study of 414 CMML patients, 27% of CMML cases harbored cytogenetic

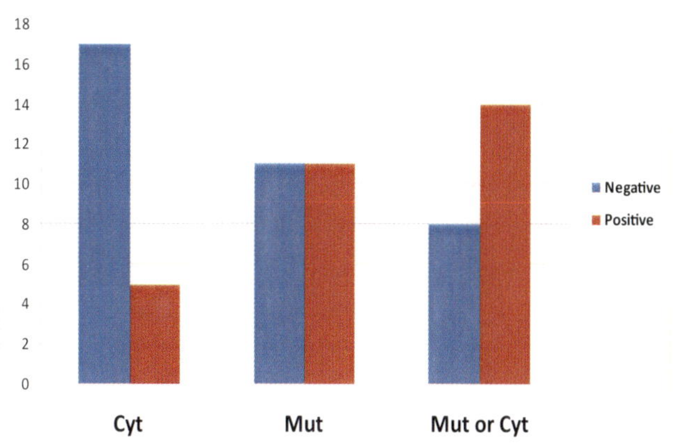

Detection rate of clonal/genetic abnormalities in 22 CMML cases, by cytogenetic testing alone (Cyt), multiplex mutation testing (Mut), and combined cytogenetic and multiplex mutation testing (Mut or Cyt)

Figure 2: Detection rate of clonal/genetic abnormalities in 22 CMML cases.

abnormalities while 73% had normal cytogenetics [6]. In this study, a three tiered cytogenetic risk stratification is described having independent prognostic significance in multivariate analysis with a five year overall survival of 35%, 26% and 4% for low, intermediate, and high risk cytogenetic groups, respectively. Similarly, in our cohort, cytogenetic analysis of 43 CMML patients detected a clonal abnormality in only 23% of cases.

Recently, a large number of recurrent gene mutations in CMML have been reported. Detection of a characteristic gene mutation may be very informative, particularly in cases where the diagnosis is not clear and there is a normal karyotype by cytogenetic analysis. In this study we genotyped CMML using a multiplex mass spectrometry based approach, and identified gene mutations in 50% of our CMML cohort. This overall incidence is lower than previously reported (75%), although prior studies also tested for genes involved in epigenetic regulation (TET2, ASXL1, EZH2) and genes involved in the splicing machinery (SRSF2), which were not analyzed in this study [9,19,20].

The incidence of specific mutations in our study, including *CBL, KRAS, NRAS, NPM, and JAK2,* is in agreement with those that have been reported in previous studies [9,19,20]. In 9 of 11 cases with gene mutations, cytogenetic analysis was normal, and in several of these cases, the initial diagnosis of CMML was difficult. As an example, one patient in our cohort was diagnosed with a peripheral blood monocytosis (3.1 K/cu mm) with a normal total white blood cell count (8.2 K/cu mm). The monocytes exhibited mature morphology and there were no distinctive dysplastic features. There was a mild anemia, but otherwise neutrophil and platelet counts were normal and cytogenetic analysis was normal. A reactive process was suspected; however gene mutation screening performed on the peripheral blood identified a CBL mutation (known to be associated with CMML) and the diagnosis was thus revised as CMML. This illustrates the diagnostic utility of mutation analysis in CMML, especially in cases with normal cytogenetics, which comprise approximately 69-73% of CMML cases [6]. Moreover, certain mutations, such as *RAS* mutations, may predict sensitivity of these tumors to drugs targeting the *RAS/RAF/MAPK* pathway [21,22]. To date, the prognostic significance of mutations in CMML is unknown, and further studies are needed.

The prognosis of CMML is still poor with only a few therapeutic options including hydroxyurea to control for myeloproliferation and hypomethylating agents to delay disease progression [23,24]. The only potentially curative therapeutic option for CMML is allogeneic stem cell transplantation, although most patients will be excluded by age and comorbidities [25]. In 2 of our CMML cases with CBL C404Y and KRAS A146T, we were able to assess the molecular status after treatment. Both patients received several cycles of a hypomethylating agent azacitidine. In both post-treatment cases, we identified the presence of the same genetic mutation, indicating the persistence of the clone after hypomethylating agent therapy. Thus, another potential utility of knowing the molecular status in CMML patients would be to monitor response to therapy and early detection of relapse in the post-transplant setting – although this indication would likely require genotyping assays with well-defined quantitative linearity and limits of detection.

Our comprehensive analysis confirms that gene mutations are common events in CMML, and revealed the presence of mutations in 50% of patients with CMML. This study shows that multiplex mutation analysis can be applied in the clinical setting and can aid in establishing a somatic genetic abnormality to confirm and monitor a diagnosis of CMML, particularly in cases with normal cytogenetics. Although our current approach using a multiplex PCR and mass-spectrometry based analysis did not include a number of recently reported mutations in epigenetic (ASXL1, TET2, EZH2) and splicing genes (SRSF2, SF3B1, U2AF35) [9,19,20], we have recently developed and validated a larger mutation panel including these (and other) genes using a next-generation sequencing approach and are now using this panel for all newly diagnosed leukemias as well as myelodysplastic syndromes. This should further improve our diagnostic sensitivity in CMML, support the development of targeted clinical trials for select patients, and help monitor disease progression and/or evolution during treatment.

Acknowledgments

We acknowledge and thank our colleagues in the Pathology Translational Research Laboratory (PTRL); Oregon Health and Science University/Knight Diagnostic Laboratories for their excellent work in the development and validation of the Sequenom Mass ARRAY system in leukemia.

References

1. Swerdlow SH, Campo E, Harris NL, Jaffe ES, Pileri SA, et al. (2008) WHO classification of tumours of hematopoietic and lymphoid tissue, IARC, Lyon, France.

2. Germing U, Gattermann N, Minning H, Heyll A, Aul C (1998) Problems in the classification of CMML--dysplastic versus proliferative type. Leuk Res 22: 871-878.

3. Vardiman JW, Thiele J, Arber DA, Brunning RD, Borowitz MJ, et al. (2009) The 2008 revision of the World Health Organization (WHO) classification of myeloid neoplasms and acute leukemia: rationale and important changes. Blood 114: 937-951.

4. Germing U, Strupp C, Knipp S, Kuendgen A, Giagounidis A, et al. (2007) Chronic myelomonocytic leukemia in the light of the WHO proposals. Haematologica 92: 974-977.

5. Parikh SA, Tefferi A (2012) Chronic myelomonocytic leukemia: 2012 update on diagnosis, risk stratification, and management. Am J Hematol 87: 610-619.

6. Such E, Cervera J, Costa D, Solé F, Vallespí T, et al. (2011) Cytogenetic risk stratification in chronic myelomonocytic leukemia. Haematologica 96: 375-383.

7. Dunbar AJ, Gondek LP, O'Keefe CL, Makishima H, Rataul MS, et al. (2008) 250K single nucleotide polymorphism array karyotyping identifies acquired uniparental disomy and homozygous mutations, including novel missense substitutions of c-Cbl, in myeloid malignancies. Cancer Res 68: 10349-10357.

8. Levine RL, Loriaux M, Huntly BJ, Loh ML, Beran M, et al. (2005) The JAK2V617F activating mutation occurs in chronic myelomonocytic leukemia and acute myeloid leukemia, but not in acute lymphoblastic leukemia or chronic lymphocytic leukemia. Blood 106: 3377-3379.

9. Meggendorfer M, Roller A, Haferlach T, Eder C, Dicker F, et al. (2012) SRSF2 mutations in 275 cases with chronic myelomonocytic leukemia (CMML). Blood 120: 3080-3088.

10. Jankowska AM, Makishima H, Tiu RV, Szpurka H, Huang Y, et al. (2011) Mutational spectrum analysis of chronic myelomonocytic leukemia includes genes associated with epigenetic regulation: UTX, EZH2, and DNMT3A. Blood 118: 3932-3941.

11. Tyner JW, Erickson H, Deininger MW, Willis SG, Eide CA, et al. (2009) High-throughput sequencing screen reveals novel, transforming RAS mutations in myeloid leukemia patients. Blood 113: 1749-1755.

12. Yoshida K, Sanada M, Shiraishi Y, Nowak D, Nagata Y, et al. (2011) Frequent pathway mutations of splicing machinery in myelodysplasia. Nature 478: 64-69.

13. Gelsi-Boyer V, Trouplin V, Adélaïde J, Bonansea J, Cervera N, et al. (2009) Mutations of polycomb-associated gene ASXL1 in myelodysplastic syndromes and chronic myelomonocytic leukaemia. Br J Haematol 145: 788-800.

14. Itzykson R, Kosmider O, Renneville A, Morabito M, Preudhomme C, et al. (2013) Clonal architecture of chronic myelomonocytic leukemias. Blood 121: 2186-2198.

15. Abdel-Wahab O, Pardanani A, Patel J, Wadleigh M, Lasho T, et al. (2011) Concomitant analysis of EZH2 and ASXL1 mutations in myelofibrosis, chronic myelomonocytic leukemia and blast-phase myeloproliferative neoplasms. Leukemia 25: 1200-1202.

16. Makishima H, Visconte V, Sakaguchi H, Jankowska AM, Abu Kar S, et al. (2012) Mutations in the spliceosome machinery, a novel and ubiquitous pathway in leukemogenesis. Blood 119: 3203-3210.

17. Dunlap J, Beadling C, Warrick A, Neff T, Fleming WH, et al. (2012) Multiplex high-throughput gene mutation analysis in acute myeloid leukemia. Hum Pathol 43: 2167-2176.

18. Bastie JN, Aucagne R, Droin N, Solary E, Delva L (2012) Heterogeneity of molecular markers in chronic myelomonocytic leukemia: a disease associated with several gene alterations. Cell Mol Life Sci 69: 2853-2861.

19. Grossmann V, Kohlmann A, Eder C, Haferlach C, Kern W, et al. (2011) Molecular profiling of chronic myelomonocytic leukemia reveals diverse mutations in >80% of patients with TET2 and EZH2 being of high prognostic relevance. Leukemia 25: 877-879.

20. Kohlmann A, Grossmann V, Klein HU, Schindela S, Weiss T, et al. (2010) Next-generation sequencing technology reveals a characteristic pattern of molecular mutations in 72.8% of chronic myelomonocytic leukemia by detecting frequent alterations in TET2, CBL, RAS, and RUNX1. J Clin Oncol 28: 3858-3865.

21. Kiessling MK, Oberholzer PA, Mondal C, Karpova MB, Zipser MC, et al. (2011) High-throughput mutation profiling of CTCL samples reveals KRAS and NRAS mutations sensitizing tumors toward inhibition of the RAS/RAF/MEK signaling cascade. Blood 117: 2433-2440.

22. Feldman EJ, Cortes J, DeAngelo DJ, Holyoake T, Simonsson B, et al. (2008) On the use of lonafarnib in myelodysplastic syndrome and chronic myelomonocytic leukemia. Leukemia 22: 1707-1711.

23. Braun T, Itzykson R, Renneville A, de Renzis B, Dreyfus F, et al. (2011) Molecular predictors of response to decitabine in advanced chronic myelomonocytic leukemia: a phase 2 trial. Blood 118: 3824-3831.

24. Costa R, Abdulhaq H, Haq B, Shadduck RK, Latsko J, et al. (2011) Activity of azacitidine in chronic myelomonocytic leukemia. Cancer 117: 2690-2696.

25. Ocheni S, Kröger N, Zabelina T, Zander AR, Bacher U (2009) Outcome of allo-SCT for chronic myelomonocytic leukemia. Bone Marrow Transplant 43: 659-661.

Stromal Tumor Microenvironment in Chronic Lymphocytic Leukemia: Regulation of Leukemic Progression

Ashima Shukla[1#], Nagendra K Chaturvedi[1#], Adam K Ahrens[1], Christine E Cutucache[1], Amit K Mittal[1], Philip Bierman[2], Dennis D Weisenburger[3], Runqing Lu[1] and Shantaram S Joshi[1*]

[1]Departments of Genetics, Cell Biology & Anatomy, Omaha, NE, USA
[2]Division of Oncology/Hematology, University of Nebraska Medical Center, Omaha, NE, USA
[3]Department of Pathology & Microbiology, University of Nebraska Medical Center, Omaha, NE, USA
[#]Indicates equal contribution to this work as co-first authors

Abstract

Chronic Lymphocytic Leukemia (CLL), the most prevalent adult leukemia in western countries, which is highly heterogeneous with a very variable clinical outcome. Emerging evidence indicates that the stromal tumor microenvironment (STME) and stromal associated genes (SAG) play important roles in the pathogenesis and progression of CLL. However, the precise mechanisms by which STME and SAG are involved in this process remain unknown. In an attempt to explore the role of STME in this process, we examined the expression levels of stromal associated genes using gene expression profiling (GEP) of CLL cells from lymph nodes (LN) (n=15), bone marrow (BM) (n=18), and peripheral blood (PB) (n=20). Interestingly, LUM, MMP9, MYLK, ITGA9, CAV1, CAV2, FBN1, PARVA, CALD1, ITGB5 and EHD2 were found to be overexpressed while ITGB2, DLC1 and ITGA6 were under expressed in LN-CLL compared to BM-CLL and PB-CLL. This is suggestive of a role for LN-mediated TME in CLL cell survival/progression. Among these genes, expression of MYLK, CAV1 and CAV2 correlated with clinical outcome as determined by time to first treatment. Together, our studies show that members of the stromal signature, particularly in the CLL cells from lymph nodes, regulate CLL cell survival and proliferation and thus leukemic progression.

Keywords: Stromal tumor microenvironment; Stromal gene signature; CLL

Introduction

Chronic lymphocytic leukemia (CLL) is a clinically heterogeneous, incurable B cell malignancy affecting elderly population in the western world. Emerging evidence suggest that CLL cells depend on complex communications with their microenvironment for survival. Due to an overt dependence of CLL cells on these interactions, their survival is greatly reduced when cultured *in vitro* by themselves. We and others [1,2] have shown that the tumor microenvironment (TME) in lymph nodes (LN) provide pro-survival/proliferation signals to CLL cells and induces host immune suppression [3]. Furthermore, prolonged survival of CLL cells in the proliferation centers in bone marrow (BM) and in LNs is mediated by several stromal micro-environmental (STME) cues; however, the precise nature of these interactions remains ambiguous. LN microenvironment is comprised of stromal and other cells along with the associated extra cellular matrix. Extra cellular matrix is comprised of proteoglycans, integrins, hyaluronic acid and reticular network. On the other hand, stromal and other cells in the lymph nodes represented by lymphatic endothelial cells, mesenchymal cells, T cells, follicular dendritic cells and monocytes-derived nurse-like cells have been shown to enhance CLL cell survival [4]. The STME helps them to escape from therapy resulting in increased relapse rate in CLL patients [4]. Once the tumor cells colonize in LNs, they shape their microenvironment to support their own survival and growth. This partly involves the activation of immune tolerance genes in CLL cells [3]. Recently Garcia-Munoz et al. have suggested that immunoglobulin gene mutated CLL cells in the LN, acquire self-reactivity for auto antigens while being tolerized with receptor editing [5]. As a consequence, the normal function and proliferation of nonmalignant B cells in the TME are also affected [5]. Lenz et al. have eloquently demonstrated that survival of diffuse large B cell lymphoma following treatment is influenced by the differences in immune cells, fibrosis and angiogenesis in the TME [6]. This conclusion was based on the analyses of stromal gene signatures in large B cell lymphomas. Orimo et al. have reported that stromal fibroblasts present in invasive human breast cancer promote tumor growth and angiogenesis through elevated SDF/CXCL12 secretion [7]. Together, these reports advocate the importance of complex interactions between CLL and other tumor cells with their microenvironment for increased proliferation leading to disease progression. In B cells, such interactions involve cytoskeletal changes possibly mediated by stromal microenvironment leading to enhanced B cell activation by BCR clustering [8,9]. Similar mechanisms may impose altered cytoskeletal changes in CLL cells leading to better survival and proliferation. Therefore, identification of molecular network involved in modification of LN microenvironment by CLL cells will lead to a better understanding of the disease. In an attempt to understand the molecular basis of stromal associated regulation of CLL progression and its prognostic implication we performed a gene expression profiling (GEP) of CLL cells from PB, BM and LN. We also performed transcriptome analysis of PB-CLL cells from patients with good versus poor prognosis to identify stromal gene signatures associated with disease aggressiveness. We identified two genes, MYLK and CAV2, whose transcript and protein expression is upregulated in patients with poor prognosis than good prognosis and significantly associated with patient's outcome.

***Corresponding author:** Shantaram S Joshi, PhD, Department of Genetics, Cell Biology and Anatomy, University of Nebraska Medical Center, 986395 Nebraska Medical Center, Omaha, NE 68198-6395, USA, E-mail: ssjoshi@unmc.edu

Methods

CLL patient information

Using an Institutional Review Board approved-protocol and informed consent, CLL samples were obtained from patients. PB (n=20), BM (n=18) and LN (n=15) samples from 53 CLL samples were collected from 37 different patients. In addition, to validate the results, additional peripheral blood CLL samples from 20 patients and another 15 patients with good prognosis (n=7) and poor prognosis (n=8) patient peripheral blood samples were also used. In this study, we included CLL patients who are untreated and who did not receive any treatment for six months prior to sample collection. For control, B cells from age matched normal donors were obtained.

The clinical information on these 72 patients are provided in tables 1a-1c.

CLL cells isolation and characterization

All CLL samples for this study were obtained using an UNMC Institutional Review Board approved protocol. CLL cells were isolated from PB and BM using density gradient centrifugation with lymphocyte separation medium, LymphoPrep, followed by negative selection using magnetic bead separation method as needed [10,11]. Frozen LN samples were obtained from the UNMC tissue bank. CLL cells were localized on frozen LN samples using immunohistochemistry by staining CD19 and CD5 positive cells. Fifteen to twenty sections of 8-10 micron thickness were made at 4°C and fixed immediately by ice-cold acetone and stained with cresyl violet (LCM Staining Kit, Ambion, TX, USA) for 30 seconds. These cells were micro dissected for RNA isolation [2]. For CLL cells isolated from PB and BM, the purity was tested by flow cytometry using the combination of CD3-FITC, CD19-PE, CD5-PE, CD38-PE and CD19-FITC (BD Biosciences, San Jose, CA, USA).

Clinical characterization of CLL patient

Patients with high CD38 positive, bulky lymphadenopathy, chromosome 11q deletion, 17p deletion and trisomy 12, unmutated IgVH and shorter time to first treatment were considered as a poor prognosis patient, whereas patients with only 13q deletion or normal karyotype, mutated IgVH and longer time to treatment were considered as a good prognosis patient [11,12].

Microarray analysis

RNA from CLL cells was extracted using TRIzol™ (Invitrogen, Grand Island, NY, USA) as per the manufacturer's instruction. Gene expression profiling was performed using a DNA microarray chip (MWG Biotech, Germany, Human 30K oligo set B) consisting of a 50-mer oligonucleotide representing 10,000 different genes. cDNAs were obtained from RNA using Stratagene manufacturer's instructions. The hybridized slides were scanned and images were collected by an Axon 4000B scanner (Axon Instruments, Grand Terrace, CA, USA). Differentially expressed stromal signature genes were identified using significance analyses of microarray (SAM).

Transcriptome analysis

RNA from peripheral blood B cells of seven good prognosis CLL patients and eight poor prognosis CLL patients was isolated as mentioned above. The mRNA levels of stromal related genes with significant p value were compared between good and poor prognosis patients. The RNA sequencing was done at the UNMC Next Generation Sequencing Core facility using Illumina HiSeq 2000 sequence analyzer. RNA sequence alignment was done by TopHat alignment software; this was followed by Picard processing for removal of duplicates. To identify differential gene expression levels among the good versus poor prognosis, Cuffdiff method was used. To determine the relative fold change the values were normalized with GAPDH. Clinical information of these 15 patients is provided in table 1d.

Patients ID	Age	Gender	Time to treatment	Fluorescence in-situ Hybridization	Bulky disease	CD 38%	IgVH Mutation status
PB12	69	M	1	NA	No lymphadenopathy	45%	NA
PB16	51	M	1	Trisomy 12; 17p-; 13q14-	Bulky adenopathy	89%	NA
PB22	66	F	Never	NORMAL	No lymphadenopathy	12%	NA
PB37	53	M	NA	NORMAL	No lymphadenopathy	4%	NA
PB82	79	M	4	Trisomy 12 , 13q14 del	BALA	92%	Unmutated
PB89	39	M	10	Trisomy 12 (23% - 56%)	Mild lymphadenopathy	3%	NA
PB90	66	F	Never	13q14 del	No lymphadenopathy	20%	NA
PB96	85	F	1	NORMAL	Mild lymphadenopathy	9%	NA
PB97	54	F	2	NORMAL	Lymphadenopathy	51%	NA
PB106	65	M	Never	13q null	No lymphadenopathy	27%	NA
PB107	58	M	2	11q22.3/ATM (96%); 13q14 deletion (96.5%)	LN (axilla, supraclavicular, mediastinal)	1.50%	NA
PB109	44	M	0.25	11q22.3/ATM (96%), 13q14 (12%), (14q32 del, 77.5%)	LN (neck and axilla)	NA	NA
PB117	80	M	48	13q14 (87.5% - 96%) IgH (12.5%)	BALA (axillary)	32.45%	NA
PB121	47	M	Never	13q14 (72%)	No lymphadenopathy	7%	NA
PB124	53	F	Never	Blood14q32 (35.5%)	No lymphadenopathy	11%	NA
PB134	57	M	82	13q nullosomy	No lymphadenopathy	23%	NA
PB141	71	M	Never	13q14 (38.5%)	No lymphadenopathy	24%	NA
PB143	69	F	Never	13q14 (53.5%), cyto-N; 13q14 (83%)	No lymphadenopathy	12%	NA
PB146	76	F	17	11q23 (84.5%), 13q14 (15.5%)	No lymphadenopathy	43%	NA
PB149	41	M	6	17p- (11%), 13q- (33%), 14q- (12%)	LN (neck)	8%	NA

Table 1A: Peripheral Blood CLL patient samples information.

Patients ID	Age	Gender	Time to treatment	Fluorescence in-situ Hybridization	Bulky disease	CD 38%	IgVH Mutation status
LN11	59	M	1	TRISOMY 12 (47%); 14q32 (25%), then 12% n 13% after that 17p del	Yes, diffuse abdominal, axilla, groin, neck LN	80%	Unmutated
LN34A	74	M	2	11q23 from 13qdel	BALA	63%	NA
LN34B	74	M	2	11q23 from 13qdel	BALA	63%	NA
LN40A	49	M	1	13q14 (68.5%),both11.5%,null 13.5%, then 17p13 in LN;	BALA	92%	Unmutated
LN40B	49	M	1	13q14 (68.5%),both11.5%,null 13.5%, then 17p13 in LN;	BALA	92%	Unmutated
LN59	62	F	108	NA	Lymphadenopathy		NA
LN64	72	F	48	17p13 *	Lymphadenopathy		NA
LN66A	61	F	11	11q22.3/ATM (78%), 13q14 (89%), 17p13.1 (3 copies in 46.3%)	BALA	84%	Unmutated
LN66B	61	F	11	11q22.3/ATM (78%), 13q14 (89%), 17p13.1 (3 copies in 46.3%)	BALA	84%	Unmutated
LN67	42	M	1	11q23, 13q14	BALA	21%	Unmutated
LN82	79	M	4	Trisomy 12 , 13q14 del	BALA	92%	Unmutated
LN83A	29	M	22	11q23 deletion (92%), 14q32 (64.5%)	BALA	98%	Unmutated
LN83B	29	M	23	11q23 deletion (92%), 14q32 (64.5%)	BALA	98%	Unmutated
LN93	50	M	1	14q-	BALA	52%	NA
LN149	41	M	6	17p- (11%), 13q- (33%), 14q- (12%)	LN (neck)	8%	NA

Table 1B: Lymph Nodes CLL patient samples information.

Patients ID	Age	Gender	Time to treatment	Karyotype	Bulky disease	CD 38%	IgVH Mutation status
BM12	69	M	1	NA	No lymphadenopathy	45%	NA
BM16	51	M	1	Trisomy 12; 17p-; 13q14-	Bulky adenopathy	89%	NA
BM32	65	F	NA	13q14	Lymphadenopathy	34%	NA
BM34	74	M	2	11q23 from 13qdel	Lymphadenopathy	63%	NA
BM37	53	M	NA	NORMAL	No lymphadenopathy	4%	NA
BM67	42	M	1	11q23, 13q14	BALA	21%	Unmutated
BM74	55	M	Never	13q13 deletion	No lymphadenopathy	5%	Mutated
BM83	29	M	22	11q23 deletion (92%), 14q32 (64.5%)	BALA	98%	Unmutated
BM89	39	M	10	Trisomy 12 (23% - 56%)	Mild lymphadenopathy	3%	NA
BM106	65	M	Never	13q null	No lymphadenopathy	27%	NA
BM117	80	M	48	13q14 (87.5% - 96%) IgH (12.5%)	BALA (axillary)	32.45%	NA
BM120	65	M	3	14q-	LN (neck)	34%	NA
BM122	50	M	17	various del, 17p del, 20q-, 7p-	No lymphadenopathy	33.50%	NA
BM124	53	F	Never	blood- normal in BM-14q32 (35.5%)	No lymphadenopathy	11%	NA
BM152	60	M	Never	13q- (48%)	No lymphadenopathy	NA	NA
BM163	70	M	Never	13q null (24%), 13q- (46%)	No lymphadenopathy	23%	NA
BM166	52	M	Never	NORMAL	LN(axillary)	28%	NA
BM168	56	F	Never	13q null (11%), 13q del (66%)	mild LA	NA	NA

Table 1C: Bone marrow CLL patient samples information.

Clinical correlation of the gene expression levels

The Kaplan Meier analysis log-rank test was used to analyze clinical correlation of gene expression levels or clinical parameters with time to first treatment. Time to treatment is the interval in months between diagnosis and initiation of the first treatment in months among the CLL patients. In some cases the CLL cells used in the study were classified based on cytogenetic chromosomal abnormality, where CLL cells 13q deletion and normal karyotype were considered as good prognosis and CLL cells with 11qdel, trisomy 12 and 17p deletion as poor prognosis group. Also CD38 low (less than 30% positive) or immunoglobulin gene mutation and CD38 high (more than 30%) or unmutated immunoglobulin gene were also grouped as good and poor prognosis, respectively.

Western blotting

The expression of MYLK, EHD2, DLC1 and CAV1 in B cells from a normal healthy donor, five good prognosis CLL patients and five poor prognosis CLL patients were determined using western blot analyses. 50 μg of protein was loaded on 10% SDS-PAGE gel, which was separated by electrophoresis, and blotted on PVDF membrane. In brief, the membrane was incubated with primary antibodies of MYLK and DLC1 (Santa Cruz Biotechnologies, Dallas, TX, USA), CAV1 (Abcam, Cambridge, MA, USA), EHD2 (homemade antibody was kindly provided by Dr. Hamid Band, UNMC) and β-actin (Sigma Aldrich, St. Louis, MO, USA). This was followed by incubation of membranes with appropriate secondary antibodies and blot was developed using Enhanced Chemiluminescence, Pierce ECL Western Blotting Substrate (Thermo Scientific, Waltham, MA, USA).

Statistical analysis

For the identification of differentially expressed genes, a significant analysis of microarray (SAM) was used. To identify the tissue specific gene signatures, analysis was performed using random variance t-test with p-value of 0.01 and false discovery rate (FDR) of 0.08. The most of analyses were performed at $p<0.05$ and $FDR<0.25$, unless specified otherwise. The Kaplan-Meier method using log-rank test was used to study the association of gene expression or clinical parameter with the clinical outcome as done previously [13].

Results

Supervised cluster analyses of differential expression of stromal signature I and II associated genes in primary CLL cells

Figure 1 shows a supervised cluster analyses of the differential expression of stromal signature I and II genes in CLL cells isolated from peripheral blood (PB), bone marrow (BM) and lymph nodes (LN) from patients in comparison to each other and with normal B cells from healthy donors (nB). In the case of stromal signature I, 119 genes were analyzed. There were in total 47 genes that are differentially expressed. Among these 47 genes, 30 genes were overexpressed and 17 genes were under expressed compared to each other. Among the 30 genes overexpressed, based on the transcript levels, we divided them into the categories of high (11 genes), medium (8 genes) and low (11 genes) expressing genes based on the fold change in their expression compared to reference as shown in table 1. In this Stromal I gene signature, these differentially expressed genes are associated with extracellular matrix, cytoskeleton maintenance, cell migration, and biosynthesis of collagen. We have recently shown that the CLL cells in the LNs induce immune tolerance against themselves to facilitate their uninhibited growth [2]. Interestingly, many of the genes including SERPINH1, SERPINF1, FBN1, APOE, PTGDS, LUM, CALD1 and MYLK were significantly overexpressed in CLL cells in the LNs compared to BM, PB and nB.

In the case of stromal II genes, there were a total of 35 genes; of these, 22 genes were differentially expressed genes. Among these 22 genes, 14 genes were overexpressed and 8 genes were under expressed in CLL cells compared to normal B cells. Among the overexpressed genes, 7 genes had high expression levels and 7 genes had medium expression levels and there were no genes in which expression was relatively low compared to other genes in the category. Stromal signature II shows the mRNA level of genes which are associated with intracellular compartment: EHD2, SDF1, PTPRB, CAV2 and CAV1 [14] were overexpressed, whereas DLC1, which is a known tumor

Patients ID	Age	Gender	Time to treatment	Fluorescence in-situ Hybridization	Bulky disease	CD 38%	IgVH Mutation status
CLL 3	61	F	98	TRISOMY 12 (65.5%)	No lymphadenopathy	83%	Unmutated
CLL 11	59	M	1	TRISOMY 12 (47%); 14q32 (25%), then 12% n 13% after that 17p del	Yes, diffuse abdominal, axilla, groin, neck LN	80%	Unmutated
CLL 29	55	F	69	11q23- (91%);13q14 mono (95.5%),13q14(60%); 14q32 (65.5%)	BALA	17%	Unmutated
CLL 30	55	F	12	Trisomy 12 (70.5%)	Lymphadenopathy	55%	Unmutated
CLL 34	74	M	2	11q23 from 13qdel	BALA	63%	NA
CLL 40	49	M	1	13q14 (68.5%),both11.5%,null 13.5%, then 17p13 in LN;	BALA	92%	Unmutated
CLL 79	62	M	15	11q22.3 (78%), 13q14 (53.5%), null13q14 (34%)	No lymphadenopathy	23%	Unmutated
CLL 82	79	M	4	Trisomy 12 , 13q14 del	BALA	92%	Unmutated
CLL10	49	F	Never	Normal	No lymphadenopathy	6%	Mutated
CLL 13	83	M	1	Normal	No lymphadenopathy	NA	NA
CLL 19	56	F	Never	13q14-	No lymphadenopathy	NA	NA
CLL 75	34	M	96	Normal	No lymphadenopathy	3%	Mutated
CLL 100	70	F	Never	13q14	No lymphadenopathy	18%	NA
CLL 108	63	M	Never	13q14 and 14q32 rearrangement	No lymphadenopathy	9%	NA
CLL 164	64	F	12	Normal	No lymphadenopathy	NA	NA

Table 1D: Patients Clinical information used for Transcriptome.

Signature	Overexpressed Genes			Under expressed Genes	
	High	Medium	Low		
Stromal 1	Apoe Clu Lum Mmp9 Mylk Robo1 Wnt2b Cxcl14 Pcolce Serpinf1 Cox7a1	Aebp1 Col4a4 Cyr61 Fbn1 Lama4 Parva Ptgds Evc	Adamdec1 Cald1 Chn1 Ctgf Ctsk Dzip1 Edg2 Itgb5 Ppa2b Rarres1 Sparc	Adra2a Angpl2 Cebpa Cspg2 Cyp27a1 Dlc1 Edil3 Gja1 Islr Maff	Pkd2 Ptprf Rab32 Rtn1 Ceecam Fap Itgb2
Stromal 2	Itga9 Saa1 Cav1 Cav2 Fabp4 Ced6 Ehd2	Col5a3 Lamb1 Prrg1 Sh3d5 Pa2ga Sparcl1 Aqp1		Sema4c Dlc1 Sdf-1 Procr Apm1 Kdr Itga6 Rbp4	

Table 2: Expression of the stromal signature 1 and 2 genes in LN-CLL compared to PB-CLL, BM-CLL and normal B-cells in gene microarray analysis. The Overexpressed genes were categorized into high (>2 fold), medium (>1.5 fold) and low (~1.5 fold) higher expressed genes compared to PB-, BM-CLL and normal B-cells.

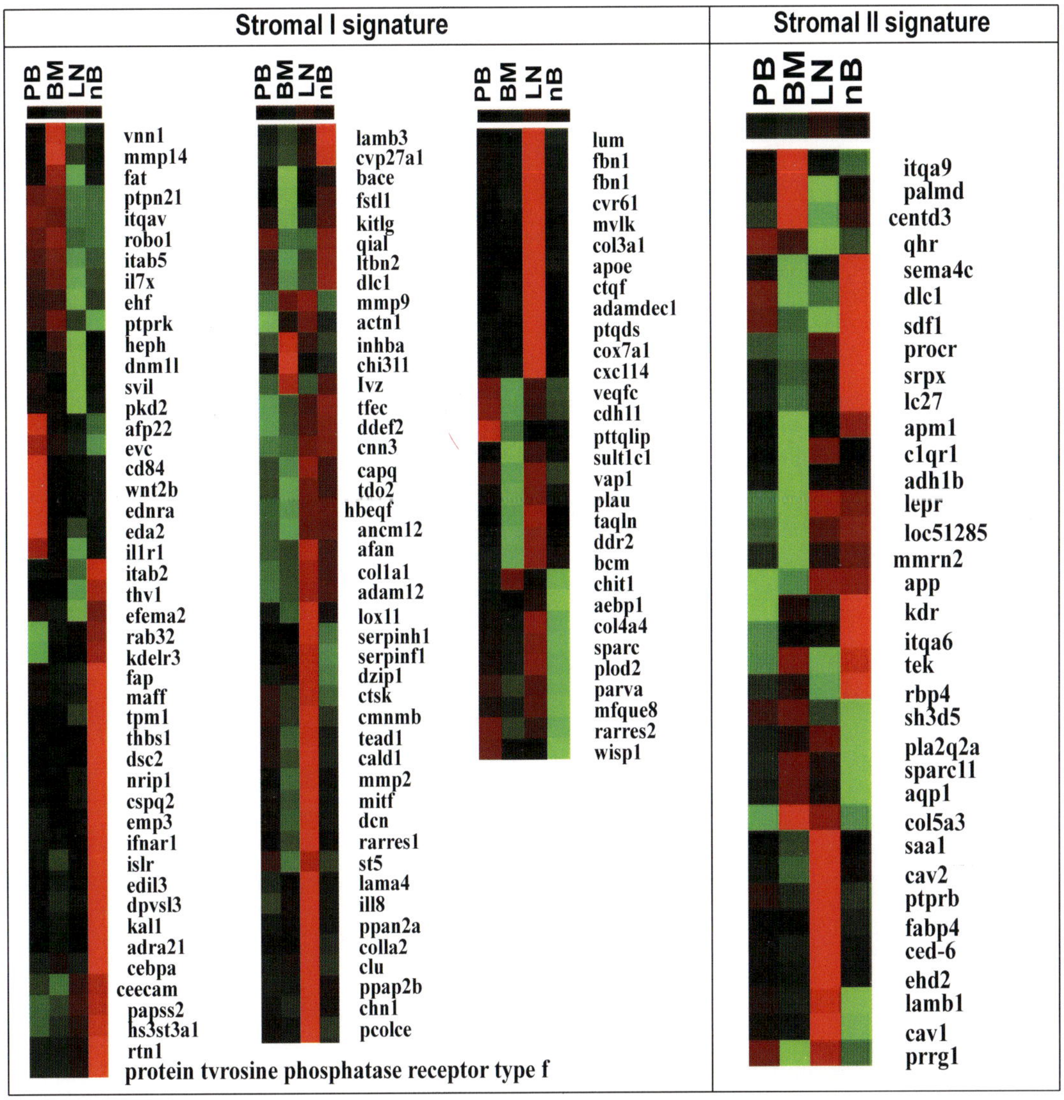

Figure 1: Differential expression of stromal signature I and II associated genes in primary CLL cells: GEP showing differential expression of Stromal Signature I & II in cells isolated from peripheral blood (PB), bone marrow (BM) and lymph nodes (LN) from CLL patients in comparison with normal B cells from healthy donors (nB). Stromal Signature I and II showing the differential gene expression in extra cellular matrix compartment and cellular components of CLL patients and healthy donors. mRNA level of some cytoskeleton related genes like MYLK, APOE and PTGDS from stroma I, EHD2, CAV2 and CAV1 from stroma II were high, whereas tumor suppressor genes like DLC1 was down regulated in both stroma I & II.

suppressor [15], was under expressed in both stromal signatures I and II.

Validation of differential expression using transcript levels of selected stromal genes in CLL cells from PB, BM and LN

We confirmed the differential expression of selected genes by evaluating the mRNA levels of each gene. In these analyses, we either compared the gene expression to the expression levels in normal B cells, and/or compared to normal B cells as well as to CLL cells from PB, BM and LNs. Figure 2 shows the results of these analyses. There was an increased expression of MYLK and decreased expression of DLC1, CSPG2/VCAN and ITGB2 in CLL B cells (Figures 2A-2D). Further comparison of these three and additional genes with CLL cells from PB, BM and LN and normal B cells showed there was a significantly increased expression ($p<0.05$) of MYLK, EHD2, CAV2 in CLL cells from the LNs compared other cells in these analyses group (Figure 2E-2G). In contrast, the expression of DLC-1 and CSPG2/VCAN were significantly decreased ($p<0.05$) in the CLL cells from the lymph nodes compared to rest of the cells in this analyses group (Figure 2H and 2I).

Validation of differential expression of selected genes at protein levels using western blotting

As further validation for higher expression of MYLK, CAV1 and EHD2 and lower expression of DLC1 seen in the transcript analyses, we performed comparison of protein expression on the basis of disease progression. The evaluation of protein levels of these genes was done using PB CLL cells from five patients with good prognosis and CLL cells from five poor prognosis and normal donor B cells. Figure 3 shows the results of these analyses. There was an increased expression of MYLK1, EHD2 and CAV2 in all five CLL patients with poor prognosis

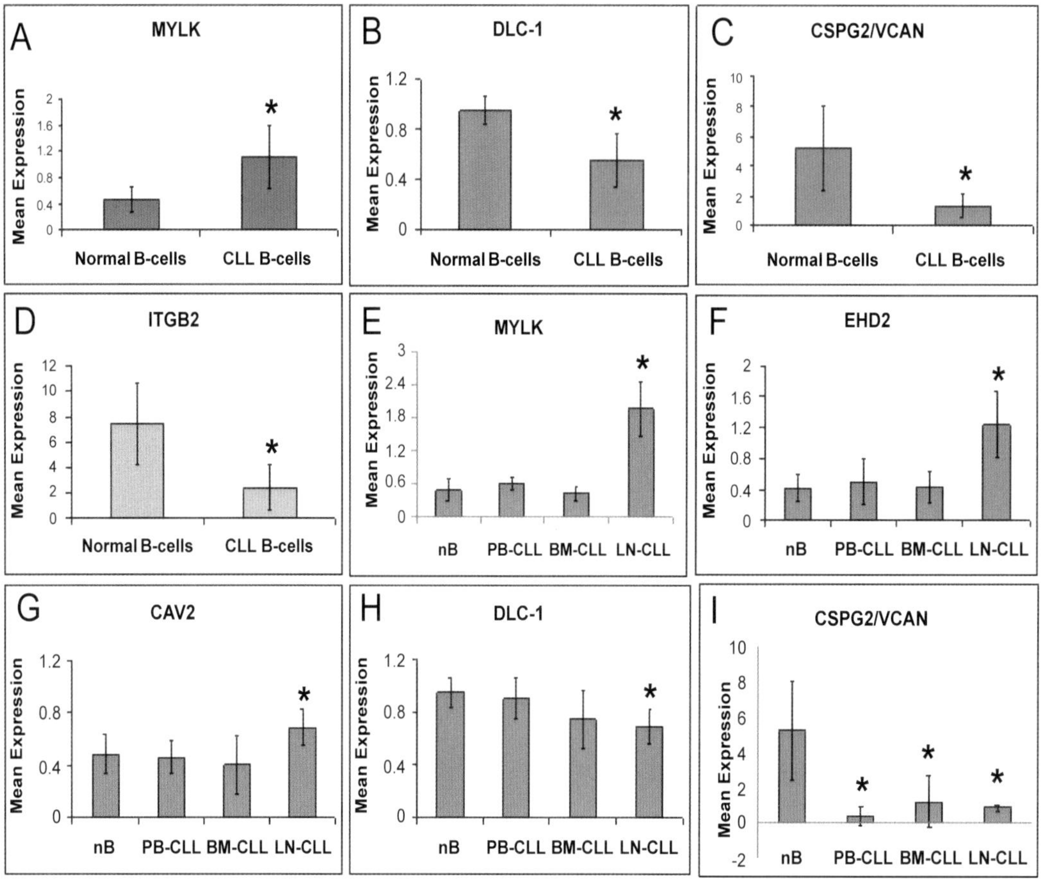

Figure 2: Expression levels of stromal genes in CLL cells from PB, BM and LN: Comparison of mRNA expression of (A) myosin light kinase (MYLK), (B) versican (VCAN), (C) deleted in liver cancer (DLC1), (D) Integrin, Beta 2 (ITGB2) in PB isolated B cells from 8 healthy donors and 20 CLL patients. mRNA expression comparison of (E) myosin light kinase (MYLK), (F) EH domain containing 2 (EHD2), (G) caveolin 2 (CAV2), (H) deleted in liver cancer (DLC1) and (I) versican (VCAN) in B cells from PB of 8 healthy donors and B cells from PB, BM and LN samples from 37 CLL patients samples. Student t-TEST was applied to determine the statistically significance among the normal healthy donors and CLL patients. "*" determine p value of ≤ 0.05. The relative expression was normalized by GAPDH.

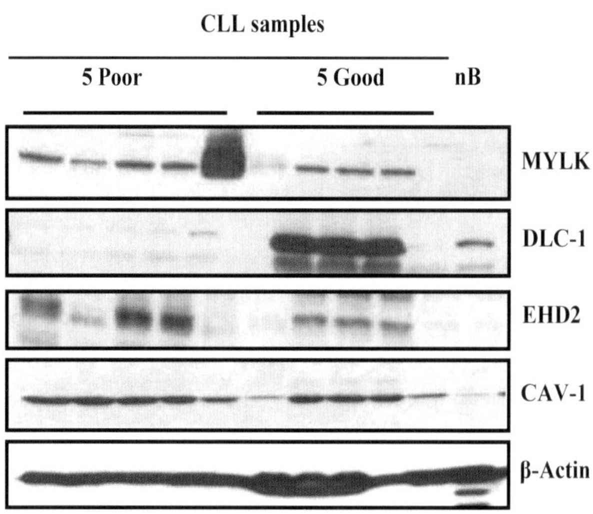

Figure 3: Analysis for protein expression: Expression of selected proteins in normal B and CLL cells from PB of 5 good prognosis and 5 poor prognosis patients using western blotting.

compared to CLL cells from five good prognosis patients, whereas the expression levels of DLC1 was significantly higher in good prognosis patients compared to CLL cells from poor prognosis patients. In these analyses, β-Actin was used as housekeeping gene control. Together these analyses confirmed the differential expression these selected genes.

Clinical significance of stromal genes

Next, in order to understand the clinical significance of the differentially expressed genes, we compared the expression levels of expression of stromal signature I associated genes whose transcript analysis were statistically significant, namely CEBPA, MYLK, APOE, RAB32, PTGDS and WNT2B and levels of expression of stromal signature II associated genes, namely DLC1, CAV2, EHD2, SDF1, RBP4 and ROBO1, with the time to first treatment in patients. Figure 4 shows the results of these analyses using Kaplan Meier analyses with log-rank test. We have previously shown that high expression CAV1 correlated with clinical outcomes; also knockdown of CAV1 impaired CLL cells to migrate and formation of immune synapse [2]. Among the 12 genes we evaluated, higher expression of MYLK and CAV2 (Figure 4) significantly correlated with poor clinical outcome. Recently Yamasaki et al., showed higher expression of CAV2 promotes cell proliferation,

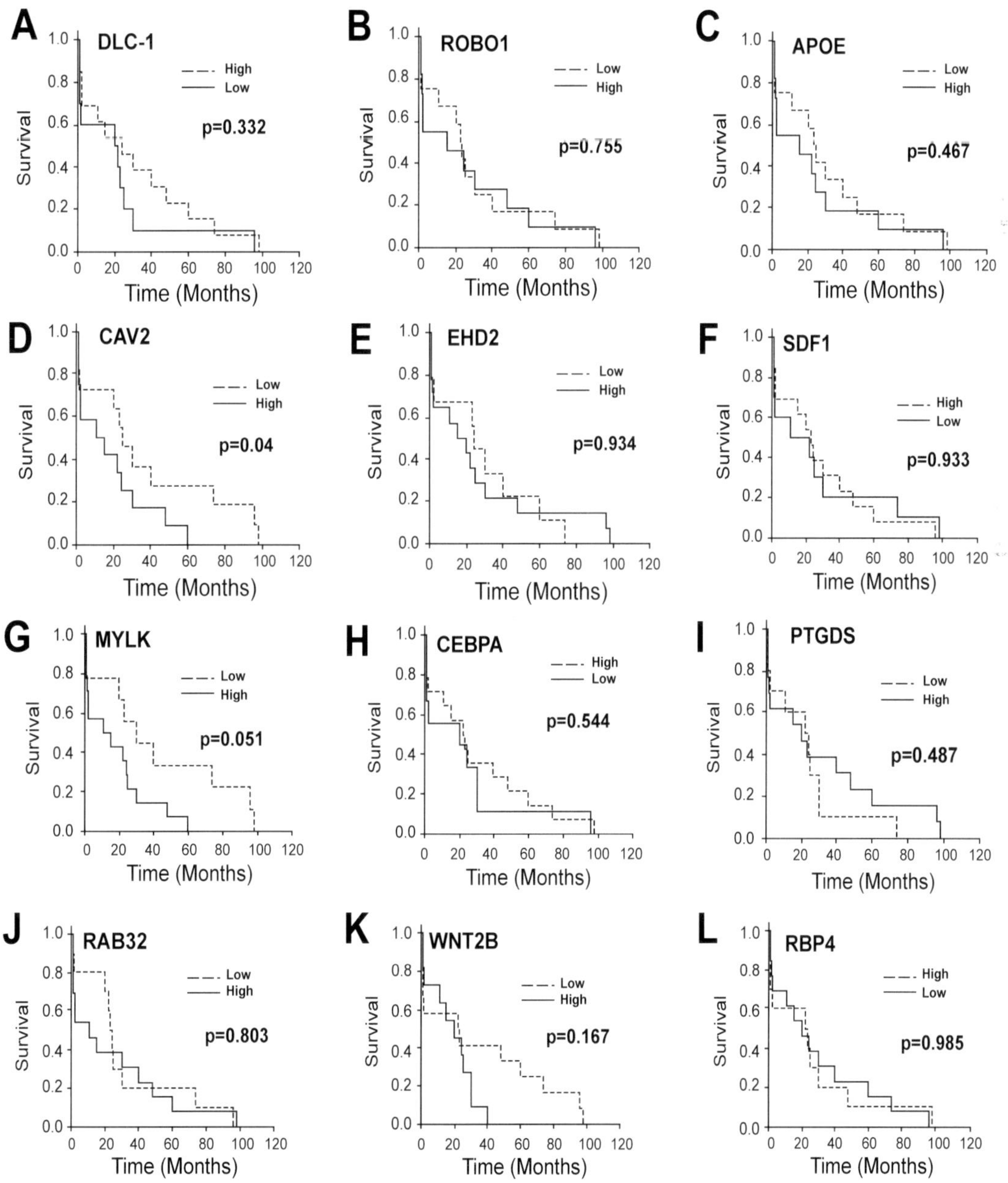

Figure 4: Clinical significance of stromal genes: Clinical correlation of expression levels of stromal signature I associated genes (CEBPA, MYLK, APOE, RAB32, PTGDS and WNT2B) and stromal signature II associated genes (DLC1, CAV2, EHD2, SDF1, RBP4 and ROBO1) in CLL patients using Kaplan Meier analyses with log-rank test. Among these genes, expression of MYLK, WNT2B, DLC1, EHD2 and CAV2 in stromal signature I and II correlated with clinical outcome as determined by time to treatment.

migration and invasion in renal cell carcinoma [16]. DLC1 is a known tumor suppressor and the western blot analysis confirmed the down regulation at the protein level which made it interesting to see the clinical outcome. However, although not statistically significant, higher expression of WNT2B and EHD2 and lower expression of DLC1 showed clinical correlation (Figure 4). The rest of genes did not show clinical correlation with time to first treatment in patients.

Gene expression levels determined by RNA sequencing

In order to identify additional genes which are associated with extracellular matrix we did comparative analysis of differential gene expression in Good Prognosis CLL and Poor prognosis CLL using RNA transcriptome analysis. The mRNA level of genes encoding for cell surface proteoglycan and glycoprotein those also associated with stromal signature (Table 2) I & II as mentioned above like VCAN and CD93 were 50 and 20 fold up-regulated respectively; inflammatory related cytokines associated genes like IL8, CXCL1 and CXCL3 were 40, 77 and 111 fold up-regulated respectively in good prognosis; and SPP1 and SERPINB2 were 955 and 1271 fold higher than poor prognosis respectively. Among these differentially expressed genes identified in our transcriptome analyses, expression levels of proteins of selected extracellular matrix genes were evaluated using Western blot analyses. There was a significantly increased protein level of VCAN, SPP1 and SERPINB2 in CLL cells from good prognosis compared to CLL cells from poor prognosis patients (Figure 5). Thus these results validated the differential expression of certain extracellular matrix associated genes as identified in transcriptome analyses.

Discussion

In this report, we have studied the nature of expression of stromal signature genes in CLL cells from PB, BM and LNs. CLL cells, particularly in the patient's body, proliferate and survive for a long time; however, they do not survive long once they are removed from the body, suggesting the role of *in vivo* microenvironment. Evidence from literature indicates that CLL cell's inability to survive *in vitro* is due to lack of complex interactions between CLL cells and the surrounding microenvironment. We and others [1,2] have shown that the tumor microenvironment (TME) in the LN provides pro-survival/proliferation signals to CLL cells leading to the formation of proliferation centers (PCs) with varied sizes from small to extensively large. It is previously demonstrated that CLL cells at the tissue sites such as LNs induce host immune suppression via differential expression of tolerogenic genes reported earlier in T cell malignancy [17]. Based on our previous studies, we believe that the CLL lymph node induced host immunosuppression significantly contributes to the leukemic progression in CLL patients [2]. However, the precise mechanism of the process and particularly the role played by stromal genes in CLL in the tissue microenvironment is not known. Therefore, the current study was undertaken.

Lenz et al. [5] have reported that in the case of diffuse large B cell lymphoma, stromal signature predicted the clinical outcome. In the present study, differentially expressed genes from both stromal I and II signatures were involved in the poor prognosis CLL with LN involvement. For example in the case of one of the overexpressed genes MYLK, a member of the stromal signature I, higher expression of this gene was correlated with poor prognosis. Similarly, CAV1 [2] and CAV2 members of the stromal II signature are overexpressed in CLL cells from LN and correlated with poor clinical outcome in patients. Furthermore, in the current study, the higher expression of CAV2 is correlated with poor prognosis. In addition, Myosin Light Chain Kinases (MLCKs) are a group of proteins found in smooth muscle and phosphorylates myosin II regulatory light chains at Ser19, allowing myosin cross bridges to bind to actin filaments and initiate contraction [18,19]. Interestingly, we have recently reported [2] that over expression of CAV1 in CLL cells in the lymph nodes might be involved in inhibiting immune synapse formation via regulating the actin polymerization. This leads us to speculate that MYLK might be involved in the CAV1 mediated inhibition of immune synapse formation of CLL cells in the LNs. Further, in-depth analyses are needed to confirm the role for MYLK in the CAV1 mediated immunosuppression specifically inhibition of immune synapse formation. In this regard, we also see the over expression of CAV2, associated with poor prognosis in CLL, might also be involved in interacting directly with G-protein alpha subunits and thus functionally regulate their activity through phosphorylation of Ser-36 to modulate mitosis in CLL cells. This might be through being a positive regulator of cellular mitogenesis of the MAPK signaling pathway.

Our transcriptome analyses of extracellular matrix associated genes revealed an over expression of VCAN, SPP1 and SERPINB2 in CLL cells from good prognosis patients. Although we do not know the significance of the elevated expression of these genes in CLL biology it is possible that these genes interact with CAV1 and CAV2 in regulating immune response towards CLL, this need to be addressed to understand the role of these overexpression genes.

In summary, differential gene expression (Table 3) of stromal signature I and II highlighted cytoskeleton associated genes like MYLK, CAV1, CAV2 and EHD2 which were significantly upregulated in CLL

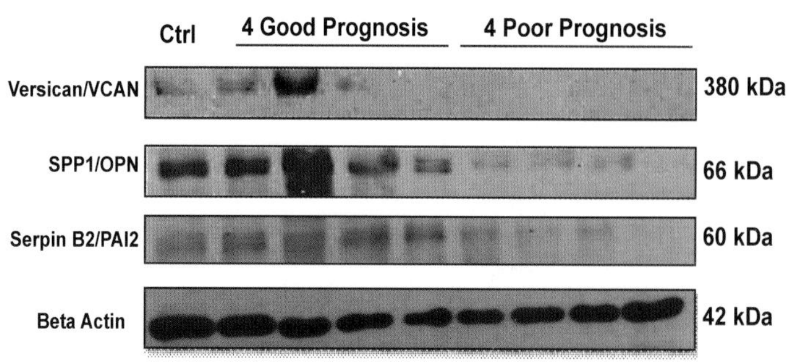

Figure 5: Validation of differentially expressed extracellular matrix associated genes in good and poor prognosis CLL samples using analyses for protein expression: Expression of selected extracellular matrix associated proteins in CLL cells from PB of 4 good prognosis and 4 poor prognosis patients using western blotting method.

Gene Symbol	Gene Name	Upregulated in Good Prognosis (Relative Fold Change)	q value
VCAN	Versican Core Protein isoform 3 precursor	50	0.00453231
SPP1	Osteopontin isoform a precursor	955	0.0463267
IL8	Interleukin-8 precursor	40	0.00027589
CD93	Complement component C1q receptor precursor	20	0.0081508
CXCL1	Growth-regulated alpha protein precursor	77	0.00492674
CXCL3	C-X-C motif chemokine 3	111	0.00090857
SERPINB2	Plasminogen activator inhibitor 2 precursor	1271	1.2298E-09

Table 3: Comparative analysis of differential gene expression of genes encoding extra cellular matrix components in Good Prognosis CLL and Poor prognosis CLL using RNA transcriptome analysis. The result shows relative fold change in the mRNA expression of particular genes states the upregulated genes in good prognosis.

cells from patient's LNs. Expression levels of stromal associated genes MYLK, DLC1, WNT2B, EHD2 and CAV2 correlated with clinical outcome. Thus, our results suggest that STME provides survival signals to CLL cells and facilitates the resistance to therapy which might be leading to leukemic progression.

In addition our transcriptome analyses showed several genes associated with extracellular matrix significantly upregulated in good prognosis. These results lay the foundation for in-depth analyses of these genes to elucidate the functional significance at the mechanistic levels of the differential expression of the relevant genes.

Acknowledgement

We thank the CLL foundation, Houston, TX and Lymphoma Research Foundation New York, NY for their financial support. We also thank Mrs. Kathryn Hyde and Mrs. Tami Houdesheldt for their help in editing the manuscript.

References

1. Herishanu Y, Pérez-Galán P, Liu D, Biancotto A, Pittaluga S, et al. (2011) The lymph node microenvironment promotes B-cell receptor signaling, NF-kappaB activation, and tumor proliferation in chronic lymphocytic leukemia. Blood 117: 563-574.
2. Gilling CE, Mittal AK, Chaturvedi NK, Iqbal J, Aoun P, et al. (2012) Lymph node-induced immune tolerance in chronic lymphocytic leukaemia: a role for caveolin-1. Br J Haematol 158: 216-231.
3. Shojaei F, Ferrara N (2008) Role of the microenvironment in tumor growth and in refractoriness/resistance to anti-angiogenic therapies. Drug Resist Updat 11: 219-230.
4. Burger JA (2012) Targeting the microenvironment in chronic lymphocytic leukemia is changing the therapeutic landscape. Curr Opin Oncol 24: 643-649.
5. García-Muñoz R, Galiacho VR, Llorente L (2012) Immunological aspects in chronic lymphocytic leukemia (CLL) development. Ann Hematol 91: 981-996.
6. Lenz G, Wright G, Dave SS, Xiao W, Powell J, et al. (2008) Stromal gene signatures in large-B-cell lymphomas. N Engl J Med 359: 2313-2323.
7. Orimo A, Gupta PB, Sgroi DC, Arenzana-Seisdedos F, Delaunay T, et al. (2005) Stromal fibroblasts present in invasive human breast carcinomas promote tumor growth and angiogenesis through elevated SDF-1/CXCL12 secretion. Cell 121: 335-348.
8. Harwood NE, Batista FD (2010) Early events in B cell activation. Annu Rev Immunol 28: 185-210.
9. Mattila PK, Feest C, Depoil D, Treanor B, Montaner B, et al. (2013) The actin and tetraspanin networks organize receptor nanoclusters to regulate B cell receptor-mediated signaling. Immunity 38: 461-474.
10. Joshi AD, Hegde GV, Dickinson JD, Mittal AK, Lynch JC, et al. (2007) ATM, CTLA4, MNDA, and HEM1 in high versus low CD38 expressing B-cell chronic lymphocytic leukemia. Clin Cancer Res 13: 5295-5304.
11. Joshi AD, Dickinson JD, Hegde GV, Sanger WG, Armitage JO, et al. (2007) Bulky lymphadenopathy with poor clinical outcome is associated with ATM downregulation in B-cell chronic lymphocytic leukemia patients irrespective of 11q23 deletion. Cancer Genet Cytogenet 172: 120-126.
12. Mittal AK, Hegde GV, Aoun P, Bociek RG, Dave BJ, et al. (2007) Molecular basis of aggressive disease in chronic lymphocytic leukemia patients with 11q deletion and trisomy 12 chromosomal abnormalities. Int J Mol Med 20: 461-469.
13. Hegde GV, Peterson KJ, Emanuel K, Mittal AK, Joshi AD, et al. (2008) Hedgehog-induced survival of B-cell chronic lymphocytic leukemia cells in a stromal cell microenvironment: a potential new therapeutic target. Mol Cancer Res 6: 1928-1936.
14. Morén B, Shah C, Howes MT, Schieber NL, McMahon HT, et al. (2012) EHD2 regulates caveolar dynamics via ATP-driven targeting and oligomerization. Mol Biol Cell 23: 1316-1329.
15. Kim TY, Vigil D, Der CJ, Juliano RL (2009) Role of DLC-1, a tumor suppressor protein with RhoGAP activity, in regulation of the cytoskeleton and cell motility. Cancer Metastasis Rev 28: 77-83.
16. Yamasaki T, Seki N, Yoshino H, Itesako T, Hidaka H, et al. (2013) microRNA-218 inhibits cell migration and invasion in renal cell carcinoma through targeting caveolin-2 involved in focal adhesion pathway. J Urol .
17. Sasaki H, Nishikata I, Shiraga T, Akamatsu E, Fukami T, et al. (2005) Overexpression of a cell adhesion molecule, TSLC1, as a possible molecular marker for acute-type adult T-cell leukemia. Blood 105: 1204-1213.
18. Connell LE, Helfman DM (2006) Myosin light chain kinase plays a role in the regulation of epithelial cell survival. J Cell Sci 119: 2269-2281.
19. Usatyuk PV, Singleton PA, Pendyala S, Kalari SK, He D, et al. (2012) Novel role for non-muscle myosin light chain kinase (MLCK) in hyperoxia-induced recruitment of cytoskeletal proteins, NADPH oxidase activation, and reactive oxygen species generation in lung endothelium. J Biol Chem 287: 9360-9375.

The History of Lymphoma Classifications with Special Consideration of Cutaneous Lymphomas

Christoph Niermann, Hans-Joachim Schulze, Christian Hallermann*

Department of Dermatology, Fachklinik Hornheide, Muenster, Germany
Parts of the presented publication have been published in German language, (Hautarzt. 2008;59(5):394-9)

Abstract

For the modern evidence based medicine classification systems are necessary to guarantee a unifying approach for therapy and for prognosis of diseases. The comparability of clinical studies depends of the usage of adequate classification systems. But because all classifications are artificial, they only mirror the technical possibilities of its area.

This review discusses the history of lymphoma classifications systems with a special focus on the topic of primary cutaneous lymphomas and the retikuloendothelial system. Furthermore special problems in terminology are discussed.

Keywords: Cutaneous lymphoma; Mycosis fungoides; Classification; Reticulosis

Introduction

Basics and background

The skin organ can be affected primarily or secondarily by a variety of neoplastic clonal B- or T-cell non-Hodgkin's lymphomas which exhibit heterogeneous clinical pictures in terms of clinical manifestations, histopathology, immunohistochemistry, cytogenetics and patterns of gene expression [1,2]. These are neoplasms of the immune system with a special tropism for skin and skin appendages [3].

If a lymphoproliferative skin disease occurs and if after completing the standard staging procedure no further extracutaneous manifestations are detectable, then a primary cutaneous lymphoma is present (PCL) [1,4]. Exclusion of a secondary skin involvement in a primary, mostly nodally located non-Hodgkin's lymphoma is prognostically and therapeutically crucial [5]. More than 30 different types of non-Hodgkin's lymphoma can affect the skin primarily or secondarily [6]. The existence of Hodgkin's disease initially displaying exclusively in the skin organ is uncertain, but would play a secondary role [7].

Depending on the inclusion criteria of the mesopharynxs and/or palatine tonsil, the skin is the second or third most commonly affected extranodal organ respectively, with increasing annual incidence. 0.3-1.0 per 100,000 people are affected, depending on the author and place / region / country of the surveys [8].

The clinical course ranges from a very good prognosis, usually without treatment such as lymphomatoid papulosis, to fatal CD4 + / CD56 + hematodermic neoplasia despite intensive treatment [9].

Considering the many and various forms of differentiation and function of lymphoid cells, the complexity of the neoplastic is also partly due to an arrested stage of development and understanding of the abnormally proliferating lymphoid cells [10]. This complexity of non-Hodgkin's lymphoma is reflected in more than 50 different classifications, in contrast to only two classifications for Hodgkin's disease [11,12].

Primary cutaneous lymphomas usually have a distinctly different clinical behavior and prognosis than histologically, cytomorphologically and immunohistochemically identical secondary cutaneous and nodal lymphomas [13]. However, for years the B-cell lymphomas in particular were divided into a classification system for nodal lymphomas which was partly not reproducible, resulting in serious consequences for treatment, which failed to meet the prognosis [13,14].

Despite the normally favorable prognosis it has to be noted that PCL, due to the movement of lymphoid cells, are usually systemic diseases with no curative therapy [15,16].

General information on classifications

Medical classifications define and describe specific and characteristic features of disease entities and arrange them in an order [10]. The classifications thus represent a central component of medical pathology and are the conceptual and clinical basis for the 1. diagnosis, 2. therapy and 3. prognosis of diseases [10]. Particularly for diseases with low case numbers, a common classification is inevitable in order to arrive at adequate comparisons regarding incidence, prevalence, prognosis and therapeutic response [17].

Classifications are a reflection of methodological possibilities [18]. Since these possibilities are subject to continuous change, there is also persistent alteration in the classification models [18]. Formulating a classification based on the latest scientific findings and showing its clinical relevance is problematic with regard to practical clinical aspects [18].

The function of classifications is to arrange the existing knowledge of a subject at any one time into understandable and reproducible

***Corresponding author:** Christian Hallermann, MD, PhD, Fachklinik Hornheide, Dorbaumstrasse 300, DE-48157 Munster, Germany,
E-mail: christian.hallermann@fachklinik-hornheide.de

categories [18]. This can be achieved either epistemologically or according to practical clinical aspects [19]. Generally, a good tumor classification requires scientific accuracy, simplicity and clinical relevance. These requirements are not easy to fulfill, as shown by numerous classifications of lymphoma in recent years [19].

Based on a well-proven norm, malignant neoplasms are sorted first by their morphology, then according to functional criteria, and lastly according to clinical significance. This also applies to malignant lymphoma [20].

Principles of attempts at classification

This section aims to give a systematic portrayal of the main criteria of the common nodal and two primary cutaneous Lymphoma classifications.

The heterogeneity of the classification approaches is presented. The classification is coded in alphabetical order as follows, for the individual classification criteria (see points 1 to 12 below) indicated in brackets in each example.

a. Rappaport classification und updated Rappaport [21]
b. Former German classification according to Lennert [22]
c. Lukes and Collins [23]
d. Kiel and updated Kiel [24]
e. Dorfman [25]
f. BNLI [26]
g. Working Formulation [26]
h. REAL [27]
i. WHO [28]
j. EORTC [29]
k. WHO-EORTC [1]
l. Isaacson [30]
m. WHO 2008 [31]

Historical

Eponyms appear in almost all classifications: Sezary (a), and Woringer Kolopp (j), Ketron and Goodman (j), Brill-Symmers (b.), Burkitt (c.), Lennert (c.), Bennet (d), Waldenstrom (m.).

Clinical

The clinical picture appears in the naming of some disease classifications and is therefore important:

Progress: aggressive behavior (i), lethal (h)

Prognosis: relative prognostic factors: low, intermediate or high (g).

Expressions: subcutaneous panniculitis-like lymphoma (j), hydroa vacciniform-like (middle), effusion (middle), mononucleosis-like (m.).

Comparisons: mycosis fungoides (d).

Local preference: leg type (j), nasal (i), mediastinal thymic (i), multilocular or unilocular (l), intestinal, hepatosplenic (i), bone (m.) CNS (m.)

Age at diagnosis: pediatric (m.)

Presence of a post-transplant status (m.)

Temporal relation to post-transplant status: early lesion (m.)

Histological

Histology and cytomorphology were and still are the gold standard in diagnosis of lymphoma [24].

Patterns: nodular versus diffuse growth technique (a).

Predominant conformation: pagetoid, granulomatous (j).

Local preference: folliculotropic (j), intravascular (j), angioimmunoblastic (i), epidermotropic (l).

Non-neoplastic cellular or noncellular accompanying reaction: T-cell-rich BCL with diffuse sclerosis (g), connective tissue proportion (d) and T-cell rich / histiocyte rich diffuse large B-cell lymphoma (i).

Composition: composite (1), mixed cellular lymphohistiocytic (g).

Imitation behavior: follicle center (j), marginal zones (j), MALTom (j).

Immunohistochemical

Thanks to immunohistochemistry, morphologically indistinguishable cells can be distinguished by their functional form:

T-cell (c.), B-cell (c.), NK-cell (h), null-cell (d), CD4 + (j), CD8 + (j), CD56 + (k), CD30 (k) Ki1 (d), ALK + (m.)

Tinctorial qualities

The tinctorial qualities are irrelevant for the nomenclature of all classifications listed in this paper except the Dorfman classification. Here the ability to transform is verified by means of the dye pyronin: Pyroninophil (e.)

Cytomorphological

Cell maturation: cytic, blastic (d.), poorly or well differentiated (a.), anaplastic (d.).

Nucleus shape: Cleav. (c.) conv. (c.) hyperchrom. (c.), cerebriform (c.) nucleus size: medium to large (c.).

Differentiation and maturity: peripheral or central (h.).

Cell size: small-cell, large-cell (g.), villous versus non-villous (i.), indicating <6.5 microns or <8 microns (d.), monomorphic or polymorphic (l.), small-medium (m.)

Imitative behavior: Follicle center cell (j.), centroblastic (d.), centrocytic (d.).

Etiological

The goal of any classification, also with PCL, should be based on a statement of etiology [31]. In neurology, this is partly realized in the classification of hereditary ataxia of the cerebellum by specifying the pathological nucleotide sequences [10].

This etiological classification feature in the form of a viral HTLV lymphoma genesis gave its name explicitly in the REAL classification. However, it was not taken up in the following classifications established by the WHO in 2001.

Etiology: HTLV-proof positive or negative (j.). This viral causal aspect could also be subsumed under the classification criterion "infectious".

WHO classification of 2008 (m) HHV 8, EBV

Molecular

The molecular-based naming of the classifications is constructed on proof of the γ/δ-configuration of the T-cell receptor. This γ/δ terminology appeared in 1994 in the REAL classification and at that time was the preferred practise of clinical study in molecular biology [10].

However, this proof can now be established by means of the βF1 monoclonal antibody.

Molecular: gamma / delta (k.), HTLV virus negative or positive (j.)

Location

Nodal versus extranodal (h.).

Lymphoma / leukemia

With or without washout lymphoid cells (b.).

Provisorily or definitely

Immunocytoma (j.); Maltom (j.).

Unclassifiable lymphomas: (g.).

From the mid-1930s until the late 1970s four different lymphoid neoplasms were distinguished: 1) lymphosarcoma, 2) reticulosarcoma, 3) giant follicular lymphoblastoma (Brill-Symmers' Disease) 4) Hodgkin's disease [22]. These concepts were not based on a uniformly accepted definition [21].

In 1964, the term non-Hodgkin's lymphoma was used for the first time [22]. Other sources report the first citation as being not until 1974 [18].

The discovery of the functional division of the immune system into B- and T-cells – along with the corresponding peripheral zones by Cooper [32] in 1964 and the morphologically reversible physiological adaptability of small lymphoid cells due to phytohemagglutinin of the green bean in large lymphoid cells by Nowell [33] in 1960 – revolutionized lymphoma research [20].

The concept of reticulosis that shaped the classification of lymphoid neoplasms for over 50 years is chronologically outlined below.

Reticuloendothelial system and reticulum cells

In 1924, Letterer [34] introduced the term "reticulosis" since the term lymphoma – referring to any swelling of a lymph node – did not seem to be sufficiently specific [22]. However, in North America the term lymphoma was largely retained [35].

At the beginning of the 20th century and based on Ehrlich's concept of vital staining, Metchnikoff observed phagocytosis through cells which he called macrophages. Metchnikoff's scientific concept was based furthermore on investigations of Aschoff [36] who introduced the functional and not primarily morphological concept of the reticuloendothelial system (RES) in 1924.

In 1930, Maximow [37] tried to provide a morphological foundation for this originally functional concept based particularly on the Marchand's [38] hypotheses from 1898.

The RES was morphologically defined as an accumulation of pluripotent mesenchymal reticular cells which were believed to be located in the vascular adventitia of the entire vascular tree. According to this definition, reticular cells had the potential of differentiation of embryonic mesenchyme and could under certain conditions differentiate in hematopoietic, lymphopoietic, reticuloendothelial and fibroblastic cells [39-44].

Siegmund [45] described the RES as "active mesenchyme" with the ability of lympho- and myelopoiesis. Extramedullary erythropoiesis by these cells would be possible as well, but rare. The RES could produce all blood cells and certain connective tissue cells [39,40].

The reticular cell was defined as a reticulin-fiber-producing support cell close to pluripotent embryonic mesenchymal cells [39].

In 1932, Pullinger [46] highlighted that there would be neoplasms of the reticular cells from their numerous offspring.

The term reticulosarcoma was introduced by Oberling [47] in 1928. In the German-speaking world it was designated by Rössle as Retothelsarkom [48].

The meaning of the term RES was specified differently in the literature. Thus Harrison [49] believed reticular cells to form channels in the form of endothelial cells. Fresen [40], however, mentioned the assumed involvement of the vascular endothelial cell layer as part of the RES [40]. Also, the term "reticular" itself has been explained using the observed tinctorially verifiable reticulin fiber formation, but also using the loose mesh-like arrangement of the cellular elements [50,51].

The RES concept was superseded partly by the reticuloendothelial system (RHS) of Fresen or the retothelian system [40].

Table 1 shows the common classification of reticuloses of the skin in the German-speaking world during the mid-1950s.

Until the late 1970s, there was no precise morphological description of the reticulum [44]. One of the most concrete definitions states that the reticulum is an "advential pluripotent reticulin-producing sustentacular cell" [44].

As opposed to Naegeli's [52] hematological dualism, the theory of a third independent leukocyte system, proposed by Schilling [53] with the reticulum cell concept, represented trialism in hematology from a genetic standpoint as well [53].

For decades, it was the common opinion that monocytes derived from reticulum cells. The RES would thus form blood monocytes and was believed to be independent of the myeloid and lymphoid system [43,54-56].

New Interpretation of the RES

Due to radioactive isotopic methods in the late 1960s, it was found that the designated reticulum cells are not stem cells [56]. Rather than from the RES, monocytes derived from the bone marrow, which is not a third hematopoietic system, but closely related to the myeloid system [56].

Thus, the RES was replaced by the mononuclear phagocyte system, which is not independent, but closely related to the myeloid system [55,56]. A third blood-cell-forming system, as previously assumed for the RES, does not exist [55-58].

New Interpretation of the reticulum

Steigleder [59] showed that the postulated reticulum cells of the skin are primarily fibroblasts, histiocytes and lymphocytes.

Proliferation	Benign	Malignant
Disseminated	Reticulosis Lymphadenosis	Reticulo-Sarcomatosis Lymphosarcomatosis
Localized	Reticuloma Lymphocytoma	Reticulosarcoma = Retothelsarkoma Lymphosarcoma

Table 1: Classification of the "reticuloendothelial system of the skin" in 1953 [40] and 1959 [41].

The reticulum cells demonstrated by Müller-Hermelink [60] in 1976 using electron microscopy and immunohistochemistry were described as interdigitating, fibroblastic, dendritic and histiocytic, having no common morphological structure with the originally designated reticulum cell [56,57,60]. However, the postulated origin of the initial cell of the CD4 + / CD56 + hematodermic neoplasm might be of interest, namely a plasmacytoid dendritic cell [1].

In some classifications neoplasia from large reticulum cells were referred to as histiocytic lymphoma, but actually mainly represent - according to the present knowledge – neoplasia of large transformed lymphoid cells, neoplasia of monocytes, or actual histiocytic proliferations [56].

The continental European usage of the term reticulosis of the skin impressed with the clinical picture of a uniform type of efflorescence, usually of multiple nodes of different sizes with a smooth surface. However, they proved to be low malignant B-cell lymphomas [56]. Likewise, the reticulosarcoma impressing clinically by a singular tumor proved to be a B-immunoblastic lymphoma and only in rare cases as neoplasia of histiocytes [56,58].

The monocytic leukemia/ reticulosarcomatosis cutis Gottron, described by Eva Gottron [61] in 1951 as a disease with paroxysmally occurring nodes proved to be – according to some authors – a skin manifestation of a myelomonocytic leukemia, while others stressed the high proportion of immunoblastic B-cell lymphomas in this disease [18].

This clinical picture shows clearly the difficulty of retrospective analysis of "reticulosis" diagnoses.

In 1978, Braun-Falco [35] suggested replacing the term reticulosis with the term "malignant lymphoma". Table 2 summarizes these results.

Methodological milestones

Each tumor classification is based on the characterization of the proliferating neoplastic cells and on the discovery of functional and cytomorphologic similarities with a physiologically postulated sister cell [11].

In the past, lymphoreticular classifications were influenced by concepts based on ideas of the reticuloendothelial or lymphoid system prevailing at the time [56].

The following six points illustrate the methodological developments.

Technical

Advancements in the field of light microscopy, electron microscopy, the "camera lucida" [23], enabled us to improve the assessment of cell morphology [62]. The reproducibility of cytomorphologic results was further improved by computer-supported morphometry [63].

In 1967, Lennert [62] succeeded in identifying the endoplasmic reticulum in reticular cells using electron microscopy.

Furthermore, by using microtomes, semithin sections could be produced which represented, in addition to optical apparative innovations, the precondition for better assessment of the slices [64].

Tinctorial

As early as the late 19th century, lymphatic cells could be distinguished from myeloid cell lines using Ehrlich's staining methods [12]. Azure-II-eosin stainings of Maximov and the industrially produced Giemsa staining represented further progress in the re-evaluation of cytomorphology [64]

Enzyme cytochemistry

Cytochemical representation of different nonspecific and specific esterases and acid phosphatases made the distinction between lymphoid cells of monocytes and histiocytes possible [64].

Cytological diagnosis of function

A so-called mitogenic stimulation with phytohemagglutinin resulted in a reversible transformation of small lymphoid cells into large blastic cells. As a result of the transformation tests, T-cell lymphocytes could be distinguished from B-cell lymphocytes [33].

Immunocytology

In a cell suspension produced from lymphoid cells by incubation with polyvalent anti-human Ig or by quantitative immunoglobulin detection, a B-cell lineage was demonstrated [65].

Through incubation with anti-human T-cell globulin, the lymphoid T cells reacted with a spontaneous rosette formation when adding sheep blood erythrocytes [56].

Kohler and Milstein [66] facilitated the production of monoclonal antibodies, which have been further optimized by the development of common paraffin antibodies. The obligatory and routine use of fresh preparations or cryostat gradually became less necessary.

The development of detection systems in the form of immunoperoxidase "bridge" technology in immunohistochemistry and newer methods for epitope demasking made retrospective assessment of paraffin preparations possible [67].

Molecular biological methods

Use of Southern-blot-hybridization and the polymerase chain reaction (PCR), placed proof of monoclonality of lymphoid infiltrates on a new methodological basis [68]. The DNA of neoplastic cells can now be selectively obtained by laser-assisted microdissection [68].

Structural chromosome aberrations, such as gene duplication or gene amplification, are often initially causally represented in a neoplastic process and are – since the REAL classification - an equal classification feature for defining entities [69]. By PCR, fluorescence in situ hybridization (FISH) and comparative genomic hybridization (CGH) these changes can be specifically detected at the chromosomal level [69].

Neoplastic cells have been characterized by pathological changes to the pattern of their gene expression [69]. Evidence of this change can

Former definition:	Autonomous atypical irreversible system-like proliferation reticulo-histiocytic cells of the reticuloendothelial system (RES)	
Contemporary sense:	1.	Neoplasms of the lymphoid tissue (usually B-cell)
	2.	Myeloproliferative diseases
	3.	Malignancies of the monocyte-histiocyte-macrophage system or the Merkel cell

Table 2: Reticuloses of the skin according to [35].

be provided at the genomic, transcriptional or proteomic level [70,71]. Due to the Human Genome Project, the semiconductor industry and bioinformatics, the characteristic expression profiles of transformed and non-transformed lymphoid cells can now be collected [70,71].

Classification of cutaneous lymphomas

Mycosis fungoides

In 1806, Alibert [72] described the "Pian fongoide", considering it a contagious European form of frambesia tropica and going on to name it mycosis fungoides (MF) in 1832. He adopted a text by Bontius [73].

According to other sources, Besnier et al. first used the term Pian fungoides in 1812 [74].

The designation was based on the similarity of the tumors of the MF with the fruiting body of certain mushroom species, such as Bovista [75]. The fact that both the fungi and the MF tumors share the characteristic feature of bursting on the "apex" reinforces the admissibility of this comparison [75,76].

Alibert [72] also distinguished at times a mycosis syphiloides and mycosis framboesoides from mycosis fungoides, assigning them all to the venereal diseases – a fact that was critically noticed by Hebra and Kaposi ten years later [77].

It was only later that a clear distinction between frambesia tropica and mycosis fungoides was made. Thus, a reference to the first description of mycosis fungoides is not possible [74]. In the following decades, mycosis fungoides was often compared to or equated with molluscum of Bateman, a disease that is now known as neurofibromatosis [74].

The initially flaky rash of mycosis fungoides has already been mentioned by Alibert. However, it was his student Bazin [78] who described the three phases of mycosis fungoides in 1870. Other sources mention the year as 1876 [75]. Bazin's student Guerard spoke of "indigenous leprosy" [74].

In 1885, Vidal and Brocq [79] described the form mycosis fungoides d'emblée as a cognisant opposition to what is now well-known as a classic MF appearance. However, it proved to be not mycosis fungoides, but probably a primary cutaneous aggressive epidermotropic $CD8^{+}$-T-cell lymphoma or cutaneous γ/δ T-cell lymphoma [1].

Ranvier and Cornill [80] in 1868 and Gillot [81] in 1869 mentioned – albeit a misconception – the relation of the MF to the lymphatic system. In 1892 Hallapeau and Besnier [82] described the erythrodermic form [65]. Other authors, however, consider Leredde [83] to be the original describer [75].

In 1874, Port [84] emphasized the sarcomatous neoplastic nature of mycosis fungoides, which Auspitz [85] however diametrically opposed to a chronic inflammatory granulomatous aspect.

There were two opinions about the assessment of malignancy of mycosis fungoides:

1. "Inflammatory granulomatous theory" by Koebner [86] ("sponge-like skin"), Paltauf and von Zumbusch because of polymorphic inflammatory cell infiltrate and
2. The primary neoplastic model by Fraser and Montgomery, also preferred by Kaposi.

Auspitz [85] acknowledged the histological chronic inflammatory granulomatous aspect so much that he suggested a renaming as granuloma fungoides. This terminology can be found until the late 1970s in the classification of Keining and Braun-Falco [87] and corresponds with PCL to the patient population of the dermatological clinic.

This abovementioned fundamental problem mirrors the still unclear issue of whether lymphoproliferative diseases of the skin are primarily a neoplastic "ab initio" or an intially inflammatory process [75]. The dermatopathologist encounters this difficulty in the differential diagnosis of "initial" mycosis fungoides or inflammatory dermatosis. In 1909, Paltauf emphasized the systemic nature of the MF [63]. Thanks to PCR T-cell receptor studies, Muche et al. [88], while detecting circulating neoplastic lymphoid cells also in the initial stages of mycosis fungoides, placed the systemic nature of the early MF on a molecular basis.

At this point, however, it has to be stressed that many benign dermatoses, such as the *Lichen ruber et planus* also partially exhibit monoclonal circulating T lymphocytes [88].

The Sézary syndrome was first described by Zumbusch [89] and in 1939 by Baccareda [90] as "reticulohistiocytosis cutanea benigna cum melanodermia" . It was Lutzner and Jordan [91] who succeeded with the electron microscopic cytologic description. However, the syndrome was named by Taswell and Winkelmann [92]. In 1964, Clendening et al. [93] described the Sezary syndrome to be a leukemic form of mycosis fungoides. In 1971, Crossen [94] not only laid the foundation for a non-lymphoid and reticuloendothelial origin of the Sézary or Lutzner cell, but also emphasized the neoplastic nature of the cells, demonstrating abnormal chromosome conditions such as in malignant cells. In 1975, the Sézary cell was characterized as belonging to the T-cell systema, and in 1978 the lymphoid cells were described as TH_2 helpers with corresponding cytokine profile [12].

As to the subtypes of mycosis fungoides, the following should be noted. The "Granulomatous slack skin syndrome" was clinically described by Bazex [95] in 1968 and eponymously coined by Ackerman [96] in 1978. Pagetoid reticulosis was described by Ketron and Goodman [97] in 1931 and in 1939 by Woringer and Kolopp [98]. However, it was named by Braun-Falco et al. [99]. The Ketron-Goodman type is defined by the WHO-EORTC classification not as pagetoid reticulosis, but as a primary cutaneous aggressive epidermotropic CD8 + T-cell lymphoma [1].

In 1984, Vakilzadeh and Brocker [100] described the syringotrope mycosis fungoides as "syringolymphoid hyperplasia with alopecia" [100].

Classification Problems

The problem of classification, as well as the temporarily divergent view of malignancy, is illustrated below using a primary cutaneous T-and B-cell lymphoma.

Example of T-cell lymphoma: Lymphomatoid papulosis

As an example, lymphomatoid papulosis may serve well: first description and naming do not coincide. Dupont [101] described the disease in 1965. It was named, however, by Mcaulay [102] in 1968. Before 1965, lymphomatoid papulosis was known as "regressive atypical histiocytosis," "atypical paradoxical reticulopathy" cutaneous Hodgkin's disease, mycosis fungoides or as T-cell pseudolymphoma [75]. In 1975, based on morphological and immunological studies, Lutzner et al. [103] mentioned the relation of LyP to the CTCL.

In 1982, histologic subtyping in A, B or C was performed in a doctoral thesis by Willemze [104]. These subtypes are included in the WHO-EORTC classification, although they exhibit–without prognostic significance – different monoclonality of the T-cell receptor depending on the type and are often represented simultaneously within one lesion [1]. Lymphomatoid papulosis is not exclusively considered as an entity, but as part of a spectrum of CD30+ lymphoproliferative diseases [105,106]. The superordinate immunohistochemical classification appears problematic because the lymphomatoid papulosis type B must "by definition" be CD30 negative [1]. Furthermore, infectious or benign dermatoses with CD30-positive cells are called "simulators" [107].

Example of B-cell lymphoma: Primary cutaneous marginal zone B-cell lymphoma

Marginal zone lymphomas were first described by Isaacson in 1984 [108]. They were designated as saltoma, immunozytome, lymphoplasmazytoide lymphoma, marginal zone lymphoma, plasmacytoma of the skin or maltome of the skin [109,110]. The distinction between immunozytomes and marginal zone lymphomas as separate entities seemed justified due to different clinical aspects (age difference, localization), histology (in the form of Dutcher or Russel bodies) and proportion of non-neoplastic cells as accompanying infiltrate [111,112]. In the WHO-EORTC classification, all of the terms mentioned above subsumed under the clinical picture, "primary cutaneous marginal zone B-cell lymphoma (PCMZL)" [1]. Many of the skin lesions formerly known as B-pseudo lymphoma retrospectically turned out to be primary cutaneous marginal zone B-cell lymphomas [109,113].

Systematic classification of cutaneous lymphomas and reticuloses

Classifications before the mid-1970s

For many decades, mycosis fungoides, Sézary syndrome, lymphomatoid papulosis and pagetoid reticulosis were the only cutaneous lymphomas that were clearly defined as entities [114,115]. Notifications of skin lymphomas which did not correspond to those mentioned above were casuistic rarities. They were referred to as malignant reticulosis or reticulum cell sarcoma, terms that were only used for forms of expression of a systemic process with an unfavorable prognosis [116].

Until the mid-1970s, cutaneous lymphomas/reticuloses were classified in visceral versus cutaneous forms, according to the nature of the skin lesion, according to the course of the disease, according to a known or unknown etiology, or histologically according to the predominance of a monomorphic or granulomatous infiltrate component [35].

Application of nodal classifications for cutaneous lymphomas

By abandoning the concept of reticulosis in favor of the lymphoma designation and by introducing and adapting nodal classifications [50] to the skin organ of Lever and Schaumburg-Lever [117] in 1974, the cutaneous lymphoma classification was placed on a new basis [11]. By immunohistochemistry, reticuloses were considered malignant lymphomas of T- or B-cell type being locked in their particular stage of differentiation, [118].

The Kiel classification was applied to the malignant lymphoma of the skin in the form of a "periodic table" [118] or simply according to a high or low degree of malignancy [118]. Furthermore, the Working Formulation was applied to skin lymphomas [119].

Further investigations led to the discovery of other B-and T-cell lymphomas differing in their clinical appearance, behavior, prognosis and histology, and subject to an inconsistent nomenclature:

1. the use of nodal classifications or
2. striking histological appearances (vascular-stressed, subcutaneous fat) or
3. immunophenotypic appearance of neoplastic cells [117].

Because of the clinical and terminological heterogeneity, reproducibility was low, which in turn led to the use of histological nodal classifications.

Modern contemporary therapeutic approaches need an adequate classification [1]. However, there was no generally accepted classification for cutaneous lymphomas.

Instead, the Rappaport classification, Kiel classification and WF were used for the systematic classification of cutaneous lymphomas, originating however in the lymph node pathology [119]. In summary, it can be stated that until the mid-1980s it was beyond dispute that malignant lymphomas not constituting mycosis fungoides/ Sézary syndrome, lymphomatoid papulosis or pagetoid reticulosis, were inevitably manifestations of systemic lymphomas [115,120].

Independent classification for cutaneous lymphomas

However, as early as a hundred years ago there was already anecdotal evidence of reticuloses, originating primarily in the skin with a long disease course, as represented by Buschke and Hirschfeld in 1911 [121].

At this point the Italian dermatologists Mariani [122], Flarer [123], Fieschi [124] and the French Sézary [125] and Cazal [126] are to be mentioned as pioneers in the recognition of primary cutaneous lymphomas.

Observations of indolent lymphomas confined for a long time to the skin organ were interpreted as casuistic rarities [127,128].

In a retrospective study by Evans et al. [129], patients who died five years after initial manifestation of the lymphoma were categorized as diseased with malignant lymphoma, while the surviving patients were classified with "lymphoid hyperplasia".

The classifications previously developed for nodal lymphoma could never fully take into account the particularities of organ-specific lymphomas with corresponding "homing" receptors. Thus, it was understandable that in dermatology many classifications were drawn up differing from nodal ones, which in turn led to a lack of understanding and recognition from the pathologists and hematopathologists [129]. As a further organ-specific classification of lymphoid neoplasms, the lymphoma of the gastrointestinal tract may be mentioned [130,131].

The concepts of classifying cutaneous lymphoma were based on anatomical structures of the lymph node, which are not represented in the skin [114,115]. Clinical pictures of the skin, such as lymphomatoid papulosis, mycosis fungoides, pagetoid reticulosis and folliculotropic mycosis fungoides, have no nodal equivalent [116]. In addition, as early as 1980 Lennert [132] mentioned the significant differences in terms of B-and T-cell proportion in nodal and cutaneous NHL [131]. Histologically, it is almost impossible to distinguish a lymphomatoid papulosis of Willemze type B from a mycosis fungoides in the plaque stage without providing clinical data [116].

Only occasionally have lymphomas of the skin been included in nodal NHL classifications: e.g. MF in the Kiel classification [18,20].

In 1975, all cutaneous lymphomas in the North American region (including mycosis fungoides, Sézary syndrome, pagetoid reticulosis) were summarized under the category "cutaneous T-cell lymphoma" (CTCL) [133]. A further subdivision was drawn up by Edelson [134] in 1980, observing the presence of an epidermotropic or non-epidermotropic infiltrate component [134]. The establishment of primary cutaneous B-cell lymphomas (PCBCL) succeeded in the early 90s [135].

It must be explicitly emphasized that no distinction was made between primary and secondary lymphomas occurring in the skin. The diametrical opposition of visceral and cutaneous form mentioned above was not supposed to express a fundamental difference in the nature of the disease, but only meant to demonstrate the chronicity and clinical aspects, as well as to provide a better prognosis in the individual case [136].

In the cytomorphologic Kiel classification, the germinal center lymphoma and anaplastic large cell lymphoma CD30 + were shown to be highly malignant. This observation was, however, contrary to the clinical observation attesting an excellent prognosis to diseases of the skin organ [115].

Furthermore, differences between histologically identical nodal and cutaneous lymphomas were discovered according to oncogenic expression, the presence of adhesion molecules, chromosomal translocations and occurrence of viral sequences proving the inadequacy of the exclusive consideration of the histology [115]. However, this was already known to dermatologists, since – as mentioned above – a mycosis fungoides can only be differentiated from a lymphomatoid papulosis type B or a small and medium cell pleomorphic T-cell lymphoma considering clinical information [136]. Furthermore, there is no nodal correspondence for numerous cutaneous lymphoid neoplastic clinical pictures, as for example for LyP, folliculotropic MF and pagetoid reticulosis [137]. Thus clinically definite entities and not histologic subtypes have been characterized [138].

In 1991, Kerl [138] classified CTCL according to the updated Kiel classification and precursor T and peripheral T-cells. The final concept was introduced three years later by the REAL classification.

In 1993, Pimpinelli et al. [139] classified CTCL in 1. MF, 2. CD 30^+ CTCL of non-MF-type and 3. CD 30^-CTCL of non-MF-type. PCBCL were viewed as a homogeneous group, without prognostic subtype [138].

Burg's [140] classification from 1994 included and arranged all cutaneous lymphomas known at that time that could affect the skin primarily and secondarily. The division was performed using the updated Kiel classification and Working Formulation [141].

A co operation between the dermatology clinics in Munich and Graz in the form of the "German-Austrian Cutaneous Lymphoma Study Group" began in 1973 [141]. In 1980, von Burg and Kerl [135] established the "EORTC cutaneous lymphoma task force" which, in 1982, now including more centers, acquired the project group status [140], whose main objectives were summarized by the Breur Committee in 1984 [141]. The classification by Willemze [114] in 1994, as a result of the Breur commission of the CTCL, represented the basis for the subsequent EORTC classification which corresponded approximately to the classification of Russell-Jones in 1996 [141]. It was based on the patient collective of all Dutch university hospitals and the university hospital of Ghent. The EORTC classification, published in 1997, was the first classification of exclusively primary cutaneous lymphomas subdividing reproducible disease entities according to clinical prognostic criteria. Pathologies that differed histologically, but not clinically with any certainty were assigned the adjective "provisional" [29].

Like any organ-specific classification, it was subject to criticism for its inability to communicate cross-disciplinarily [75]. A uniform communication is essential, however, especially for primary cutaneous lymphomas, as not only dermatologists and pathologists, but also hematology oncologists are involved in diagnosis, therapy and treatment [75].

The REAL classification, published in 1994 by the "International Lymphoma Study Group" (ILSG) [27] and based on the fundamental principles of the updated Kiel classification, contained numerous primary, but also secondary cutaneous lymphoma entities, and no histological subtypes. Thus, as already mentioned, it was the first joint classification of NHL, created by 24 experts from North America and Europe [27].

In 2001, the REAL classification was superseded by the WHO classification, which also contained defined clinical pictures not yet known to the EORTC classification in 1997 [30].

The main benefit of the EORTC classification for the hematopathologists was the awareness of the clinical features of primary cutaneous lymphomas with similar histo-and cytomorphology [141-143].

Table 3 [138,144-158] illustrates the significant systematic classifications of reticuloses of the skin and cutaneous lymphomas.

WHO-EORTC classification

Being subject-specific, the EORTC classification consisted

Year	Authors/Main Proponents	Year	Authors/Main Proponents
1949	De Graciansky and Paraf [143]	1976	Burg and Braun-Falco [153]
1956	Lindner and Meyer [144]	1976	Pinkus and Mehregan [154]
1957	Degos et al. [145], Winkelmann and altman [147]	1978	Lever and Schaumburg [117]
1958, 1957	Gans and Steigleder [148]	1979	Kerl et al. [155]
1960	Gottron [149]	1991	Kerl et al. [155], Pimpinelli et al. [139]
1962	Gertler [150]	1994	Willemze et al. [115], Isaacson [30]
1964	Cazal [151]	1994	Burg et al. [139], Slater [158]
1966,1967	Musger [152]	1996	Knobler et al. [141]
1969, 1961	Keining and Braun-Falco [87]	1997	EORTC [29]
1975	Lutzner [103]	2005	WHO-EORTC [1]

Table 3: Overview of systematic attempts at classification of lymphomas and reticuloses of the skin.

exclusively of lymphomas initially emerging in the skin organ. According to the WHO classification, primary cutaneous lymphomas are partially classified in the general classification context by denomination as special entities [1]. However, as mentioned above, even within the same academic institution different classifications were used [1]. Thus, as with nodal classifications, studies and therapy results could not be compared.

The differences between the two classifications were not only linguistic, but also represented fundamentally different conceptions. The WHO classification assigned the sum of diffuse large B-cell lymphomas of the skin organ to the category of DLBCL, frequently implicating the therapeutic measure of chemotherapy [159]. Lymphomas comprising follicular structures were classified as follicular lymphomas of the type "follicle center", usually not requiring chemotherapeutic treatment [1,159].

In contrast, according to the EORTC classification PCFCL consists of germinal center cells with diffuse, diffuse and follicular, or only follicular structure, normally not requiring chemotherapeutic intervention [29].

By means of two consensus conferences, in Lyon in September 2003 and in Zurich in January 2004, the first common classification for primary cutaneous lymphomas was adopted: the WHO-EORTC classification [1].

According to Burg et al. [160], the current WHO-EORTC classification represents only a working basis for a further increase in knowledge through prospective gene expression pattern analyses, epigenetic and proteomic analyses also influencing the classification of PCL [160-162].

References

1. Willemze R, Jaffe ES, Burg G, Cerroni L, Bert E, et al. (2005) WHO-EORTC classification for cutaneous lymphomas. Blood 105: 3768-3785.
2. Zinzani PL, Quaglino P, Pimpinelli N, Berti E, Baliva G, et al. (2006) Prognostic factors in primary cutaneous B-cell lymphoma: the Italian Study Group for Cutaneous Lymphomas. J Clin Oncol 24: 1376-1382.
3. Kerl H, Volkenandt M, Cerroni L (1994) Malignant lymphoma of the skin. Hautarzt 45: 421-443.
4. Kim YH, Willemze R, Pimpinelli N, Whittaker S, Olsen EA, et al. (2007) TNM classification system for primary cutaneous lymphomas other than mycosis fungoides and sezary syndrome: A proposal of the international society for cutaneous lymphomas (ISCL) and the cutaneous lymphoma task force of the European organization of research and treatment of cancer (EORTC). Blood 110: 479-484.
5. Kaudewitz P, Sander CA, Flaig MJ (2000) Maligne Lymphome. Empfehlungen zur Diagnostik, Therpie und Nachsorge, W. Zuckerschwerdt Verlag München Bern Wien New York 146-155.
6. Kazakov DV, Burg G, Dummer R, Kempf W (2002) Cutaneous Lymphomas and Pseudolymphomas: Newly described entities. Recent Results in Cancer Research 160: 283-293.
7. Guitart J, Fretzin D (1998) Skin as the primary site of Hodgkin's disease: a case report of primary cutaneous Hodgkin's disease and review of its relationship with non-Hodgkin's lymphoma. Am J Dermatopathol 20: 218-222.
8. d'Amore F, Christensen BE, Brincker H, Pedersen NT, Thorling K, et al. (1991) Clinicopathological features and prognostic factors in extranodal non-Hodgkin lymphomas. Danish LYFO Study Group. Eur J Cancer 27: 1201-1208.
9. Cerroni L (2006) Lymphoproliferative lesions of the skin. J Clin Pathol 59: 813-826.
10. Hiddemann W, Dreyling M, Stein H (2004) Lymphome. Neue Erkenntnisse und Therapiestrategien, Thieme Verlag, Stuttgart 30-36.
11. Aisenberg AC (2000) Historical review of lymphomas. Br J Haematol 109: 466-476.
12. Dorfman RF (1994) Hematopatology: A crescendo of sholarly activity.Mod Pathol 7: 226-241.
13. Sander CA, Flaig MJ, Jaffe ES (2001) Cutaneous manifestations of lymphoma: a clinical guide based on the WHO classification. World Health Organization. Clin Lymphoma 2: 86-100.
14. Pandolfino TL, Siegel RS, Kuzel TM, Rosen ST, Guitart J (2000) Primary cutaneous B-cell lymphoma: Review and current concepts. J Clin Oncol 18: 2152-2168.
15. Koh HK, Jacobson JO, Foss F, Lew RA (1995) Is cutaneous T-cell lymphoma curable? Arch Dermatol 131: 1081-1082.
16. Harris NL (1987) Lymphoma 1987. An interim approach to diagnosis and classification. Pathol Annu 22 Pt 2: 1-67.
17. Dehner LP (1995) Here we go again: a new classification of malignant lymphomas. A viewpoint from the trenches. Am J Clin Pathol 103: 539-540.
18. Lennert K (2006) History of European Association for Haematopathology. Springer Verlag, Berlin Heidelberg.
19. Isaacson PG (2000) The current status of lymphoma classification. Br J Haematol 109: 258-266.
20. Lennert K (1992) [Non-Hodgkin's lymphomas: principles and application of the Kiel classification]. Verh Dtsch Ges Pathol 76: 1-13.
21. Rappaport H (1964) Classification of neoplastic diseases of the reticular system. Symposium on lymphoreticular tumours in Africa. Karger, Basel New York 394-404.
22. Lennert K (1967) Classification of malignant lymphomas (European concept). In: Rüttimann A., Progress in lymphology.Thieme Verlag, Stuttgart.
23. Lukes RJ (1979) The immunologic approach to the pathology of malignant lymphomas. Am J Clin Pathol 72: 657-669.
24. Lennert K, Stein H, Kaiserling E (1975) Cytological and functional criteria for the classification of malignant lymphomata. Br J Cancer Suppl 2: 29-43.
25. Dorfman RF (1974) Letter: Classification of non-Hodgkin's lymphomas. Lancet 1: 1295-1296.
26. (1985) Classification of non-Hodgkin's lymphomas. Reproducibility of major classification systems. NCI non-Hodgkin's Classification Project Writing Committee. Cancer 55: 91-95.
27. Harris NL, Jaffe ES, Stein H, Banks PM, Chan JK, et al. (1994) A revised European-American classification of lymphoid neoplasms: a proposal from the International Lymphoma Study Group. Blood 84: 1361-1392.
28. Harris NL, Jaffe ES, Diebold J, Flkandrin G., Muller-Hermelink HK et al (1997) The World Health Organization classification of neoplasms of the hematopoetic and lymphoid tissues: report of the Clinical Advisory Committee meeting – Airlie House, Virginia, Hematol J., 1: 53-66.
29. Willemze R, Kerl H, Sterry W, Berti E, Cerroni L, et al. (1997) EORTC classification for primary cutaneous lymphomas: a proposal from the Cutaneous Lymphoma Study Group of the European Organization for Research and Treatment of Cancer. Blood 90: 354-371.
30. Issacson PG, Norton AJ (1994) Extranodal lymphomas.Churchill Linvigstone, Edinburgh, London, Madrid, Melbourne, New York, Tokio.
31. Swerdlow SH, Campo E, Harris NL (2008) WHO classification of tumours of haematopoetic and lymphoid tissues (4thedn.) IARC, Lyon France.
32. Cooper MD, Peterson RDA, Gabrielson (1966) Early suggestion of immunolological relationship to lymphomas.Cancer Res 26: 1165
33. Nowell PC (1960) Phytohemagglutinin: an initiator of mitosis in cultures of normal human leukocytes. Cancer Res 20: 462-466.
34. Letterer E (1924) Acute reticulosis of infancy.Frank Z Pathol 30: 377.
35. Braun-Falco O, Burg G, Schmoeckel C (1978) Klassifikation von malignen Hautlymphomen. Hautarzt 28: 37-45.
36. Aschoff L (1924) Account of the reticulo-endothelialsystem.Erg Inn Med Kinderheilkd 26: 1.
37. Maximov AA (1932) Lymphocyte types. Special Cytology (2ndedn). Hoeber, New York, 602.
38. Marchand FJ (1913) Nature of lymphoid follicles.Verh Dtsch Ges Patholg 16: 5.

39. Robb-Smith AHT, Taylor CR (1982) Lymph Node Biopsy: 223-262.

40. Fresen O (1953) Pathological anatomy and differentiation of hemoblastosis and reticulosis. Strahlentherapie 91: 1-34.

41. Knoth W (1959) Zur Cyto- und Histiogenese und zur klinischen Einteilung der reticulo-histiocytären Erkrankungen der Haut.Arch Klin Exp Dermatol, 209: 130-170.

42. Taylor CR, Classification of lymphoma."New Thinking" and old Thoughts.

43. Taylor CR (1978) Classification of lymphoma. Arch Pathol Lab Med 102: 549-554.

44. Kimming J, Jänner M (1969) Retikulosen (S. 583-602), Handbuch der Haut- und Geschlechtskrankheiten, Ergänzungswerk. Springer Verlag, Berlin Heidelberg New York.

45. Siegmund H (1927) Reticuloendothel und aktives Mesenchym.Berlin (Urban Schwarzenberg).

46. Pullinger BD (1932) Histology of Hodgkin s disease.In: Gordon MH, Rose Research of lymphadenoma.John Wright and Sons, Bristol: 117.

47. Oberling C (1928) Reticilosarcomas.Bull Cancer 17: 259.

48. Rössle R (1939) Das Rethothelsarkom der Lymphdrüsen. Seine Formen und Verwandschaften.Beitr Path Anat, 103: 385-415.

49. Harrison CV (1956) An introduction to the reticuloses. Practitioner 177: 123-132.

50. Gall EA (1955) Enigmas in lymphoma; reticulum cell sarcoma and mycosis fungoides. Minn Med 38: 674-681.

51. Symmers WS (1951) Some comments on the pathology of the reticuloses. Br J Radiol 24: 469-475.

52. Naegeli O (1919) Blutkrankheiten und Blutdiagnostik. Lehrbuch der klinischen Hämatologie.Vereinigung wissenschaftlicher Verleger, Berlin. 62.

53. Schilling V (1950) [Clinical aspects of reticuloendotheliosis and monocytosis]. Z Gesamte Inn Med 5: 506-520.

54. Trümper LH, Brittinger G, Diehl V, Harris NL (2004) Non Hodgkin s lymphoma: A history of classification and clinical observations. Lippincott, Williams and Wilkans, New York, NY, USA.

55. Taylor CR (1980) Changing concepts in the classification of lymphoma. Malignant lymphoproliferative diseases.Leiden Universtity Press, The Hague Boston London.

56. Lennert K (2006) History of European Association for Haematopathology. Springer Verlag, Berlin Heidelberg.

57. Leder LD (1978) On the terms "reticulosis" and "reticulum cell sarcoma" with regard to the modern concept of the monocyte macrophage system. Klin Wochenschr 56: 1091-1096.

58. Kerl H, Kresbach H (1979):Lymphoreticuläre Hyperplasien und Neoplasien der Haut, Histopathologie der Haut, Teil 2. Springer-Verlag Berlin Heidelberg

59. Steigleder GK (1976) Benign and malignant proliferative response. Dermal infiltration, origin and importance. Acta Derm Venereol 56: 33-41.

60. Müller-Hermelink HK, Heusermann U, Kaiserling E, Stutte HJ (1976) Human lymphatic microecology - specificity, characterization and ontogeny of different reticulum cells in the B cell and T cell regions. Adv Exp Med Biol 66: 177-182.

61. Gottron E (1951) So called reticulosarcomatose of the skin.Hautarzt 2: 42.

62. Lennert K (1978) Classification of Non-Hodgkins lymphoma. Handbuch der speziellen pathologischen Anatomie und Histologie. Springer Verlag, Berlin Heidelberg New York.

63. Burg G, Braun-Falco O (1977) Morphological and functional differentiation and classification of cutaneous lymphomas. Bull Cancer 64: 225-240.

64. Taylor CR (1978) Classification of lymphoma. Arch Pathol Lab Med 102: 549-554.

65. Jaffe ES, Braylan RC, Frank MM, Green I, Berard CW (1976) Heterogeneity of immunologic markers and surface morphology in childhood lymphoblastic lymphoma. Blood 48: 213-222.

66. Köhler G, Milstein C (1975) Continuous cultures of fused cells secreting antibody of predefined specificity. Nature 256: 495-497.

67. Mason DY, Cordell JL, Abdulaziz Z, Naiem M, Bordenave G (1982) Preparation of peroxidase: antiperoxidase (PAP) complexes for immunohistological labeling of monoclonal antibodies. J Histochem Cytochem 30: 1114-1122.

68. Southern EM (1975) Detection of specific sequences among DNA fragments separated by gel electrophoresis. J Mol Biol 98: 503-517.

69. Flaig MJ, Schuhmann K, Sander CA (2000) Impact of molecular analysis in the diagnosis of cutaneous lymphoid infiltrates. Semin Cutan Med Surg 19: 87-90.

70. Catalano A, Iland H (2005) Molecular biology of lymphoma in the microarray era. Pathology 37: 508-522.

71. Becker B, Landthaler M, Vogt T (2005) Profiling methods in dermatology. J Dtsch Dermatol Ges 3: 448-462.

72. Alibert JLM (1806) Tableau du pian fongoide. Description des maladies de la peau, observees a l Hospital Saint-Louis et exposition des meilleurs methods suivies pour leur traitement.Barrois L Aine Fils, Paris France.

73. Bontius (1642) De medicina indorum libri IV.Piso.

74. Besnier, Doyon, Kaposi (1891) Pathologie et traitement des maladies de la peau. Paris.

75. Burg G, Kempf W, Dummer R (2002) Kutane Lymphome, Ein Rücklick auf 50 Jahre anlässlich des 80. Geburtstages von Herrn Professor Dr. med. Dr.hc. mult. Otto Braun-Falco (S. 33-51).Steinkopff, Darmstadt.

76. Reid J (1904) Case report mycosis fungoides, Brit Med Journal: 482

77. Hebra F, Kaposi M (1874) Lehrbuch der Hautkrankheiten.In: Virchow R: Handbuch der speciellen Pathologie und Therapie.Enke, Erlangen.

78. Bazin (1862) Lecons sur les affections cutanees.Paris.

79. Vidal, Brocq (1895) Etude sur le mycosis fungoides.France med, Nr. 79-85.

80. Ranvier L, Cornill L (1868) Manuel d histology pathologique.Paris.

81. Gillot X (1869) Etude sur une affection de la peau decrite sous le nome de Mycosis fungoides.Thesis de Paris.

82. Hallapeau H, Besnier E (1892) The forms of mycosis fungoides. Br J Dermatol 4: 318 .

83. Leredde E (1894) Contribution a l etude histologique du mycosis fungiede. Ann Dermatol Venerol, 104: 509-516.

84. Port D (1874) Mycosis fungoides.Arch f Klin Med 184 .

85. Auspitz A (1885) Ein Fall von Granuloma fungoides,Arch f. Dermat.

86. Köbner (1864) Über multiple beerenschwammähnliche Papillargeschwülste. Klin. U. Exper. Mitt. Dermat. U. Syph., Erlangen.

87. Keining E, Braun-Falco O (1979) Dermatologie und Venerologie.Lehamm, München Germany.

88. Muche JM, Lukowsky A, Asadullah K, Gellrich S, Sterry W (1997) Demonstration of frequent occurrence of clonal T cells in the peripheral blood of patients with primary cutaneous T-cell lymphoma. Blood 90: 1636-1642.

89. Zumbusch von L (1926) Atlas der Hautkrankheiten. (2ndedn). With G. Riehl. Verlag Vogel, Leipzig.

90. Baccaredda A (1939) Reticulohistiocytosis cutanea hyperplastica benigna cum melanodermia.Arch Dermatol Syphilol, 179: 209-256.

91. Lutzner MA, Jordan HW (1968) The ultrastructure of an abnormal cell in Sézary's syndrome. Blood 31: 719-726.

92. TASWELL HF, WINKELMANN RK (1961) Sezary syndrome--a malignant reticulemic erythroderma. JAMA 177: 465-472.

93. Clendenning WE, Brecher G, Vanscott EJ (1964) Mycosis Fungoides. Relationship to malignant cutaneous reticulosis and the s'ezary syndrome. Arch Dermatol 89: 785-792.

94. Crossen PE, Mellor JE, Finley AG, Ravich RB, Vincent PC, et al. (1971) The Sézary syndrome: cytogenetic studies and identification of the Sézary Cell as an abnormal lymphocyte. Am J Med 50: 24-34.

95. Bazex A, Dupré A, Christol B (1968) [Chalazodermic Besnier-Boeck-Schaumann disease?]. Bull Soc Fr Dermatol Syphiligr 75: 448-449.

96. Ackerman AB (1978) Granulomatous slack skin, Histologic diagnosis of inflammatory diseases, Lea and Fibiger, Philadelphia.

97. Ketron LW, Goodman MH (1931) Multiple lesions of the skin apparently of epithelial origin resembling clinically mycosis fungoides. Arch Dermatol 24: 758-785.

98. Woringer F, Kolopp P (1939) Lesion erythemato-squameuse polycylique de l avant-bras evoluant depuis 6 ans chez ungarconnet de 13 ans.Ann Dermatol Syphilol, 10: 945-958.

99. Braun-Falco O, Marghescu S, Wolff HH (1973) [Pagetoide reticulosis--Woringer-Kolopp's disease]. Hautarzt 24: 11-21.

100. Vakilzadeh F, Bröcker EB (1984) Syringolymphoid hyperplasia with alopecia. Br J Dermatol 110: 95-101.

101. Dupont A (1965) Slowly developing and clinically benign reticulopathy with extremely malignant histological structure. Hautarzt 16: 284-286.

102. Macaulay WL (1968) Lymphomatoid papulosis. A continuing self-healing eruption, clinically benign--histologically malignant. Arch Dermatol 97: 23-30.

103. Lutzner M, Edelson R, Schein P, Green I, Kirkpatrick C, et al. (1975) Cutaneous T-cell lymphomas: the Sézary syndrome, mycosis fungoides, and related disorders. Ann Intern Med 83: 534-552.

104. Willemze R, Meyer CJ, Van Vloten WA, Scheffer E (1982) The clinical and histological spectrum of lymphomatoid papulosis. Br J Dermatol 107: 131-144.

105. Slater DN (2005) The new World Health Organization-European Organization for Research and Treatment of Cancer classification for cutaneous lymphomas: a practical marriage of two giants. Br J Dermatol 153: 874-880.

106. Kempf W, Burg G, Kazakov DV (2005) Lymphomatoide Papulosis, Cutaneous lymphomas, Taylor Francis, Boca Raton, USA 165-172.

107. Kempf W, Kazakov DV, Burg G. (2005) Clonal T-cell Disorders. Cutaneous lymphomas, Taylor Francis, Boca Raton, USA 367-371.

108. Isaacson P, Wright DH (1983) Malignant lymphoma of mucosa-associated lymphoid tissue. A distinctive type of B-cell lymphoma. Cancer 52: 1410-1416.

109. Kerl H, Cerroni L (2006) Primary cutaneous B-cell lymphomas: then and now. J Cutan Pathol 33 Suppl 1: 1-5.

110. Kerl H, Kodama K, Cerroni L (2004) Diagnostic principles and new developments in primary cutaneous B-cell lymphomas. J Dermatol Sci 34: 167-175.

111. Kazakov DV, Burg G, Kempf W (2005) Primary cutaneous Plasmacytoma, Cutaneous lymphomas Taylor Francis, Boca Raton, USA 243-247.

112. Kempf W, Kazakov DV, Burg G (2005) Primary cutaneous Marginal Zone B-cell lymphoma. Cutaneous lymphomas, Taylor Francis, Boca Raton, USA 231-236.

113. Isaacson P (1979) Middle East lymphoma and alpha-chain disease. An immunohistochemical study. Am J Surg Pathol 3: 431-441.

114. Willemze R (1995) New concepts in the classification of cutaneous lymphomas. Arch Dermatol 131: 1077-1080.

115. Willemze R, Beljaards RC, Meijer CJ, Rijlaarsdam JR (1994) Classification of primary cutaneous lymphomas. Historical overview and perspectives. Dermatology 189 Suppl 2: 8-15.

116. Willemze R, Meijer CJLM (1998) Classification of cutaneous lymphomas: crosstalk between pathologist and clinican.Curr Diagn Pathol 5: 23-33.

117. Lever WF, Schaumburg-Lever G (1975) Histopathology of the skin.Lippingcott, Philadelphia USA.

118. Lennert K, Feller AC (1990) Histopathologie der Non-Hodgkin-Lymphome (rach der aktuaPirienton Kiel-klassifikation),Springer Verlag, Berlin Heidelberg New York.

119. Vonderheid EC, Diamond LW, van Vloten WA, Scheffer E, Meijer CJ, et al. (1994) Lymph node classification systems in cutaneous T-cell lymphoma. Evidence for the utility of the Working Formulation of Non-Hodgkin's Lymphomas for Clinical Usage. Cancer 73: 207-218.

120. Willemze R, Meijer CJ (2006) Classification of cutaneous T-cell lymphoma: from Alibert to WHO-EORTC. J Cutan Pathol 33 Suppl 1: 18-26.

121. Buschke A, Hirschfeld H (1911) Über Leucosarcomatosis cutis.Folia haemat (Lpz) 12: 73.

122. Mariani G (1914) Klinischer und pathologisch-anatomischer Beitrag zum Studium der kutanen Leukämie der fibroepitheloiden Polylymphomatosen (Hodgkinsche rankheit) und der Mycosis fungoides. Arch Dermat Syph 120: 781-869.

123. FLARER F (1951) [Current orientation of clinical dermosyphilology]. Minerva Dermatol 26: 141-143.

124. Fieschi A (1936) Vergangene und moderne Forschungen im Lichte ätioüathologischer Probleme, Erg Inn Med 51: 386.

125. Sezary A (1941) Classification des reticuloendothelioses, 49: 655.

126. Cazal P (1912) Les reticulopathies et le systeme reticulohistiocytaire, Vigot Freres, Paris

127. Smith NP, Levene A (1978) An unusual presentation of cutaneous malignant lymphoma. Clin Exp Dermatol 3: 167-172.

128. Davis TH, Morton CC, Miller-Cassman R, Balk SP, Kadin ME (1992) Hodgkin's disease, lymphomatoid papulosis, and cutaneous T-cell lymphoma derived from a common T-cell clone. N Engl J Med 326: 1115-1122.

129. Evans HL, Winkelmann RK, Banks PM (1979) Differential diagnosis of malignant and benign cutaneous lymphoid infiltrates: a study of 57 cases in which malignant lymphoma had been diagnosed or suspected in the skin. Cancer 44: 699-717.

130. Banks PM (2007) Gastrointestinal lymphoproliferative disorders. Histopathology 50: 42-54.

131. Hall PA, Jass JR, Levison DA, Morson BC, Shepherd NA, et al. (1988) Classification of primary gut lymphomas. Lancet 2: 958.

132. Lennert K (1980) [Malignant lymphomas of the skin from the viewpoint of lymph node pathology]. Z Hautkr 55: 1257-1259.

133. Edelson RL (1977) Recent advances in the cutaneous T cell lymphomas. Bull Cancer 64: 209-224.

134. Edelson RL (1980) Cutaneous T-cell lymphoma. J Dermatol Surg Oncol 6: 358-368.

135. Kerl H, Burg G (1979) Immunozytome und immunoblastische Lymphome der Haut. Hautarzt 30: 662- 672.

136. Willemze R, Meijer CJ (1999) Classification of primary cutaneous B-cell lymphomas: EORTC classification or REAL classification? Br J Dermatol 141: 350-352.

137. Russell-Jones R (1998) Primary cutaneous B-cell lymphoma: how useful is the new European Organization for Research and Treatment of Cancer (EORTC) classification? Br J Dermatol 139: 945-949.

138. Kerl H, Cerroni L, Burg G (1991) The morphologic spectrum of T-cell lymphomas of the skin: a proposal for a new classification. Semin Diagn Pathol 8: 55-61.

139. Pimpinelli N, Santucci M, Giannotti B (1993) Cutaneous lymphoma: a clinically relevant classification. Int J Dermatol 32: 695-700.

140. Burg G, Dummer R, Kerl H (1994) Classification of cutaneous lymphomas. Dermatol Clin 12: 213-217.

141. Knobler R, Burg G, Whittaker S, Baila L (2002) EORTC cutaneous lymphoma task force. European Organisation for Research and Treatment of Cancer. Eur J Cancer 38 Suppl 4: S60-64.

142. Russell-Jones R, Spittle MF (1996) Management of cutaneous lymphoma. Baillieres Clin Haematol 9: 743-767.

143. Niermann C, Schulze HJ, Hallermann C (2008) Classification of NHL with special emphasis on cutaneous lymphoma. Hautarzt 139- 142.

144. De Graciansky P, Paraf H (1949) Les hematodermies.Masson, Paris.

145. Lindner H, Meyer R (1956) [Not Available]. Arch Klin Exp Dermatol 203: 409-432.

146. Degos R, Ossipovski B, Civatte J, Touraine R (1957) Ann Dermatol Syphiligr (Paris) 84: 125-152.

147. Altman J, Winkelmann RK (1960) Lymphosarcoma of the skin and testis. Arch Dermatol 82: 943-947.

148. Gans O, Steigleder GK (1956) Milestones in dermatology. XVI. Skin diseases with malignant growth of juvenile connective tissue cells. Excerpta Med (Dermatol) 10: 139-141.

149. Gottron HA (1960) Retikulosen der Haut, Dermatologie und Venerologie, Thieme, Stuttgart Germany 501-590.

150. Gertler W (1962) Retikulosen der Haut. Dermatologie und Venerologie, Band 1Thieme, Stuttgart Germany.

151. Cazal P (1966) [Cytologic and histologic diagnosis of malignant lymphoreticulopathies]. Rev Prat 16: 837-857.

152. Musger A (1967) [On the etiology and pathogenesis of cheiropompholyx (dyshidrosis)]. Dermatol Wochenschr 153: 111-119.

153. Burg G, Braun-Falco O (1975) Classification and differentiation of cutaneous lymphomas. Enzyme-cytochemical and immunocytological studies. Br J Dermatol 93: 597-599.

154. Pinkus H, Mehregan AH (1969, 1976) A guide to dermatohistopathology. Meredith Corporation, Des Moines.

155. Kerl H, Rauch HJ, Hödl ST (1982) Cutaneous B-cell lymphomas, Lymphoproliferative disease of the skin 179-191.

156. Kerl H, Cerroni L, Burg G (1991) The morphologic spectrum of T-cell lymphomas of the skin: a proposal for a new classification. Semin Diagn Pathol 8: 55-61.

157. Isaacson PG (1994) Gastrointestinal lymphoma. Hum Pathol 25: 1020-1029.

158. Slater D (2001) Histopathological aspects of cutaneous lymphoma. J R Soc Med 94: 337-340.

159. Jaffe ES, Harris NL, Stein H, Vardimman JK (2001) WHO classification of tumors.IARC Press 2001, Lyon.

160. Burg G, Kempf W, Cozzio A, Döbbeling U, Feit J, et al. (2006) Cutaneous malignant lymphomas: update 2006. J Dtsch Dermatol Ges 4: 914-933.

161. Morgensztern D, Lossos IS (2005) Molecular prognostic factors in diffuse large B-cell lymphoma. Curr Treat Options Oncol 6: 269-277.

162. Alizadeh AA, Eisen MB, Davis RE, Ma C, Lossos IS, et al. (2000) Distinct types of diffuse large B-cell lymphoma identified by gene expression profiling. Nature 403: 503-511.

Therapeutic Value of Silymarin as Iron Chelator in Children with Beta Thalassemia with Iron Overload

Adel A Hagag* and Mokhtar Abd Elfatah
Department of Pediatrics, Faculty of Medicine, Tanta University, Egypt

Abstract

Beta thalassemia is an inherited hemoglobin disorder resulting in chronic hemolytic anemia. The most common treatment for thalassemia is blood transfusion which is necessary to provide the patients with healthy red blood cells containing normal hemoglobin. Repeated blood transfusion leads to iron overload. Excess iron is deposited in body organs as liver, heart and endocrine glands causing organ damage. Iron chelation therapy is the main way to treat iron overload in beta thalassemia major. Silymarin and its biologically active component Silybin are strong antioxidant and have documented iron chelating activities in patients with beta-thalassemia major. The aim of this review was to spotlight on the therapeutic value of silymarin as iron chelator in children with beta thalassemia major with iron overload.

Keywords: Thalassemia; Silymarin; Iron overload

Introduction

Thalassemias are heterogeneous group of inherited anemias that collectively represents the most common monogenic disorders. β-thalassemia are characterized by absent or reduced synthesis of β-globin chains of hemoglobin, caused by mutations of β-globin gene cluster resulting in reduced hemoglobin in RBCs, decreased RBCs production and anemia [1]. In Egypt, β-thalassemia is the commonest cause of chronic hemolytic anemia and represents a major public health problem. It was estimated that 1000/1.5 million per year live birth suffer from thalassemia disease in Egypt with carrier rate of 9-10% [2,3].

The most common treatment for thalassemia is blood transfusion which is necessary to provide the patients with healthy red blood cells containing normal hemoglobin. Repeated blood transfusion leads to iron overload [4]. Excess iron is deposited in body organs as liver, heart and endocrine glands causing organ damage [5].

Iron loading in thalassemia depends on volume of transfused blood and amount accumulated from gut absorption. In β-thalassemia increased gastrointestinal iron absorption is mediated by down-regulation of hepcidin and up-regulation of ferroportin [6].

Role of Hepcidin Ferroportin System in Iron Overload

Hepcidin is a key regulatory hormone of iron homeostasis produced by hepatocytes, in response to iron loading [7]. Increased hepcidin release in thalassemia major generates a negative feedback loop [8] that inhibits intestinal iron absorption and iron release from hepatic stores and from macrophages [9]. Increased hepcidin in thalassemia major could be explained by transfusion therapies in thalassemia major, which suppress the erythropoietic drive and increase body iron load, both of which increase hepcidin level [10] or it might reflect the effects of concomitant minor infections or other inflammatory stimuli that increase hepcidin level [11].

Hepcidin deficiency in thalassemia intermedia may be the key factor allowing excessive iron absorption and development of iron overload in this milder form of anemia that remain mostly transfusion independent, but develop iron overload [12-16]. Hepcidin production is suppressed by pathological signal from an expanded population of erythrocyte precursors that fail to mature to fully differentiated erythrocytes or hypoxia which suppresses hepcidin directly in hepatocyte as patients with thalassemia intermedia had lower oxygen delivery to tissues due to lower hemoglobin concentration and high proportion of fetal hemoglobin [14-16] (Figure 3).

The sole known molecular target of hepcidin is the protein ferroportin which acts as transmembrane conduit for the transfer of cellular iron to plasma. The binding of hepcidin to ferroportin on the membranes of iron-exporting cells induces the endocytosis and proteolysis of ferroportin and thereby decreases the delivery of iron to plasma. In iron-overload disorders, ferroportin is hyperactive, stimulating intestinal iron absorption and the release of iron from macrophages, and causing an increase in plasma iron concentrations, transferrin saturation, and iron deposition in the liver and other organs [17,18] (Figure 1).

Mechanism of Iron Toxicity

Iron is highly reactive and easily alternating between ferrous (Fe^{2+}) and ferric (Fe^{3+}) states in a process which results in the gain and loss of electrons generating harmful free radicals (atoms or molecules with unpaired electrons). These can damage lipid membranes, organelles and DNA causing cell death and the generation of fibrosis [5].

In healthy human, iron is absorbed by duodenal enterocytes and circulates in the plasma bound to transferrin. Then iron is stored in monocyte-macrophage system and parenchymal cells of liver [5]. So iron is 'kept safe' by binding to molecules as transferrin in blood and storage in the form of ferritin inside cells [19].

In iron overload, excess iron is sequestered in the cells of the monocyte-macrophage system and then the liver [20]. But when these organs get filled up and have no ability to store more iron, it is bound to transferrin and when the capacity of transferrin is saturated, iron

***Corresponding author:** Adel A Hagag, Department of Pediatrics, Faculty of Medicine, Tanta University, Egypt, E-mail: adelhagag20@yahoo.com

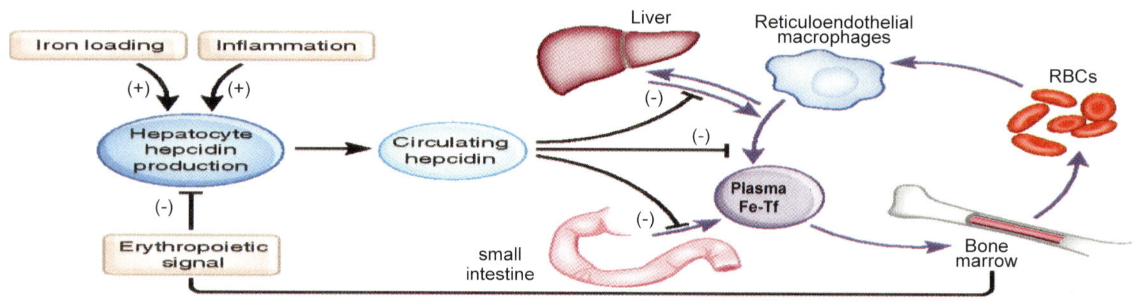

Figure 1: Role of hepcidin in iron overload [18].

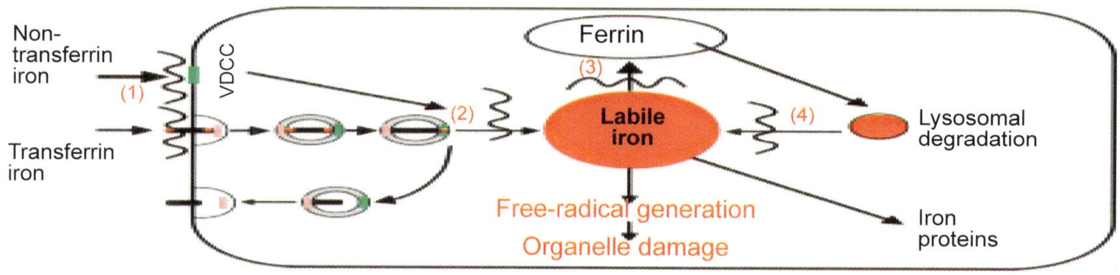

Figure 2: Mechanism of iron toxicity in iron overload [23].

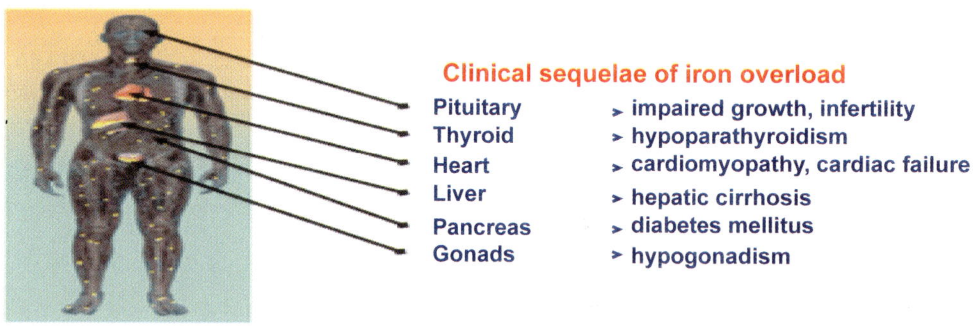

Figure 3: Clinical Sequelae of iron overload [29].

circulates in the bloodstream as extracellular non-transferrin-bound iron (NTBI) which is very toxic [21]. There is labile plasma iron (LPI) or 'free iron' which is a directly chelatable component of NTBI. It is highly toxic as it can catalyze and form harmful free hydroxyl radicals [22].

LPI is detected in patients with transfusional iron overload. It isn't detected in healthy person [10]. LPI is thought to be the iron that loads cells via a mechanism other than the transferrin receptor. Voltage-dependent calcium channels have been hypothesized as the route of entry of LPI. LPI is taken up excessively by cells leading to iron-overload pathologies. This raises the cell labile iron pool (LIP) [23]. With sustained iron loading, the iron deposits can exceed the storage and detoxification capacity of ferritin and might eventually also transform into hemosiderin. When LIP levels exceed the cell antioxidant capacity they evoke the formation of reactive oxygen species (ROS) that lead to cell damage by affecting lipids, proteins and nucleic acids. The resulting 'free iron' damages many tissues in the body and is fatal unless treated by iron chelation therapy [24] (Figure 2).

Clinical Feature of Iron Overload

Excess iron is deposited in major organs especially liver, heart, pancreas, thyroid, pituitary gland and other endocrine organs resulting in organ damage [25]. Liver is the principal site for iron storage and has the largest capacity for excess iron storage with resulting collagen deposition and portal fibrosis within 2 years from the start of transfusion regimen [26]. When liver capacity is exceeded, iron is deposited in other organs. In the heart, iron collects in the cardiac muscle fiber particularly in the ventricular wall, septum, papillary muscles and the epicardium. Signs of myocardial damage due to iron overload present as arrhythmia, cardiomegaly, heart failure and pericarditis [27]. Iron loading of the anterior pituitary can disrupt sexual maturation. Many patients suffer growth failure due to growth hormone deficiency or defective synthesis of insulin-like growth factor. Excess iron can also damage thyroid, parathyroid and adrenal glands. It can cause skin hyperpigmentation and diabetes [28].

Investigations for Assessment of Iron Overload

Serum markers

I-Serum ferritin: Ferritin is the iron-storage protein [5]. Serum ferritin assay is easy to perform, well established, generally correlating with body iron stores. Inflammation, hepatitis, liver damage, hemolysis and ineffective erythropoiesis may falsely increase ferritin while vitamin C deficiency may depress it. A sudden and unexpected rise in ferritin should prompt a search for hepatitis, other infections or inflammatory conditions [29,30].

II-Transferrin saturation (TS): It is usually extremely high in regularly transfused patients and its level may suggest the site of iron accumulation (reticuloendothelial iron overload alone is associated with normal TS, whereas parenchymal iron overload leads to a high TS) [31]. TS above 50% is suggestive of high iron load [32].

Tissue Iron Concentration or Distribution

I-Liver iron concentration (LIC): LIC is now regarded as the reference standard for estimating body iron load and can accurately predict total body iron stores using the formula: Total body iron stores in mg/kg = 10.6 x LIC (in mg/g dry weight). Normal LIC values are up to 1.8 mg/g dry weight [19]. LIC is particularly useful when new chelating regimes are being used [33].

Liver biopsy: Inadequate sample size (<1 mg/g dry weight or about 2.5 cm core length) or uneven distribution of iron, as in case of cirrhosis, may give misleading results [34].

Superconducting quantum interference device (SQUID): LIC can also be measured accurately using SQUID. Only four machines are currently available worldwide. SQUID is very expensive and require trained staff [33].

Hepatic MRI: LIC can also now be measured using MRI. This technique can be applied with little training at any center with a reasonably up-to-date MRI machine [34].

Cardiac iron concentration (CIC):

Heart function: Regular monitoring of left ventricular ejection fraction is essential. Mild reductions in left ventricular function were used as the basis to intensify iron chelation therapy. Left ventricular function can be assessed using MRI, MUGA or echocardiography [31].

Cardiac MRI: Estimation of myocardial iron using MRI is becoming increasingly available. T2 value in tissues shortens as iron concentration increases. Myocardial T2 <20 ms indicates increased myocardial iron and is associated with decreased LV function [30].

Iron load of other tissues and organs:

Assessment of iron load in pancreas and pituitary gland using MRI is currently available. An increase in pancreas R2 indicates iron overload and needs modification of chelation therapy even if cardiac and hepatic iron estimates are stable [35].

Iron toxicity markers

Plasma non-transferrin bound iron (NTBI) and Labile plasma iron (LPI): NTBI or LPI promotes the formation of free hydroxyl radicals and peroxidation of membrane lipids and are directly involved in iron induced tissue toxicity [36,37].

Other markers of oxidative damage: Malondialdehyde is increased, while a wide range of antioxidants are depleted [19].

Measurement of urinary and fecal iron excretion: Urinary iron excretion can assist in evaluation of desferrioxamine effects (about half of total iron excreted in urine) or deferiprone (over 80% of iron excreted in urine) while fecal iron excretion can assist in evaluation of deferasirox [19].

Treatment of iron overload

Iron chelation therapy: Iron chelation therapy is the main way to treat iron overload in beta thalassemia major. The goals of iron chelation therapy are to prevent iron stores from reaching levels at which tissue damage occurs and to remove excess iron already present, thereby reversing tissue/organ dysfunction [23]. Effective protection against iron toxicity requires detoxification of both extracellular iron stores (non-transferrin bound or labile plasma iron) and intracellular iron stores (labile iron pool). NTBI and LPI appear within minutes of clearing of the iron chelator from the body. Once low levels of iron have been achieved, it is theoretically more appropriate to reduce the dose than to interrupt or decrease the frequency of iron chelator [38].

Types of iron chelators

Conventional iron chelators: 1-Desferrioxamine (DFO) is the major iron-chelating treatment of transfusional iron overload [39]. The standard recommended dose is 20-40 mg/kg by slow subcutaneous (SC) infusion over 8-12 hours using an infusion pump for 6 nights a week [40]. SC bolus of desferrioxamine twice daily may be indicated when an infusion pump is not available or when 10-hour infusions are not tolerated [41] and may be also considered if the patient is not at high risk of heart disease [19]. Intravenous desferrioxamine in high-risk β-thalassemia can be used in either 24-hour continuous infusion or intermittent high dose for 8-10 hours per day [42].

2-Deferiprone was first licensed for use in thalassaemia in India, followed by European Union and other countries outside US and Canada, in 1990s [43]. According to official European licensing agency (EMEA), Deferiprone could be used as a second line drug for removing iron in patients who are unable to use Desferrioxamine or in whom DFO therapy has proven ineffective [8]. Deferiprone daily dose that had been evaluated most thoroughly is 75 mg/kg/day in three divided doses [44].

3-Deferasirox had been licensed as first-line monotherapy for thalassemia major in over 70 countries worldwide including the US and the EU [45]. The drug is taken orally, once daily, preferably before meal and is dissolved in water (or apple juice) using a non-metallic stirrer. A recommended dose is 20-30 mg/kg [46].

Silymarin as new era in iron chelation: Silymarin is a flavonolignan complex isolated from Silybin marianum which is already being used for the treatment of liver disorders characterized by degenerative necrosis and functional impairment [47]. It protects hepatocytes from injury caused by ischemia, radiation, iron overload, and viral hepatitis [48].

Besides its hepatoprotective activity, several studies have shown that silymarin is a strong antioxidant that is capable of scavenging both free radicals and reactive oxygen species. By inhibiting lipid peroxidation, silymarin protects against hepatic toxicity induced by a wide variety of agents [47].

In beta thalassemia with iron overload a wide range of antioxidants are depleted and there is an interest in the use of antioxidants

	Gharagozloo et al. [50]	**Moayedi et al.** [51]	**Hagag et al.** [52]	**Adibi et al.** [54]
Number and age of studied patients	59 patients aged 12 years or older divided into 2 groups	97 patients aged 12 years or older divided into 2 groups	40 patients aged 2.5-6 years divided into 2 groups	37 patients aged 12 years or older divided into 2 groups
Method used for assessment of iron overload	Serum ferritin, serum iron, TIBC, glutathione levels of RBCs and liver functions	Serum ferritin, iron, TIBC, soluble transferrin receptor, hepcidin and liver functions	Serum ferritin, serum iron, TIBC, renal and liver functions	Liver iron concentration by MRI
Duration of the study	3 months	9 months	6 months	6 months
Dose of silymarin	140 mg three times per day	140 mg three times per day	140 mg three times per day	140 mg three times per day
Drug used with silymarin	Desferroxamine	Desferroxamine	Deferasirox	Desferroxamine
Effects of silymarin in iron overload	Significantly reduced serum iron and ferritin with Significant improvement in liver alkaline phosphatase and glutathione levels of red blood cells	Significantly reduced serum iron, ferritin, hepcidin, soluble transferrin receptor with significant improvement in liver functions	Significantly reduced serum iron and serum ferritin with no detectable abnormalities in complete blood count, liver or renal functions	No significant changes in liver iron concentration after silymarin use for 6 months

Table 1: Comparison of silymarin values in iron chelation in different studies.

or naturally occurring products with antioxidant properties in thalassemia syndromes with iron overload [19]. Silymarin has also iron chelating activities however but little is known about the biochemical mechanisms of action of these substances [49]. There are some studies designed to investigate the therapeutic activity of silymarin in patients with thalassemia major under conventional iron chelation therapy [50-52].

Gharagozloo et al. [50] investigated the therapeutic activity of oral silymarin in patients with thalassemia major under conventional iron chelation therapy in 3 months randomized, double-blind, clinical trial in 59 beta-thalassemia major patients who were randomized to receive a silymarin tablet (140 mg) three times per day plus desferrioxamine (group I) or desferrioxamine and placebo (group II). Clinical and laboratory tests were assessed at the beginning and the end of the trial. This study revealed that combined therapy of silymarin and desferrioxamine were well tolerated and more effective than desferrioxamine and placebo in reducing serum ferritin level. Significant improvement in liver alkaline phosphatase and glutathione levels of red blood cells was also observed in silymarin-treated beta-thalassemia patients.

Moayedi et al. [51] studied therapeutic effects of silymarin in β-thalassemia major patients in randomized double-blind, placebo-controlled study. Patients were treated with combination of desferrioxamine and silymarin (n= 49) or desferrioxamine and placebo (n=48) for 9 months. The serum levels of ferritin, iron, total iron-binding capacity, soluble transferrin receptor, hepcidin and liver function were determined at the baseline and after 9 months therapy. Serum ferritin levels decreased significantly from the beginning to the end of silymarin treatment (3028.8 ± 2002.6 vs. 1972.2 ± 1250.6 ng/mL); however, no significant changes in serum ferritin was observed in the patients receiving placebo (2249.0 ± 1304.2 vs. 2015.6 ± 1146.8), significantly reduced serum iron, serum hepcidin and soluble transferrin receptor and significant improvement in liver function tests was observed in silymarin group in comparison with placebo and they concluded that silymarin is effective at reducing iron overload in patients when used in conjunction with desferrioxamine.

Hagag et al. [52] studied the therapeutic value of combined therapy with deferasirox and silymarin on iron overload in children with beta thalassemia. Patients were treated with combination of silymarin and deferasirox (n=20) or deferasirox and placebo (n=20) for 6 months. They found that, serum ferritin and serum iron were significantly lower in patients who received silymarin and deferasirox than patients who received deferasirox and placebo with no detectable abnormalities in complete blood count, liver or renal functions due to silymarin use and they concluded that combined therapy of silymarin and deferasirox depleted iron stores more successfully than deferasirox alone and so they recommended to use combination of silymarin and deferasirox in treatment of iron overloaded thalassemic children.

Despite the iron chelating activity of silymarin suggests its possible application in chelation therapy of iron overload [53]; little is known about the biochemical mechanisms of action of these substances [49]. The biological effects of silymarin are different from other iron chelators, probably due to antioxidant activity of silymarin, which causes pro-oxidant effect via iron-catalyzed oxidation with subsequent generation of reactive oxygen species [53].

On the other hand Adibi et al. [54] 2012 studied the therapeutic effects of deferoxamine and silymarin versus deferoxamine alone in β-thalassemia major based on findings of liver MRI in 37 cases of thalassemia major older than 12 years in 6 months treatment. Patients included in this study were divided into 2 groups; group I included 22 patients who were treated with desferroxamine and placebo and group II included 15 patients who were treated with desferroxamine and silymarin. The mean liver iron concentrations before therapy were 290 ± 62 μmol/g and 328 ± 27.8 μmol/g in group I and group II respectively while the mean liver iron concentrations after 6 months of intervention were 290.4 ± 65.4 μmol/g in group I and 334.6 ± 27.9 μmol/g in group II. No group experienced a significant inter group differences in LIC before and after the 6-months trial (p=0.43). They concluded that administration of silymarin did not cause significant changes in liver iron concentration and recommended evaluating a longer course of treatment with this drug to clarify their effects on reduction of liver iron concentration.

Table 1 shows comparison between different studies that were done to evaluate the therapeutic values of silymarin in iron chelation; three studies found that silymarin has good therapeutic effects as iron chelator through reduction of serum iron and serum ferritin while one study found that silymarin has no effect on reduction of liver iron concentration.

Toxicity of silymarin

Although silymarin has low oral absorption, oral dosages of 420 mg/day have shown some therapeutic potential, with good tolerability and largely free of adverse effects [54]. An average daily dose of silymarin (420 mg/day for 41 months) was found to be non-toxic, relative to placebo, in clinical trials [55]. Drug-drug interaction and liver toxicity by interference with co-drugs by induction or inhibition of cytochrome- P450 is a major concern for the use of silymarin [56]. Studies were performed to investigate the potential for hepatotoxicity, cytochrome-P450 isoenzymes induction and inhibition on dry extract from *S. marianum*. The results indicated that interference or hepatotoxicity of the dry extract from *S. marianum* at the recommended maximum daily dose of 420 mg/day of silymarin which is equivalent to 210 mg silybin is unlikely and is considered safe [57].

Conclusion

From this review we concluded that, silymarin can be used as iron chelator in iron-loaded thalassemic children at the recommended safe daily dose of 420 mg/day of silymarin especially if combined with traditional iron chelating agents as desferroxamine or deferisorax.

Recommendations

From this review we can recommend extensive multicenter studies in large number of patients with longer duration of follow up and more advanced methods of assessment of iron status to clarify the exact role of silymarin in reduction of iron over load in thalassemic children and long term side effects due to lifelong use of iron chelators.

References

1. Galanello R, Origa R (2010) Beta-thalassemia. Orphanet J Rare Dis 5: 11.
2. El-Beshlawy A, Youssry I (2009) Prevention of hemoglobinopathies in Egypt. Hemoglobin 33 Suppl 1: S14-20.
3. Soliman OE, Yahia S, Shouma A, Shafiek HK, Fouda AE, et al. (2010) Reverse hybridization StripAssay detection of beta-thalassemia mutations in northeast Egypt. Hematology 15: 182-186.
4. Pathare A, Taher A, Daar S (2010) Deferasirox (Exjade) significantly improves cardiac T2* in heavily iron-overloaded patients with beta-thalassemia major. Ann Hematol 89: 405-409.
5. Kohgo Y, Ikuta K, Ohtake T, Torimoto Y, Kato J (2008) Body iron metabolism and pathophysiology of iron overload. Int J Hematol 88: 7-15.
6. Gardenghi S, Marongiu MF, Ramos P, Guy E, Breda L, et al. (2007) Ineffective erythropoiesis in beta-thalassemia is characterized by increased iron absorption mediated by down-regulation of hepcidin and up-regulation of ferroportin. Blood 109: 5027-5035.
7. Park CH, Valore EV, Waring AJ, Ganz T (2001) Hepcidin, a urinary antimicrobial peptide synthesized in the liver. J Biol Chem 276: 7806-7810.
8. Ramos E, Kautz L, Rodriguez R, Hansen M, Gabayan V, et al. (2011) Evidence for distinct pathways of hepcidin regulation by acute and chronic iron loading in mice. Hepatology 53: 1333-1341.
9. Ganz T (2004) Hepcidin in iron metabolism. Curr Opin Hematol 11: 251-254.
10. Papanikolaou G, Tzilianos M, Christakis JI, Bogdanos D, Tsimirika K, et al. (2005) Hepcidin in iron overload disorders. Blood 105: 4103-4105.
11. Nemeth E, Roetto A, Garozzo G, Ganz T, Camaschella C (2005) Hepcidin is decreased in TFR2 hemochromatosis. Blood 105: 1803-1806.
12. Nemeth E, Ganz T (2006) Regulation of iron metabolism by hepcidin. Annu Rev Nutr 26: 323-342.
13. Nemeth E, Ganz T (2006) Hepcidin and iron-loading anemias. Haematologica 91: 727-732.
14. Nicolas G, Chauvet C, Viatte L, Danan JL, Bigard X, et al. (2002) The gene encoding the iron regulatory peptide hepcidin is regulated by anemia, hypoxia, and inflammation. J Clin Invest 110: 1037-1044.
15. Gardenghi S, Grady RW, Rivella S (2010) Anemia, ineffective erythropoiesis, and hepcidin: interacting factors in abnormal iron metabolism leading to iron overload in Î²-thalassemia. Hematol Oncol Clin North Am 24: 1089-1107.
16. Tanno T, Bhanu NV, Oneal PA, Goh SH, Staker P, et al. (2007) High levels of GDF15 in thalassemia suppress expression of the iron regulatory protein hepcidin. Nat Med 13: 1096-1101.
17. Ganz T, Nemeth E (2011) The hepcidin-ferroportin system as a therapeutic target in anemias and iron overload disorders. Hematology Am Soc Hematol Educ Program 2011: 538-542.
18. Kroot JJ, Tjalsma H, Fleming RE, Swinkels DW (2011) Hepcidin in human iron disorders: diagnostic implications. Clin Chem 57: 1650-1669.
19. Cappellini MD, Cohen A, Eleftheriou A, Piga A, Porter J, et al. (2008) Guidelines for the clinical management of thalassemia. Thalassemia International Federation 3: 33-40.
20. Rachmilewitz EA, Giardina PJ (2011) How I treat thalassemia. Blood 118: 3479-3488.
21. Wood JC (2007) Diagnosis and management of transfusion iron overload: the role of imaging. Am J Hematol 82: 1132-1135.
22. Kruszewski M (2004) The role of labile iron pool in cardiovascular diseases. Acta Biochim Pol 51: 471-480.
23. Porter JB (2007) Concepts and goals in the management of transfusional iron overload. Am J Hematol 82: 1136-1139.
24. Poggiali E, Cassinerio E, Zanaboni L, Cappellini MD (2012) An update on iron chelation therapy. Blood Transfus 10: 411-422.
25. Cazzola M, Della Porta MG, Malcovati L (2008) Clinical relevance of anemia and transfusion iron overload in myelodysplastic syndromes. Hematology Am Soc Hematol Educ Program .
26. Rechavi G, Rivella S (2008) Regulation of iron absorption in hemoglobinopathies. Curr Mol Med 8: 646-662.
27. Wood JC, Claster S, Carson S, Menteer JD, Hofstra T, et al. (2008) Vitamin D deficiency, cardiac iron and cardiac function in thalassaemia major. Br J Haematol 141: 891-894.
28. Delvecchio M, Cavallo L (2010) Growth and endocrine function in thalassemia major in childhood and adolescence. J Endocrinol Invest 33: 61-68.
29. Gabutti V, Piga A (1996) Results of long-term iron-chelating therapy. Acta Haematol 95: 26-36.
30. Kwiatkowski JL (2011) Management of transfusional iron overload - differential properties and efficacy of iron chelating agents. J Blood Med 2: 135-149.
31. Piga A, Roggero S, Longo F (2009) Evaluation and treatment of secondary iron overload. In: Beaumont C, Béris P, Beuzard Y, et al (Eds). The handbook on disorders of erythropoiesis, erythrocytes and iron metabolism. New revised edition. European school of haematology. Paris.; 25: 584-605.
32. Hershko C (2010) Pathogenesis and management of iron toxicity in thalassemia. Ann N Y Acad Sci 1202: 1-9.
33. Taher A, Cappellini MD (2009) Update on the use of deferasirox in the management of iron overload. Ther Clin Risk Manag 5: 857-868.
34. Hoffbrand AV, Taher A, Cappellini MD (2012) How I treat transfusional iron overload. Blood 120: 3657-3669.
35. Noetzli LJ, Panigrahy A, Hyderi A, Dongelyan A, Coates TD, et al. (2012) Pituitary iron and volume imaging in healthy controls. AJNR Am J Neuroradiol 33: 259-265.
36. Taher AT, Musallam KM, Inati A (2009) Iron overload: consequences, assessment, and monitoring. Hemoglobin 33 Suppl 1: S46-57.
37. Koonrungsesomboon N, Chattipakorn SC, Fucharoen S, Chattipakorn N (2013) Early detection of cardiac involvement in thalassemia: From bench to bedside perspective. World J Cardiol 5: 270-279.
38. Piga A, Gaglioti C, Fogliacco E, Tricta F (2003) Comparative effects of deferiprone and deferoxamine on survival and cardiac disease in patients with thalassemia major: a retrospective analysis. Haematologica 88: 489-496.
39. Daar S, Pathare AV (2006) Combined therapy with desferrioxamine and deferiprone in beta thalassemia major patients with transfusional iron overload. Ann Hematol 85: 315-319.
40. Giardina PJ, Rivella S (2012) Thalassemia syndromes. Churchill Livingstone Elsevier. Philadelphia.; Ch.41: 505-535.
41. Yarali N, FiÅŸgin T, Duru F, Kara A, Ecin N, et al. (2006) Subcutaneous bolus injection of deferoxamine is an alternative method to subcutaneous continuous infusion. J Pediatr Hematol Oncol 28: 11-16.
42. Hershko C (2006) Oral iron chelators: new opportunities and new dilemmas. Haematologica 91: 1307-1312.
43. Kwiatkowski JL (2008) Oral iron chelators. Pediatr Clin North Am 55: 461-482, x.

44. Cappellini MD, Musallam KM, Taher AT (2009) Overview of iron chelation therapy with desferrioxamine and deferiprone. Hemoglobin 33 Suppl 1: S58-69.

45. Romzan M, Yadav SP, Sachedeva A (2012) Management of beta- thalassemia major. In: Sachdeva. Practical pediatric hematology. 2nd edn. JAYPEE.; Ch. 10: 78-80.

46. Dubey AP, Sudha S, Parakh A (2007) Deferasirox: the new oral iron chelator. Indian Pediatr 44: 603-607.

47. Gazák R, Walterová D, Kren V (2007) Silybin and silymarin--new and emerging applications in medicine. Curr Med Chem 14: 315-338.

48. Stickel F, Schuppan D (2007) Herbal medicine in the treatment of liver diseases. Dig Liver Dis 39: 293-304.

49. Valenzuela A, Garrido A (1994) Biochemical bases of the pharmacological action of the flavonoid silymarin and of its structural isomer silibinin. Biol Res 27: 105-112.

50. Gharagozloo M, Moayedi B, Zakerinia M, Hamidi M, Karimi M, et al. (2009) Combined therapy of silymarin and desferrioxamine in patients with beta-thalassemia major: a randomized double-blind clinical trial. Fundam Clin Pharmacol 23: 359-365.

51. Moayedi B, Gharagozloo M, Esmaeil N, Maracy MR, Hoorfar H, et al. (2013) A randomized double-blind, placebo-controlled study of therapeutic effects of silymarin in ß-thalassemia major patients receiving desferrioxamine. Eur J Haematol 90: 202-209.

52. Hagag AA, Elfrargy MS1, Gazar RA1, El-Lateef AE2 (2013) Therapeutic value of combined therapy with deferasirox and silymarin on iron overload in children with Beta thalassemia. Mediterr J Hematol Infect Dis 5: e2013065.

53. Gharagozloo M, Khoshdel Z, Amirghofran Z (2008) The effect of an iron (III) chelator, silybin, on the proliferation and cell cycle of Jurkat cells: a comparison with desferrioxamine. Eur J Pharmacol 589: 1-7.

54. Adibi A, Azin SH, Behjat SM, Marjan J, Seyed Mohammad JM, et al. (2012) Therapeutic effects of deferoxamine and silymarin versus deferoxamine alone in ß-thalassemia major based on findings of liver MRI. Journal of Research in Medical Sciences 1: 873-878.

55. Tamayo C, Diamond S (2007) Review of clinical trials evaluating safety and efficacy of milk thistle (Silybum marianum [L.] Gaertn.). Integr Cancer Ther 6: 146-157.

56. Izzo AA, Ernst E (2009) Interactions between herbal medicines and prescribed drugs: an updated systematic review. Drugs 69: 1777-1798.

57. Doehmer J, Weiss G, McGregor GP, Appel K (2011) Assessment of a dry extract from milk thistle (Silybum marianum) for interference with human liver cytochrome-P450 activities. Toxicol In Vitro 25: 21-27.

Protective Effect of *Nigella sativa* Oil against Methotrexate Induced Hepatotoxicity in Children with Acute Lymphoblastic Leukemia

Adel A Hagag*, Ahmed M Abd Elaal, Ayman Elsheik and Enas Arafa Elzamarany

Department of Paediatrics and Clinical Pathology, Faculty of Medicine, Tanta University, Egypt

Abstract

Background: Acute Lymphoblastic Leukemia (ALL) is the most common childhood malignancies representing about one third of all pediatric cancers. Adding methotrexate to leukemia treatment protocols has been associated with an increased survival rate in children with ALL. The efficacy of this agent is often limited by its toxicity which can be reduced if supplemented with anti-oxidants. *Nigella sativa* has antioxidant property through different mechanisms.

Objective: The aim of this work was to study the role of *Nigella sativa* oil in the protection against hepatotoxicity induced by methotrexate therapy in children with ALL and the impact on the treatment outcome.

Patients and methods: The present study was conducted in the period between July 2010 and July 2013 on 40 children with newly diagnosed ALL including 28 males and 12 females, with mean age value of 9.17 ± 3.81 years and they were divided into 20 patients of ALL under methotrexate therapy included in ALL treatment protocol, delayed leukovorin rescue (10 mg/m^2 orally or IV every 6 hours for five doses beginning 48 hours after start of methotrexate infusion and *Nigella sativa* oil in form of soft gelatin capsule 450 mg in dose of 80 mg/kg/day on three divided doses for one week after each methotrexate dose (Group II) and 20 patients of ALL under methotrexate therapy included in ALL treatment protocol, delayed leukovorin rescue (10 mg/m^2 orally or IV every 6 hours for five doses beginning 48 hours after start of methotrexate infusion and placebo for one week after each methotrexate dose (Group III). This study also included 20 healthy children as a control group (11 males and 9 females) with their mean age value of 9.1+ 2.9 (Group I). All patients included in the study were subjected to the following investigations: Complete blood picture, bone marrow aspiration, cytochemistry, immunophenotyping and liver function testes.

Results: There were no significant difference in serum bilirubin, alanine aminotransferase, aspartate amino-transferase, alkaline phosphase levels and prothrombin time between group II and group III but there was significant difference between group II and group III compared to controls. There was no significant difference in total protein, albumin, globulin levels, and albumin globulin ratio between studied groups. There were non-significant increase in total, direct and indirect serum bilirubin, serum ALT, AST, and alkaline phosphatase levels and prothrombin time in group II after methotrexate and *Nigella sativa* oil therapy but there was significant increase in group III after treatment with methotrexate and placebo with significant difference between group II and III after therapy. There were significant differences in overall and disease free survival between group II and group III.

Conclusion: Oral administration of *Nigella sativa* oil in leukemic children can prevent MTX hepatotoxicity and improved survival in patients with ALL.

Recommendations: *Nigella sativa* oil is recommended adjuvant drug as hepatoprotective agent in patients with ALL who received methotrexate therapy.

Keywords: Acute lymphoblastic leukemia; Hepatotoxicity; Methotrexate; Thymoquinone; *Nigella sativa* oil

Introduction

ALL is the most common childhood malignancies, representing nearly one third of all pediatric cancers [1]. Among children with ALL, 75%-85% survive free of leukemia recurrence at least 5 years from diagnosis with current treatment that incorporate systemic combination chemotherapy with or without cranial radiation [2].

Methotrexate (MTX) is a key drug in the curative regimen of children with ALL [3]. Hepatotoxicity is a common complication of long term treatment with MTX and is defined as an injury of the liver associated with impaired liver function caused by exposure to the drug [4]. Methotrexate hepatotoxicity causes discontinuation of chemotherapy and may affects the overall prognosis and outcome of the disease [5]. In children with cancer, dose reduction or withdrawal of therapy in case of abnormal liver function tests might be more harmful than continuing treatment [6].

The underlying mechanism of MTX hepatotoxicity remains unclear. However, it was reported that MTX causes oxidative stress in liver tissue. MTX is metabolized and stored in hepatocytes in polyglutamated form. The presence of higher levels of polyglutamates causes a longer intracellular presence of the drug which was suggested as a mechanism for hepatotoxicity [7]. There is a debate about the concurrent use of antioxidants with chemotherapy [5] *Nigella sativa* is the black cumin herb belongs to Ranunculaceae family of flowering plants and genus of about 14 species [8] Thymoquinone (TQ) is the main active constituent of volatile oil of the black seed [9].

The oil of *N. sativa* and TQ are known to possess strong antioxidant

***Corresponding author:** Adel A Hagag, Department of Paediatrics and Clinical pathology, Faculty of Medicine, Tanta University, Egypt,
E-mail: adelhagag20@yahoo.com

activities. TQ has been shown to inhibit non-enzymatic peroxidation in ox brain phospholipid liposomes also it has extremely high superoxide anion radical-scavenging abilities as effective as Superoxide Dismutase (SOD) [10].

Nigella sativa might protect the liver against the ischemia reperfusion injury. An excessive production of oxygen free radicals has been reported in ischemic re-perfused liver, leading to tissue damage [11].

Also hepatotoxicity caused by acetaminophen as shown by significant increases in alanine aminotransferase (ALT), total nitrate/nitrite, and lipid peroxide and decreased glutathione was prevented by 5 days of 2 mg/kg/day of oral TQ in mice [12].

Aim of the Work

The aim of this work was to study the role of the *Nigella sativa* oil (NSO) in the protection against hepatotoxicity induced by methotrexate therapy in children with acute lymphoblastic leukemia and the impact on the treatment outcome.

Study Design

After research ethical committee approval and informed written parental consent from all participants in this research, this study was carried out on 40 patients of newly diagnosed ALL (28 males and 12 females). They were attendants to Oncology Unit, Pediatric Department, Tanta University Hospital in the period between July 2010 and July 2013. Their ages ranged from 4-13 years with mean value of 9.17 ± 3.81 years and they were divided into 20 patients of ALL under methotrexate therapy included in ALL treatment protocol, delayed leukovorin rescue (10 mg/m^2 orally or IV every 6 hours for five doses beginning 48 hours after start of methotrexate infusion and *Nigella sativa* oil in form of soft gelatin capsule 450 mg (Baraka; Pharco Pharmaceuticals) in dose of 80 mg/kg/day on divided doses for one week after giving methotrexate therapy (Group II) and 20 patients of ALL under methotrexate therapy included in ALL treatment protocol, delayed leukovorin rescue (10 mg/m^2 orally or IV every 6 hours for five doses beginning 48 hours after start of methotrexate infusion and placebo for one week after giving methotrexate therapy (Group III). This study also included 20 healthy children as a control group (11 males and 9 females) with their age ranged from 6-15 years and mean age value of 9.1 ± 2.9 (Group I). Diagnosis and classification of ALL were made according to French–American–British (FAB) criteria and immunophenotype analyses. The immunophenotyping was pre-B (CD19, CD22, CD10-), common ALL (CD19, CD22, CD10-), and T-ALL (CD3, CD5, CD7). The clinical data from all patients were obtained, including age at diagnosis, sex, presence of fever, pallor, purpura, bone ache, hepatomegaly, splenomegaly and lymphadenopathy. All patients were subjected to follow up for two year to evaluate their prognosis.

Protocol of Treatment

Induction (6 weeks)

Vincristine 1.5 mg/kg/m^2/week IV (days 0, 7, 14, 21, 28, 35), Doxorubicin 25 mg/m^2/ week IV infusion (days 0, 7, 14, 21, 28, 35), L-Asparginase 6000 μ/m^2 SC on alternate days for 10 doses, and Prednisone 40 mg/m^2/day for 6weeks orally. On day 21, bone marrow aspiration was done. In non-responding cases, we add Etopsoide 100 mg/m^2/dose IV (days 22, 25, 29), Cyclophosphamide 750 mg/ m^2/dose IV infusion (days 22, 25, 29), Aracytin 100/m^2/dose IV (days 22, 25, 29), and high dose methotrexate 5 g/m^2 over 4 hours on day 28 [13].

Consolidation (9 weeks)

IV methotrexate 1 gm/m^2/dose over 24 hour infusion on days 0, 21, 42 and 63, Mercaptopurine 60 mg/m^2 orally daily on days 0-13 and 28-41, Vincristine 1.5 mg/m^2 IV on days 14, 21, 42 and 49, PEG Asparaginase 2,500 units/m^2 IM on days 14 and 22, Cyclophosphamide 750 mg/m^2/dose IV infusion on days 0 and 28, Aracytin 100/m^2/dose IV on days 1-4, 8-11, 29-32 and 36-39 and age-adjusted intrathecal methotrexate on days 1,8,15 and 22 [14,15].

Interim maintenance (6 weeks)

Vincristine 1.5 mg/m^2 per day IV on days 0, 10, 20, 30, 40, IV methotrexate starting dose of 100 mg/m^2/dose over 10-15 minutes on day 0 thereafter escalate by 50 mg/m^2/dose on days 10, 20, 30 and 40, PEG Asparaginase 2,500 units/m^2 IM on days 1 and 21 and age-adjusted IT Methotrexate on days 0 and 30 [15].

Delayed –intensification (6 weeks)

Oral dexamethasone (10 mg/m^2/day on days 1-7 and 14-21, IV vincristine 1.5 mg/m^2 on days 0, 7 and 14, IM or IV pegylated L-asparaginase 2500 u/m^2 on day 4, doxorubicin 25 mg/m^2 IV push on days 0, 7 and 14, IV cyclophosphamide 1 gm/m^2 over 30 minutes on day 28, oral 6-thioguanine 60 mg/m^2 on days 28 to 41, cytarabine 75 mg/m^2 on days 29-32 and 36-39 and age-adjusted intrathecal methotrexate on day 28 [16].

Maintenance (30 months)

Weekly IV Methotrexate 20 mg/m^2 in B cell and 30 mg/m^2 in T cell ALL, Prednisone 120 mg/m^2/day for 5 days every 3 weeks, Vincristine 2 mg/m^2 IV every 3 weeks, 6-mercaptopurine 50 mg/m^2/day orally for 14 days every 3 weeks and age-adjusted IT Ara-C and methotrexate every 18 weeks [17].

Inclusion criteria

Children with newly diagnosed ALL who were treated with MTX based protocol.

Exclusion criteria

1. Patients with ALL who were positive for hepatitis A, B, C.
2. ALL patients who received medications, other than chemotherapy, that may affects the liver functions.

For all patients the following Laboratory investigations were done including:

Complete Blood Count (CBC).

One ml venous blood was collected in EDTA tubes from each patient for CBC [18].

Bone marrow examination with morphological, cytochemistry and immunophenotypic classification:

One ml BM for BM morphologic, cytochemistry and immunophenotyping [18].

Liver function tests to assess methotrexate hepatotoxicity

3.8 ml venous blood was collected from each patient, and delivered into two tubes. 1.8 ml blood into tube containing 0.4 ml sodium citrate for prothrombin time and activity and 2 ml into a plain tube for assessment of other liver function tests including total, direct and indirect serum bilirubin, total serum protein and its fractions albumin and globulin, albumin globulin ratio (A/G ratio), serum alkaline phosphatase, serum Alanine Aminotransferase (ALT) and serum Aspartate Aminotransferase (AST) [19-25].

Statistics

Data were collected and analyzed using Statistical Package for Social Science (SPSS) (version 12). All Data were expressed as in terms of mean values ± SD. Comparisons of parameters among groups were made using paired t test. Two-group comparisons were performed nonparametrically using Mann-Whitney U test. All statistical tests were two tailed, and $P<0.05$ was considered statistically significant.

Results

- The most common presenting clinical manifestations in studied patients were pallor, purpura and fever followed by hepatomegaly, splenomegaly and lymphadenopathy with no significant difference between group II and III (Table1).
- There was no significant difference in immunophenotyping between group II and group III (Table 2).
- There were no significant differences in total serum bilirubin, ALT, AST, alkaline phosphase levels and prothrombin time between group II and group III at time of diagnosis but there was significant difference between group II and group III compared to control (Table 3).
- There were no significant differences in total protein, albumin, globulin levels, and albumin globulin ratio between studied groups at time of diagnosis.
- There were non-significant increase in total, direct and indirect serum bilirubin, serum ALT, AST, and alkaline phosphatase levels and prothrombin time in group II after methotrexate and *Nigella sativa* oil therapy but there was significant increase in group III after treatment with methotrexate and placebo with significant difference between group II and III after therapy (Table 4).
- There was no significant difference in total serum protein, serum albumin, globulin levels and A/G ratio in group II and group III before and after methotrexate therapy with no significant difference between group II and III after therapy (Table 4).
- There was significant difference in prognosis regarding complete remission, relapse, death, disease free survival and Overall survival between group II and group III (Figures 2 and 3, Table 5).

Clinical manifestations	Group II	(20 patients)	Group III	(20 patients)	X2	P
	N	%	N	%		
Fever	15	75	16	80	0.140	0.704
Pallor	16	80	15	75	0.140	0.704
Purpura	16	80	15	75	0.140	0.704
Bone ache	6	30	5	25	0.130	0.723
Hepatomegaly	13	65	12	60	0.110	0.743
Splenomegaly	12	60	12	60	0.000	1.00
Lymphadenopathy	10	50	9	45	0.100	0.751

Table 1: Clinical manifestations of the studied patients.

Immunophynotyping	Group II (20 patients)		Group III (20 patients)		T	P
	N	%	N	%		
Early pre-B	6	30	5	25	0.668	0.745
Pre-B	11	55	12	60	0.968	0.558
T-cell	3	15	3	15	0.000	1.00

Table 2: Immunophenotyping of the studied patients.

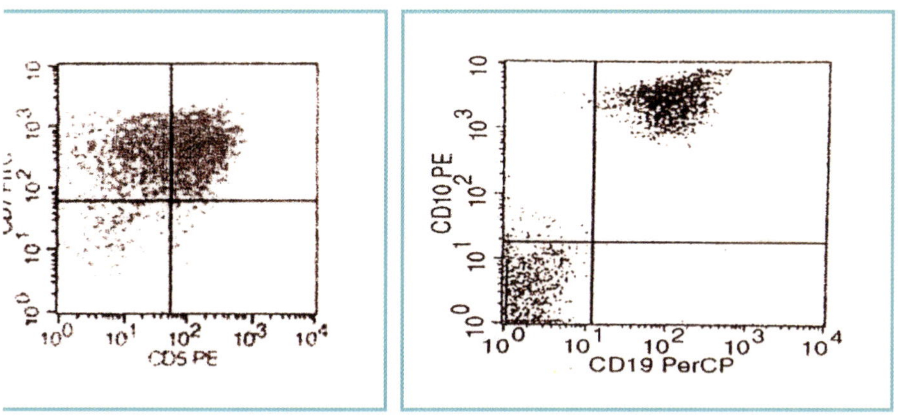

Figure 1: Immunophenotyping of some patients included in this study, to the left, a case T-cell ALL with CD 7 and CD 5 positive and to the right, a case of B-cell ALL with CD19 positive and CD 10 negative.

Parameters		Group I (No= 20)	Group II (No= 20)	Group III (No= 20)
Total serum bilirubin (mg/dl)	Mean ± SD	0.70 ± 0.09	0.82 ± 0.22	0.80 ± 0.12
	P - Value	0.034 ‡	0.635 ★	0.031♠
Serum ALT (u/l)	Mean ± SD	17.85 ± 4.06	57.69 ± 17.63	60.10 ± 20.36
	P - Value	0.001‡	0.068 ★	0.001♠
Serum AST(u/l)	Mean ± SD	25.75 ± 7.97	74.4 ± 28.06	59.65 ± 20.36
	P - Value	0.001‡	0.89 ★	0.002♠
Alkaline phosphatase (u/l)	Mean ± SD	189 ± 85.41	221.09 ± 59.63	231.8 ± 87.24
	P - Value	0.042‡	0.635 ★	0.039♠
Total serum protein (gm/dl)	Mean ± SD	6.99 ± 0.70	6.74 ± 1.13	7.32 ± 0.64
	P - Value	0.448‡	0.524 ★	0.335♠
Serum albumin (gm/dl)	Mean ± SD	4.10 ± 0.34	3.83 ± 0.52	3.93 ± 0.37
	P - Value	0.589‡	0.447 ★	0.665♠
Serum globulin (gm/dl)	Mean ± SD	2.91 ± 0.459	2.89 ± 0.71	3.17 ± 0.63
	P - Value	0.102‡	0.269 ★	0.223♠
Albumin globulin ratio	Mean ± SD	1.40 ± 0.34	1.40 ± 0.32	1.20 ± 0.21
	P - Value	1.00‡	0.086 ★	0.096♠
Prothrombin time (seconds)	Mean ± SD	13.99 ± 0.81	14.68 ± 1.05	14.37 ± 0.48
	P - Value	0.034‡	0.886 ★	0.049♠

Significant *p-value*<0.05, non-significant *p-value*>0.05
‡ Between Group I & Group II,
♠ Between Group I & Group III, ★Between Group II & Group III

Table 3: Comparison between patients and control group regarding liver function tests at time of diagnosis.

Parameters	Group II (No= 20)	Group III (No= 20)	t. test	P. value
Total serum bilirubin (mg/dl)				
Pre-treatment	0.8 ± 0.12	0.82 ± 0.29	0.47	0.64
Post-treatment	0.83 ± 0.14	2.21 ± 0.83	7.4	0.000*
t. test	1.2	7.38		
P. value	0.23	0.000*		
Direct bilirubin (mg/dl)				
Pre-treatment	0.22 ± 0.04	0.23 ± 0.05	-1.17	0.25
Post-treatment	0.23 ± 0.04	1.08 ± 0.51	-7.35	0.000*
t. test	1.00	7.38		
P. value	0.33	0.000*		
Indirect bilirubin (mg/dl)				
Pre-treatment	0.56 ± 0.17	0.58 ± 0.27	0.39	0.69
Post-treatment	0.58 ± 0.19	1.13 ± 0.35	6.5	0.000*
t. test	0.92	6.00		
P. value	0.36	0.000*		
Serum ALT (u/l)				
P re-treatment	55.85 ± 9.48	54.75 ± 8.27	1.57	0.13
Post-treatment	57.1 ± 6.53	103.6 ± 24.39	8.8	0.000*
t. test	0.44	8.78		
P. value	0.66	0.000*		
Serum AST(u/l)				
Pre-treatment	56.9 ± 9.21	58.15 ± 6.42	0.77	0.44
Post-treatment	59.9 ± 5.09	99.85 ± 17.43	9.5	0.000*
t. test	1.8	10.45		
P. value	0.78	0.000*		
Alkaline phosphatase (u/l)				
Pre-treatment	213.5 1 ± 5.74	215.15 ± 27.81	0.29	0.77
Post-treatment	220.85 ± 25.03	482.8 ± 29.47	7.9	0.000*
t. test	1.27	8.00		
P. value	0.21	0.000*		
Prothrombin time (seconds)				
Pre-treatment	14.77 ± 1.12	15.12 ± 1.33	1.58	0.13
Post-treatment	14.92 ± 0.97	16.18 ± 1.14	4.05	0.01*
t. test	1.83	3.24		
P. value	0.83	0.04*		
Total serum protein (gm/dl)				
Pre-treatment	6.74 ± 1.13	7.32 ± 0.64	0.558	0.524
Post-treatment	7.13 ± 0.79	7.24 ± 0.71	0.668	0.550
t. test	0.652	0.358		
P. value	0.428	0.210		

Serum albumin (gm/dl)				
Pre-treatment	3.83 ± 0.52	3.93 ± 0.37		
Post-treatment	3.95 ± 0.38	3.80 ± 0.31	0.887	0.589
t. test	0.963	0.612	0.753	0.158
P. value	0.811	0.258		
Serum globulin (gm/dl)				
Pre-treatment	2.89 ± 0.61	3.38 ± 0.53		
Post-treatment	3.05 ± 0.64	3.41 ± 0.65	2.114	0.125
t. test	0.899	0.774	0.841	0.637
p. value	0.335	0.621		
Albumin globulin ratio				
Pre-treatment	1.40 ± 0.32	1.20 ± 0.21		
Post-treatment	1.37 ± 0.38	1.12 ± 0.23	1.587	0.086
t. test	0.214	0.635	0.244	0.336
P. value	0.330	0.447		

**Significant when p-value<0.05, non-significant when p-value>0.05. ®Liver function is the main value of peaked level determined on successive days after giving each methotrexate dose. Persistent elevation of liver enzymes more than 2 folds for one month warrants a reduction of or discontinuation of methotrexate therapy* [25]

Table 4: Mean values of liver function tests before and after MTX therapy® in group II and III during follow up period.

Prognosis		Group		Total
		GII	GIII	
Complete remission	N	13	10	23
	%	65	50	57.5
Relapse	N	5	7	12
	%	25	35	30
Died	N	2	3	5
	%	10	15	12.5
Total	N	20	20	40
	%	100	100	100
Chi-Square	X^2	3.552		
	P-value	0.029*		

**significant.*

Table 5: Prognosis of patients after follow up for two years.

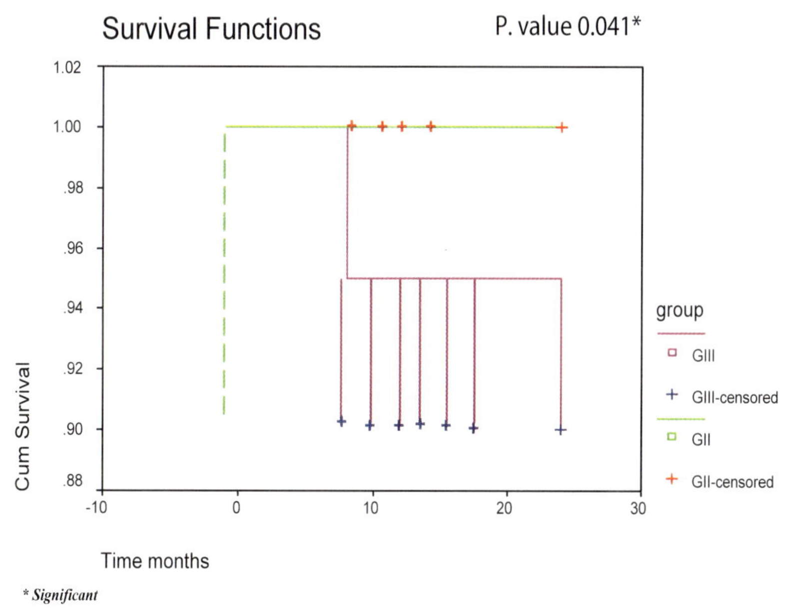

Figure 2: Disease free survival in group II and group III.

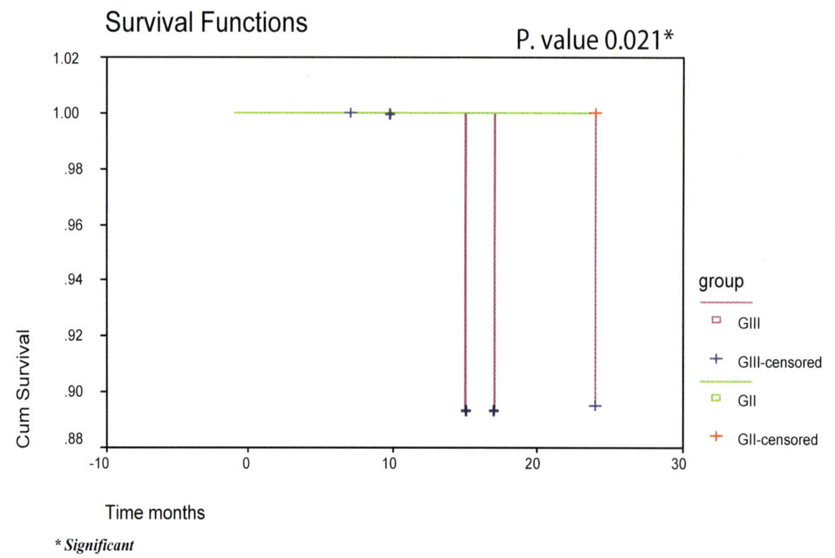

Figure 3: Overall survival in group II and group III.

Discussion

MTX is a folic acid antagonist that can cause unpredictable serious side effects [26]. Daily combination therapy of folic acid with MTX has been widely suggested as it reduces hepatic toxicity of MTX however; it is still controversial whether the use of folic acid reduces therapeutic efficiency of MTX or not [27]. Therefore, new antioxidant agents have been put on experimental trials against systemic oxidative damage caused by MTX [28].

The oil of *N. sativa* and TQ are known to possess strong antioxidant activities. TQ has been shown to inhibit non-enzymatic peroxidation in ox brain phospholipid liposomes also it has extremely high superoxide anion radical-scavenging abilities as effective as Superoxide Dismutase (SOD) [10]. The present study aimed to evaluate the protective effect of *Nigella sativa* oil on liver of children with ALL during treatment with MTX in oncology unit, Pediatric department, Tanta university hospital to helps these patients to complete the course of treatment without interruption and improve the prognosis and outcome of the disease.

In this study, the most common presenting clinical manifestations in studied patients were pallor, purpura and fever followed by hepatomegaly, splenomegaly and lymphadenopathy with no significant difference between group II and III. This is consistent with Biswas et al., [29] and Karimi et al., [30] who found the same results. Fever in ALL patients may be caused by pyrogenic cytokines released from leukemic cells, including interleukin-1, tumor necrosis factor and interleukin-6, but in about 30% of patients, fever is caused by infection [31].

In this study there was significant lower hemoglobin level and platelet count and significant higher white blood cell count in group II and group III compared to control with no significant difference between group II and III. This is consistent with Silverman and Sallan 2003 who found anemia and thrombocytopenia in the majority of cases with ALL at diagnosis (32) and Biswas et al., 2009, who found leucocytosis in 88% of their studied patients (29).

There was a significant higher serum bilirubin, ALT, AST and alkaline phosphatase levels and prothrombin time in group II and group III compared with control with no significant difference between group II and group III. After therapy there were non-significant increase in total, direct and indirect serum bilirubin, serum ALT, AST, and alkaline phosphatase levels and prothrombin time in group II but there was significant increase in group III with significant difference between group II and III after therapy.

These results were in agreement with Dogar et al., who investigate the efficacy of *Nigella sativa* seeds in ALL and found that no significant increase in ALT, AST, total serum bilirubin and alkaline phosphatase, in group received *Nigella sativa* oil in comparison with group not received [33] Ilham and Firas, [34], who investigate the effect of maintenance therapy for childhood ALL on the liver and found that seven of 30 children with ALL receiving daily oral 6–mercaptopurine and weekly methotrexate developed both hepatocellular destruction and intrahepatic cholestasis with abnormally elevated levels of serum aminotransferases enzymes, alkaline phosphatase and total serum bilirubin that mainly indicate biliary tract disorder [34] and El-Gharieb et al., who studied the hepatoprotective effect of NSO and vitamin E on liver of liver of workers exposed to organophosphorus insecticide, there was a significant reduction in serum hepatic transaminases in group received NSO [35] .

There was no significant difference in the total serum protein, albumin, globulin levels, and A/G ratio between group II and group III compared to control, also there is no significant difference between group II and group III after MTX therapy. This is in agreement Ilham and Firas [34] who found the same results. This could be explained this by the ability of the liver to increase protein, albumin biosynthesis during diseases associated with protein loss, or in presence of liver cell damage or injury induced by cytotoxic drugs, until the parenchymal damage or loss is severe [36].

Conclusion

Our study showed that oral administration of *Nigella sativa* oil in leukemic children prevented the side effects of MTX treatment on the liver in patients with ALL which lead to improvement in OAS and DFS.

Recommendations

Nigella sativa oil and its active constituent thymoquinone is recommended adjuvant drug as hepatoprotective agent in patients with ALL who received MTX therapy.

References

1. Ribera JM, Oriol A (2009) Acute lymphoblastic leukemia in adolescents and young adults. Hematol Oncol Clin North Am 23: 1033-1042.
2. Pui CH, Campana D, Pei D, Bowman WP, Sandlund JT, et al. (2009) Treating childhood acute lymphoblastic leukemia without cranial irradiation. N Engl J Med 360: 2730-2741.
3. Styczynski J, Wysocki M (2001) Methotrexate resistance in acute leukemias. Pol Merkur Lekarski 11: 175-179.
4. Navarro VJ, Senior JR (2006) Drug-related hepatotoxicity. N Engl J Med 354: 731-739.
5. Moss RW (2006) Should patients undergoing chemotherapy and radiotherapy be prescribed antioxidants? Integr Cancer Ther 5: 63-82.
6. Najjar TA, al Fawaz IM (1993) Pharmacokinetics of methotrexate in children with acute lymphocytic leukemia. Chemotherapy 39: 242-247.
7. Hemeida RA, Mohafez OM (2008) Curcumin attenuates methotraxate-induced hepatic oxidative damage in rats. J Egypt Natl Canc Inst 20: 141-148.
8. Aggarwal BB, Kunnumakkara AB, Harikumar KB, Tharakan ST, Sung B, et al. (2008) Potential of spice-derived phytochemicals for cancer prevention. Planta Med 74: 1560-1569.
9. El-Dakhakhny M (1963) Studies on chemical constitution of Egyptian Nigella sativa L. seeds. The essential oil. Planta Medica 11: 465-470.
10. Muhtasib HG, El-Najjar N, Regine SS (2006) The medicinal potential of Nigella sativa and its components. Advances in Phytomedicine 133-153.
11. Hassan-Khabbar S, Cottart CH, Wendum D, Vibert F, Clot JP, et al. (2008) Postischemic treatment by trans-resveratrol in rat liver ischemia-reperfusion: a possible strategy in liver surgery. Liver Transpl 14: 451-459.
12. Nagi MN, Almakki HA, Sayed-Ahmed MM, Al-Bekairi AM (2010) Thymoquinone supplementation reverses acetaminophen-induced oxidative stress, nitric oxide production, and energy decline in mice liver. Food Chem Toxicol 48:2361-2365.
13. Lichtman MA, Beulter E, Seligsonn U, Kipps TO, Kaushansky K, et al. (2006) Acute lymphoplastic leukemia: Overview. William textbook of Hematology. (17thedn). McGraw-Hill Companies, Inc. New York.
14. Chauvenet AR, Martin PL, Devidas M, Linda SB, Bell BA, et al. (2007) Antimetabolite therapy for lesser-risk B-lineage acute lymphoblastic leukemia of childhood: a report from Children's Oncology Group Study P9201. Blood 110: 1105-1111.
15. Seibel NL, Steinherz PG, Sather HN, Nachman JB, Delaat C, et al. (2008) Early postinduction intensification therapy improves survival for children and adolescents with high-risk acute lymphoblastic leukemia: a report from the Children's Oncology Group. Blood 111: 2548-2555.
16. Lanzkowsky PH (2011) Leukemias, Lanzkowsky Philip Manual of Pediatric Hematology and Oncology. (4thedn) Churchill livingstone. Nek, London, Madrid.
17. Goldberg JM, Silverman LB, Levy DE, Dalton VK, Gelber RD, et al. (2003) Childhood T-cell acute lymphoblastic leukemia: the Dana-Farber Cancer Institute acute lymphoblastic leukemia consortium experience. J Clin Oncol 21: 3616-3622.
18. Catovsky D, Hoffbrand AV (2005) Acute myeloid leukaemia. In:Hoffbrand AV and Lewis SM (Eds.), Postgraduate Haematology, (5thedn) Reed Educational and Professional Publishing Ltd. 509-524.
19. Young DS, Pestaner LC, Gibberman V (1975) Effects of drugs on clinical laboratory tests. Clin Chem 21: 1D-432D.
20. Peters T Jr (1968) Proposals for standardization of total protein assays. Clin Chem 14: 1147-1159.
21. Doumas BT, Watson WA, Biggs HG (1997) Albumin standards and the measurement of serum albumin with bromcresol green. Clin. Chem Acta 258: 21-30.
22. Gella FJ, Olivella T, Cruz Pastor M, Arenas J, Moreno R, et al. (1985) A simple procedure for the routine determination of aspartate aminotransferase and alanine aminotransferase with pyridoxal phosphate. Clin Chim Acta 153: 241-247.
23. Yang DT, Robetorye RS, Rodgers GM (2004) Home prothrombin time monitoring: a literature analysis. Am J Hematol 77: 177-186.
24. Belfield A, Goldberg DM (1971) Revised assay for serum phenyl phosphatase activity using 4-amino-antipyrine. Enzyme 12: 561-573.
25. Cash JM, Klippel JH (1994) Second-line drug therapy for rheumatoid arthritis. N Engl J Med 330: 1368-1375.
26. Miyazono Y, Gao F, Horie T (2004) Oxidative stress contributes to methotrexate-induced small intestinal toxicity in rats. Scand J Gastroenterol 39: 1119-1127.
27. Figueiredo JC, Grau MV, Haile RW, Sandler RS, Summers RW, et al. (2009) Folic acid and risk of prostate cancer: results from a randomized clinical trial. J Natl Cancer Inst 101: 432-435.
28. Ladas EJ, Jacobson JS, Kennedy DD, Teel K, Fleischauer A, et al. (2004) Antioxidants and cancer therapy: a systematic review. J Clin Oncol 22: 517-528.
29. Biswas S, Chakrabarti S, Chakraborty J, Paul PC, Konar A, et al. (2009) Childhood acute leukemia in West Bengal, India with an emphasis on uncommon clinical features. Asian Pac J Cancer Prev 10: 903-906.
30. Karimi M, Mehrabani D, Yarmohammadi H, Jahromi FS (2008) The prevalence of signs and symptoms of childhood leukemia and lymphoma in Fars Province, Southern Iran. Cancer Detect Prev 32: 178-183.
31. Dinarello CA, Bunn PA Jr (1997) Fever. Semin Oncol 24: 288-298.
32. Silverman LB, Sallan SE (2003) Newly diagnosed childhood acute lymphoblastic leukemia: update on prognostic factors and treatment. Curr Opin Hematol 10: 290-296.
33. Dogar MZ, Humaira A, Muhammad S (2009) Prelimiary assessment of efficacy of Nigella sativa seeds in acute lymphoblastic leukemia local children. Pharmacologyonline 2: 769-777.
34. Ilham AFF, Firas ST (2005) Effect of maintenance therapy for childhood with acute lymphoblastic leukaemia by combination of methotrexate and 6-mercaptopurine on the liver. Al-Mustansiriyah Journal for Pharmaceutical Sciences 2: 18-23.
35. El-Gharieb MA, El-Masry TA, Emara AM (2010) Potential hepatoprotective effects of vitamin E and Nigella sativa oil on hepatotoxicity induced by chronic exposure to malathion in human and male albino rats. Toxicol Environ Chem 92: 391-407.
36. Philip D (1994) Clinical Chemistry in Diagnosis and Treatment. In: Andrew D, Philip M, Philip DM (Eds.), (6thedn) USA, Oxford University press Inc., 284-85, 295-297.

Abnormal Free Light Chain Ratios are Significantly Associated with Clinical Progression in Chronic Lymphocytic Leukemia

Johannes Matschke[1]*, Lewin Eisele[1], Ludger Sellmann[1], Naser Kalhori[2], Arnd Nusch[2], Ulrich Dührsen[1], Jan Dürig[1] and Holger Nückel[1]

[1]*Department of Hematology, Medical Faculty, University of Duisburg-Essen, Germany*
[2]*Gemeinschaftspraxis für Hämatologie und Onkologie, Velbert, Germany*

Abstract

Serum Free Light Chains (FLC) have prognostic significance in diverse plasma cell dyscrasias. Although monoclonal protein secretion is a typical feature of these diseases, it can also be detected in other B cell malignancies including chronic lymphocytic leukemia. Recent data suggests a significant correlation between abnormal ratio of FLC and outcome. Therefore, we investigated the role of FLC in a large cohort of 135 patients and the correlation to immunofixation (IF) and flow cytometry. Abnormal FLC ratios were found in 78 patients (58%) whereas the IF was positive in only 32 cases (24%). In 55 cases the FLC ratio was positive while IF was negative and in only 9 cases IF was positive while the FLC ratio was normal. In 52 of 98 patients (53%) light chain restriction determined by flow cytometry was concordant with the monoclonal FLC whereas in 5 patients they did not agree. In 41 of 98 patients (42%) a normal ratio of FLC was observed while the immunophenotype was positive for lambda or kappa.

Patients with an abnormal FLC ratio for lambda had a significantly shorter time to first therapy (TFT) than patients with an abnormal ratio for kappa FLC or with a normal FLC ratio (median TFT: 34 versus 76 versus 88 months, p for trend=0.039). Additionally, monoclonal FLC had a significantly shorter time to first treatment compared to polyclonal normal and abnormal FLC ratios (p for trend=0.0489). As expected, polyclonal sFLC correlated significantly with normal and abnormal serum-creatinine (p<0.0001). Future studies are warranted to elucidate the role of FLC as biomarkers of disease and as a prognostic factor for response.

Keywords: Chronic lymphocytic leukemia; Free light chains; Monoclonal protein; Prognostic marker

Introduction

Chronic Lymphocytic Leukemia (CLL) has a variable clinical course. Some patients have an excellent prognosis never requiring treatment, whereas in others survival is short despite early initiation of therapy. Staging systems devised by [1] and [2] are useful for predicting survival and treatment requirements in patients with CLL. However, these staging systems are of limited prognostic value in early stages of the disease (Binet A or Rai stage 0 to II) which today applies to most of the patients at first diagnosis. During the last few years there has been a continuous effort to identify novel prognostic factors in B-CLL which may help define patient subgroups that may benefit from early therapeutic intervention.

Molecular markers like IGVH mutation status, CD38 or ZAP70 expression are able to provide this information. However, the limitations of these new molecular markers are the cost and complexity of the technical procedures, the limitation in clinical use and the necessity for further standardization. Due to these limitations the focus of research has recently changed to new simple prognostic markers allowing wide-spread clinical practice. Currently, the prognostic influence of the number of smudge cells in CLL has been demonstrated [3,4].

Although secretion of monoclonal immunoglobulins is a typical feature of plasma cell dyscrasias, it can also be detected in other B cell malignancies including CLL [5]. Serum Free Light Chains (FLC) have prognostic significance in monoclonal gammopathy of undetermined significance, solitary plasmocytoma of bone, smouldering myeloma, multiple myeloma, Waldenstroms macroglobulinaemia and AL amyloidosis [5-8]. Thus, we were intrigued by three recent studies showing a significant correlation between abnormal ratio of FLC or sFLC levels and outcome in patients with CLL [9-12]. In this study we investigated the role of abnormal ratio of FLC in a large, well characterized cohort of 135 CLL patients. Moreover, we investigated the correlation of FLC ratio to immunofixation and flow cytometry.

Patients and Methods

Study population and CLL patients

Between 1999 and 2011, 135 patients with B-CLL were enrolled in this retrospective analysis and analyzed with regard to several biological and clinical characteristics: Binet stage, age, gender, CD38 and ZAP-70 status, IGHV status, β2-microglobulin, time from diagnosis to first treatment and overall survival. The diagnosis of B-CLL required a persistent B cell lymphocytosis of more than 5.0×10^9/l and a typical CD19+, CD20+ CD5+, CD23+, Ig light chain (κ or λ light chain) restricted immunophenotype as revealed by flow cytometry of peripheral blood cells. Comprehensive clinical information including treatment histories was available for all patients. Patient selection was based on the availability of cryopreserved plasma samples in our CLL cell bank collected at the time before the initiation of therapy or six months after finishing therapy.

Standard clinical criteria were used for the initiation of chemotherapy [13]. CD38 and ZAP-70 expression were determined by flow cytometry as recently described [14,15]. In Table 1 the clinical and laboratory data are shown.

***Corresponding author:** Johannes Matschke, Department of Hematology, Medical Faculty, University of Duisburg-Essen Hufelandstr. 55, D-45122 Essen, Germany, E-mail: Johannes.Matschke@uk-essen.de

	All patients no. (%), n=135		Normal FLC ratio no. (%), n=57		Abnormal FLC-ratio (involving kappa) no. (%), n=60		Abnormal FLC-ratio (involving lambda) no. (%), n=18		p-value
Age at diagnosis years (median), range	60	(30-84)	61	(43-84)	61	(36-80)	56	(30-84)	0.027*
Sex (M/F ratio)	135	(100)	57	(42.2)	60	(44.4)	18	(13.3)	
M	94	(69.6)	41	(72.0)	40	(66.7)	13	(72.2)	
F	41	(30.4)	16	(28.0)	20	(33.3)	5	(27.8)	0.8
Binet stage	124	(100)	52	(41.9)	54	(43.6)	18	(14.5)	
A	77	(62.1)	33	(63.5)	36	(66.7)	8	(44.4)	
B	31	(25.0)	14	(26.9)	13	(24.1)	4	(22.2)	
C	16	(12.9)	5	(9.6)	5	(9.3)	6	(33.3)	0.09
IGVH status	63	(100)	24	(38.1)	29	(46.0)	10	(15.9)	
Unmutated	30	(47.6)	10	(41.7)	14	(48.3)	6	(60.0)	
Mutated	33	(52.4)	14	(58.3)	15	(51.7)	4	(40.0)	0.62
ZAP-70	75	(100)	30	(40.0)	33	(44.0)	12	(16.0)	
Positive	39	(52.0)	18	(60,0)	17	(51.5)	4	(33.3)	
Negative	36	(48.0)	12	(40.0)	16	(48.5)	8	(66.6)	0.29
CD38	125	(100)	54	(43.2)	54	(43.2)	17	(13.6)	
Positive	73	(58.4)	33	(61.1)	35	(64.8)	5	(29.4)	
Negative	52	(41.6)	21	(38.9)	19	(35.2)	12	(70.6)	0.03
ß2M	124	(100)	55	(44.4)	55	(44.4)	14	(11.3)	
Normal	27	(21.8)	20	(36.4)	6	(10.9)	1	(7.2)	
Abnormal	97	(78.2)	35	(63.6)	49	(89.1)	13	(92.9)	0.002
Immunofixation	133	(100)	56	(42.1)	60	(45.1)	17	(12.8)	
Positive	32	(24.1)	9	(16.0)	18	(30.0)	5	(29.4)	
Negative	101	(75.9)	47	(84)	42	(70.)	12	(70.6)	0.18
Creatinine	123	(100)	56	(45.5)	54	(43.9)	13	(10.6)	
Normal	60	(48.9)	24	(42.9)	26	(48.2)	10	(77.0)	
Abnormal	63	(51.2)	32	(57.1)	28	(51.8)	3	(23.0)	0.09

*Kruskal Wallis Test

Table 1: Patient characteristics. All three groups have been statistically analyzed and compared with each other

The levels of serum FLC were assessed using commercially available immunoassays (FREELITE, The Binding Site, UK) and quantified nephelometrically with the BNII analyzer (Siemens, Germany). These tests detect κ or λ FLC at a low concentration of 3 to 4 mg/L. An abnormal κ:λ ratio was defined as <0.26 or >1.65 [16]. Moreover, in all cases we evaluated the M band on Immunofixation (IF) using an approach combining standard serum electrophoresis with screening immunofixation (Hydragel 12IF, Sebia, Fulda, Germany). The screening IF uses a pentavalent antiserum that is electrophoresed in parallel to the standard electrophoresis on the same gel. Whenever a monoclonal protein was detected, confirmatory IF with classification of the monoclonal protein followed. A normal serum-creatinine was defined for women 0.6 to 1.1 mg/dl and men 0.6 to 1.3 mg/dl, as well as β2-microglobulin 0.8 to 2.4 mg/l. In Table 1 the characteristics of all treated and untreated patients are shown. The samples of 88 patients were taken before treatment, 42 samples were taken after treatment (at least 6 months interval from last therapy). In 5 samples therapy status was unknown.

Statistical analysis

The primary endpoint of this analysis was time to first treatment (TFT). TFT was calculated from the date of first diagnosis until first therapy. Times of patients who never got treated were censored. We used Kaplan-Meier survival analysis, the log-rank test and the log-rank test for trend to investigate the prognostic importance of FLC. Prognostic factors for TFT were analyzed using Cox's proportional hazards regression. Comparison of clinical or laboratory parameters between patient subgroups was performed using the non-parametric Mann-Whitney-U test for continuous variables, the Kruskal-Wallis test and the χ^2 test for categorical data. An effect was considered as statistically significant if the p-value of its corresponding test statistic was not larger than <0.05. All statistical computations were done using GraphPad Prism 3.0 (**GraphPad Software,** San Diego, CA, USA) or SPSS version 17 (SPSS, Chicago, IL, USA).

Results

Correlation of tumor cell immunophenotype, abnormal FLC ratio and immunofixation

First we correlated the clonal light chain of the CLL cells according to tumor cell immunophenotype with the ratio of the free light chains and IF. In 98 patients all parameters were available. In 52 of 57 patients (91%), excluding those patients with normal FLC ratio (41 patients), we observed the same clonal light chain in tumor cell immunophenotype as well as in the ratio of FLC whereas in 5 patients the clonal light chain did not agree. There was an association between light chain restriction determined by flow cytometry and serum FLC ratio (p<0.0001). However, a significant correlation between FLC ratio and tumor cell immunophenotype was not evident (p=0,18). Only 27 of 98 patients (28%) were positive in IF (Table 2).

Correlation between abnormal FLC ratio and immunofixation

Abnormal FLC ratios were found in 78 of 135 patients (58%) (Figure 1) whereas the IF was positive in only 32 cases (24%). In 54 cases the FLC ratio was abnormal while IF was negative and in 9 cases the IF was positive while the FLC ratio was normal. In total, 23 patients had both a positive IF and an abnormal FLC ratio (Table 3).

Light chain restriction by flow cytometry	Normal FLC-ratio	Abnormal FLC-ratio (involving kappa)	Abnormal FLC-ratio (involving lambda)	IF positive
Kappa	19	42	2	20
Lambda	22	3	10	7

Table 2: Association between light-chain restriction by flow cytometry and serum FLC ratio Correlation of the light chain restriction determined by flow cytometry with the ratio of the free light chains and immunofixation. In 98 patients the results of the clonal light chain in CLL patients were evaluable. There was an association between light chain restriction determined by flow cytometry and serum FLC-ratio (p<0.0001).

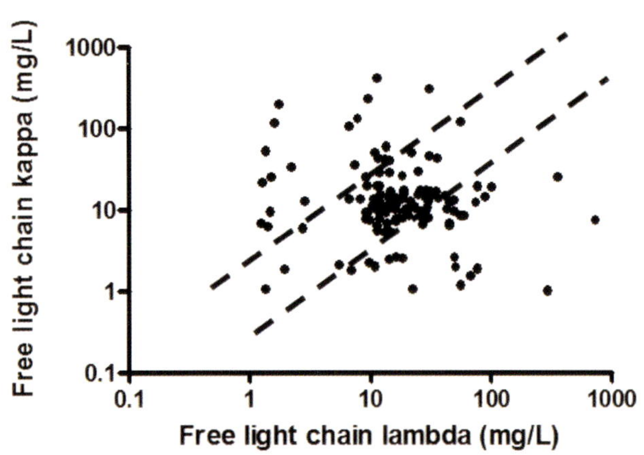

Figure 1: A scatterplot showing serum free kappa and lambda levels for 135 CLL patients In 42% of cases a normal FLC ratio (between the dashed lines) was demonstrated.

	All patients no. (%)		Normal FLC-ratio, no. (%)		Abnormal FLC-ratio, no. (%)	
Immunofixation	133	(100)	56	(42.1)	77	(57.9)
Positive	32	(24.1)	9	(28.2)	23	(71.9)
Negative	101	(75.1)	47	(46.5)	54	(53.5)

Table 3: Association between immunofixation and FLC ratio.

Association of abnormal FLC ratio and treatment free survival

Patients with an abnormal FLC ratio involving λ FLC had a significantly shorter Time To First Treatment (TFT) than patients with an abnormal ratio for κ and those with a normal FLC ratio (median TFT: 34 versus 76 versus 88 months, p for trend=0.039) (Figure 2a). Additionally, monoclonal FLC ratios had a significantly shorter time to first treatment compared to polyclonal normal and abnormal FLC ratios (p for trend=0.0489) (Figure 2b). Additionally, the trend in untreated (88 patients) and treated patients (42 patients) was nearly identical, but the p value was not significant due the small patient number. Therefore, we analyzed both patient groups together.

Multivariate analysis

Using multivariate Cox regression analysis, we compared the abnormal ratio of FLC with other prognostic factors - namely, age, gender, early and advanced clinical stage (Binet stage A vs. B/C), CD38 (cut off 30%) and ZAP-70 expression (cut off 20%) and genomic aberrations (deletion 17p and 11q). High risk cytogenetics (Hazard ratio (HR) 3.2; 95% Confidence interval (CI) 1.8-5.6; p=0.0001), positive CD38 status (HR 3.5; CI 1.7-7.3; p=0.001) and advanced stage according to Binet (HR 3.1; CI 1.7-5.5; p=0.0001) had independent power predicting an unfavorable prognosis.

Association of abnormal FLC ratio and established prognostic markers

As shown in Table 1 we could find an association of abnormal sFLC ratios and the established markers CD38 (p=0.03) and β2-microglobulin (p=0.002). However, there was no association between ZAP-70 (p=0.29) and IGHV (p=0.62).

Moreover, we analyzed the correlation between sFLC and serum-creatinine. In this CLL-cohort, in 13 of 123 patients (11%) we found both an abnormal FLC-ratio and renal dysfunction. A significant correlation between abnormal sFLC and renal damage was not evident (p=0.58) (data not shown). However, for polyclonal FLC´s a significant higher serum-creatinine was demonstrated (p<0.0001) (data not shown).

Combined analysis of abnormal FLC ratio with CD38 and ZAP-70

By summing the number of risk factors defined as abnormal FLC ratio, ZAP-70 and CD38 we separated the cohort into four subgroups (Figure 3). For those patients with no risk factor the TFT was not reached, for patients with one of the three markers the median TFT was 119 months, with two prognostic factors markers 43 months, and with all three markers 26 months (p<0.0001, Figure 3).

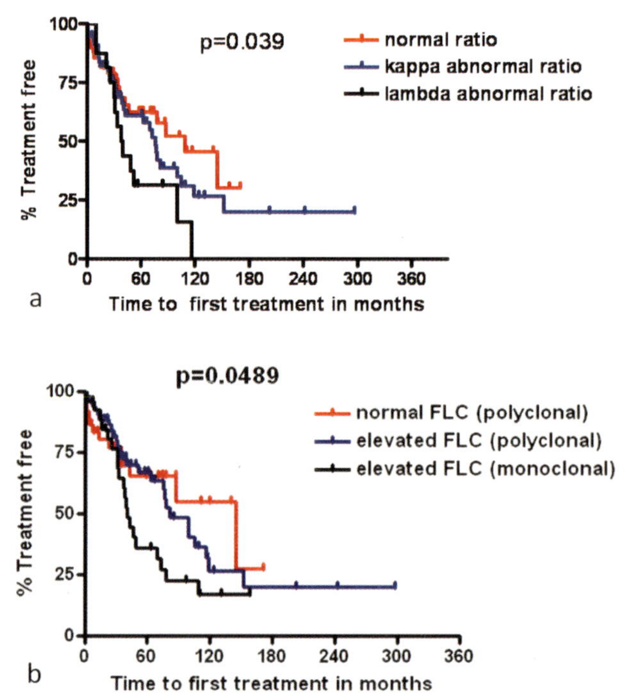

Figure 2: Association of Time to first treatment (TFT) and sFLC ratio Patients with an abnormal FLC ratio involving l FLC had a significantly shorter TFT than patients with an abnormal ratio for k and those with a normal FLC ratio (median TFT: 34 versus 76 versus 88 months, p for trend=0.039) (a). Monoclonal FLC had a significantly shorter time to first treatment compared to polyclonal elevated FLC and normal polyclonal FLC (p for trend=0.0489) (b). Differences in survival times were compared with the log-rank test and the log-rank test for trend.

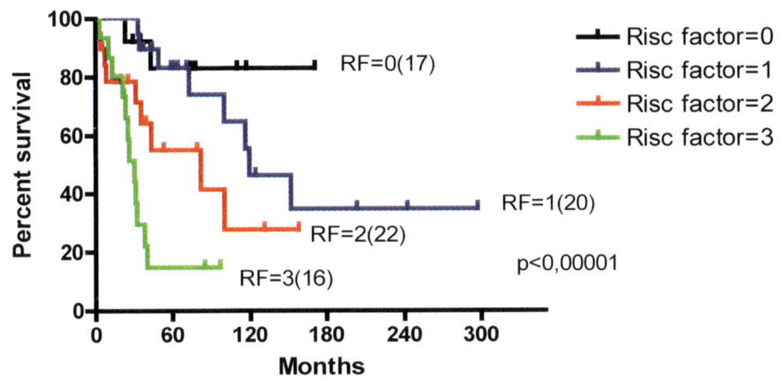

Figure 3: Time to first Treatment (TFT) survival curves in relation to combined analysis of abnormal FLC ratio with CD38 and ZAP-70
Kaplan Meier curves for TFT survival: median time to first treatment not reached (RF=0), 119 months (RF=1), 43 months (RF=2), 26 months (RF=3). Statistical analysis was performed using the log-rank test. RF=risk factor.

Discussion

So far, analyses of abnormal free light chain ratios were explored in multiple myeloma, monoclonal gammopathy of undetermined significance, solitary plasmocytoma, Waldenstrom´s macroglobulinemia and AL amyloidosis [5-8,17]. However, sFLC can be also detected in a substantial fraction of patients with CLL in about 30-40%. Recently, the first evaluation of non-plasma cell B-cell lymphoid malignancies using sFLC assays was reported from the Mayo Clinic. They demonstrated an abnormal sFLC ratio in 44% of a low number of 18 CLL patients [18]. However, [9] could show an abnormal sFLC ratio in 100 out of 259 CLL patients (39%). Moreover, they demonstrated a poor overall survival for patients with an abnormal sFLC ratio. Furthermore, Perdigao presented a correlation between an abnormal sFLC ratio, time to first treatment, IGHV status and overall survival in 84 patients with CLL [19,20]. Studied 34 CLL patients at various disease stages and found an abnormal sFLC ratio in 18 out of 34 patients (53%).

Recently, [10] also showed an abnormal ratio in 30 patients out of 101 CLL patients (30%) with shorter overall survival. Actually, Maurer et al. demonstrated an association of monoclonal FLC and polyclonal FLC with poor overall survival compared to patients with normal FLC [11].

Therefore, we investigated the role of an abnormal ratio of FLC in a large, well characterized cohort of 135 patients and also analyzed the association with immunofixation and light-chain restriction determined by immunophenotyping.

Firstly, we were able to confirm an abnormal FLC ratio in 78 of 135 CLL patients (58%), but interestingly, in only 53% of patients we found both the same clonal B-cell light chain restriction by flow cytometry and the involved FLC of an abnormal ratio. The IF was positive in only 32 of 134 patients and among the 32 patients 23 (17%) patients had both an abnormal FLC-ratio and a positive IF. One reason for the discrepancy can be explained by the fact that some M-proteins could not be detected despite existing FLC`s in the serum. Tsai et al. found a similar result [21]. The other reason is the higher sensitivity of the FLC assay compared to immunofixation. CLL patients with an abnormal FLC-ratio had a detectable M-protein in 15% of cases.

In 5 of 98 patients (5%) we observed a disagreement of the clonal light chain in tumor cell immunophenotype and the abnormal ratio of FLC. A similar result was specified by [23]. (8%) and Ruchlemer et al. (15%) [20]. However, monoclonal gammopathy of undetermined significance (MGUS) is expected in 3-5% of the normal population over 50 years [22] suggesting that the differences in tumor cell immunophenotype and abnormal FLC ratio could be explained by an underlying MGUS in these patients in addition to the CLL. Moreover, the differences could be produced by false positive FLC results.

Secondly, in this retrospective study we observed that patients with an abnormal FLC ratio involving lambda FLC are significantly associated with a worse TFT than kappa and normal ratio (median TFT for abnormal lambda: 34 months; for abnormal kappa 76 months and for normal ratio 88 months; $p=0.039$) confirming the results of [23].

Concerning high FLC serum-concentrations, it has been shown in Multiple Myeloma that a reduced renal function causes a higher serum FLC [24]. It has also been shown that in chronic kidney disease increasing levels of polyclonal κ and λ sFLC correlate with declining kidney function. Further, studies revealed an extended FLC ratio of 0.37 to 3.1 in patients with renal dysfunction [16,25]. We therefore analyzed the correlation between FLC and serum-creatinine. 13 of 123 patients had renal dysfunction and an abnormal FLC ratio. 4 patients had abnormal FLC ratio for lambda and a renal dysfunction. A significant correlation between high sFLC and renal damage was not found ($p=0.332$) and polyclonal sFLC correlated significantly with normal and abnormal serum-creatinine ($p=<0.0001$), as expected (data not shown).

Following the aforementioned analysis we investigated the influence of abnormal sFLC ratio in the different risk groups like ZAP-70 status, CD38, and IGVH status. We could partly find a correlation between FLCs and these CLL prognostic factors. However, there was an association between CD38 and β2-microglobulin.

Furthermore, we could not confirm abnormal sFLC ratio as an independent prognostic factor in multivariate analysis [23]. And also Maurer [11] describe the abnormal sFLC ratio as an independent prognostic factor analyzed by Cox regression analysis. However, the correlation of CD38 and abnormal FLC (Table 1) and the strong impact of CD38 on TFT could explain this fact in our cohort.

Finally, we investigated whether combining information on the expression of CD38, ZAP-70 and abnormal FLC could help refine the prognostic information provided by any of the three factors alone. By summing the number of risk factors, this approach allowed for separation of our patient cohort into four subgroups which differed significantly with regard to their clinical outcome. Summarized, our results confirm the results of the other studies and demonstrate the pivotal role of abnormal FLC in CLL prognosis. Furthermore, we demonstrate for the first time the correlation of FLC and IF in CLL.

Follow-up studies are warranted to elucidate the role of FLC as biomarkers of disease and as a predictive factor for response.

References

1. Rai KR, Sawitsky A, Cronkite EP, Chanana AD, Levy RN, et al. (1975) Clinical staging of chronic lymphocytic leukemia. Blood 46: 219-234.
2. Binet JL, Lepoprier M, Dighiero G, Charron D, D'Athis P, et al. (1977) A clinical staging system for chronic lymphocytic leukemia: prognostic significance. Cancer 40: 855-864.
3. Johansson P, Eisele L, Klein-Hitpass L, Sellmann L, Dührsen U, et al. (2010) Percentage of smudge cells determined on routine blood smears is a novel prognostic factor in chronic lymphocytic leukemia. Leuk Res 34: 892-898.
4. Nowakowski GS, Hoyer JD, Shanafelt TD, Zent CS, Call TG, et al. (2009) Percentage of smudge cells on routine blood smear predicts survival in chronic lymphocytic leukemia. J Clin Oncol 27: 1844-1849.

5. Dingli D, Kyle RA, Rajkumar SV, Nowakowski GS, Larson DR, et al. (2006) Immunoglobulin free light chains and solitary plasmacytoma of bone. Blood 108: 1979-1983.

6. Dispenzieri A, Lacy MQ, Katzmann JA, Rajkumar SV, Abraham RS, et al. (2006) Absolute values of immunoglobulin free light chains are prognostic in patients with primary systemic amyloidosis undergoing peripheral blood stem cell transplantation. Blood 107: 3378-3383.

7. Kyrtsonis MC, Vassilakopoulos TP, Kafasi N, Sachanas S, Tzenou T, et al. (2007) Prognostic value of serum free light chain ratio at diagnosis in multiple myeloma. Br J Haematol 137: 240-243.

8. Rajkumar SV, Kyle RA, Therneau TM, Melton LJ 3rd, Bradwell AR, et al. (2005) Serum free light chain ratio is an independent risk factor for progression in monoclonal gammopathy of undetermined significance. Blood 106: 812-817.

9. Pratt G (2008) The evolving use of serum free light chain assays in haematology. Br J Haematol 141: 413-422.

10. Yegin ZA, Ozkurt ZN, Yagci M (2010) Free light chain: a novel predictor of adverse outcome in chronic lymphocytic leukemia. Eur J Haematol 84: 406-411.

11. Maurer MJ, Cerhan JR, Katzmann JA, Link BK, Allmer C, et al. (2011) Monoclonal and polyclonal serum free light chains and clinical outcome in chronic lymphocytic leukemia. Blood 118: 2821-2826.

12. Morabito F, De Filippi R, Laurenti L, Zirlik K, Recchia AG, et al. (2011) The cumulative amount of serum-free light chain is a strong prognosticator in chronic lymphocytic leukemia. Blood 118: 6353-6361.

13. Hallek M, Cheson BD, Catovsky D, Caligaris-Cappio F, Dighiero G, et al. (2008) Guidelines for the diagnosis and treatment of chronic lymphocytic leukemia: a report from the International Workshop on Chronic Lymphocytic Leukemia updating the National Cancer Institute-Working Group 1996 guidelines. Blood 111: 5446-5456.

14. Dürig J, Naschar M, Schmücker U, Renzing-Köhler K, Hölter T, et al. (2002) CD38 expression is an important prognostic marker in chronic lymphocytic leukaemia. Leukemia 16: 30-35.

15. Dürig J, Nückel H, Cremer M, Führer A, Halfmeyer K, et al. (2003) ZAP-70 expression is a prognostic factor in chronic lymphocytic leukemia. Leukemia 17: 2426-2434."

16. Katzmann JA, Clark RJ, Abraham RS, Bryant S, Lymp JF, et al. (2002) Serum reference intervals and diagnostic ranges for free kappa and free lambda immunoglobulin light chains: relative sensitivity for detection of monoclonal light chains. Clin Chem 48: 1437-1444.

17. van Rhee F, Bolejack V, Hollmig K, Pineda-Roman M, Anaissie E, et al. (2007) High serum-free light chain levels and their rapid reduction in response to therapy define an aggressive multiple myeloma subtype with poor prognosis. Blood 110: 827-832.

18. Martin W, Abraham R, Shanafelt T, Clark RJ, Bone N, et al. (2007) Serum-free light chain-a new biomarker for patients with B-cell non-Hodgkin lymphoma and chronic lymphocytic leukemia. Transl Res 149: 231-235.

19. Perdigao J, Cabrai MJ, Costa N, Carrao C, Rodrigues T, et al. (2008) Prognostic factors in CLL: Is serum free light chain ratio a new biological marker? Annals of Oncology 19: 204-410.

20. Ruchlemer R, Reinus C, Paz E, Cohen A, Melnikov N, et al. (2007) Free light chains, monoclonal proteins and chronic lymphocytic leukaemia. Blood 110: 4697.

21. Tsai HT, Caporaso NE, Kyle RA, Katzmann JA, Dispenzieri A, et al. (2009) Evidence of serum immunoglobulin abnormalities up to 9.8 years before diagnosis of chronic lymphocytic leukemia: a prospective study. Blood 114: 4928-4932.

22. Eisele L, Dürig J, Hüttmann A, Dührsen U, Assert R, et al. (2012) Prevalence and progression of monoclonal gammopathy of undetermined significance and light-chain MGUS in Germany. Ann Hematol 91: 243-248.

23. Pratt G, Harding S, Holder R, Fegan C, Pepper C, et al. (2009) Abnormal serum free light chain ratios are associated with poor survival and may reflect biological subgroups in patients with chronic lymphocytic leukaemia. Br J Haematol 144: 217-222.

24. Drayson M, Begum G, Basu S, Makkuni S, Dunn J, et al. (2006) Effects of paraprotein heavy and light chain types and free light chain load on survival in myeloma: an analysis of patients receiving conventional-dose chemotherapy in Medical Research Council UK multiple myeloma trials. Blood 108: 2013-2019.

25. Hutchison CA, Plant T, Drayson M, Cockwell P, Kountouri M, et al. (2008) Serum free light chain measurement aids the diagnosis of myeloma in patients with severe renal failure. BMC Nephrol 9: 11."

Therapeutic Combination of Nanoliposomal Safingol and Nanoliposomal Ceramide for Acute Myeloid Leukemia

Timothy J Brown[1,2], Aileen M. Garcia[3,4], Lindsey N Kissinger[1,2], Sriram S Shanmugavelandy[4], Xujung Wang[1,2], Myles C Cabot[5], Mark Kester[2,4], David F Claxton[1,2] and Brian M Barth[1,2,4*]

[1]*Department of Medicine, Division of Hematology and Oncology, Penn State College of Medicine, Hershey, PA, USA*
[2]*Penn State Hershey Cancer Institute, Hershey, PA, USA*
[3]*Department of Biomedical Science, Inter American University of Puerto Rico, Ponce, PR, USA*
[4]*Department of Pharmacology, Penn State College of Medicine, Hershey, PA, USA*
[5]*John Wayne Cancer Institute, Santa Monica, CA, USA*

Abstract

Novel approaches to enhancing the efficacy of ceramide-based therapeutics are of interest for the treatment of acute myeloid leukemia (AML). Ceramide is a bioactive sphingolipid that has long been established as an inducer of apoptosis. We have pioneered the effort to develop nanoliposomal C6-ceramide (Lip-C6) as an anticancer therapeutic and recently have engaged in efforts to enhance its therapeutic efficacy. Ceramide catabolism by acid ceramidase and subsequently sphingosine kinase 1 yields the metabolite oncogenic sphingosine-1-phosphate (S1P). Therefore, in the present study we hypothesized that targeting of this metabolic pathway with the sphingosine kinase 1 inhibitor safingol would augment the anti-AML efficacy of Lip-C6. We generated and evaluated nanoliposomes encapsulating safingol (Lip-Saf), in combination with Lip-C6 using AML cell lines and primary AML patient samples. This combination exerted synergistic therapeutic efficacy using HL-60 and KG-1 cells, and additive efficacy using HL-60/VCR cells. In contrast, the combination of Lip-C6 and Lip-Saf yielded an antagonistic effect using the murine AML cell line C1498 and this effect was correlated with an increase in autophagy as a potent leukemia survival mechanism. Intriguingly, by using an inhibitor of ceramide glycosylation, nanoliposomal tamoxifen, we observed synergistic anti-AML efficacy using the C1498 cell line demonstrating that unique manipulations of ceramide metabolism may be prevalent in different AMLs. Lastly, we evaluated both favorable prognosis and poor prognosis primary patient AML samples and observed combinatorial efficacy of Lip-C6 and Lip-Saf. This was reflected by a decrease in autophagy and concomitant increase in apoptosis, as well as the ability to block colony forming capacity. Altogether, these results demonstrated that the efficacy of Lip-C6 as an experimental anti-AML therapy can be dramatically enhanced through combination with inhibitors of ceramide metabolism.

Keywords: Nanoliposome; Ceramide; Safingol; Tamoxifen; Autophagy; Apoptosis; Acute myeloid leukemia; Sphingosine kinase, Glucosylceramide synthase; P-Glycoprotein

Introduction

Acute myeloid leukemia (AML) is a growing public health problem in the United States with approximately 12,000 new cases of AML and nearly 9,000 deaths occurring yearly. In spite of substantial efforts, therapeutic progress has been limited. AML is a highly heterogeneous disease and the 2008 WHO classification, which incorporates known karyotypic data of prognostic importance, has been accepted for its clinical classification [1-3]. New drugs are urgently needed as a large majority of patients with AML have an unfavourable outlook illustrated by relapse and multidrug resistance.

One promising avenue of therapeutic development has been liposomal encapsulation of drugs. This approach has augmented the efficacy of several chemotherapeutics, while simultaneously decreasing toxicity [4,5]. In addition to protecting therapeutics from degradation and augmenting systemic retention, liposomal formulations also offer the prospect of delivering highly insoluble molecules such as lipids [4,5]. Recently, our group has developed nanoliposomal C6-ceramide (Lip-C6) for the treatment of both solid tumor malignancies and hematological malignancies [4,5]. Ceramide is a naturally occurring bioactive sphingolipid that has been well-established as an inducer of apoptosis and regulator of cell stress [4-10]. Ceramide has also been shown to exert therapeutic efficacy in a variety of *in vitro* and *in vivo* models of cancer, and endogenous ceramides have also been documented to increase in response to chemotherapy [5,7,10]. As a very insoluble lipid, the utility of ceramide as a standalone therapeutic was limited until its formulation into nanoliposomes [4,5]. A significant obstacle to effective ceramide-based therapy is the inherent ability of some malignant cells to detoxify ceramide by metabolism that often yields oncogenic metabolites [6,7]. In one metabolic pathway, ceramide can be converted to sphingosine-1-phosphate (S1P) by the action of acid ceramidase and sphingosine kinase (SphK) [8-10]. S1P is a potent bioactive sphingolipid that can bind to specific S1P receptors which mediate its vast array of mitogenic and oncogenic effects [11,12]. Alternatively, ceramide can be metabolized to glucosylceramide by the coordinated action of glucosylceramide synthase (GCS) and P-glycoprotein (P-gp) [8-10]. In this pathway, the drug efflux pump P-gp is located at the Golgi where it is responsible for moving newly synthesized glucosylceramide into the Golgi thereby promoting further metabolism and preventing product inhibition of GCS [8-10].

***Corresponding author:** Brian M Barth, Ph.D. Department of Medicine, Division of Hematology and Oncology, Penn State Hershey Cancer Institute, Penn State College of Medicine, 500 University Drive, PO Box 850, CH46 Hershey, PA 17033, USA, E-mail: bmb14@psu.edu, bbarth1@hmc.psu.edu

As both the SphK and GCS/P-gp pathways are upregulated in many malignanices, these enzymes have gained substantial attention as targets for the development of cancer therapeutics [10]. Furthermore, second generation development of ceramide as a therapeutic has included strategies to block either the SphK or GCS/P-gp pathways [10].

Recently, a liposomal formulation of the SphK inhibitor Safingol was described and tested in a model of leukemia [13]. Safingol, also known as L-threo-dihydrosphingosine, competitively inhibits SphK1 and has been shown to induce autophagy in pancreatic, colon, and breast cancer cell lines by the generation of reactive oxygen species [14,15]. Autophagy is a cellular self-eating process where intracellular vacuoles sequester organelles and other cellular components. These vacuoles fuse with lysosomes to form autophagosomes that ultimately consume these organelles for the production of energy [16,17]. It was originally suggested that autophagy was a cellular mechanism to avoid starvation during times of nutrient deprivation, but recently autophagy is also implicated as a mechanism of inducing cell death in a caspase-independent fashion [15-17]. Research has suggested that autophagy not only can be a process by which malignant cells overcome nutrient starvation but also a mechanism of therapy resistance [18,19]. Accordingly, studies have demonstrated that inhibition of autophagy can be used to sensitize malignant cells to chemotherapy [18-20]. In contrast, recent studies have also demonstrated conflicting evidence that autophagy may play a role in apoptosis of tumor cells [19,21]. Therefore, it is important to recognize that pharmacological blockade of autophagy remains a questionable proposition without further mechanistic understanding of the roles of autophagy in cancer. Comparatively, pharmacological inhibition of sphingolipid metabolism provides a reasonable therapeutic target because the generation of bioactive sphingolipid metabolites, such as S1P, is readily linked to oncogenesis [4-15].

In the present study, we designed nanoliposomal safingol (Lip-Saf) to specifically combine with Lip-C6 for the treatment of AML. In particular, we utilized Lip-Saf as a means to augment the efficacy of Lip-C6 in AML cell lines and AML patient samples that otherwise were less sensitive to Lip-C6 alone. Furthermore, we evaluated autophagy and apoptosis and demonstrated that efficacy of combining Lip-Saf with Lip-C6 is lost when autophagy is upregulated. However, in this case the combinatorial efficacy of Lip-C6 can be achieved by instead blocking the GCS/P-gp pathway with nanoliposomal tamoxifen (Lip-Tam). Altogether, this study demonstrated the anti-AML efficacy of combining Lip-C6 with nanoliposomal formulations that block its metabolism. This study is highly significant because safingol has recently entered clinical trials for the treatment of solid tumor malignancies [22].

Materials and Methods

Cell culture

Human HL-60, HL-60/VCR, and murine C1498 cells, were maintained at 37°C, and 5% CO2, in RPMI-1640 supplemented with 10% fetal bovine serum (FBS) and 1% penicillin/streptomycin. Human KG-1 likewise maintained, in IMDM supplemented with 20% FBS and 1% penicillin/streptomycin. Patient AML samples were prepared from peripheral blood obtained under informed consent and approved by the Penn State College of Medicine Institutional Review Board. These samples were maintained in RPMI-1640 supplemented with 10% FBS.

Nanoliposomal preparation and characterization

Nanoliposomes were prepared by the Penn State College of Medicine Drug Discovery Core following previously established methods with minor changes for the new Lip-Saf formulation. All lipids were obtained from Avanti Polar Lipids (Alabaster, AL). Ghost nanoliposomes (Lip-Ghost), Lip-C6, and Lip-Tam, were prepared as previously described [7,23,24]. Briefly, lipids dissolved in chloroform, or other organic solvents, were combined in specific molar ratios. For Lip-

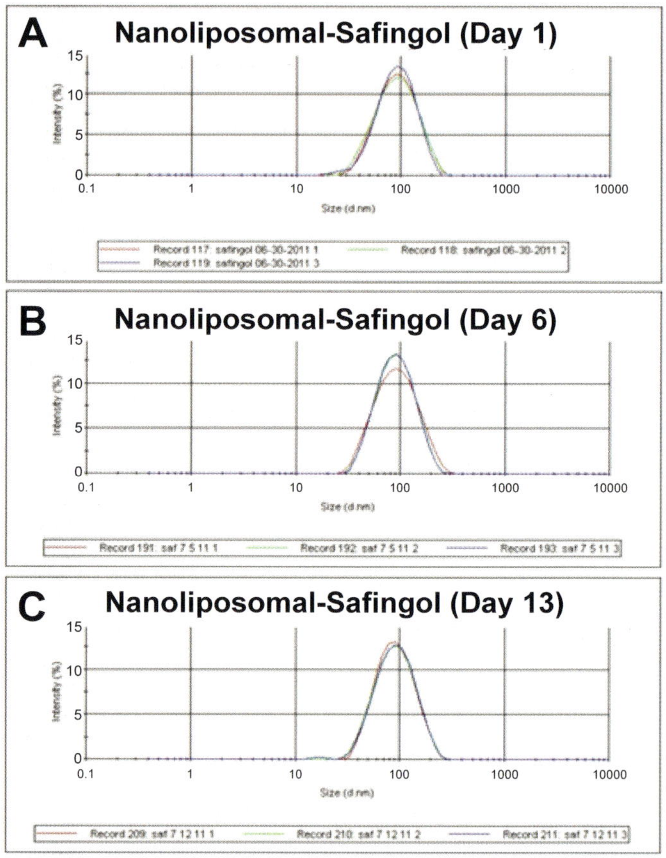

Figure 1: Stability of Lip-Saf. Dynamic light scattering was used to verify the size and stability of Lip-Saf after (A) one day, (B) six days, and (C) thirteen days.

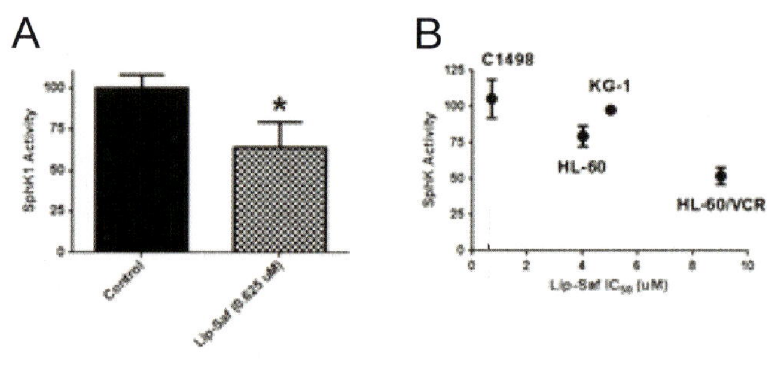

Figure 2: SphK activity. (A) Lip-Saf inhibited recombinant SphK1 activity in a cell-free inhibitor screening assay (t-test, *p<0.05, n=5). Error bars represent standard deviation from the mean. (B) SphK activity was determined and compared for the C1498, KG-1, HL-60, and HL-60/VCR cell lines. Activity was determined by dividing fluorescence (SphK activity) by the total amount of protein assayed for a given sample. Activity was plotted versus the Lip-Saf IC50 for each cell line. The Pearson correlation coefficient was -0.89, but was not significant as p = 0.11. Error bars represent standard deviation from the mean.

Saf, aliquots of DSPC (1,2-distearoyl-sn-glycero-3-phosphocholine), DOPE (1,2-dioleoyl-sn-glycero-3-phosphoethanolamine), DSPE-PEG2000 (1,2-distearoyl-sn-glycero-3-phosphoethanolamine-N-[methoxy(polyethylene glycol)- 2000]), and safingol, were made in a 4.66:2.37:1.47:1.5 molar ratio. Solutions were dried to a film under a stream of nitrogen, and then hydrated by addition of 0.9% NaCl. Solutions were sealed, heated at 60°C (60 min), and subjected to vortex mixing and sonicated until light no longer diffracted through the suspension. The lipid vesicle-containing solution was quickly extruded at 60°C by passing the solution 10 times through 100 nm polycarbonate filters in an Avanti Mini-Extruder. Nanoliposomal size was determined using a Malvern Zetasizer Nano ZS at 25°C. Nanoliposome solutions were stored at room temperature until use. Lip-Saf was stable for at least two weeks (Figure 1).

Cell viability assay

Cells were plated at 2.5×10^4 cells per well in 96-well tissue culture plates and treated for 48 hours. Following treatment, cellular viability was assessed using a Cell Titer 96 AQueous Non-Radioactive Cell Proliferation Assay according to the manufacturer's instructions (Promega, Madison, WI). Viability was determined by measuring absorbance at 490 nm using a microplate reader and normalizing to the viability observed under control conditions.

Flow cytometry detection of autophagy and apoptosis

Cells were treated for 48 hours prior to autophagy or apoptosis detection. Autophagy was detected using the Cyto-ID Autophagy Kit (Enzo Life Sciences, Farmingdale, NY) according to the manufacturer's protocol [24]. Apoptosis was detected by Annexin V and 7-AAD staining. Patient AML samples were also stained with anti-CD34 and anti-CD38 antibodies to evaluate autophagy or apoptosis within leukemia progenitor populations (CD34+CD38-). All antibodies and apoptosis detection reagents were obtained from BD Biosciences (San Jose, CA). Samples were evaluated at the Penn State College of Medicine Flow Cytometry Core using a LSR II flow cytometer and BD FACS Diva software.

Colony forming assay

Patient AML was prepared in MethoCult H4434 according to the manufacturer's instructions (Steem Cell Technologies, Vancouver, BC, Canada). Colonies were propagated for two weeks, and blast colonies were counted in a blinded manner using a light microscope.

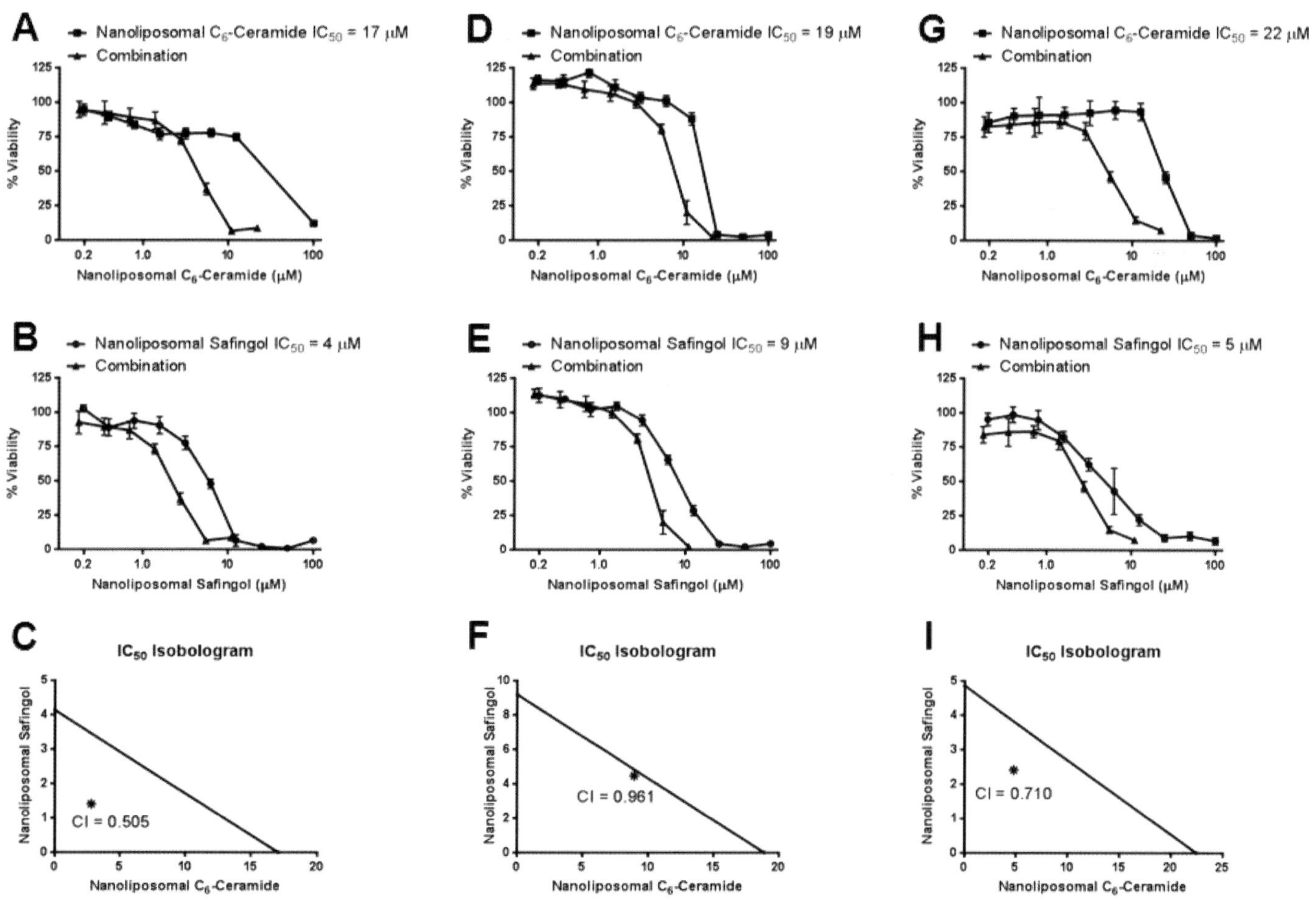

Figure 3: Combinatorial efficacy of Lip-C6 and Lip-Saf in human AML cell lines. Cellular viability was evaluated and IC50 values were determined for Lip-C6 (Nanoliposomal C6-Ceramide), Lip-Saf (Nanoliposomal Safingol), or the combination (2;1 ratio, respectively). Calcusyn software was used to determine CI values. Isobolograms depict the combinatorial dose needed to achieve the IC50, with points under the line being synergistic, points on the line being additive, and points over the line being antagonistic. (A-C) HL-60 cells. (D-F) HL-60/VCR cells. (G-I) KG-1 cells. Error bars represent standard error from the mean.

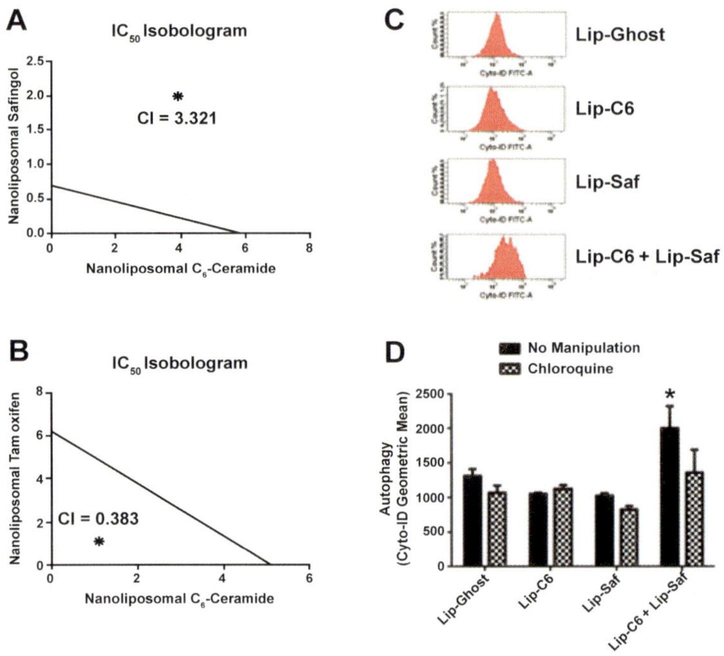

Figure 4: Increased autophagy mediates resistance of murine AML cells to the combination of Lip-C6 and Lip-Saf. The combination of Lip-C6 and Lip-Saf was evaluated using the murine AML cell line C1498. (A) Isobologram analysis revealed that the combination of Lip-C6 and Lip-Saf was antagonistic despite individual treatments being effective. (B) Isobologram analysis showed that the combination of Lip-C6 with Lip-Tam was highly synergistic using C1498 cells. (C) The Cyto-ID Autophagy Detection Kit was used to visualize autophagy by flow cytometry using C1498 cells. The combination of Lip-C6 (4 μM) and Lip-Saf (0.75 μM) augmented the Cyto-ID signal, indicating an upregulation of autophagy. (D) Quantification of Cyto-ID autophagy analysis. Alternatively, the autophagy blocker chloroquine was added thirty minutes prior to Cyto-ID addition to verify that the signal observed was due to an increase in autophagy. 1-way ANOVA, *$p<0.05$ compared to all treatments. Error bars represent standard deviation from the mean.

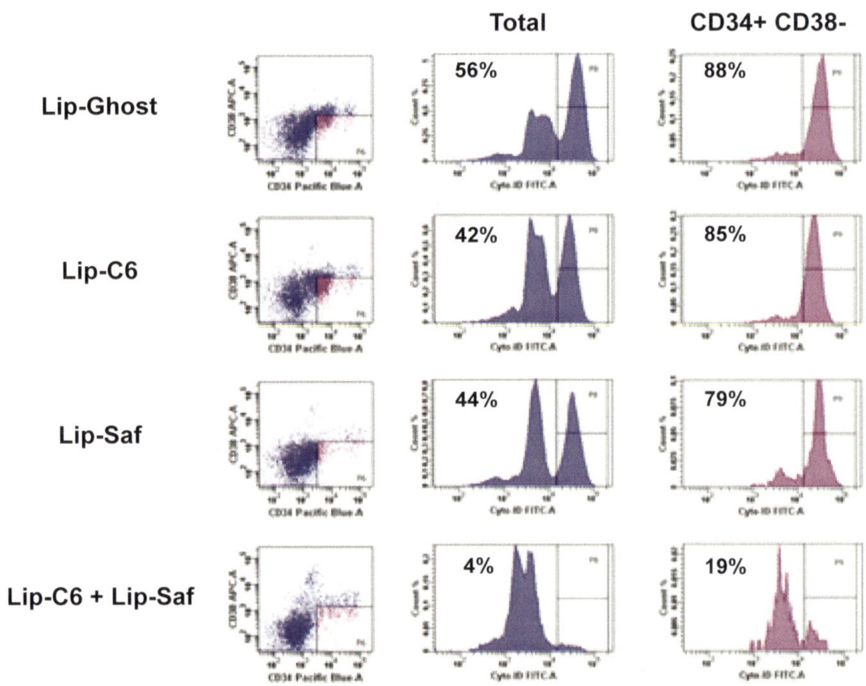

Figure 5: Therapeutic efficacy of Lip-C6 and Lip-Saf using human patient AML is reflected by a decrease of autophagy. The Cyto-ID Autophagy Detection Kit was used to visualize autophagy by flow cytometry using a favorable-prognosis human AML patient sample characterized as having translocation 8;21 (patient 632). Cells were also stained to analyze the leukemia progenitor population (CD34+CD38-). The combination of Lip-C6 (10 μM) and Lip-Saf (5 μM) dramatically decreased autophagy. Percentages displayed are for cells undergoing the highest level of autophagy. The intermediate stained population, not gated as positive, corresponds to normal lymphocytes.

Sphingosine kinase assay

The Sphingosine Kinase 1 Inhibitor Screening Assay kit was used according to the manufacturer's instructions (Cayman Chemical Company, Ann Arbor, MI). To determine SphK activity of cell lines, 10 µl of cells lysed in 1% Triton X-100 was substituted for 10 µl of recombinant SphK1 in the normal kit procedure. Activity was standardized based on total protein content of the lysates determined by BCA assay (Thermo Fisher Scientific, Waltham, MA).

Combinatorial analysis

CalcuSyn Software (Biosoft, Cambridge, UK) was used to determine combinatorial effects of treatments [7]. Cellular viability data was used for this analysis, and a combination index (CI) less than or equal to 0.9 was considered synergistic. CI values greater than or equal to 1.1 were considered antagonistic, whereas CI values between 0.9 and 1.1 were considered additive.

Statistical analysis

One-way analysis of variance (ANOVA) was used to determine statistically significant differences between treatments ($p<0.05$). At least three independent experiments were performed for each condition. Post hoc comparisons of specific treatments were performed using either Tukey's or Bonferroni test. For the SphK inhibitor assay a student's t-test was used to determine significance. All statistical analyses were carried out using GraphPad Prism 4 software (La Jolla, CA).

Sample	Karyotype	NPM1	FLT3-ITD	Prognosis	Combination % Apoptosis	Combination % Autophagy
329	inv3, -7	ND	ND	Unfavorable	ND	ND
632	t8;21	ND	ND	Favorable	62	4
663	Normal (prior MDS)	ND	ND	Unfavorable	46	12
664	Complex	ND	ND	Unfavorable	ND	77
667	inv16	Neg	Neg	Favorable	60	54
668	Complex	Neg	Neg	Unfavorable	96	3
669	Normal	Pos	Pos	Unfavorable	22	86

Table 1: Individual information for human clinical AML samples used to evaluate the combinatorial efficacy of Lip-C6 and Lip-Saf in apoptosis, autophagy, and colony forming assays. ND: Not determined.

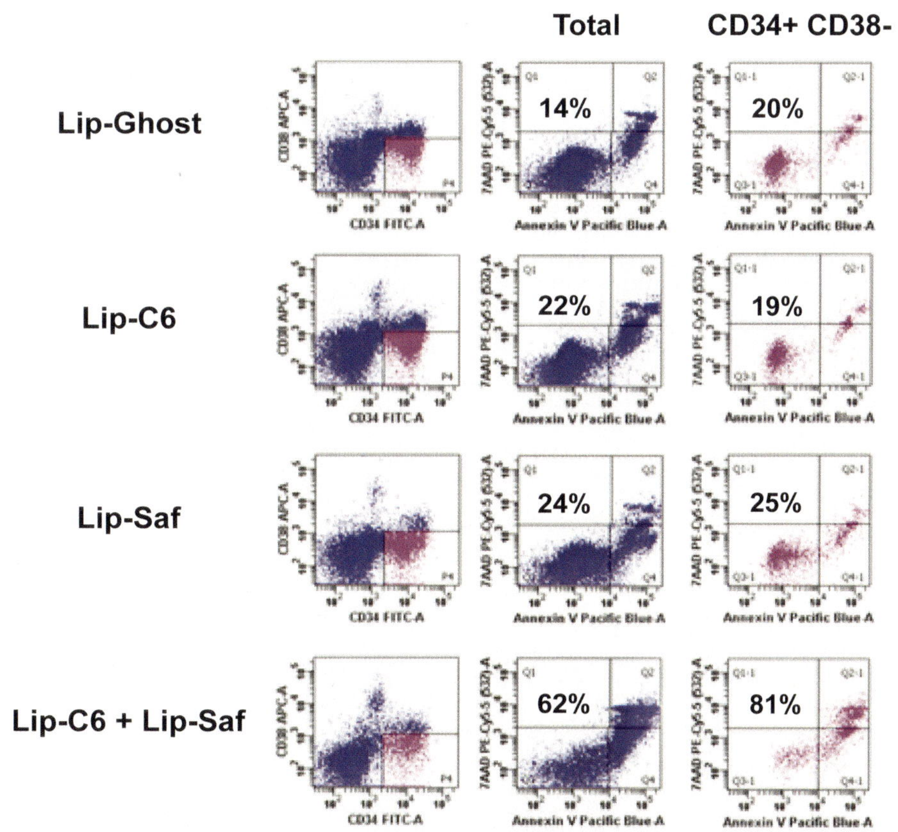

Figure 6: Therapeutic efficacy of Lip-C6 and Lip-Saf using human patient AML is reflected by an increase in apoptosis. Annexin V and 7-AAD staining were used to visualize apoptosis by flow cytometry using a favorable-prognosis human AML patient sample characterized as having translocation 8;21 (patient 632). Cells were also stained to analyze the leukemia progenitor population (CD34+CD38-). The combination of Lip-C6 (10 µM) and Lip-Saf (5 µM) dramatically augmented apoptosis. Percentages displayed are for Annexin V+ cells (upper and lower right quandrants combined).

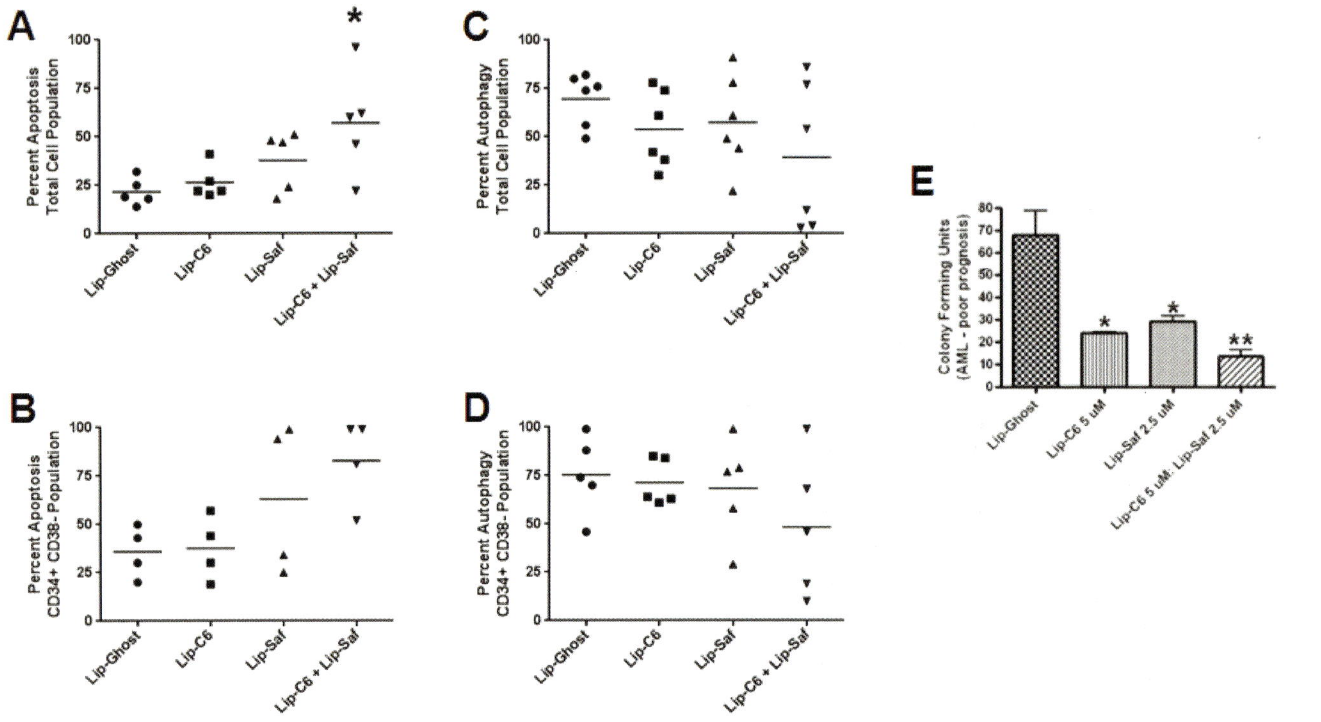

Figure 7: The combination of Lip-C6 and Lip-Saf induce cell death and decrease autophagy of human patient AML. Annexin V and 7-AAD staining were used to determine apoptosis of primary AML samples exposed to the control (Lip-Ghost), Lip-C6, Lip-Saf, or the combination. Alternatively, the Cyto-ID Autophagy Detection Kit was used to visualize autophagy. (A, C) Total cellular population. 1-way ANOVA, *p<0.05 compared to Lip-Ghost. (B, D) CD34+ CD38- LSC fraction. (E) Colony forming capacity was evaluated using a poor-prognosis human AML patient sample characterized as having inversion 3 and monosomy 7 (patient 329). Lip-C6, Lip-Saf, or the combination of both, was shown to block colony forming capacity after a two week growth period. 1-way ANOVA, *p<0.05 compared to Lip-Ghost, **p<0.05 compared to all treatments. Error bars represent standard error from the mean.

Results and Discussion

Our group is engaged in an effort to augment the efficacy of Lip-C6 for the treatment of cancer. In a previous study evaluating pancreatic cancer, we generated a nanoliposomal formulation that combined C6-ceramide with an inhibitor of GCS to prevent its metabolism to C6-glucosylceramide [7]. In the current study, we generated Lip-Saf to block the catabolism of C6-ceramide to S1P by SphK1, and validated these nanoliposomes using *in vitro* models of AML. Using a SphK1 inhibitor screening assay, we confirmed that Lip-Saf inhibited SphK1 at 0.625 μM (Figure 2A). Next, we adapted this same assay to determine the SphK activity in four AML cell lines. The AML cell lines that we studied, C1498, KG-1 HL-60, and HL-60/VCR (vincristine-resistant variant), were readily stratified from highest to lowest SphK activity, respectively (Figure 2B). We next expanded our evaluation of the three human cell lines, which are noteworthy of being representative of drug-resistant and poor prognosis AML, to evaluate specific sensitivity to Lip-C6 and Lip-Saf (Figure 3). In general, these three cells lines were more resistant to Lip-C6 than others we have previously evaluated (Lip-C6 IC50: HL-60=17 μM, HL-60/VCR=19 μM, KG-1=22 μM) [10]. These AML cell lines were collectively more sensitive to Lip-Saf than Lip-C6 (Lip-Saf IC50: HL-60=4 μM, HL-60/VCR=9 μM, KG-1=5 μM). Most notably, the combination of Lip-C6 and Lip-Saf resulted in synergistic efficacy using HL-60 and KG-1 cell lines, and additive efficacy using the HL-60/VCR cell line. These results demonstrated that the blockade of SphK1 using Lip-Saf can enhance the anti-AML efficacy of Lip-C6.

In contrast, while the murine AML cell line C1498 is highly sensitive to either Lip-C6 (5.8 μM) or Lip-Saf (0.7 μM) individually, the combination of these two experimental therapeutics did not result in a synergistic effect (Figure 4A). However, it is important to note that while the combinatorial effect was not synergistic the IC50 of the combination was achieved with Lip-C6 (3.9 μM) and Lip-Saf (2 μM) concentrations that were still very low. This is important because this demonstrates that the C1498 cell line is much more sensitive to individual treatments of Lip-C6 or Lip-Saf than HL-60, HL-60/VCR, or KG-1 cells. To further explore the antagonistic effects of Lip-C6 and Lip-Saf, and to offer a therapeutic alternative, we first investigated if blockade of another ceramide metabolic pathway other than SphK1 would be beneficial for the treatment of C1498 cells. Indeed, the combination of Lip-C6 with Lip-Tam induced a highly synergistic effect against C1498 cells (Figure 4B). The individual IC50 for Lip-Tam was 6.2 μM. Tamoxifen is an inhibitor of P-gp and therefore blocks the glycosylation of ceramide [6,23,25-27]. We have separately evaluated the sphingolipidome of C1498 cells and have observed a strong propensity to convert C6-ceramide to C6-glucoyslceramide (data not shown). This corroborates our current findings that the combination of Lip-C6 and Lip-Tam can exert synergistic efficacy against C1498 cells. We further evaluated a mechanistic reason why the combination of Lip-C6 and Lip-Saf yielded an antagonistic effect using C1498 cells. Previous reports suggested that safingol could induce autophagy in some cancer models [14,15]. Furthermore, it has been suggested that autophagy is a mechanism by which cells can overcome stress conditions including chemotherapy [16,17,28]. For these two reasons, we evaluated autophagy as a possible reason why the combination of

Lip-C6 and Lip-Saf induced an antagonistic effect in C1498 cells. We observed that he combination of Lip-C6 and Lip-Saf, but not individual treatments, induced autophagy in C1498 cells (Figures 4C and 4D). Altogether, these results suggest that up-regulation of autophagy is a mechanism that some AML cells may use to overcome the combination of Lip-C6 and Lip-Saf. Moreover, alternative approaches blocking the metabolism of C6-ceramide, such as blockade of the GCS/P-gp pathway, can effectively be used for anti-AML therapy in these cases.

We lastly evaluated the combination of Lip-Saf and Lip-C6 using primary human patient AML samples. We evaluated several cases of AML spanning from favorable to unfavourable prognosis outlooks (Table 1). As a model case, we demonstrated using a case of favorable prognosis AML (translocation 8;21), that the combination of Lip-C6 and Lip-Saf blocked autophagy in both the total AML population as well as the CD34+CD38- AML progenitor population (Figure 5). We next showed that the combination augmented apoptosis using the same case (Figure 6, indicating that apoptosis is induced concomitantly as autophagy is down-regulated. For the entire cohort of samples evaluated, the combination of Lip-C6 with Lip-Saf significantly stimulated apoptosis in the total AML population (Figure 7A; Table 1). Apoptosis was also induced by the combination of Lip-C6 and Lip-Saf in many of the primary sample CD34+ CD38- LSC fractions (Figure 7B), and this was often associated with a decrease in autophagy in either the total or LSC fractions (Figures 7C and 7D; Table 1). We also observed a similar result using a colony forming assay to evaluate the combination of Lip-C6 and Lip-Saf when evaluating a poor prognosis case of AML (inversion 3, monosomy 7). In this situation, we observed efficacy for the individual treatments, but a significantly more efficacious anti-AML effect with the combination (Figure 7E). Collectively, these results demonstrate that the combination of Lip-C6 and Lip-Saf can exert combinatorial anti-AML efficacy using primary clinical samples.

Finally, it is noteworthy that sensitivity to ceramide-based therapeutics is not necessarily reflective of the standard risk assessment for human AML. It is hypothesized that sensitivity to ceramide-based therapeutics such as Lip-C6, Lip-Saf, Lip-Tam, or combinations of these therapeutics, is directly related to the ability of a given AML to metabolize ceramide and specifically by what pathways. In-depth sphingolipid metabolic analysis would fully reveal the utility of ceramide-based therapeutics for the treatment of AML by identifying sensitivity to specific therapeutics. More so, ceramide metabolism in AML could be further explored as a means to enhance risk stratification. The further advancement of the preclinical development of ceramide-based therapeutics has the potential to ultimately improve the outcomes of AML patients that otherwise may have unfavourable outcomes with standard chemotherapy.

Acknowledgements

This study was funded in part by the Penn State University Kiesendahl Family Endowed Leukemia Research Fund, the Kenneth Noel Memorial Fund, and PA Tobacco Settlement funds. The Penn State Research Foundation has licensed ceramide nanoliposomes, and other nonliposomal technology, to Keystone Nano, Inc. (State College, PA). M.K. is Chief Medical Officer of Keystone Nano, Inc.

References

1. Baldus CD, Mrózek K, Marcucci G, Bloomfield CD (2007) Clinical outcome of de novo acute myeloid leukaemia patients with normal cytogenetics is affected by molecular genetic alterations: a concise review. Br J Haematol 137: 387-400.
2. Becker H, Marcucci G, Maharry K, Radmacher MD, Mrózek K, et al. (2010) Favorable prognostic impact of NPM1 mutations in older patients with cytogenetically normal de novo acute myeloid leukemia and associated gene- and microRNA-expression signatures: a Cancer and Leukemia Group B study. J Clin Oncol 28: 596-604.
3. Kottaridis PD, Gale RE, Frew ME, Harrison G, Langabeer SE, et al. (2001) The presence of a FLT3 internal tandem duplication in patients with acute myeloid leukemia (AML) adds important prognostic information to cytogenetic risk group and response to the first cycle of chemotherapy: analysis of 854 patients from the United Kingdom Medical Research Council AML 10 and 12 trials. Blood 98: 1752-1759.
4. Zolnik BS, Stern ST, Kaiser JM, Heakal Y, Clogston JD, et al. (2008) Rapid distribution of liposomal short-chain ceramide *in vitro* and *in vivo*. Drug Metab Dispos 36: 1709-1715.
5. Watters RJ, Kester M, Tran MA, Loughran TP Jr, Liu X (2012) Development and use of ceramide nanoliposomes in cancer. Methods Enzymol 508: 89-108.
6. Chapman JV, Gouazé-Andersson V, Messner MC, Flowers M, Karimi R, et al. (2010) Metabolism of short-chain ceramide by human cancer cells--implications for therapeutic approaches. Biochem Pharmacol 80: 308-315.
7. Jiang Y, DiVittore NA, Kaiser JM, Shanmugavelandy SS, Fritz JL, et al. (2011) Combinatorial therapies improve the therapeutic efficacy of nanoliposomal ceramide for pancreatic cancer. Cancer Biol Ther 12: 574-585.
8. Hannun YA, Obeid LM (2008) Principles of bioactive lipid signalling: lessons from sphingolipids. Nat Rev Mol Cell Biol 9: 139-150.
9. Morad SA, Cabot MC (2013) Ceramide-orchestrated signalling in cancer cells. Nat Rev Cancer 13: 51-65.
10. Barth BM, Cabot MC, Kester M (2011) Ceramide-based therapeutics for the treatment of cancer. Anticancer Agents Med Chem 11: 911-919.
11. Pyne NJ, Pyne S (2010) Sphingosine 1-phosphate and cancer. Nat Rev Cancer 10: 489-503.
12. Stevenson CE, Takabe K, Nagahashi M, Milstien S, Spiegel S (2011) Targeting sphingosine-1-phosphate in hematologic malignancies. Anticancer Agents Med Chem 11: 794-798.
13. Tan KB, Ling LU, Bunte RM, Chng WJ, Chiu GN (2012) *In vivo* efficacy of a novel liposomal formulation of safingol in the treatment of acute myeloid leukemia. J Control Release 160: 290-298.
14. Ling LU, Tan KB, Lin H, Chiu GN (2011) The role of reactive oxygen species and autophagy in safingol-induced cell death. Cell Death Dis 2: e129.
15. Coward J, Ambrosini G, Musi E, Truman JP, Haimovitz-Friedman A, et al. (2009) Safingol (L-threo-sphinganine) induces autophagy in solid tumor cells through inhibition of PKC and the PI3-kinase pathway. Autophagy 5: 184-193.
16. Neufeld TP (2012) Autophagy and cell growth--the yin and yang of nutrient responses. J Cell Sci 125: 2359-2368.
17. Gozuacik D, Kimchi A (2004) Autophagy as a cell death and tumor suppressor mechanism. Oncogene 23: 2891-2906.
18. Rabinowitz JD, White E (2010) Autophagy and metabolism. Science 330: 1344-1348.
19. White E (2012) Deconvoluting the context-dependent role for autophagy in cancer. Nat Rev Cancer 12: 401-410.
20. Amaravadi RK, Lippincott-Schwartz J, Yin XM, Weiss WA, Takebe N, et al. (2011) Principles and current strategies for targeting autophagy for cancer treatment. Clin Cancer Res 17: 654-666.
21. Wang RC, Wei Y, An Z, Zou Z, Xiao G, et al. (2012) Akt-mediated regulation of autophagy and tumorigenesis through Beclin 1 phosphorylation. Science 338: 956-959.
22. Dickson MA, Carvajal RD, Merrill AH Jr, Gonen M, Cane LM, et al. (2011) A phase I clinical trial of safingol in combination with cisplatin in advanced solid tumors. Clin Cancer Res 17: 2484-2492.
23. Morad SA, Madigan JP, Levin JC, Abdelmageed N, Karimi R, et al. (2013) Tamoxifen magnifies therapeutic impact of ceramide in human colorectal cancer cells independent of p53. Biochem Pharmacol 85: 1057-1065.
24. Lee JS, Lee GM (2012) Monitoring of autophagy in Chinese hamster ovary cells using flow cytometry. Methods 56: 375-382.
25. Liu YY, Han TY, Giuliano AE, Hansen N, Cabot MC (2000) Uncoupling ceramide glycosylation by transfection of glucosylceramide synthase antisense reverses adriamycin resistance. J Biol Chem 275: 7138-7143.

26. Morad SA, Levin JC, Shanmugavelandy SS, Kester M, Fabrias G, et al. (2012) Ceramide--antiestrogen nanoliposomal combinations--novel impact of hormonal therapy in hormone-insensitive breast cancer. Mol Cancer Ther 11: 2352-2361.

27. Chapman JV, Gouazé-Andersson V, Cabot MC (2010) Expression of P-glycoprotein in HeLa cells confers resistance to ceramide cytotoxicity. Int J Oncol 37: 1591-1597.

28. Mahoney E, Lucas DM, Gupta SV, Wagner AJ, Herman SE, et al. (2012) ER stress and autophagy: new discoveries in the mechanism of action and drug resistance of the cyclin-dependent kinase inhibitor flavopiridol. Blood 120: 1262-1273.

Permissions

All chapters in this book were first published in JL, by OMICS International; hereby published with permission under the Creative Commons Attribution License or equivalent. Every chapter published in this book has been scrutinized by our experts. Their significance has been extensively debated. The topics covered herein carry significant findings which will fuel the growth of the discipline. They may even be implemented as practical applications or may be referred to as a beginning point for another development.

The contributors of this book come from diverse backgrounds, making this book a truly international effort. This book will bring forth new frontiers with its revolutionizing research information and detailed analysis of the nascent developments around the world.

We would like to thank all the contributing authors for lending their expertise to make the book truly unique. They have played a crucial role in the development of this book. Without their invaluable contributions this book wouldn't have been possible. They have made vital efforts to compile up to date information on the varied aspects of this subject to make this book a valuable addition to the collection of many professionals and students.

This book was conceptualized with the vision of imparting up-to-date information and advanced data in this field. To ensure the same, a matchless editorial board was set up. Every individual on the board went through rigorous rounds of assessment to prove their worth. After which they invested a large part of their time researching and compiling the most relevant data for our readers.

The editorial board has been involved in producing this book since its inception. They have spent rigorous hours researching and exploring the diverse topics which have resulted in the successful publishing of this book. They have passed on their knowledge of decades through this book. To expedite this challenging task, the publisher supported the team at every step. A small team of assistant editors was also appointed to further simplify the editing procedure and attain best results for the readers.

Apart from the editorial board, the designing team has also invested a significant amount of their time in understanding the subject and creating the most relevant covers. They scrutinized every image to scout for the most suitable representation of the subject and create an appropriate cover for the book.

The publishing team has been an ardent support to the editorial, designing and production team. Their endless efforts to recruit the best for this project, has resulted in the accomplishment of this book. They are a veteran in the field of academics and their pool of knowledge is as vast as their experience in printing. Their expertise and guidance has proved useful at every step. Their uncompromising quality standards have made this book an exceptional effort. Their encouragement from time to time has been an inspiration for everyone.

The publisher and the editorial board hope that this book will prove to be a valuable piece of knowledge for researchers, students, practitioners and scholars across the globe.

List of Contributors

Ayad A, Kababri M, Kili A, Hsissen L and Khattab M
Pediatric Hematology and Oncology Center (CHOP), Rabat children's hospital, Morrocco

Xiaohong I. Wang, Xinyan Lu, C. Cameron Yin, Lian Zhao, Carlos E. Bueso-Ramos, L. Jeffrey Medeiros and Pei Lin
Department of Hematopathology, The University of Texas MD Anderson Cancer Center, Houston, Texas, 77030, USA

Shaoying Li
Department of Pathology, Vanderbilt University School of Medicine, Nashville, Tennessee, 37235, USA

J. Rogers and Eric D. Hsi
Department of Clinical Pathology, Cleveland Clinic Foundation, Cleveland, Ohio, 44195, USA

Patricia Kropf
Fox Chase Cancer Center, Philadelphia, PA, USA

Gisoo Barnes, Boxiong Tang and Ashutosh Pathak
Global Health Economics and Outcomes Research, Teva Pharmaceuticals, Frazer, PA, USA

Jean-Pierre Issa
Fels Institute for Cancer Research, Temple University School of Medicine, Philadelphia, PA, USA

Manar M. Ismail and Morsi Heba K
Laboratory Medicine Department, Faculty of Applied Medical Science, Umm Al Qura University, KSA

Manar M. Ismail and Abdulateef Nahla AB
Clinical Pathology Department, National Cancer Institute, Cairo University, Egypt

Amal Zaghloul
Hematology and Immunology Department, Faculty of Medicine, Umm Al Qura University, KSA,
Clinical Pathology Department, Faculty of Medicine, Ain Shams University, Egypt

Abdulateef Nahla AB
Laboratory and Blood Bank Department, KAMC, Makkah, KSA

Morsi Heba K
Medical Biochemistry Department, Faculty of Medicine, Mansoura University, Egypt

Elżbieta Pels
Department of Paedodontics, Medical University of Lublin, Poland

Zuli Yang, Yajuan Zheng, Fan Hu, Zhang Zhang, Fukun Zhao and Shifu Zhang
College of Life Sciences, Zhejiang Sci-Tech University, Hangzhou, China

Yoshiko Hashii
Department of Pediatrics, Osaka University Graduate School of Medicine, Osaka, Japan

Yoshiyuki Kosaka
Department of Hematology and Oncology, Children's Cancer Center, Hyogo Prefectural Kobe Children's Hospital, Hyogo, Japan

Kenichiro Watanabe
Department of Hematology and Oncology, Shizuoka Children's Hospital, Shizuoka, Japan

Koji Kato
Department of Pediatrics, Japanese Red Cross Nagoya Daiichi Hospital, Aichi, Japan

Masue Imaizumi
Department of Hematology and Oncology, Miyagi Children's Hospital, Miyagi, Japan

Takashi Kaneko
Department of Hematology/Oncology, Tokyo Metropolitan Children's Medical Center, Tokyo, Japan

Shosuke Sunami
Department of Pediatrics, Japanese Red Cross Narita Hospital, Chiba, Japan

Arata Watanabe
Department of Pediatrics, Nakadori General Hospital, Akita, Japan

Hidefumi Hiramatsu
Department of Pediatrics, Graduate School of Medicine, Kyoto University, Kyoto, Japan

Yuhki Koga
Department of Pediatrics, Graduate School of Medical Sciences, Kyushu University, Fukuoka, Japan

Masahiro Hirayama
Department of Pediatrics, Mie University Graduate School of Medicine, Mie, Japan

Takafumi Nakao
Department of Hematology, Osaka City General Hospital, Osaka, Japan

Tomoko Hata
Department of Hematology, Atomic Bomb Disease Institute, Nagasaki University, Nagasaki, Japan

Naoyuki Uchida
Department of Hematology, Toranomon Hospital, Tokyo, Japan

Ken Ishiyama
Department of Hematology, Kanazawa University Hospital, Ishikawa, Japan

Kinuko Mitani
Department of Hematology and Oncology, Dokkyo Medical University, School of Medicine, Tochigi, Japan

Michihiro Hidaka
Department of Hematology, National Hospital Organization Kumamoto Medical Center, Kumamoto, Japan

Kunio Kitamura
Division of Hematology, Ichinomiya Municipal Hospital, Aichi, Japan

Hiroko Tsunemine
Department of Hematology, Shinko Hospital, Hyogo, Japan

Yasunori Ueda
Department of Haematology/Oncology, Transfusion and Haemapheresis Center, Kurashiki Central Hospital, Okayama, Japan

Atsuko Mugitani
Department of Hematology, Seichokai Fuchu Hospital, Osaka, Japan

Kensuke Usuki
Department of Hematology, NTT Medical Center, Tokyo, Japan

Yoshinobu Kanda
Division of Hematology, Department of Medicine, Jichi Medical University, Tochigi, Japan

Yoshihide Miyazaki
Diagnostic Division, Otsuka Pharmaceutical Co., Ltd., Tokushima, Japan

Kiyotoshi Imai
Department of Hematology, Sapporo Hokuyu Hospital, Sapporo, Japan

Tomoki Naoe
National Hospital Organization Nagoya Medical Center, Aichi, Japan

Katsuyoshi Koh
Department of Hematology/Oncology, Saitama Children's Medical Center, Saitama, Japan

Haruo Sugiyama
Department of Cancer Immunotherapy, Osaka University Graduate School of Medicine, Osaka, Japan

Keizo Horibe and Yoshiko Hashii
Clinical Research Center, National Hospital Organization Nagoya Medical Center, Aichi, Japan

Jiehao Zhou, Anupama Tewari, Mehdi Nassiri and Magdalena Czader
Department of Pathology and Laboratory Medicine, Indiana University, Indianapolis, IN 46202, USA

Kumar Saurabh, Michael T Scherzer, Amy Song, Chi Li and Levi J Beverly
James Graham Brown Cancer Center, University of Louisville, Louisville, KY 40202, USA

Levi J Beverly
Department of Medicine, Division of Hematology and Oncology, University of Louisville, School of Medicine, Louisville, KY 40202, USA

Chi Li and Levi J Beverly
Department of Pharmacology and Toxicology, University of Louisville School of Medicine, Louisville, KY 40202, USA

Michael T Scherzer
Department of Bioengineering, University of Louisville, Louisville, KY 40292, USA

Kenneth W Yip and John C Reed
Sanford-Burnham Medical Research Institute, La Jolla, CA, 92037, USA

Kenneth W Yip
Sanford-Burnham Medical Research Institute, La Jolla, CA, 92037, USA

Victor Pernin, Sofia Zefkili, Dominique Peurien, Alain Fourquet and Youlia M Kirova
Department of Radiation Oncology, Institute Curie, Paris, France

Merav Bar
Division of Clinical Research, Fred Hutchinson Cancer Research Center, USA

Department of Medicine, University of Washington, Seattle, WA, USA

Nassima Messali, Pierre Génin and Robert Weil
Institut Pasteur, Unité de Signalisation Moléculaire et Activation Cellulaire, CNRS URA 2582, 75724 Paris Cedex 15, France

Mohamed Z Abd Elrahman, Dalia Ahmad Nigm and Azza Abo Elfadle
Department of Clinical Pathology, Assiut University, Egypt

Muthu Sivaramakrishnan and Andrew Affleck
Department of Dermatology, Ninewells Hospital and Medical School, Dundee, UK

Ronald Kerr
Department of Haematology, Ninewells Hospital and Medical School, Dundee, UK

Alan Evans
Department of Histopathology, Ninewells Hospital and Medical School, Dundee, UK

Farhan S and Anjum F
Senior Medical Residents, Section of Hematology, Department of Medicine, College of Medicine and King Khalid University Hospital, King Saud University, Riyadh, Saudi Arabia

Al-Qahtani FS
Assistant Professor and Consultant Hemato-pathologist, Division of Hematopathology, Department of Pathology, King Khalid University Hospital, King Saud University, Riyadh, Kingdom of Saudi Arabia

Al-Anazi KA
Consultant Hemato-Oncologist, Section of Adult Hematology and Oncology, Department of Medicine, College of Medicine and King Khalid University Hospital, King Saud University, Riyadh, Saudi Arabia

Shingo Yanagiya
Junior resident of Asahikawa Kosei Hospital, 1-24, Asahikawa, 078-8211, Japan

Kazuya Sato, Nodoka Tsukada and Junki Inamura and Takaaki Hosoki
Department of Hematology/Oncology, Asahikawa Kosei Hospital, Japan

Satoshi Ito and Motohiro Shindo
Division of Gastroenterology and Hematology/Oncology, Department of Medicine, Asahikawa Medical University, Japan

Keisuke Sato and Koji Sakurai
Department of Pathology, Asahikawa Kosei Hospital, 1-24, Asahikawa, 078-8211, Japan

Shiozawa, Toshiko Yamochi and Hidekazu Ota
Department of Pathology and Laboratory Medicine, Showa University School of Medicine, Japan

Gaza F Salih
Department of Biology, University of Sulaimania, Sulamania, KRG, Iraq

Mehmet Yilmaz
SANKO University School of Medicine, Department of Hematology Gaziantep, Turkey

Salih Sertac Durusoy
Gaziantep University Department of Hematology, Gaziantep, Turkey

Alperen Kizikli, Salih Subari and Azer Abiyev
Gaziantep University Department of Internal Medicine, Gaziantep, Turkey

Mahmut Yeral and Ilknur Kozanoglu
Baskent University School of Medicine Department of Hematology Adana, Turkey

Sibel Cangi
Gaziantep University Department of Pathology, Gaziantep, Turkey

Hatem E Sabaawy
Department of Medicine, Rutgers-Robert Wood Johnson Medical School, USA
Department of Cellular and Molecular Pharmacology, Rutgers-Robert Wood Johnson Medical School, USA
Rutgers Cancer Institute of New Jersey, New Brunswick, NJ 08903-2681, USA

Olaniyi John A and Ogundeji Peter S
University College Hospital, Ibadan, Nigeria

Ogbaro Daniel D
Babcock University, Ilisan-Remo, Ogun State, Nigeria

Azza M Kamel, Nahla M El-Sharkawy and Eman K Abd El-Fattah
Department of Clinical Pathology, NCI, Cairo University, Egypt

Raafat M Abd El-Fattah, Mohammed A Samra and Hossam K Mahmoud
Department of Medical oncology, NCI, Cairo University, Egypt

Paul K Wallace
Flow Cytometry Lab, Roswell Park Cancer Institute, USA

Yi Zhang, Yan Zhao and Ikuo Murohashi
Hematology, Center for University-Wide Education, School of Health and Social Services, Saitama Prefectural University, Koshigaya-City, Saitama 343-8540, Japan

Kazuma Miyahara, Mai Shimada and Noriko Ihara
Department of Health Sciences, School of Health and Social Services, Saitama Prefectural University, Koshigaya-City, Saitama 343-8540, Japan

Ken-ichi Tanaka
Physiology, Center for University-Wide Education, School of Health and Social Services, Saitama Prefectural University, Koshigaya-City, Saitama 343-8540, Japan

Hiroyuki Hayashi
Anatomy, Center for University-Wide Education, School of Health and Social Services, Saitama Prefectural University, Koshigaya-City, Saitama 343-8540, Japan

Ashley E Rosko, Paolo F Caimi and Clark W Distelhorst
Division of Hematology-Oncology, University Hospitals Case Medical Center, Cleveland, Ohio, USA

Karen S McColl, Fei Zhong, Christopher B Ryder, Ming-Jin Chang, Paolo F Caimi and Clark W Distelhorst
Division of Hematology-Oncology, Case Western Reserve School of Medicine, Cleveland, USA

Abdus Sattar
Department of Epidemiology and Biostatistics, Case Western Reserve University, Cleveland, OH, USA

Brian T Hill
Department of Hematologic Oncology and Blood Disorders, Cleveland Clinic, Cleveland, Ohio, USA

Sayer Al-Harbi
Department of Cancer Biology, Lerner Research Institute, Cleveland Clinic, Cleveland, Ohio, USA

Paolo F Caimi, Brian T Hill, Alexandru Almasan and Clark W Distelhorst
Case Comprehensive Cancer Center, Case Western Reserve University School of Medicine, Ohio, USA

Ashley E Rosko
Division of Hematology, Department of Medicine, Ohio State University College of Medicine, Columbus, Ohio, USA

Yihui He and Xiaoyan Chen
Department of Pathology, Fujian Provincial Hospital, Fuzhou, Fujian 350001, China

Lingying Kong
Department of Pathology, Affiliated People's Hospital of Fujian University of Traditional Chinese Medicine, Fuzhou, Fujian 350004, P.R. China

Salem Akel, Daniel Bertolette and Francis W Ruscetti
Leukocyte Biology Section, Laboratory of Experimental Immunology, Center for Cancer Research, NCI, Frederick, Maryland

Salem Akel
St. Louis Blood Bank and Cellular Therapy Laboratory, Cardinal Glennon Children's Medical Center, St. Louis, MO

Gonul Hicsonmez
Faculty of Medicine, Department of pediatric Hematology, Hacettepe University, Ankara 06100, Turkey

Nicolas Batty and Meir Wetzler
Department of Medicine, Roswell Park Cancer Institute, Buffalo, NY, USA

Joseph Shatzel, Samuel Wiles, Mathew Kabalan, Rohit Sharma, Jonathan Pang, David Yi, Iris Alatovic, Sana Saif, Anthony Troitino, Michael Weinstein, Eric Murawski, Mathew Valerio and Yong Yin
State University of New York at Buffalo, Buffalo, NY, USA

Rohit Sharma, Joseph LaPenna and Kristopher Attwood
Erie County Medical Center, Buffalo, NY, USA

Adel A Hagag, Mohamed S Elfrargy, Mokhtar Abd Elfatah
Department of Pediatrics and Clinical Pathology, Tanta University, Egypt

Aml Ezzat Abd El-Lateef
Department of Medicine, Tanta University, Egypt

Yasser H Elnahass
Department of Clinical Pathology, BMT Lab Unit, National Cancer Institute, Cairo University, Egypt

Hossam K Mahmoud and Mohamad Abdel Moaty Samra
Department of Hematology and BMT, National Cancer Institute, Cairo University, Egypt

Fahmy T Ali, Mohamed R Mohamed, Mahmoud M Said and Mohamed AM Ali
Department of Biochemistry, Faculty of Science, Ain Shams University, Egypt

Amir Salem
Department of Pathology, National Research Center, Cairo, Egypt

Wafaa H ElMetnawy
Clinical Oncology Center, School of Medicine, Cairo University, Egypt

Jooeun Bae, Derin B Keskin, Kristen Cowens, Glen Dranoff, Nikhil C Munshi and Kenneth C Anderson
Harvard Medical School, Boston, Massachusetts, USA

Ann-Hwee Lee
Weill Cornell Medical College, New York, NY, USA

Nikhil C Munshi
VA Boston Healthcare System, Boston, Massachusetts, USA

Ota Fuchs
Institute of Hematology and Blood Transfusion, Prague, Czech Republic

Anna Jonasova and Radana Neuwirtova
Department of Medicine, Department of Hematology, General University Hospital, Charles University, Prague, Czech Republic

Sara Charmsaz and Andrew W Boyd
Leukaemia Foundation Research Unit, Queensland Institute of Medical Research, 300 Herston Road, Herston, Queensland 4006, Australia

Andrew W Boyd
Department of Medicine, University of Queensland, Herston, Queensland 4006, Australia

Irina Shipounova, Natalia Petinati, Alexey Bigildeev, Nina Drize, Tamara Sorokina, Larisa Kuzmina, Elena Parovichnikova and Valery Savchenko
FGBU Hematological Scientific C enter, M inistry of Health, Russia

Daphne Ang, Guang Fan, Nicky Leeborg, Marc Loriaux, Ken Gatter, Rita M. Braziel, Christopher L. Corless, Richard Press and Jennifer Dunlap
Department of Pathology, Oregon Health and Science University

Andrea Warrick, Carol Beadling, Susan Olson, Christopher L. Corless and Richard Press
Knight Cancer Institute, Oregon Health and Science University

Elie Traer, Tibor Kovacsovics and Carol Beadling
Division of Hematology and Medical Oncology, Oregon Health and Science University

Susan Olson
Department of Molecular and Medical Genetics, Oregon Health and Science University

Ashima Shukla, Nagendra K Chaturvedi, Adam K Ahrens, Christine E Cutucache and Amit K Mittal
Departments of Genetics, Cell Biology and Anatomy, Omaha, NE, USA

Philip Bierman
Division of Oncology/Hematology, University of Nebraska Medical Center, Omaha, NE, USA

Dennis D Weisenburger
Department of Pathology and Microbiology, University of Nebraska Medical Center, Omaha, NE, USA

Christoph Niermann, Hans-Joachim Schulze and Christian Hallermann
Department of Dermatology, Fachklinik Hornheide, Muenster, Germany

Adel A Hagag and Mokhtar Abd Elfatah
Department of Pediatrics, Faculty of Medicine, Tanta University, Egypt

Adel A Hagag, Ahmed M Abd Elaal, Ayman Elsheik and Enas Arafa Elzamarany
Department of Paediatrics and Clinical Pathology, Faculty of Medicine, Tanta University, Egypt

Johannes Matschke, Lewin Eisele, Ludger Sellmann, Ulrich Dührsen, Jan Dürig and Holger Nückel
Department of Hematology, Medical Faculty, University of Duisburg-Essen, Germany

Naser Kalhori and Arnd Nusch
Gemeinschaftspraxis für Hämatologie und Onkologie, Velbert, Germany

Timothy J Brown, Lindsey N Kissinger, Xujung Wang, David F Claxton and Brian M Barth
Department of Medicine, Division of Hematology and Oncology, Penn State College of Medicine, Hershey, PA, USA

Timothy J Brown, Lindsey N Kissinger, Xujung Wang, Mark Kester, David F Claxton and Brian M Barth
Penn State Hershey Cancer Institute, Hershey, PA, USA

Aileen M. Garcia
Department of Biomedical Science, Inter American University of Puerto Rico, Ponce, PR, USA

Aileen M. Garcia, Sriram S Shanmugavelandy and Sriram S Shanmugavelandy
Department of Pharmacology, Penn State College of Medicine, Hershey, PA, USA

Myles C Cabot
John Wayne Cancer Institute, Santa Monica, CA, USA

Index